## DATE DUE

# Flexible
# Bronchoscopy

*To today's students and tomorrow's bronchoscopists*

# Flexible Bronchoscopy

EDITED BY

## Ko-Pen Wang MD, FCCP

Director
Chest Diagnostic Center and Lung Cancer Center
Harbor Hospital Part-time Faculty of Interventional
Pulmonology
Johns Hopkins Hospital
Baltimore, MA, USA

## Atul C. Mehta MB, BS, FACP, FCCP

Professor and Staff Physician
Respiratory Institute
Cleveland Clinic
Cleveland, OH, USA

## J. Francis Turner Jr. MD FACP FCCP FCCM

Section Head
Interventional Pulmonary and Critical Care Medicine
Professor of Medicine
Nevada Cancer Institute and University of Nevada School of Medicine
Las Vegas, NV, USA

## THIRD EDITION

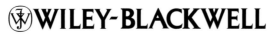

WILEY-BLACKWELL

A John Wiley & Sons, Ltd., Publication

*Registered office:* John Wiley & Sons, Ltd, The Atrium, Southern Gate, Chichester, West Sussex, PO19 8SQ, UK

*Editorial offices:* 9600 Garsington Road, Oxford, OX4 2DQ, UK

The Atrium, Southern Gate, Chichester, West Sussex, PO19 8SQ, UK

111 River Street, Hoboken, NJ 07030-5774, USA

For details of our global editorial offices, for customer services and for information about how to apply for permission to reuse the copyright material in this book please see our website at www.wiley.com/wiley-blackwell

*Library of Congress Cataloging-in-Publication Data*
Flexible bronchoscopy / edited by Ko-Pen Wang and Atul C. Mehta and J. Francis Turner Jr. – 3rd ed.
      p. ; cm.
  Includes bibliographical references and index.
  ISBN-13: 978-1-4051-7587-6 (hardcover : alk. paper)
  ISBN-10: 1-4051-7587-7 (hardcover : alk. paper)
  1. Bronchoscopy.  I. Wang, Ko Pen.  II. Mehta, Atul C.  III. Turner, J. Francis.
  [DNLM: 1. Bronchial Diseases–diagnosis.  2. Bronchoscopy–methods.  3. Bronchial Diseases–therapy.  WF 500]
  RC734.B7F54 2011
  616.2'307545–dc22
                    2011011048

A catalogue record for this book is available from the British Library.

Wiley also publishes its books in a variety of electronic formats. Some content that appears in print may not be available in electronic books.

Set in 9/12 pt Meridien by Toppan Best-set Premedia Limited
Printed and bound in Malaysia by Vivar Printing Sdn Bhd
01  2011

# Contents

Contents

# List of Contributors

**Fumihiro Asano** MD, FCCP
Director
Department of Pulmonary Medicine and
Bronchoscopy
Gifu Prefectural General Medical Center
Gifu
Japan

**Heinrich D. Becker** MD, FCCP
Professor
Internal Medicine and Pulmonology
Interdisciplinary Endoscopy
Thoraxclinic-Heidelberg
University School of Medicine
Heidelberg
Germany

**Robert F. Browning Jr.** MD, FCCP
Director of Interventional Bronchoscopy
National Naval Medical Center
Bethesda MD
USA

**Alex Chen** MD
Director of Interventional Pulmonology
Washington University School of Medicine
St Louis MO
USA

**Erik M. Folch** MD, MSc
Director of the Medical Procedure Service
Division of Thoracic Surgery and Interventional
Pulmonology
Beth Israel Deaconess Medical Center
Harvard Medical School
Boston MA
USA

**Mario Gomez** MD
Internal Medicine Physician
Pulmonary and Sleep Center
West Laco
Texas TX
USA

**Sara R. Greenhill** MD, FCCP
Director
Interventional Pulmonology Fellowship
Chicago Chest Center
Elk Grove Village IL
USA

**Richard Helmers** MD
Thoracic Diseases
Mayo Clinic Scottsdale
Scottsdale AZ
USA

**Taichiro Ishizumi** MD, PhD
Assistant Professor
Department of Thoracic Surgery
Tokyo Medical University
Tokyo
Japan

**Prasoon Jain** MD, FCCP
Staff Physician
Louis A Johnson VA Medical Center,
Clarksburg WV
USA

**Michael A. Jantz** MD
Associate Professor of Medicine
Director of Interventional Pulmonology
University of Florida
Division of Pulmonary and Critical Care
Medicine
University of Florida
Gainesville FL
USA

**Harubumi Kato** MD, PhD, FCCP, FIAC
Honorary President
Niizashiki Chuo General Hospital
and
Professor Emeritus
Tokyo Medical University
Tokyo
Japan

**Yasufumi Kato** MD, PhD
Staff Doctor
Department of Surgery
Tokyo Medical University
Tokyo
Japan

**Mani S. Kavuru** MD
Division Director and Professor
Division of Pulmonary & Critical Care Medicine
Co-Director, Jefferson Center for Critical Care
Thomas Jefferson University & Hospital
Philadelphia PA
USA

**Marian H. Kollef** MD, FACP, FCCP
Director
Medical ICU Respiratory Care Services
Washington University School of Medicine
St Louis MO
USA

**Kevin L. Kovitz** MD, MBA, FACP, FCCP
Director
Chicago Chest Center
Elk Grove Village IL
USA

**Noriaki Kurimoto** MD, PhD, FCCP
Professor
Division of Chest Surgery
St Marianna University School of Medicine
Kanagawa
Japan

**Navatha Kurugundla** MD
Division of Pulmonary and Critical Care Medicine
New York Methodist Hospital
Brooklyn NY
USA

**Stephen C. T. Lam** MD, FRCPC
Professor of Medicine
University of British Columbia
and
Chair
Provincial Lung Tumor Group
British Columbia Cancer Agency
Vancouver BC
Canada

**Xicheng Liu** MD
Professor of Pediatrics
Center for Pediatric Bronchoscopy
Beijing Children's Hospital
Capital Medical University
Beijing
China

**Adnan Majid** MD, FCCP
Director, Interventional Pulmonology
Beth Israel Deaconess Medical Center
and
Assistant Professor of Medicine
Harvard Medical School
Boston MA
USA

## List of Contributors

**Samir Makani** MD
Director
Interventional Pulmonology and Bronchoscopy
University of California
and
VA San Diego Health Care System
San Diego CA
USA

**Praveen N. Mathur** MB, BS
Professor of Medicine
Division of Pulmonary, Critical Care and
Occupational Medicine
Department of Medicine
Indiana University Medical Center
Indianapolis IN
USA

**Atul C. Mehta** MB, BS, FACP, FCCP
Professor and Staff Physician
Respiratory Institute
Cleveland Clinic
Cleveland OH
USA

**Teruomi Miyazawa** MD, PhD, FCCP
Professor and Chairman
Division of Respiratory and Infectious Diseases
St Marianna University School of Medicine
Kanagawa
Japan

**Peter J. Mogayzel** Jr MD PhD
Associate Professor of Pediatrics
Director, Cystic Fibrosis Center
Johns Hopkins School of Medicine
Johns Hopkins Cystic Fibrosis Center
Baltimore MD
USA

**Ali I. Musani** MD, FCCP, FACP
Associate Professor of Medicine and Pediatrics
Director, Interventional Pulmonology Program
National Jewish Health
Associate Professor of Medicine
University of Colorado
Denver CO
USA

**Brian Palen** MD
Mayo Clinic Scottsdale
Thoracic Diseases
Scottsdale AZ
USA

**Rajesh R. Patel** MD
Fellow in Pulmonary and Critical Care Medicine
Mayo Clinic
Rochester MN
USA

**Sunit R. Patel** MD, FCCP, DABSM
Associate Clinical Professor
UC Davis Medical Center and Touro University
and
Medical Director of California Sleep Center and
Medical Director of ICU & Respiratory Therapy
Mercy Medical Center Merced CA
USA

**Luis F. Riquelme** MS CCC-SLP, BRS-S
Director
Center for Swallowing and Speech-Language
Pathology
New York Methodist Hospital
Brooklyn
and
Assistant Professor
New York Medical College
Valhalla NY
USA

**Navreet Sandhu Sindhwani** MD
Fellow
Division of Pulmonary, Allergy, and Critical Care
Medicine
Duke University Medical Center
Durham NC
USA

**Scott L. Shofer** MD, PhD
Assistant Professor of Medicine
Interventional Pulmonology
Division of Pulmonary, Allergy & Critical Care
Medicine
Duke University Medical Center
Durham NC
USA

**Gerard A. Silvestri** MD, MS
Professor of Medicine
Department of Internal Medicine
Division of Pulmonary, Critical Care, Allergy
and Sleep Medicine
Medical University of South Carolina
Charleston SC
USA

**Michael J. Simoff** MD FCCP
Associate Professor of Medicine, FTA
Director, Bronchoscopy and Interventional
Pulmonology
Henry Ford Hospital
Wayne State University School of Medicine
Detroit MI
USA

**James K. Stoller** MD, MS
Chair, Education Institute
Head, Cleveland Clinic Respiratory Therapy
Jean Wall Bennett Professor of Medicine
The Cleveland Clinic Foundation
Cleveland OH
USA

**Arthur Sung** MD, FCCP
Director of Interventional Pulmonology and
Bronchoscopy
Beth Israel Medical Center
New York NY
USA

**J. Francis Turner** Jr
Section Head
Interventional Pulmonary and Critical Care
Medicine
Professor of Medicine
Nevada Cancer Institute and University of
Nevada School of Medicine
Las Vegas NV
USA

**Jitsuo Usuda** MD, PhD
Assistant Professor
Department of Surgery
Tokyo Medical University
Tokyo
Japan

**James P. Utz** MD
Associate Professor of Medicine
Pulmonary and Critical Care Medicine
Mayo Clinic
Rochester MN
USA

**Momen M. Wahidi** MD MBA
Director
Interventional Pulmonology and Bronchoscopy
Division of Pulmonary, Allergy and Critical Care
Medicine
and
Associate Professor of Medicine
Duke University Medical Center
Durham NC
USA

**Ko-Pen Wang**
Director
Johns Hopkins Bayview Medical Center
Division of Pulmonary Medicine
Harbor Medical Center
Baltimore MA
USA

**Shunying Zhao** MD
Associate Professor of Pediatrics
Department of Respiratory Medicine
Beijing Children's Hospital
Capital Medical University
Beijing
China

# Preface to the Third Edition

Almost a half-century ago Professor Shigeto Ikeda invented the Fiberoptic Bronchoscope. We introduce the third edition of *Flexible Bronchoscopy* on the dawn of this fifth decade of international experience with great enthusiasm. In his book *Never Give Up,* Professor Ikeda reviews the groundbreaking work in the development of the bronchoscope, initially proposed in 1964, with the first use of the apparatus in 1966 by Professor Ikeda, which was manufactured by the Machida Corporation.

Since the invention of the fiberscope, the advances in technology have led to improvements not only in the basic instrument, but also with the accessories to improve the endoscopic image, maneuverability and tissue acquisition. The third edition of *Flexible Bronchoscopy* builds on the prior editions with emphasis on the fundamental techniques of bronchoscopy with expanded information on newer technologies at the bronchoscopists' disposal.

As the armamentarium of diagnostic and therapeutic options expand, we revisit the challenges outlined in the second edition; that being, elimination of non-diagnostic bronchoscopy, minimizing any potential complications and application of therapeutic techniques in a selective, aggressive, and yet cautious approach to ensure optimal Quality of Life for our patients.

To meet the above challenges, we urge our fellow bronchoscopists to review the historical aspects of bronchoscopy and it's diagnostic and therapeutic applications; for it is in the understanding of the development and history of this art and science that true mastery will develop.

Finally, as the practice of medicine becomes more technology oriented, we as specialists must always act as the ultimate advocates for our patients. Professor Ikeda overcame several physical challenges during his lifetime; with his philosophy being "it is necessary for me to have my best mental power and belief to live my life of Never Give Up . . . and do as much work as I can for the public."

It is our hope as the editors that the following text aids readers in an understanding of flexible bronchoscopy and Professor Ikeda's spirit of *Never Give Up* in the pursuit of excellence in the art and science of bronchology.

Ko-Pen Wang
Atul C. Mehta
J. Francis Turner Jr.
February 2012

# 1

# Fundamentals of Bronchoscopy

# 1 Bronchoscopy in the New Millennium

## Noriaki Kurimoto and Teruomi Miyazawa

St Marianna University, Kawasaki, Japan

The development of flexible bronchoscopy was started by Ikeda *et al.* in 1965. In the history of flexible bronchoscopy, there have been several developments and improvements as a result of higher resolutions and finer scopes. Higher-resolution bronchoscopes have mainly been used for bronchial lesions in central lung cancer, which can be observed by bronchoscopy, while thinner bronchoscopes have been used to reach peripheral lung lesions that cannot be directly observed. With high resolution images, the properties of the tracheal surface and microvessels can be evaluated with the use of fluorescence bronchoscopy to diagnose epithelial thickness via the attenuation of autofluorescence, and narrowband imaging (NBI), which results in narrow bands at wavelengths that are absorbed by hemoglobin [1]. Large absorption peaks exist near 415 nm and 540 nm due to the absorption characteristics of hemoglobin. Light at 415 nm and 540 nm, which is readily absorbed by hemoglobin, is used for high-contrast images to determine whether blood or blood vessels are present. As the wavelength of light becomes shorter, transmission depth becomes shallower, and thus the presence or absence of blood is more strongly reflected with narrowband light than with broadband light.

When bronchoscopy is conducted for the diagnosis of central lung cancer following examination for bloody sputum and sputum cytology abnormalities, fluorescence bronchoscopy, which can show attenuation of autofluorescence emitted from bronchial walls at lesion sites, is very useful in addition to regular white light bronchoscopy [2]. Diagnosis of the range and depth is essential in determining whether central lung cancer can be treated by photodynamic therapy (PDT) rather than surgery. In diagnosing the extent of central lung cancer, the border between diseased and healthy tissue can be observed with fluorescence bronchoscopy. Special optical observation with NBI has also proven to be effective in identifying the margin of lesions and evaluating microvessels on the lesion surface.

Endobronchial ultrasound (EBUS) can depict five to seven structural layers in bronchial walls, and it has been useful in diagnosing invasion depth [3]. In lesions that do not extend beyond the third layer with EBUS, that is tumors that have not gone beyond the collar of cartilage, there is a possibility of complete recovery with PDT. Moreover, the possibility of using NBI to diagnose invasion depth based on the pattern of surface vessels in the lesion area is currently being investigated.

Of great importance is the careful insertion and withdrawal of bronchoscopes while investigating whether there are also lesions in the nasal cavity, pharynx, and larynx, as the bronchoscope passes through these areas. Careful observation should also be made, particularly among heavy smokers and heavy drinkers, for the presence of pharyngeal and laryngeal cancer.

In cases of advanced central lung cancer, flexible bronchoscopy is used in histological diagnosis by direct-vision biopsy, in assessing the patency of the airway lumen in cases of intervention, and in assessing whether there is pressure invasion of lesions within the airway walls or from outside the walls.

Rapid advances are also being made in the diagnosis of peripheral lung cancer using flexible bronchoscopy. Lesions are reached from the bronchial lumen, and cells or tissue are collected using techniques such as exfoliative or lavage cytology, transbronchial biopsy, and transbronchial needle aspiration (TBNA) from the lesion area. These cells or tissue are then presented for histopathological examination.

Until recently, the bronchi involved in lesions were judged by the doctor while looking at segmental, subsegmental, and sub-subsegmental bronchi on chest plain films or chest CT, while considering anatomy. With recent advances in CT, it has become possible to see the length of bronchi up to the peripheral lesions before any tests are performed through the use of virtual bronchoscopy [4,5]. Thus, there is little

*Flexible Bronchoscopy*, Third Edition. Edited by Ko-Pen Wang, Atul C. Mehta, J. Francis Turner.
© 2012 Blackwell Publishing Ltd. Published 2012 by Blackwell Publishing Ltd.

difference between doctors in reading CTs, and there is a greater likelihood that the lesion can be reached.

Procedures are performed under fluoroscopy in order to help determine whether a lesion has been reached. However, some lesions are difficult to see under fluoroscopy, and it has become possible to depict lesions present in the lung by guiding the thin ultrasound probe of EBUS into lesions from the bronchi [6]. Moreover, a method has appeared in which the thin ultrasound probe is covered with a sheath [7] in order to ensure a route to the lesion, and then exfoliative or lavage cytology is performed, or cells or tissue are collected through transbronchial biopsy (Fig. 1.1).

There has also been an increase in shadows presenting ground glass opacity (GGO). As pure GGO cannot be seen on radioscopy or EBUS in confirming whether the lesion has been reached, there have been reports of bronchoscopy under CT guidance. Exposure and other problems with this

method have been pointed out, but this is a trend that should be followed in the future.

Staging is an important issue in diagnosing lung cancer. There has been dependence on CT, PET, and other diagnostic imaging techniques, particularly in diagnosing lymph node metastasis, but diagnostic imaging has its own limitations. In the past, surgery and mediastinoscopy were necessary for cytohistological diagnosis of mediastinal lymph node metastasis, and the burden on patients was great. In 2003, the use of ultrasound bronchoscopy with a convex ultrasound probe fixed to the tip of the bronchoscope became possible. This technique makes it possible to obtain cross-sectional images in the longitudinal direction around the trachea and bronchi, and ultrasound imaging and transbronchial needle aspiration (TBNA) with a guide are now being performed. EBUS-TBNA conducted under local anesthesia has made cytological and histological diagnosis easier, and this technique has

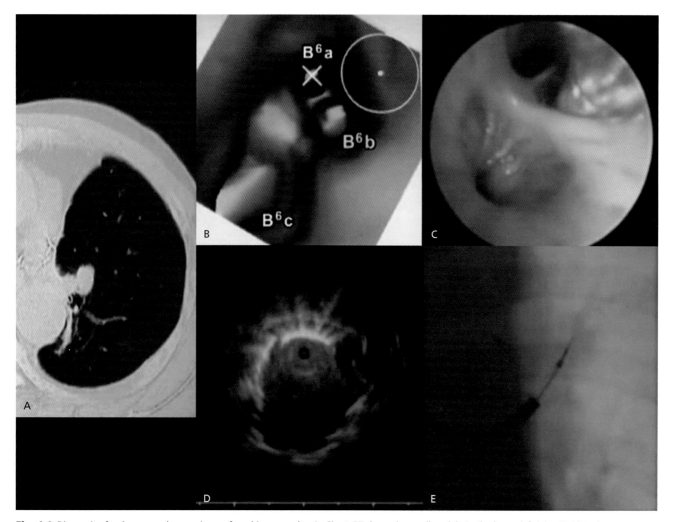

**Fig. 1.1** Diagnosis of pulmonary adenocarcinoma from biopsy results. A. Chest CT showed a small nodule in the lower left lobe. B. Virtual bronchoscopic navigation (VBN), in combination with C. EBUS-GS confirmed the location of the nodule at B6b. D. A 20 MHz probe could clearly visualize the internal structure of the lesion. E. Fluoroscopy was used to guide the probe to the site of the lesion.

spread rapidly worldwide [8]. While mediastinoscopy has the advantage of enabling tissue collection from numerous lymph nodes, the advantages of EBUS-TBNA in comparison with mediastinoscopy are: (i) it can be performed under local anesthesia; (ii) it is possible to observe the interior of the lymph node and avoid aspiration of necrotic areas; (iii) it is possible to puncture lymph nodes from the left and right main bronchi (nodes #10, 11, and 12); and (iv) there are few serious complications such as severe hemorrhage.

The future outlook for flexible bronchoscopy includes the application of NBI and cytological evaluation by high-magnification bronchoscopy for airway lesions, development of easy-to-use tools such as navigation screens interfaced with bronchoscope screens for peripheral lesions, and evaluation of lymph node regions with high-resolution ultrasound images, blood analysis with pulsed Doppler, and adjustment of collected tissue with puncture needle modifications in EBUS-TBNA.

## References

1 Shibuya K, Hosino H, Chiyo M, *et al.* High magnification bronchovideoscopy combined with narrow band imaging could detect capillary loops of angiogenic squamous dysplasia in heavy smokers at high risk for lung cancer. *Thorax* 2003; **58**: 989–95.

2 Miyazu YM, Miyazawa T, Hiyama K, *et al.* Telomerase expression in noncancerous bronchial epithelia is a possible marker of early development of lung cancer. *Cancer Res* 2005; **65**: 9623–7.

3 Miyazu Y, Miyazawa T, Kurimoto N, *et al.* Endobronchial ultrasonography in the assessment of centrally located early-stage lung cancer before photodynamic therapy. *Am J Respir Crit Care Med* 2002; **165**: 832–7.

4 Asano F, Matsuno Y, Shinagawa N, *et al.* A virtual bronchoscopic navigation system for pulmonary peripheral lesions. *Chest* 2006; **130**: 559–66.

5 Asano F, Matsuno Y, Tsuzuku A, *et al.* Diagnosis of pulmonary peripheral lesions using a bronchoscope insertion guidance system combined with endobronchial ultrasonography with a guide sheath. *Lung Cancer* 2008; **60**: 366–73.

6 Kurimoto N, Murayama M, Yoshioka S, Nishisaka T. Analysis of the internal structure of peripheral pulmonary lesions using endobronchial ultrasonography. *Chest* 2002; **122**: 1887–94.

7 Kurimoto N, Miyazawa T, Okimasa S, *et al.* Endobronchial ultrasonography using a guide sheath increases the ability to diagnose peripheral pulmonary lesions endoscopically. *Chest* 2004; **126**: 959–65.

8 Yasufuku K, Chiyo M, Sekine Y, *et al.* Real-time endobronchial ultrasound guided transbronchial needle aspiration of mediastinal and hilar lymph nodes. *Chest* 2004; **126**: 122–8.

# Infection Control and Radiation Safety in the Bronchoscopy Suite

**Prasoon Jain[1] and Atul C. Mehta[2]**
[1] Louis A Johnson VA Medical Center, Clarksburg, WV, USA
[2] Respiratory Institute, Cleveland Clinic, Cleveland, OH, USA

Bronchoscopy is the premier diagnostic procedure in pulmonary medicine. The procedure is remarkably safe with about 1–3% complication rate. Most physicians are familiar with immediate complications of bronchoscopy such as bleeding, pneumothorax, and hypoxemia. Although less common, bronchoscopy can also transmit infection, either from one patient to another or from an environmental source to the patient. In addition to patients, there is also some risk of transmission of infection to the health-care workers during bronchoscopy. In the first part of this chapter, we discuss the infection control issues surrounding bronchoscopy. We will address the scope of the problem, the current guidelines on reprocessing of bronchoscopes, and discuss how to minimize the risk of transmitting infection during bronchoscopy.

Another less recognized complication of bronchoscopy is excessive radiation exposure to the patient and operators when fluoroscopy is used during the procedure. In the second part of this chapter, we will discuss potential health risks of radiation exposure to the patients and the health-care workers during bronchoscopy. We will also discuss the practical guidelines to minimize the radiation exposure to the patients and the operators during bronchoscopy.

## Transmission of infection

Bronchoscopy-related infections have been reported sporadically ever since the procedure was introduced in clinical practice. However, the issue has taken the center stage with the recent publication of several high-profile reports of infections after bronchoscopy [1,2]. These reports provide ample evidence that bronchoscope can act as a vector in transmission of infection. Clinically, the bronchoscopy-related infections are classified as true infections and pseudoinfections [3,4]. True infection is said to occur when an organism transmitted during bronchoscopy causes a new illness in patient after the procedure. Most of the true infections are caused by highly pathogenic organisms. Patients with immunocompromised state are at highest risk of developing true bronchoscopy-related infection. These infections are generally difficult to treat and may be associated with considerable morbidity and mortality. Pseudoinfection refers to the isolation of an organism in the bronchoscopy specimen without any clinical evidence of infection. Most of the pseudoinfections arise when a specimen such as bronchoalveolar lavage is contaminated due to an inadequately disinfected bronchoscope. Even though patients do not develop clinical illness, pseudoinfections cause several indirect harms to the patients [5,6]. Isolation of a microbial agent causes diagnostic confusion leading to incorrect diagnosis and treatment. Pseudoinfections cause delay in diagnosis that can have serious implications. For example, cases have been reported in which early diagnosis of lung cancer was missed because acid-fast bacilli were isolated from the bronchoscopy specimen. Furthermore, due to incorrect diagnosis, patients may receive unnecessary antibiotic or antitubercular therapy, exposing them to potential adverse effects of these medications. Then there are important cost implications, not only for the individual patients, but also for the institutions because the epidemiological investigation of an outbreak is an expensive affair. Finally, pseudoinfections in a bronchoscopy facility represent a critical failure in reprocessing protocol and until the cause is found and corrected, all patient undergoing bronchoscopy are at risk of developing infection after the procedure.

### Scope of the problem

Transmission of infection by bronchoscope is uncommon. However, the problem is possibly under-recognized and under-reported. Accurate estimations are difficult to make because routine microbiological studies are not performed on bronchoscopy specimen and the majority of bronchos-

*Flexible Bronchoscopy*, Third Edition. Edited by Ko-Pen Wang, Atul C. Mehta, J. Francis Turner.

copy facilities do not have a system for prospective surveillance. Most of the information on this subject is derived from retrospective case series. In an extensive review of the literature in 2003, Culver and coworkers identified 953 patients who had either pseudoinfection or true infection after flexible bronchoscopy [7]. Only 3–4% of these patients had true infections after bronchoscopy. The overwhelming majority of reported patients had pseudoinfections. The relative paucity of infectious complications after bronchoscopy is reassuring considering the hundreds of thousand procedures performed every year worldwide. However, these data provide no basis for complacency in this matter. Every infectious complication after bronchoscopy should be considered a serious potential threat to a patient's well-being. In fact, bronchoscopy-related infections have possibly contributed to three deaths in recent reports [1,2].

## Microbial agents

A wide variety of bacteria, mycobacteria, and fungal agents have been implicated in bronchoscopy-related outbreaks (Table 2.1). *Pseudomonas aeruginosa* and *Serratia marcescens*

**Table 2.1** Organisms implicated in bronchoscopy-related infections

**Bacterial agents**
*Pseudomonas aeruginosa**
*Serratia marcescens**
*Klebsiella pneumonia*
*Legionella pneumophilia*
*Burkholderia pseudomallei**
*Proteus*
*Bacillus*
*Methylobacterium mesophilicum*
*Morganella morganii*

**Mycobacterial agents**
*Mycobacterium tuberculosis**
*M. chelonae**
*M. avium-intercellulare*
*M. xenopi*
*M. fortuitum*
*M. gordonae*
*M. abscessus*

**Fungal agents**
*Rhodotorula rubra*
*Aureobasidium* sp.
*Blastomyces dermatidis*
*Trichosporon cutaneum*
*Penicillium* sp.
*Cladosporium* sp.
*Phialospora* sp.

*Organisms reported to cause true bronchoscopy-related outbreaks.

have caused the majority of both pseudoinfections and the true infections. Environmental mycobacteria have also caused a large number of outbreaks [8]. Of these, the most common is *M. chelonae* which has caused several pseudo-outbreaks after bronchoscopy [9–15]. True infection due to environmental mycobacteria is very rare [16]. The risk of transmission of tuberculosis via bronchoscopy is well established. Fortunately, there are only a handful of cases in which *M. tuberculosis* was transmitted by the bronchoscope [17–22]. The majority of fungal outbreaks reported in the literature are pseudoinfections due to environmental fungi. *Rhodotorula rubra* is the most common fungal agent involved in these cases [23–25]. Human immunodeficiency virus (HIV) RNA can be isolated from a bronchoscope after it is used in an HIV infected patient [26]. However, adequate reprocessing is highly effective in eliminating any traces of the virus and there are no reports of HIV transmissions via bronchoscopy. Similarly, there are no known cases of hepatitis B or hepatitis C transmission after bronchoscopy.

## Terms used in infection control

In the recent years, nosocomial infections have emerged as an important threat to the hospitalized patients and patients undergoing invasive procedures. Medical devices including endoscopes have become the leading cause of nosocomial infections. All health-care workers are responsible for making maximum efforts to reduce the transmission of infections during bronchoscopy. A sound knowledge of the principles of infection control is essential prerequisite to achieve this goal. To start, all health-care workers, including bronchoscopists, must have a clear understanding of basic terms used in infection control, such as sterilization, high-level disinfection, intermediate-level disinfection, and low-level disinfection. The definitions and the common methods used to achieve the different levels of disinfection are summarized in Table 2.2.

Depending on the risk of transmission of infection, Spaulding classified medical devices into three categories: critical, semicritical, and non-critical [27,28] (Table 2.3). According to this classification, a bronchoscope is classified as a semicritical device. The minimal recommended level of disinfection for a semicritical medical device is high-level disinfection. On the other hand, the accessories used during bronchoscopy are classified as critical devices because mucosal breach always occurs during transbronchial needle aspiration (TBNA) or bronchoscopic lung biopsy. The minimum recommended level of disinfection for the accessory instruments is sterilization. Standard methods to disinfect the medical devices such as bronchoscopes are highly effective in reducing the transmission of infection. The problem usually arises when instead of using validated guidelines, health-care workers use non-standard methods and protocols to reprocess the medical devices. In some

**Table 2.2** Levels of disinfection

| Level | Definition | Common agents | Uses in bronchoscopy |
|---|---|---|---|
| Sterilization | Destroys all forms of microbial life including bacterial spores | Steam<br>Ethylene oxide | Reusable biopsy forceps, cleaning brushes, atomizers |
| High-level disinfection (HLD) | Destroys all form of microbial life and reduces but not eliminate all bacterial spores | 2% glutaraldehyde for 20 min<br>1% Peracetic acid for 30 min<br>0.55% | Bronchoscopes |
| | By definition, HLD achieves 6 log reduction of mycobacteria | Orthophthaaldehyde for 12 min | |
| Intermediate-level disinfection | Destroys vegetative bacteria, mycobacteria, most fungi, and most viruses but not bacterial spores | Chlorhexidine<br>Chloroxylenol<br>Iodophores | Not FDA approved for critical or semicritical devices<br>Useful as skin antiseptic agents and for cleaning non-critical objects such as bronchoscopy cart, side-railings with visible blood |
| Low-level disinfection | Destroys vegetative bacteria, some fungi, some virus but not mycobacteria and bacterial spores | Quaternary ammonium compounds e.g. benzalkonium chloride | Useful for non-critical objects without visible blood |

**Table 2.3** Spaulding classification of medical devices

| Device | Definition | Examples in bronchoscopy | Recommended cleaning method |
|---|---|---|---|
| Critical | Enter sterile tissues or vascular spaces | Biopsy forceps, needles for transbronchial needle aspiration procedure | Sterilization |
| Semicritical | Come in contact with sterile mucus membranes but do not penetrate sterile tissues | Bronchoscopes | High-level disinfection |
| Non-critical | Do not contact patients or contact only intact skin | Stethoscopes, blood pressure cuffs, bronchoscopy cart | General precautions and intermediate to low-level disinfection |

instances this happens due to human error, and in others it is caused by lack of knowledge and training.

The potential for cross infection has increased due to increasing use of bronchoscopy in high-risk patients with advanced age, multiple medical problems, cancers, organ transplantation, and other immunocompromised states. On one hand, these patients are more likely to harbor resistant organisms and on the other hand, these patients also have poor host defenses. Due to this reason, bronchoscopy with an inadequately reprocessed bronchoscope can cause a serious systemic infection in these patients.

Our understanding regarding causes and mechanisms of reprocessing failures has greatly expanded in recent years. Exciting new developments are taking place in the field of molecular techniques for diagnosis and investigation of infection outbreaks. In the past decade, an impressive amount of new information has also emerged on the role of biofilms in endoscopy-related infections.

## Role of biofilms

Biofilms play a central role in infections secondary to contaminated medical devices and prostheses [29]. Many bronchoscopy outbreaks have now been traced back to biofilms in the bronchoscopes or the automatic endoscopic reprocessors (AER). A biofilm is a community of microbial agents encased within a hydrated matrix of polysaccharides and proteins (Figs 2.1, 2.2) Bacteria in the biofilms exhibit several physiological properties that are different from corresponding free-living organisms. The bacteria in biofilms are firmly attached to the surface and to each other, forming microcolonies. The individual cells in the microcolonies respond to one-another and seem to function in a highly coordinated manner. This property, called quorum sensing, is thought to be an integral part of the formation and survival of biofilms. The extracellular matrix allows free circulation of water and serves as a nutrient storage facility for the bacteria. Even though the bacteria in

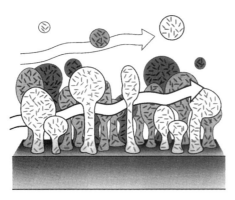

**Fig. 2.1** Biofilms arise when micro-organisms adhere to solid surfaces, forming structures composed of colonies and extracellular material. Liquid flow through the biofilm provides nutrients and removes waste. (Published with permission from Wang, Mehta, and Turner; Flexible Bronchoscopy 2003; Blackwell publishing Ltd.)

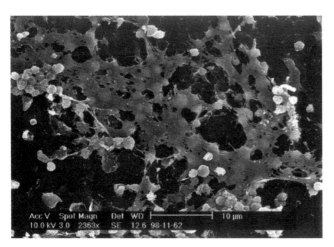

**Fig. 2.2** Electron micrograph of a biofilm. Courtesy of Drs Rodney Dolan and Janice Carr, Centers for Disease Control, Atlanta, GA.

**Table 2.4** Mechanism of resistance in biofilm

Extracellular polymeric substance:
  diffusion barrier
  neutralizes antimicrobial agent
Slow growth rate of bacteria
Stored nutrition
Inactivation of antimicrobial agent by bacterial surface molecules
Change in membrane transport system
Production of catalase
Persister cells with high resistance to antimicrobial agents
Plasmid-mediated resistance

biofilms do not have a higher degree of intrinsic virulence than the free-living organisms, from an evolutionary standpoint, biofilms provide a clear survival advantage for the resident bacteria.

Once formed, biofilm is very difficult to eradicate with the conventional antimicrobial agents and disinfectants. Several mechanisms are proposed to explain the high degree of resistance of bacteria in biofilm [30] (Table 2.4). By creating a diffusion barrier and neutralizing certain antimicrobial agent, extracellular polymeric substances play a critical role in increasing bacterial resistance in biofilm. Interestingly, bacterial resistance to disinfection is greater in those biofilms that are formed on a rough surface. This may explain a high propensity for formation of biofilms in the working channels of endoscopes that are damaged during the procedures. Studies are needed to clarify whether microscopic damage

and normal wear and tear of the working channel also promote development of biofilm.

Several reports have linked biofilms on bronchoscopes with pseudoinfection or true infection. For instance, two recent outbreaks of *Pseudomonas aeruginosa* and *Serratia marcescens* infections after bronchoscopy were traced to the biofilms formed on the threads of the biopsy port and inside the cap of the biopsy port [1,2]. Biofilms can also develop in the inner channel of the endoscopes. For example, Pajkos and coworkers examined inner channels of 13 endoscopes for the presence of biofilm and bacteria by scanning electron microscopy. Biological deposits were detected on all samples tested. Biofilms were found on the suction or biopsy channels of five of 13 instruments. Bacterial microcolonies were often associated with surface defects on the tubing but many were also present on channels that had no visible damage [31]. By design, a bronchoscope is an easy target for the formation of biofilm. The instrument has a complex structure with long and narrow inner channels that are soiled with bacteria and organic matter with each procedure. Direct visual inspection of inner channels is not possible and therefore it is difficult to determine the adequacy of initial cleaning or the early stages of development of biofilms. A thorough initial mechanical cleaning prior to the disinfection remains the most effective method to prevent the development of biofilms. Unfortunately, several detergents commonly used for cleaning endoscopes are not very effective in removing the established biofilms [32]. Finding an ideal agent for this purpose remains an area of active research [33].

Biofilm may also form inside the automated endoscope reprocessors. Alvarado and coworkers reported contamination of endoscopes with *Pseudomonas aeruginosa* due to heavy biofilms in the detergent holding tank, inlet water hose, and air vents of the AER [34]. Disinfection of AER using the protocol specified by the manufacturer did not resolve the problem. In another report, Fraser and coworkers isolated *Mycobacterium chelonae* from endoscopic or bronchial washings in 14 patients [12]. The source was found to be the rinse water of the AER. The problem could not be resolved with attempted disinfection of the AER, presumably because of the presence of a biofilm inside the machine. Once biofilm is formed, the AER is difficult to disinfect and, in many instances, replacement of the entire unit is needed to resolve the problem [35].

## Reprocessing of bronchoscopes

Several features inherent to the design of flexible bronchoscopes increase the risk of contamination and colonization of the device. The bronchoscope has a long and narrow working channel, angulations, and matted surfaces, all of which make the internal cleaning more difficult. Because the instrument is heat-sensitive, steam sterilization cannot be used. The current models of bronchoscopes are not com-

patible with certain chemical agents used for sterilization and disinfection. In addition, poorly designed biopsy ports and suction ports may become reservoirs, causing serious cross infections.

Recommendations for reprocessing of bronchoscopes are summarized in Table 2.5. Generally, high-level disinfection of bronchoscopes is highly effective when these recommendations are strictly followed. In fact, outbreak investigations nearly always reveal important breaches in reprocessing protocol. Therefore, it is essential that all personnel involved in bronchoscopy are thoroughly aware of the current reprocessing guidelines [36–38]. In the following section, we briefly discuss the rationale of individual steps of bronchoscope reprocessing and describe how failure to follow the recommended guidelines can lead to transmission of bronchoscopy-related infections.

**Table 2.5** Steps in reprocessing of flexible bronchoscopes

| Step | Main purpose | Process | Comments |
|---|---|---|---|
| Mechanical cleaning | To prevent drying of organic material on the internal and external surfaces of bronchoscope | Wipe outer surface of insertion tube with a gauze piece soaked in detergent solution<br><br>Suction of detergent solution through working channel<br><br>Detach suction ports and biopsy attachments and discard disposable items<br><br>Instrument is now ready for leak testing | |
| Leak testing | To detect damage to the working channel or to the outer sheath<br><br>Bronchoscope with positive leak test cannot be adequately disinfected | Pressurize the instrument with leak tester<br><br>Fully immerse the instrument in water<br><br>Look for escape of air bubbles<br><br>Gently flex and extend the bending section to detect minor leak of air bubbles<br><br>Instrument is now ready for cleaning with enzymatic detergent | Do not use damaged bronchoscope<br><br>Return the bronchoscope to the manufacturer for repair<br><br>Label bronchoscope sent for repairs as a contaminated medical device |
| Detergent cleaning | To further reduce the organic matter and prevent formation of biofilm | Soak bronchoscope in water and enzymatic detergent for 5 min<br><br>Clean and wipe external surface of bronchoscope with enzymatic detergent<br><br>Clean all ports and working channel of bronchoscope with sterile brush<br><br>Flush working channel repeatedly to remove loose material<br><br>Rinse the external and internal surfaces with water to remove the detergent residues<br><br>The instrument is now ready for high-level disinfection | Thorough cleaning achieves 3.5 to 4 log reduction in bacterial load<br><br>Use either disposable cleaning brushes or mechanically cleaned and sterilized brushes |

*Continued*

**Table 2.5** *Continued*

| Step | Main purpose | Process | Comments |
|------|-------------|---------|----------|
| High-level disinfection | To destroy remaining microbial agents as much as possible | The process can be manual or fully automated (using AER)<br><br>Both methods are equally effective when procedural guidelines are strictly followed<br><br>Ethylene oxide sterilization is highly effective but causes logistic difficulties and delays in reprocessing<br><br>Further sterilization is no more effective than HLD in reducing the transmission of infection via bronchoscope<br><br>Instrument is ready for rinsing and drying after HLD | Make sure that bronchoscope is compatible with AER model<br><br>Verify appropriate connection of working channel with AER tubing<br><br>Failure to do so may lead to inadequate exposure of the working channel to the liquid disinfectant<br><br>Strictly follow the HLD protocol as recommended by the manufacturer<br><br>Maintain AER according to manufacturer's recommendation |
| Final rinsing and drying | Removes residual liquid disinfectant from the working channel and external surface<br><br>Moisture in working channel during storage promotes recontamination of bronchoscopes with microbial agents | Rinse working channel and external surface with sterile or filtered tap water<br><br>Instrument is dried by purging the working channel with 70% alcohol or dried air | Tap water should not be used for final rinsing<br><br>The rinsing and drying takes place in most models of AER The quality of rinse water in AER should be monitored<br><br>Do not reuse rinse water<br><br>Do not use the same sink for initial cleaning and final rinsing |
| Storage | Improperly stored instrument may cause recontamination with potentially pathogenic organisms | Store in well-ventilated cabinets<br><br>Drying cabinet using a desiccant is optional<br><br>Store in hanging position<br><br>Do not re-attach any disposable or detachable parts during storage | Do not store in original carrying case |

AER, automated endoscopic reprocessor; HLD, high-level disinfection.

## Cleaning

A thorough initial cleaning of bronchoscopes reduces the organic soil, decreases infective burden, and prevents formation of biofilms in the bronchoscopes. Contamination of the instrument with upper airway secretions is inevitable during bronchoscopy. After a routine procedure, the bronchoscope is contaminated with as many as $6.4 \times 10^4$ CFU/mL of bacteria [39]. Most commonly isolated organisms are streptococci and other oral commensal agents. The risk of contamination of bronchoscopes with virulent organisms is greater when the procedure is performed in high-risk patients, such as organ transplant recipients and HIV-infected patients with pulmonary infiltrates.

The purpose of mechanical cleaning is to remove the infected secretions and organic matter from the exposed surfaces of the bronchoscope. A thorough mechanical cleaning immediately after bronchoscopy is shown to reduce the bacterial burden by 3.5 to 4 logs [40]. Inadequate cleaning also leaves organic matter in the working channel that significantly reduces the effectiveness of disinfecting agents. In addition, inadequate mechanical cleaning also promotes formation of biofilm, which becomes an important reservoir for future infections.

Current guidelines strongly emphasize a thorough manual cleaning of bronchoscopes prior to high-level disinfection (Table 2.5). The cleaning process is labor intensive and requires at least 15 minutes of operator time. It is therefore not surprising that external reviews have shown poor compliance with the recommended cleaning guidelines. For example, manufacturers recommend a minimum of 5 minutes contact between the enzymatic detergent and the endoscope but this recommendation is frequently ignored [41]. Newer, automated endoscopic reprocessors with the capability to clean the bronchoscopes prior to high-level disinfection are now available. These instruments are intended to replace the manual cleaning and brushing with an automated and standard process that is less prone to human errors. The US Food and Drug Administration has approved the labeling of these instruments as "washer-disinfectors". Currently, independent data on the efficacy of automated washers are rather limited but some encouraging information has started to emerge. For example, in a recent study, an automated disinfector was found to be as effective as manual cleaning for artificially soiled bronchoscopes [42]. While these results are encouraging, further work is needed to confirm these results. For now, a thorough manual cleaning of bronchoscopes prior to high-level disinfection remains the standard operating procedure.

Proper cleaning of bronchoscopes requires disconnection and disassembly of all detachable components, such as biopsy ports and suction valves. Disposable components should be discarded. Reusable valves, if still used, should undergo thorough cleaning and high-level disinfection or sterilization according to manufacturer's recommendations. The current American College of Chest Physicians (ACCP) guidelines recommend using disposable bronchoscopic valves because failure to adequately reprocess the reusable valves has caused several outbreaks [1,2,19,43].

Leak testing is an essential component of bronchoscope reprocessing. Leak test detects internal damage to the working channel, which is otherwise difficult to detect. Damage to the inner channel promotes development of biofilm and, once developed, a reliable high-level disinfection of these instruments cannot be guaranteed. Several outbreaks have occurred due to failure to perform leak test and detect damage to the working channel. Among these, most serious was the transmission of tuberculosis to several patients due to use of a damaged bronchoscope contaminated with *M. tuberculosis* [17]. In this report, a hole in the working channel precluded adequate disinfection of the bronchoscope after it was used in a confirmed case of tuberculosis. The damage to the bronchoscope was not detected because the leak test was not routinely performed after each procedure.

The enzymatic detergent used for cleaning the bronchoscopes should be discarded after a single use. Similarly, water used for rinsing the bronchoscopes after detergent cleaning should not be reused for cleaning other bronchoscopes.

## High-level disinfection

Bronchoscopes are semicritical devices and high-level disinfection is required after every procedure. The process involves immersion of the entire bronchoscope in an approved disinfectant for a specified period of time. The process is highly effective, as long as adequate precleaning is performed and recommended guidelines are followed. The Food and Drug Administration has approved several chemical agents for high-level disinfection of endoscopes. A com-

plete list of the approved disinfectants, recommended concentration, contact time, and the maximum reuse days was updated in March 2009 and can be accessed from http://www.fda.gov/cdrh/ODE/germlab.html [44]. The most commonly used agents for high-level disinfection are 2% glutaraldehyde, peracetic acid, and orthophthaldehyde. The advantages, disadvantages and adverse effects of these agents are summarized in Table 2.6 and have been reviewed elsewhere [45,46]. Although Food and Drug Administration (FDA) guidelines are somewhat more stringent, the ACCP expert committee recommends bronchoscope disinfection for 20 minutes in 2% alkaline glutaraldehyde at 20°C for high-level disinfection after the scopes are adequately precleaned according to the recommended techniques [38]. This recommendation is based on results from several validated sources. Multisociety guidelines have made similar recommendation for high-level disinfection of flexible gastrointestinal endoscopes [47]. High-level disinfection can be accomplished either by manual methods or with the use of AERs (Fig. 2.3). When done properly, both methods are equally effective for high-level disinfection of endoscopes [48]. Advantages and disadvantages of each method are listed in Table 2.7. The most important concern with the manual method of high-level disinfection is health risks to the bronchoscopy staff due to occupational exposure to glutaraldehyde. For this reason, an increasing number of bronchoscopy facilities have adopted the use of AER for high-level disinfection. Regardless of which method is used, it is important to make sure that all components of the bronchoscope, including the inner channel, are adequately perfused with the disinfectant solution and there is adequate contact time between the disinfectant and the bronchoscope. When a manual method is used, the working channel needs to be

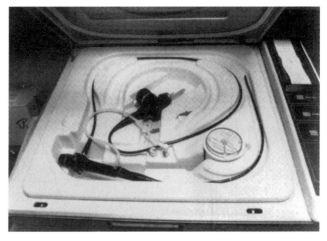

**Fig. 2.3** Steris system automated endoscope reprocessor (Steris Corp, Mentor, OH) with bronchoscope in place in preparation for automated chemical sterilization.

**Table 2.6** Common agents used for high-level disinfection of bronchoscopes

| Agent | Advantages | Disadvantages | Adverse effects | Comments |
|---|---|---|---|---|
| 2% Glutaraldehyde | Inexpensive | High incidence of adverse effects | Pungent odor | Interferes with DNA, RNA, and protein synthesis of microbial agents |
| | Easily available | Requires optimal pH (7.5–8.5) to be effective | Respiratory irritant | Check pH and concentration at the beginning of every day and maintain a written record |
| | Extensive experience | Shelf-life limited to 14 days due to spontaneous polymerization and loss of free aldehyde groups | May cause occupational asthma | 20-2-20 rule: a minimum of 20 min exposure, 2% concentration at a minimum of 20°C needed for adequate HLD |
| | No damage to the bronchoscopes | May coagulate blood and fix organic material to the surface if initial cleaning is poor | Skin and eye irritation | All external and internal surfaces should come in contact with the agent |
| | | Becomes diluted with repeated use | Contact dermatitis | Precautions to minimize exposure to the health-care workers are essential |
| | | Mucosal irritation and inflammation if traces of agent are left in the working channel due to incomplete final rinse | | Ambient glutaraldehyde concentration should be <0.05 ppm |
| | | *M. chelonae, Trichosporon*, fungal ascospores are resistant to disinfection | | Area should be well-ventilated |
| | | | | 7–15 air exchanges per hour |
| | | | | Use ducted exhaust hoods or ductless fume-absorbent hoods to reduce exposure |
| Peracetic acid | Environmentally friendly without toxic by-products | More expensive than glutaraldehyde | No major adverse effects under normal conditions | Used in fully automated systems such as Steris system 1 |
| | Good sporicidal activity | May cause serious skin and eye burns if accidentally spilled | | Requires contact time of 30–45 min |
| | May facilitate removal of organic material from working channel | | Fumes can cause irritation of nose, throat, and lungs | Single use eliminates need for routine concentration monitoring |
| | Does not coagulate blood or fix organic material to the surface | | | |
| Orthophthaldehyde | Fast-acting high-level disinfectant | More expensive than glutaraldehyde | Eye irritation with contact | Less commonly used in the US |
| | Excellent stability over a pH range 3–9 | Slower sporicidal action | | |
| | Does not coagulate blood or fix organic material to the surface | | | |
| | No odor | | | |

**Table 2.7** Advantages and disadvantages of manual and automated endoscopic reprocessors for high-level disinfection

|  | Manual method | Automated endoscopic reprocessors |
|---|---|---|
| Advantages | Low cost | Requires less operator time |
|  | Less complicated | Ensures standard disinfectant concentration and appropriate contact period |
|  | No risk of mechanical failure | Less health risks to operators |
|  |  | Less prone to human errors |
| Disadvantages | Time-consuming | High initial cost |
|  | Health risks to operators due to vapors, chemical spills | More complicated than manual method |
|  | Need to check concentration of glutaraldehyde every day | Risk of mechanical failure |
|  | Inadequate contact time due to human factors | Potential for improper connections |
|  | Potential to reuse the solution for more than recommended period | Potential for contamination of detergent tank |
|  |  | Contamination of waterlines and water filters |
|  |  | May need expensive repairs or replacement once contaminated |

filled with the disinfectant using a syringe containing the solution. When using the AER, it is critical to ensure that the instrument and the bronchoscope model are compatible and that proper channel connectors are used as recommended by the manufacturer. Failure to do so may result in inadequate flow of the disinfectants through the bronchoscope, resulting in suboptimal or insufficient high-level disinfection [49].

Contamination of AERs has caused several bronchoscopy-related outbreaks. These include true infections as well as pseudoinfections due to non-tubercular mycobacteria, *Pseudomonas aeruginosa*, and several other microbial agents [8,35,50]. As discussed above, biofilm is the cause of recurring infections in many cases and, once formed, it is difficult to remove with the conventional disinfection methods. Regular maintenance of AER according to manufacturer's recommendations is essential for reliable functioning of the machines. In-line water filters should be changed on a regular basis as recommended. Failure to do so has led to *M. chelonae* pseudo-outbreaks [50].

**Rinsing, drying, and storage**

The next important step in reprocessing after high-level disinfection is rinsing of the bronchoscope and its working channel with either sterile or filtered water. Rinsing is done to remove the residual disinfectant agent from the bronchoscope before it is used for the next procedure. Ideally, rinsing should be done with sterile water but, in practical terms, filtered tap water may be acceptable. Use of tap water for this purpose is unacceptable because of risk of contamination with non-tubercular mycobacterium and other pathogenic bacteria. Because several outbreaks have been traced

back to an inadequate quality of rinse water, some authors have suggested routine microbiologic sampling of the rinse water used for endoscope reprocessing [51–53]. However, due to lack of studies showing efficacy of this practice in reducing outbreaks, and due to the cost and resource utilization issues, routine monitoring of rinse water remains a debatable issue.

After rinsing with water, the insertion tube and working channel should be thoroughly dried at the completion of every reprocessing cycle [54]. Moist environment inside the working channel promotes bacterial growth and can lead to outbreaks after bronchoscopy. Drying of the working channel is best achieved by first rinsing it with 70% alcohol, followed by forcing compressed air through the channel. Apart from drying, rinsing with alcohol also inhibits the growth of microbial agents. Rinsing with 70% alcohol and drying with air are essential between use of bronchoscope for each patient and before final overnight storage of the instruments.

Proper storage is important in preventing the recontamination of the bronchoscopes. After thorough drying, the bronchoscopes should be stored in an upright hanging position in a roomy drying cabinet that uses a desiccant to reduce relative humidity. The suction and biopsy ports should not be reassembled prior to storage. In one report, replacement of the suction biopsy valve immediately after cleaning allowed moisture to accumulate in these areas which caused contamination of the bronchoscope with *Rhodotorula rubra* [23]. Storing the bronchoscope in the carrying cases or in a coiled position is inappropriate and may increase the risk of outbreaks of infections after bronchoscopy [55].

### Reprocessing of accessory instruments

Unlike bronchoscopes, many accessory instruments used during bronchoscopy are critical medical devices from an infection control view point. Because breach of mucosal lining and bleeding are inevitable, only sterile biopsy forceps can be used during bronchoscopic lung biopsies. Contaminated biopsy forceps have been implicated in transmitting infections in patients undergoing colonoscopy. After every use, the biopsy forceps should be thoroughly cleaned with a detergent. The complex design of the distal part of biopsy forceps and the spiral wound configuration of its shaft limit the efficacy of manual detergent cleaning. Use of a medical-grade ultrasonic cleaner is highly effective in cleaning the soiled biopsy forceps and is the preferred method for this purpose [56]. After thorough cleaning, the forceps should be sterilized. Being heat stable, steam autoclaving according to the manufacturer's recommendations is the most commonly used method to sterilize the reusable biopsy forceps. Ethylene oxide sterilization is equally effective and may also be used. Sometimes a single-use biopsy forceps is reused after steam sterilization. However, the safety of this practice is not established and should be strongly discouraged. Similarly, needles such as those used during TBNA cannot be adequately sterilized. These needles are intended for single patient use and any attempt to sterilize them for reuse is unacceptable.

A related issue is the potential for malfunctioning biopsy forceps to damage the inner channel of the bronchoscope. Damage to the inner channel compromises the adequacy of reprocessing, even when all guidelines are strictly followed. Damage to the inner channel by defective biopsy forceps was recently implicated in several cases of bronchoscopy-related *Pseudomonas aeruginosa* infections and pseudoinfections [57]. Therefore all malfunctioning biopsy forceps should be discarded.

Another potential source of infection during bronchoscopy is a contaminated atomizer. After a single use, the atomizer lumen and the fluid reservoir frequently get contaminated with micro-organisms [58]. A cluster of cases of tuberculosis has been linked to improper sharing of an atomizer for administering topical anesthesia in patients undergoing bronchoscopy [20]. Therefore, use of the same atomizer for more than one patient should be strictly prohibited. After using on an individual patient, an atomizer should be thoroughly cleaned and steam sterilized. The blocked nozzles of atomizer are difficult to clean and should be discarded. A presterilized single-use or disposable atomizer is another good option.

A pseudo-outbreak of *Aureobasidium* species after bronchoscopy has been reported due to reuse of plastic three-way stopcocks on different patients during bronchoalveolar lavage [59]. After every use, the sterilization of stopcocks was attempted by placing them in an automated disinfection machine designed for bronchoscopes. This process failed and

the cultures from the stopcocks showed heavy growth of the fungus. This report illustrates several important points. First, isolation of an unusual organism should raise suspicion of a breakdown in the reprocessing or infection control practices during bronchoscopy. Second, it reinforces that reuse of single-use items during bronchoscopy is not a safe practice. Finally, it highlights the importance of using only standard and validated methods to sterilize medical devices. The disinfection machines designed for bronchoscopes cannot guarantee disinfection of other medical instruments unless clearly specified by the manufacturer.

Attention should also be paid to cleaning brushes as the potential source of bronchoscopy-related infections. These brushes can become highly contaminated after a single use. In one report, failure to adequately disinfect and sterilize the cleaning brushes led to a pseudo-outbreak of *Rhodotorula rubra* [24]. Disposable cleaning brushes are cheap and are recommended for cleaning the inner channels of the bronchoscopes. Non-disposable cleaning brushes should undergo thorough cleaning with detergent, followed by high-level disinfection or sterilization after every use.

### Prevention of outbreaks
### Education and training

A close look at the underlying cause of an outbreak nearly always reveals a significant deviation from standard reprocessing methods. Most of the problems arise from a lack of proper education in the principles of disinfection and sterilization and practical training in reprocessing methods. External reviews and postal surveys have similarly shown major deficiencies in the manner endoscopes are reprocessed in many institutions. For example, an onsite survey of fiberoptic endoscope reprocessing in 18 Massachusetts hospitals showed a considerable within and interhospital variability in reprocessing practices [60]. Investigators identified several problems, such as less than recommended contact time with the disinfectant solution, inadequate disinfection of the inner channel, improper final rinsing of the endoscopes with tap water, and inadequate sterilization of the biopsy forceps. Interestingly, in several instances, methods for reprocessing endoscopes used in patients known to be infected with human immunodeficiency virus, hepatitis, or tuberculosis were different from those used after an endoscopy on non-infected patients. Interviews with the employees designated to perform reprocessing showed that lack of knowledge of the principles that govern high-level disinfection was an important cause of discrepancies between written policies and actual practice. Several deficiencies were also found in a survey on disinfection practices in 107 North Carolina hospitals [61]. In this study, 44% of hospitals reported immersing the endoscope in disinfectant solution for less than 10 minutes and 55% reported using tap water for the final rinse. Striking problems with adherence to national guidelines was also reported in a large-scale postal survey from 159 bronchoscopy units in the United Kingdom [62]. In this study, 35% of units were using less than minimum recommended disinfection time after bronchoscopy. More troubling was the finding that no disinfection was performed in 34% of units before emergency bronchoscopies. Further, 43% of units did not use sterile or filtered water for the final rinse. This study raises serious questions regarding adequacy of reprocessing after an emergency bronchoscopy performed during off-hours when the usual bronchoscopy staff is not available. Clearly, there is a strong case for all hospitals to designate well-trained and proficient employees who can adequately reprocess endoscopes in off hours and weekends. A recent survey further illustrates serious problems with the familiarity and knowledge base of the health-care workers involved in reprocessing bronchoscopes [63]. In this survey, 65% of respondents, including 55% of the medical directors of the bronchoscopy facility, were not aware of nationally accepted, published reprocessing guidelines. Nearly 40% did not know the reprocessing method and 35% did not know which disinfectant is used at their own institution. About 50% of participants did not keep the record of which bronchoscope was used in each patient. Thirty percent of respondents reported doing routine periodic bronchoscope cultures to detect persistent contamination of bronchoscopes after reprocessing. Only one-third of respondents reported some form of surveillance of bronchoscopy culture results. The knowledge regarding specific reprocessing steps was deficient in many areas.

All of these studies point to an unacceptable lack of knowledge and training in reprocessing of bronchoscopes. These studies also make a strong case for all bronchoscopy facilities to implement an educational initiative for all personnel involved in reprocessing of bronchoscopes.

## Oversight

Unfortunately, the health-care providers have historically shown some degree of complacency towards infection control practices. Endoscopic reprocessing is no exception. Although a very powerful tool, education alone may not be sufficient in improving adherence to the guidelines. A good-quality control program also requires periodic review of reprocessing policies and a careful oversight of the actual practice. Unannounced site visits may also play a role in this regard.

## Environmental sampling

Routine environmental sampling is sometimes recommended on the premise that it will provide an early warning and prevents of bronchoscopy-related infections [5,49]. However, no study has specifically looked into the value of periodic cultures of bronchoscopes or environmental sources to prevent bronchoscopy-related outbreaks. There are no guidelines as to how to perform such a surveillance program,

how often to obtain cultures, and how to interpret the positive results. Also, the cost of such a program is likely to be prohibitive. Due to these reasons, routine microbiological environmental surveillance is not recommended for prevention of bronchoscopy-related outbreaks. Similarly, the current guidelines do not recommend routine microbiological monitoring of the water used for final rinsing of bronchoscopes after high-level disinfection.

## Surveillance

On the contrary, careful surveillance of positive cultures from bronchoscopy is highly useful in the early detection of outbreak. The majority of outbreaks reported in the literature were detected after an unusual or unexpected increase in the isolation rate of certain microbial agent had been detected [64]. Early detection of an outbreak is essential for reducing the size of the outbreak. Therefore, a formal mechanism for surveillance of isolates from bronchoscopy specimens is highly recommended. Unfortunately, many bronchoscopy facilities have no such mechanism in place and no formal surveillance of microbiological data from bronchoscopy specimens is done. The problem is further compounded when several bronchoscopists are sharing the same facility. We strongly recommend designating someone with an infection control background to take charge of such a surveillance program.

The clinician should maintain a high index of suspicion for possible transmission of infection after bronchoscopy. For example, in one report, an unexpected occurrence of *Pseudomonas aeruginosa* lung infection soon after major thoracic surgeries led to an epidemiological investigation [64]. Contaminated bronchoscopes used during single lung anesthesia were found to be the cause of infection. Clearly, observations of astute clinicians played a critical role in curtailing the outbreak at an early stage.

Several other indicators should alert health-care workers regarding a possible breakdown in reprocessing of bronchoscopes. These include isolation of a rare organism, clusters of tuberculosis, isolation of environmental mycobacteria, and an unexpected isolation of organisms such as *Pseudomonas aeruginosa* or *Serratia marcescens* from patients who have no clinical evidence of infection.

## Outbreak investigation

Transmission of infection due to a breach in infection control during bronchoscopy has serious implications for patients, bronchoscopy personnel, and the institution. Once an outbreak of infection is suspected, several simultaneous actions may be needed. Depending on the severity of the situation, the director or physician in charge of the bronchoscopy facility may be forced to temporarily close down the facility until the full extent and the cause(s) of the problem are identified and the corrective actions are taken. Ignoring or willfully overlooking the problem is never appropriate and will only worsen the situation.

## Team approach

A thorough investigation of an outbreak in bronchoscopy facility needs a team of health-care providers. The members of the team should include the director or in-charge of bronchoscopy facility, infection control specialist, infectious disease consultant, laboratory personnel trained in microbiology and molecular techniques, epidemiologist, staff from biomedical engineering, and bronchoscopy assistants. An early involvement of representatives from manufacturers of the bronchoscope, AER, and disinfectants is also useful in many circumstances.

## Data collection

The investigation starts with careful review of all procedures performed during the period of the outbreak. To back-track the data on individual patients, all facilities performing bronchoscopy should maintain a careful record of the patient's name and medical record number, bronchoscopist who performed the procedure, and the serial number or other unique identifier of the bronchoscope used for each procedure [36,38]. A record of the bronchoscopy assistant for each procedure should also be maintained. Without this information, a meaningful epidemiological investigation is impossible to conduct. The information should include the indication for bronchoscopy, clinical and radiological findings, procedures performed during bronchoscopy, microbiological results from bronchoscopy specimens, and results of other relevant microbiological tests such as sputum and blood cultures. The outcome of all patients undergoing bronchoscopy during the outbreak needs to be determined by thorough chart reviews, telephone contact, clinical evaluation, and relevant radiological and laboratory testing. The microbiological results from the bronchoscopy specimens during the outbreak should be compared with the data from preceding months to confirm whether or not there is an actual increase in the infection rate. Using these data, the investigating team should try to identify a link between the infections and a common identifiable variable such as the same bronchoscope, same date of procedure, etc.

The next important step is to thoroughly review the reprocessing practices of the facility in the preceding months. The panel should thoroughly look into all potential breaches in reprocessing that are known to cause contamination (Table 2.8). One should not forget that more than one mechanisms of contamination may be involved in the outbreak [65]. Every staff member designated for reprocessing bronchoscopes should be contacted and interviewed. How the accessory instruments are reprocessed should be recorded. Note should be made of any reuse of an accessory instrument intended for single use. Records of routine maintenance of AER, results of routine surveillance of glutaraldehyde

**Table 2.8** Sources of contamination during bronchoscopy

**Inadequate cleaning**
Inadequate manual cleaning
Biofilm in inner channel
Damaged inner channel
Failure to perform leak test
Loose suction valve
Biopsy port

**Inadequate high-level disinfection**
Inappropriate agent
Incorrect disinfectant concentration

**Contamination of disinfectant solution**
Use of improper connectors to reprocessors
Inadequate flow of disinfectant through inner channel
Mechanical failure of reprocessor

**Contamination of reprocessors**
Biofilm formation
Rinsing tank
Tubing
Filters

**Contamination after high-level disinfection**
Use of tap water for final rinse
Contamination of water filters
Reuse of sterile water for rinsing
Failure to dry bronchoscopes
Reassembly of suction and biopsy port before storage
Storage in coiled position

**Contamination of accessory instruments**
Cleaning brushes
Biopsy forceps
Reuse of three-way stopcocks
Reuse of atomizer without sterilization
Contaminated local anesthetic solution

concentration, change of water filters, etc. should be reviewed. Any deviation from manufacturer's recommended guidelines should be recorded.

## Environmental sampling

Cultures from environmental sources and the bronchoscopes and its components play a critical role in the epidemiological investigation of an outbreak. Cultures should be obtained from detergents bottles and wash basin, disinfectant solution, AER tanks, tap water, filtered water used for final rinse, bronchoscopes, cleaning brushes, multidose medication vials, atomizers, and reusable bronchoscopic accessories. Cultures from the bronchoscope should be obtained in both an anterograde and retrograde manner. An anterograde culture specimen is obtained by flushing 50 mL of sterile saline through the biopsy port into a sterile container. Retrograde culture is obtained by aspirating about one-half of this volume through the endoscope and collecting it into a suction trap. Swabs of biopsy and suction ports should also be obtained.

## Molecular techniques

An outbreak is usually suspected when a pathogen is isolated at a rate higher than expected. Isolation of organisms with similar phenotypic characteristics, such as biotype, serotype, or a unique pattern of antimicrobial susceptibility, provides an early warning of nosocomial infections due to bronchoscopy. While the phenotypic analysis is important in early identification of an epidemic, it has low discriminatory power, limiting its value in further epidemiological investigation. Phenotypic similarity between an organism isolated from an environmental source and the bronchoscopic specimen may be coincidental. Molecular techniques have a greater accuracy in establishing the relatedness of isolates recovered from different sources during investigation of bronchoscopy-related outbreaks. The majority of recent studies looking into bronchoscopy-related outbreaks have used genotypic analysis to identify the source of infection. The most widely used genotypic method for this purpose is pulsed-field gel electrophoresis (PFGE) [66]. In this technique, restriction enzymes are used to digest the chromosomal DNA of the isolates into fragments of different sizes. The DNA fragments are then separated using agarose gel electrophoresis. The analysis of the PFGE pattern is performed using software programs. The results are charted in the form of dendrograms, which provide a visual representation of genetic similarities or differences between isolates from different sources. The PFGE analysis is very reproducible and has a high discriminatory power in epidemiological investigation of an outbreak. Another commonly used technique is polymerase chain reaction (PCR). Several investigators have successfully used PCR-based techniques in epidemiological investigations of bronchoscopy outbreaks. For example, random arbitrary polymorphic DNA PCR was used to identify the bronchoscopes as the source of a *Pseudomonas aeruginosa* outbreak in a Spanish intensive care unit [67]. Recently, repetitive sequence based polymerase chain reaction (REP-PCR) was effectively used to identify the incoming water supply of the automated bronchoscopic washer as the source of an *M. chelonae* pseudo-outbreak [68]. These studies make a strong case for routine application of molecular techniques in bronchoscopy-related outbreak investigation.

## Corrective measures

The corrective measures depend on the underlying cause of the outbreak. In some instances, the solution may be as simple as flushing the working channel with 70% alcohol after final rinse or ensuring proper storage of instruments. In other cases, drastic and potentially very expensive measures, such as replacement of entire AER system, are needed. The epidemiological investigation does not end with implementation of corrective measures. It is critical to continue surveillance of cultures and oversight of reprocessing methods for several weeks to months after the appropriate changes are made.

## Notification

All bronchoscopy-related outbreaks should be notified to the infection control department, local and state health departments, CDC, FDA, and manufacturers of bronchoscopes, AER, and disinfectants. The patients and bronchoscopy personnel who were potentially exposed to infection during the outbreak should also be notified.

## Risk of infection to bronchoscopy staff

The aerosols generated during bronchoscopy have the potential to transmit serious respiratory infections such as tuberculosis, chicken pox, measles, and other respiratory viruses to the bronchoscopy staff. Fortunately, except for a single case of adenovirus infection [69], active respiratory tract infections from exposure during bronchoscopy have not been reported. Still, there is considerable anxiety among health-care workers regarding exposure to tuberculosis during bronchoscopy. This is a valid concern and there are some indirect data to support it. For example, exposure to tuberculosis as determined by the tuberculin skin test conversion rate is shown to be higher among pulmonary fellows than the infectious disease fellows [70]. This discrepancy is postulated to be due to greater risk of exposure to *M. tuberculosis* during bronchoscopy among pulmonary fellows. Another indirect line of evidence comes from a report in which bronchoscopy and endotracheal intubation were linked to a tuberculosis outbreak in a dialysis unit [71]. Bronchoscopists can take several preventive measures to reduce the risk of spreading tuberculosis during bronchoscopy. First, bronchoscopy should be avoided in patients with tuberculosis as much as possible. At least three satisfactory sputum samples should be examined for acid-fast bacilli before considering bronchoscopy. Examination of gastric lavage and urine samples for acid-fast bacilli may be considered in selected situations. When the diagnosis remains elusive, the need to perform bronchoscopy should be carefully weighed against the risk of transmission to the bronchoscopy staff. When the procedure is unavoidable, certain precautions may reduce the risk of transmission and increase the safety of procedure. The procedure should be performed in a negative pressure room. The air should either be discharged outside or pass through high efficiency particulate air (HEPA) filtration before it is recirculated (Fig. 2.4). As much as possible, the patient should wear a mask throughout the procedure. Adequate topical anesthesia and antitus-

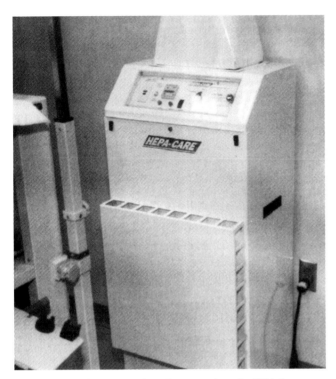

**Fig. 2.4** High-efficiency particle exchanger, such as the HEPA-Care (Abatement Technologies Inc, Atlanta, GA), which cycles room-volume air at least 14 times/hour.

sive medications should be administered to minimize the coughing spells during the procedure. All bronchoscopy personnel should wear a power air-purifying respirator hood that has high efficacy in reducing transmission of tuberculosis [72]. Unfortunately, these devices may not be readily available. The N95 particulate respirator is a minimally acceptable alternative to a power air-purifying respirator hood. Use of a simple surgical mask is inadequate for this purpose.

Needle-stick injury is another potential mechanism for transmission of infection during bronchoscopy. Transmission of hepatitis B infection has been reported after an operator received a needle-stick injury while trying to retrieve the specimen from biopsy forceps using a hypodermic needle [73]. This practice should be strictly prohibited.

Human papilloma virus DNA has been recovered from the smoke plume of the skin lesions treated with carbon dioxide laser and with electrocoagulation [74]. This has raised some occupational safety concerns with endobronchial treatments of human papilloma virus infections. To date, there are no reported cases of transmission of HPV from patients to bronchoscopy staff. Nevertheless, respiratory precautions, such as wearing respiratory masks, are prudent for all staff members performing these procedures. Tight-fitting surgical masks are highly effective in protecting the operators from potential inhalation exposure to papilloma virus. Adequate

facility for the exhaust of smoke generated during these procedures also reduces the exposure to the operators. Similar concerns have also been raised regarding potential transmission of HIV infections. Till date, no bronchoscopy operator is known to have developed HIV seroconversion as a direct result of exposure during bronchoscopy.

Compliance with universal precautions is the single most effective measure to prevent the transmission of infection from the patients to the operators. All health-care workers involved in bronchoscopy should wear full barrier clothing including gowns, gloves, masks, and eye shields [36–38]. Similar barrier precautions are also essential for the staff members delegated to clean and reprocess the bronchoscopes after completion of the procedure. Unfortunately, surveys have shown a very poor compliance with the recommended universal precautions measures during bronchoscopy [62].

## Reprocessing in specific situations
### Mycobacterial diseases
Standard reprocessing methods are highly effective in disinfection of bronchoscopes used in patients with suspected or proven case of tuberculosis [75,76]. No special precautions are needed as long as reprocessing guidelines are strictly followed [36,38].

### Viral diseases
As discussed above, bronchoscope is invariably contaminated with HIV virus after use in AIDS patients [26]. However, current methods of reprocessing are very effective in eliminating all traces of HIV virus. In an experimental study, immersion of contaminated bronchoscope for 2 minutes in glutaraldehyde solution removed all traces of HIV virus [77]. No cases of patient-to-patient transmission of HIV virus has been known to occur due to a contaminated or inadequately reprocessed bronchoscope. Similarly, no cases of hepatitis B and C have been reported after bronchoscopy. Studies from gastrointestinal endoscopy literature indicate that current methods are highly effective in eliminating all traces of hepatitis B and hepatitis C virus from endoscopes [78]. However, adequate mechanical precleaning is essential for effective removal of hepatitis viruses from the working channel. Failure of adequate precleaning has been linked to transmission of hepatitis C after colonoscopy [79].

### Other agents
Anthrax spores are resistant to high-level disinfection. However, transmission of anthrax from patient-to-patient via bronchoscope is not a major concern since spores are produced only in soil and dead tissues and not in blood or living tissues. Therefore, high-level disinfection of bronchoscopes is adequate after use in patients with suspected or proven cases of anthrax [7]. A more complicated

problem is use of bronchoscope in patients with suspected or proven Creutzfeldt–Jacob disease (CJD). According to expert opinion, no special precautions are necessary for reprocessing bronchoscopes after use in suspected or proven cases of CJD [7,80]. In contrast, the European Society of Gastrointestinal Endoscopy (ESGE) has suggested avoiding endoscopy in these patients as much as possible and, when unavoidable, using an endoscope that is approaching the end of its useful life [81]. The endoscope used in CJD patient should then be destroyed or quarantined for future use only for patients with proven CJD. In the absence of any literature on this subject, the physicians may elect to follow the same guidelines when bronchoscopy is required in patients with suspected CJD.

## Novel approaches

Reprocessing a bronchoscope is a labor intensive process needing a minimum of 30 to 60 minutes of downtime before the bronchoscope can be used for the next procedures. Due to this limitation, many bronchoscopy facilities require several ready-to-use bronchoscopes at all times. Further, as discussed above, the cleaning and disinfection are highly prone to errors, leading to breakdown in infection control during bronchoscopy. To overcome some of these shortcomings, a novel bronchoscope that uses a presterilized, single-use endoscope sheath system has been introduced. The sheath completely covers the bronchoscope and prevents any contact between the body secretions and the surfaces of the bronchoscope. The bronchoscope used in this system has no working channel. Instead, the system uses a 2.1-mm working channel that is built into the disposable sheath. Proper placement of the sheath over the bronchoscope requires some training and about 5 minutes of operator time. The sheath is discarded after completion of the procedure. This device is approved by the FDA. In a preliminary report involving 24 patients, the initial experience with this device was generally satisfactory [82]. Some of the limitations were difficulty in inserting a slip tip syringe, lower handing comfort, and less than ideal image quality in some instances. A larger French study has reported some difficulty with the suction capability and the maneuverability of the bronchoscope [83]. However, this system may find useful application when bronchoscopy is performed in off-sites such as intensive care units, in off-hours such as nights and weekends, and in high-risk patient such as those who are suspected to have multidrug resistant tuberculosis.

## Radiation protection in bronchoscopy

### Background

Fluoroscopy is an important source of occupational radiation exposure among non-radiology medical personnel. Bronchoscopists use fluoroscopy during a variety of diagnostic

**Table 2.9** Common procedures using fluoroscopy

| |
| --- |
| Transbronchial biopsy |
| Cytology brush specimens from peripheral lung masses |
| Peripheral transbronchial needle aspiration |
| Localization of radiopaque foreign body |
| Brachytherapy |
| Airway stent placement |
| Postprocedure to rule out pneumothorax |

and therapeutic procedures (Table 2.9). It is assumed that the benefit with these procedures is greater than the risk from radiation exposure. While it is correct in most cases, the magnitude of risk is difficult to estimate because there is no practical method to determine the radiation dose to the patients during these procedures. Radiation exposure is associated with several potential health problems. Most feared is the future risk of cancer due to low-level radiation exposure. This is a valid concern not only for the patients but also for the health-care professionals such as bronchoscopists, pulmonary fellows, nurses, bronchoscopy assistants, and other support staff who receive scattered radiation during the procedure [84]. As a matter of common sense, every effort should be made to minimize the radiation doses used during bronchoscopy. This will not only reduce the risk to the patients but will also reduce the radiation exposure to the health-care workers. However, a sound knowledge of radiation protection principles is needed to achieve this goal.

Although the cumulative low-dose radiation exposure over a prolonged period is a serious concern, the dose used in a single diagnostic and therapeutic procedure seldom causes any immediate problem. Because of the absence of any acute effects, health-care workers generally underestimate the radiation hazards, and frequently ignore the radiation hygiene practices. To make the matter worse, the majority of health-care workers who use diagnostic radiation outside the radiology departments have never received any formal training in radiation physics or the principles of radiation protection. Included in this category are bronchoscopists, who are ultimately responsible for the radiation safety of their patients and the staff members present in the bronchoscopy room.

In this section, we will discuss radiation terminology and the possible health risks associated with diagnostic radiation. We will discuss how fluoroscopy works and how to minimize the radiation exposure to the patients and the bystanders when using fluoroscopy. We will also discuss the radiation monitoring and safety procedures for all personnel who perform or assist with fluoroscopy during flexible bronchoscopy.

## Radiation terminology

Practicing physicians and health-care providers are unfamiliar with several technical terms used in radiation medicine. In this section, we provide a simplified explanation of some commonly used terms. For a more in-depth discussion, readers are referred to recent reviews on this subject [85,86].

**X ray** is a type of ionizing radiation, consisting of high-energy photons. When X rays strike the human body, some photons penetrate the tissues and others are reflected in different directions. A fraction of these photons are absorbed by the tissues and the remaining photons pass through the body. The fraction that passes through the tissues carries the diagnostic information. One of the quantities used to describe the intensity or the strength of X rays generated by the source is **exposure**, which is measured by the ionization produced by X rays in a unit mass of air. Exposure is defined strictly for air and it quantifies the amount of radiation directed towards the photographic film or the image intensifier. Exposure by itself does not quantify the radiation-induced health risk to the patient because many other factors determine how much damaging radiation is absorbed by the tissues. In Systeme Internationale d'Unites (SI units), the radiation exposure is expressed as coulombs per kilogram (C/kg). The conventional unit of radiation exposure is the roentgen (R). One R is equal to $2.58 \times 10^{-4}$ C/kg. A better parameter to quantify the intensity of an X ray beam is **kerma**, which stands for kinetic energy released per unit mass. Kerma quantifies the amount of energy transferred from the X ray photons to the charged particles in the medium, which could be either air or other media such as human tissues. The unit of kerma is the gray (Gy). One Gy is equal to 1 joule of energy transferred from X rays to the charged particles per kilogram of the medium. Exposure and kerma are the measures of intensity of X ray beam. Since the tissues absorb only a fraction of incident X ray beam, these quantities do not measure the absorbed dose of radiation. The **absorbed dose** is the amount of energy imparted to a unit mass of the medium by the ionizing radiation. The SI unit of absorbed radiation dose is the gray (Gy). One gray is equal to 1 joule/kg. The old unit of absorbed dose is radiation absorbed dose or rad. One gray is equal to 100 rads. Another important parameter, especially relevant to fluoroscopy is absorbed dose rate, which is the radiation dose absorbed by the tissues per unit time. It is measured in Gy/min.

The degree of tissue damage depends not only on quantity of radiation but also on the biological effectiveness of the type of radiation in causing damage and on the tissue's susceptibility to radiation damage. Some types of radiation are more damaging to tissues than others. For instance, for a given absorbed dose, a beam of neutrons will cause more damage to the tissues than a beam X rays. The **equivalent dose** is a measure of the absorbed dose of a type of radiation weighted for its potential to cause tissue injury. The SI unit

of equivalent dose is sievert (Sv). The old unit of equivalent dose is rem. One Sv is equal to 100 rem. The quantity that defines the damaging potential of different types of radiation is called the radiation weighting factor ($W_r$). The equivalent dose is calculated as follows:

Equivalent dose (Sv) = Absorbed dose (Gy) $\times W_r$

The International Commission on Radiological Protection (ICRP) has recently revised the $W_r$ values for the different types of radiations [87]. For X rays, the radiation-weighting factor is equal to one; so the equivalent dose in Sv units is equal to the absorbed dose in Gy.

Health-care workers receive different radiation exposures to different parts of the body during procedures involving diagnostic radiation. All parts of the body are not equally susceptible to the damaging effects of radiation. Different tissues have been assigned a tissue weighting factor ($W_t$) depending on their sensitivity to the damaging effect of radiation. To take into account the amount of dose and individual susceptibility of each organ to radiation damage the concept of the **effective dose** (ED) has been introduced to assess overall risk to the body from radiation. The ED is the sum of the equivalent doses to all tissues each weighted for the radiosensitivity of that tissue:

$$\text{Effective dose (Sv)} = \sum_{T} D_T \, W_t$$

$D_T$ is the equivalent dose received by each organ or tissue, and $W_t$ is the tissue-weighting factor.

ED is the best indicator of the radiation risk to patients and health-care workers who are exposed to radiation during their professional duties. It measures the overall risk of radiation exposure to the human body. Radiation protection guidelines use ED to define the radiation dose limits for the public and professionals who are exposed to radiation. The SI unit of ED is the sievert (Sv). The old unit of ED is roentgen-equivalent-man (rem). One Sv is equal to 100 rem.

## Health risks from radiation

Biologic risks of radiation are well known. The damaging effect of radiation is primarily mediated by ionization in the tissues. Ionization is the process of adding or subtracting electron(s) from atoms or molecules, creating negatively or positively charged ions. Water molecules are the primary target of radiation-induced ionization in human cells. The hydroxyl radicals generated by this reaction cause breaks in the continuity of DNA chains that can involve either single or both strands. The single-strand breaks in the DNA are rapidly repaired. The double-strand breaks are more difficult to repair. Inadequate repair of DNA causes point mutations and various other chromosomal aberrations. These changes in the genetic material are linked to future induction of

**Table 2.10** Adverse health effects of radiation

**Deterministic effects**
Erythema
Desquamation
Skin necrosis
Bone marrow suppression
Organ atrophy
Low fertility
Cataract

**Stochastic effects**
Cancer
Germ cell DNA defects

cancer. Severe damage to chromosomal DNA can lead to cell death.

The harmful effects of radiation on the human body are divided into deterministic and stochastic effects (Table 2.10). The fundamental mechanism of deterministic effects is radiation-induced cell death. Deterministic effects have a dose threshold; the degree of tissue injury is a function of the radiation dose. Below the threshold dose, the damage to the tissues is not clinically evident. Above this threshold dose, the severity of damage to the tissues is proportional to the radiation dose. Large radiation doses, typically in the range 1–2 Gy, are required to cause deterministic changes. The skin exposure during certain lengthy interventional procedures, such as difficult angioplasty procedures and vascular stenting, may approach this dose [88]. Deterministic effects due to radiation use have not been reported with fluoroscopy use in bronchoscopy.

With stochastic effects, the probability of an adverse event increases with higher doses, but the intensity of the adverse effect does not. A typical example of a stochastic effect is the induction of cancer by radiation exposure. Carcinogenic potential of high doses of radiation is well accepted. However, the association between low-level occupational radiation exposure and the risk of cancer in humans has caused a considerable debate [89]. Estimates of cancer risks from low-level exposure to radiation are largely derived either from extrapolation of results from experimental studies that used high-dose exposure [90] or from long-term follow-up of atomic bomb survivors [91]. According to one estimate, 1% of all cases of leukemia and less than 1% of all cases of breast cancer result from diagnostic radiation [92]. Recent analyses have revealed good evidence of increased risk of cancer for individuals exposed to more than 50–100 mSv of radiation dose over a protracted period of time [93].

Due to the serious nature of the illness, health-care workers are rightly concerned about the future risk of cancer due to occupational radiation exposure. Indeed, most

experts, including the Committee on the Biological Effect of Ionizing Radiation in their 1990 report (BEIR V), have taken a conservative stand on this issue and proposed that the risk of a radiation-induced malignancy should be assumed to have a linear dose–response curve with a perceptible risk whenever exposure is higher than zero [94]. This makes a strong case for limiting occupational radiation exposure to as low as possible.

### Limiting radiation exposure

The natural sources of radiation are responsible for about 85% of the lifetime radiation exposure to human beings. Artificially produced radiation accounts for the remaining 15% of exposure [87]. Most of the latter comes from diagnostic and interventional radiology procedures. The health benefits from appropriate use of these procedures cannot be disputed. The real challenge is to minimize the radiation exposure during these procedures without sacrificing the health benefits. In this context, it is important to note the wide variation in the amount of radiation exposure between different radiological procedures and within the same radiological procedure performed by different operators. Clearly, there is scope for a decrease in radiation dose without affecting the quality of the procedure.

In recent years, concern about the possibility of excessive radiation exposure to health-care workers has increased [95]. Numerous studies among intervention radiologists [96], invasive cardiologists [97], orthopedic surgeons [98], urologists [99], anesthetists [100], and physicians from various other specialties have found the occupational radiation exposures to be well below the accepted upper limits. These data have greatly assured medical personnel about the safety of their work environment. Although similar information for health-care workers involved in bronchoscopy is unknown, there is no reason to suspect that radiation exposure to bronchoscopists is any greater than radiation exposure to medical personnel in other specialties who use fluoroscopy.

A number of national and international scientific committees and regulatory agencies are working together to establish limits for the radiation exposure to anyone who is at high risk of radiation exposure. In addition to collecting and analyzing data on radiation, these organizations have proposed upper limits of safe radiation exposure in occupational settings. The ICRP has recommended that in occupational setting, the average ED over 5 years should not exceed 20 mSv per year. The committee also recommends that ED should not exceed 50 mSv in any single year [87,101]. Organ-specific upper limits are summarized in Table 2.11.

While much has been discussed regarding the risk of radiation to health-care workers, the importance of reducing exposure to the patient has not received adequate attention from the scientific community. However, this trend is changing and in recent years experts have started to raise concern

**Table 2.11** Dose limits for occupational radiation exposure

| Effective dose | 20 mSv/year, on average over 5 years |
| | 50 mSv in any 1 year |
| Organ-specific dose: | |
| lens | 150 mSv |
| skin | 500 mSv |
| hand and feet | 500 mSv |

about excessive radiation exposure to the patients due to the overuse of radiological procedures [102,103]. With the assumption of net benefit with diagnostic radiation use, no regulatory agency has set limits for the radiation dose to the patients during imaging and interventional procedures. Instead, the ICRP and other experts in this area have advised physicians to follow the principles of justification, optimization, and dose reduction whenever using diagnostic radiation in patient care [101,104]. All health-care providers, including bronchoscopists, should have a clear understanding of these principles.

The principle of justification refers to a careful risk–benefit analysis before a procedure. The diagnostic use of radiation is justified when the benefits from the procedure clearly outweigh the risks. The physician ordering a radiological procedure must have an unequivocal justification for the request. Periodic external validation through audits is an essential tool to establish the appropriateness of these procedures. A second and perhaps a higher level of justification is to judge whether a procedure using radiation should become a part of medical practice at all. This is an important question for professional medical organizations, which provide guidelines to the physicians and set standards of practice. This can be best explained by the following example. The conventional TBNA has a high diagnostic yield in patients with mediastinal lymph node enlargement due to lung cancer. The TBNA yield is further increased with endobronchial ultrasound guidance (EBUS). No radiation is involved in conventional or EBUS-guided TBNA. Some studies have also looked into the potential role of CT-fluoroscopy guidance during TBNA [105]. In a small study, the diagnostic yield from TBNA was higher with the CT-fluoroscopy-guided procedure than the conventional procedure, but the difference did not reach statistical difference. Thus, without a clear advantage over standard TBNA procedure, radiation exposure to the patient with CT-fluoroscopy-guided TBNA cannot be justified. The principle of justification in radiation use requires the professional organization to consider radiation risks before endorsing such a procedure in practice guidelines.

The principle of optimization refers to the choice of examination, imaging technique, and equipment so that the desired goal of imaging or intervention is achieved with the

minimum radiation dose. This is also called the ALARA (as low as reasonably achievable) principle [106]. Some of its essential components are strong quality-assurance programs, audits, and planned replacement of outdated or suboptimal equipment. An example of optimization is the comparison of fluoroscopy time for a given procedure among different operators within a department. Such information is easy to obtain. This may allow early intervention through education and training to the outliers who consistently use longer fluoroscopy time than their peers for a given procedure.

Successful application of these principles requires all end users to be trained and educated in the basic principles that govern the radiation use during diagnostic procedures. Since fluoroscopy is the leading source of mostly unmonitored radiation exposure to the patients, it is critical for all operators to learn the technical and operational aspects of fluoroscopy machines. This can significantly reduce the patient and staff exposure without compromising the quality and outcome of the procedure.

**Fluoroscopy**

Fluoroscopy is designed to display the real-time images of the internal organs. The essential components of all fluoroscopic systems are an X-ray tube and an image intensifier attached to a video camera unit (Fig. 2.5). The X rays are produced by accelerating electrons from a cathode to an anode within an evacuated glass tube, which is covered by a shield of lead and steel. The X rays are produced when the electron beam is abruptly blocked by a tungsten metal target. The **primary X-ray beam** exits through a small opening in the shield called the **radiation port**. When the primary beam strikes the human body, a fraction of it is fully absorbed

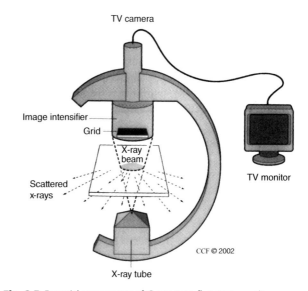

**Fig. 2.5** Essential components of C-arm type fluoroscopy units. (Published with permission from Wang, Mehta, and Turner; Flexible Bronchoscopy 2003; Blackwell publishing Ltd.)

by the tissues, another fraction is partially absorbed, changes directions and exits as scattered radiation, and the rest passes through the body and is received by the image intensifier. The tissue type and density determine the extent to which each of these processes occurs. Diagnostic information is provided by the fraction of the primary beam that passes through the patient and enters the image intensifier. The image intensifier converts the X rays into a visible image which is captured by the television camera and displayed on a monitor. In a typical C-arm fluoroscopy system, the X-ray tube is located under the table and the image intensifier is above the patient. These are called undercouch systems and are strongly preferred over the overcouch systems where the X-ray source is in front of the patient and the image intensifier is under the table. Overcouch systems give higher radiation dose to the patients and the staff than undercouch systems [107]. The harmful effect of radiation to the patient is mainly from the fraction that is absorbed in the tissues. Modern fluoroscopy systems have several features that can reduce this fraction without significantly affecting the image quality. **Scattered radiation** is the portion of the X-ray beam that changes direction and exits from all sides of the patient. Scattered radiation is the chief hazard to health-care workers present in the room. Several effective methods are available to minimize radiation exposure to the health-care workers during fluoroscopy use [108,109].

### Characteristics of the X-ray beam

The electron flow inside the glass tube is called the tube current and it is expressed in milliamperes (mA). The intensity of the X rays produced is proportional to the tube current. Intensity of X rays increases with increase in the tube current. The increase in tube current improves the quality of the image. However, it comes at a cost of greater radiation exposure to the patients and the by-standers. For most interventional procedures including bronchoscopy, the higher image quality with high mA tube current is not needed. Therefore, the tube current in mA should be lowered as much as possible during fluoroscopic examination. Typical tube currents used in routine fluoroscopy systems range from 1 to 5 mA.

The energy of the primary X-ray beam is determined by the tube voltage, expressed in kilovolt peak (kVp). The voltage of the beam affects the intensity and penetrating power of the X rays. Higher kVp increases the penetrating power of the X rays and allows fluoroscopy to operate at low tube current. An X-ray beam of high voltage (kVp) and low current (mA) gives a lower radiation dose to the patient than a beam with low voltage and high current. Using X rays of high kVp and low mA is particularly important in overweight and large patients who tend to have a greater amount of radiation exposure during fluoroscopy. The voltage during fluoroscopy varies from 60 to 125 kVp. The goal is to keep the kVp as high as possible. The main disad-

vantage of using high kVp is a decrease in image contrast, but this is not a major problem during most bronchoscopic procedures. Most modern fluoroscopy systems have automatic dose-rate control (ADRC) and automatic brightness control (ABC) capabilities, which are made possible by predefined adjustments in the mA and kVp. Many systems have preset low, medium, and high dose-rate settings for ADRC. High dose rate setting gives high quality images but it also increases radiation dose. Low ADRC setting gives least amount of radiation dose to the patient, but the images tend to have a snowy quality. For general purposes, low dose-rate setting for ADRC is adequate in most cases and should be used as much as possible. Older fluoroscopic instruments require manual adjustment of mA and kVp. The bronchoscopists using these machines should learn how to make adjustments to achieve the images of acceptable quality using least the mA and highest kVp. Those working with older fluoroscopy machines should also consider upgrading to newer generation systems as much as possible.

### Filters

The X rays produced in the fluoroscopy tube have variable amounts of energy. Low-energy X rays in the primary beam are mostly absorbed in the tissues and may contribute to adverse effects without contributing to the image. Most fluoroscopy systems are equipped with a metal sheet or foil that covers the radiation port of the X-ray tube and filters the low energy X rays from the primary beam. Removal of low-energy X rays from the primary beam reduces the radiation dose to the patient. It also allows the use of high current and low voltage X rays without affecting the radiation dose or the image contrast. Different types of filters differ in their capacity to block the low energy beam. The operators should be aware of this feature in the fluoroscopy system they are using.

### Collimators

In modern fluoroscopy systems, the size and shape of the primary beam can be adjusted to minimize the area of the radiation field. This is made possible by the collimators, which are X-ray blockers outside the X-ray tube. The operator adjusts the collimator blades through the control panel to limit the area of the image to a minimum. This not only reduces the radiation dose to the patient but also decreases the image-degrading radiation scatter, thus improving the image quality. The radiation scatter in the room and exposure to health-care workers are also reduced when the volume of irradiated tissue is reduced with tight collimation.

### Source to skin distance

The intensity of X rays rapidly decreases as the distance from the X-ray source to the target is increased. By increasing the distance from the X-ray source to patient, it is possible to significantly reduce the dose to the skin and reduce the potential for radiation injury to the skin. The image quality may slightly deteriorate by increasing this distance but it has no major implications in bronchoscopic procedures. There is some concern about greater scatter but with proper collimation, the radiation scatter in the room is not significantly changed. International guidelines mandate a minimum separation of 30 cm from the radiation port to the skin. The mobile C-arms are equipped with separator cones that are placed on top of X-ray tubes to maintain this distance.

### Image intensifier to skin distance

The image intensifier should be kept as close to the patient as possible. This simple precaution significantly reduces the radiation dose to both the patient as well as the operators. Most mobile C-arms have a fixed distance between the X-ray source and the image intensifier (source to image distance [SID]). In these systems, when the image intensifier is moved closer to the patient, the X-ray source automatically moves farther away, thus reducing the skin radiation dose to the patient. Reducing this distance decreases the radiation dose to the operators because the image intensifier absorbs a large proportion of X rays exiting from the patient, thus acting as a radiation shield for the operators.

### Grid

The grid is a flat plate device placed in front of the image intensifier that blocks the image-degrading radiation but allows the image-forming radiation to pass through the image intensifier. As a result, grids improve the image contrast, but their use also increases the radiation dose to the patient and the personnel performing the procedure. In most situations, removal of grids decreases the radiation dose to the patients and operators by one-third to one-half without significantly compromising the image quality. Removal of grids is especially useful when the image intensifier cannot be brought close to the patients. In some systems, grids are retracted with an automatic mechanism by pressing a button on the control panel whereas in other systems grids can only be removed manually. Grids can be removed during most bronchoscopic procedures performed under fluoroscopy.

### Beam on-time

Fluoroscopy should only be used when the operator is actively using the image on the monitor to perform the task at hand. For this, the operator needs to have full control on when to engage and disengage the fluoroscopic exposure. In most machines, the beam on-time is controlled either by a button on control panel or by a foot pedal. The X-ray exposure occurs only when the button or the foot pedal is pressed. During bronchoscopy, the operators typically use foot pedals to control fluoroscopy use during the procedure. In most systems, there are two side-by-side foot pedals: one controls normal-dose fluoroscopy and other controls high-

dose fluoroscopy. The bronchoscopist should only use the normal-dose and not the high-dose fluoroscopy pedal during the procedures. The bronchoscopists should learn to limit the beam on-time to a minimum. This will greatly reduce the overall radiation exposure both to the patient as well as the staff.

### Last image hold

In most modern fluoroscopy systems, the last image can be digitally frozen. This is a very useful feature because it allows the operator to review the image and plan the next move without additional radiation exposure. This feature can significantly reduce radiation exposure to the patients during bronchoscopy. We find this feature very useful while teaching bronchoscopy to fellows.

### Pulsed fluoroscopy

Another new feature in modern systems that can reduce the radiation dose is pulse fluoroscopy [110]. As opposed to conventional fluoroscopy, where a continuous stream of X rays are generated, the X rays are emitted in short bursts during pulsed fluoroscopy. In a typical pulse fluoroscopy system, the images are acquired at a rate of 15 frames per second as compared to 30 frames per second with continuous fluoroscopy. This results in 25–30% dose reduction to the patient. Further lowering of frames per second is feasible but it causes the images from moving organs to become choppy.

### Image magnification

Another newer feature in fluoroscopy systems is the ability to magnify images. Larger images improve visibility during the procedure but it also gives higher radiation dose. The image magnification can be geometric or electronic. Geometric magnification is accomplished by changing the position of the patient relative to the X-ray tube or image intensifier. Images can be magnified either by increasing the distance between the patient and the image intensifier or by decreasing the distance between the patient and the X-ray tube. In both instances, the radiation dose to the patient will increase, as discussed above. Another disadvantage of geometric magnification is decrease in the spatial resolution of images. Electronic magnification is another option available in many newer fluoroscopy systems. The operators can select one of the several electronic magnification options on the control panel. In general, the increase in radiation dose with electronic magnification is less that that with geometric magnification. Regardless, the magnification option should be used sparingly during interventional procedures.

### Reducing exposure during bronchoscopy

Several measures can be taken to minimize the radiation exposure during interventional procedures performed under fluoroscopic guidance [111]. Because scattered radiation is

**Table 2.12** Measures to reduce radiation exposure during bronchoscopy

**General measures**
Educate all health-care workers potentially exposed to radiation
Avoid unnecessary procedures
Minimize fluoroscopy time
Maintain as much distance from patient as possible
Avoid direct exposure to radiation beam
Wear lead aprons at all times
Wear thyroid shield
Proper calibration and maintenance of fluoroscopy system

**Specific measures**
Use lowest possible tube current (mA)
Use highest possible voltage (kVp)
Use low or medium automatic dose-rate control settings
Keep X-ray source as far away from patient as possible
Keep image intensifier as close to patient as possible
Use filters
Proper collimation
Remove grid
Use beam on-time
Use last image hold
Use pulse fluoroscopy
Avoid magnification

the chief source of radiation to medical personnel, limiting radiation exposure to patients automatically reduces radiation exposure to the staff. Education in the optimal use of fluoroscopy systems and knowledge of radiation hygiene practices are essential in this regard. Comprehensive education programs on proper fluoroscopy are highly effective in reducing the radiation exposure to both patients and the staff members [112]. Education and training decrease the variation in fluoroscopy use and improve compliance with safety guidelines. For example, in one study, a comprehensive education program resulted in a decrease in the average fluoroscopy exposure time from 121.5 seconds to 41.7 seconds for transbronchial biopsies without affecting the complication rate or ability to establish a diagnosis [113]. Strategies shown to reduce the radiation exposure to the patient and the staff are summarized in Table 2.12.

### Avoid unnecessary procedures

A clear indication should exist for all bronchoscopic procedures that require fluoroscopy guidance. Radiation exposure should be avoided whenever a safer alternative is available.

### Maintain distance

According to the inverse square law, the radiation dose is inversely proportional to the square of the distance [114]. For health-care workers, scattered radiation is the source of the radiation. By doubling the distance from the patient, health-care workers would reduce their radiation exposure by one-fourth. This may not be possible for the primary operators but other personnel not directly involved in the procedure should maintain the maximum possible distance from the patient whenever fluoroscopy is in use. The operators should keep their hands away from the primary beam as much as possible.

### Optimal use of the fluoroscopy system

As discussed above, proper use of the fluoroscopy system can reduce the radiation exposure to patients and staff by several fold (Table 2.12). All bronchoscopy staff must be familiar with the operational aspects of the fluoroscopy system they are using and should receive appropriate training in the principles of radiation protection.

### Limit fluoroscopy time

The duration of fluoroscopy varies according to the complexity of the case and the experience of the bronchoscopist. In our experience, pulmonary fellows in the early part of their training tend to overuse fluoroscopy during transbronchial biopsy. The supervising physician should strongly emphasize the need to reduce the total duration of fluoroscopy use.

### Wear shielding devices

Lead aprons are the most effective means of reducing radiation exposure during fluoroscopic procedures. The protective value of lead aprons is expressed as millimeters of lead equivalent. Typical aprons have a lead-equivalent thickness of 0.5 mm, which shield the operators from at least 90% of scattered radiation. Many of these aprons are heavy and can cause fatigue and back pain if worn over an extended period of time. Some workers find the lighter 0.25-mm lead equivalent thickness aprons more comfortable, but attenuation of the radiation beam by these aprons is less effective than the standard 0.5-mm lead equivalent aprons [115]. Special aprons are available for use during pregnancy to further reduce radiation doses to the abdominal and pelvic areas.

Standard lead aprons do not protect the thyroid gland. Because thyroid cancer is clearly linked to prior radiation exposure, it is important to avoid excessive radiation exposure to the neck. This is best achieved by wearing thyroid collars, which are inexpensive and are comfortable to wear. Thyroid collars reduce radiation exposure to the thyroid gland at least 20-fold [116]. Unfortunately, in our experience, medical personnel often fail to use the thyroid shield during diagnostic procedures, a practice that should be strongly discouraged.

Because excessive radiation exposure to eyes may lead to premature cataract formation, some physicians routinely wear eye protection during fluoroscopy. Ordinary eye glasses do provide some protection. The best protection, however, is provided by 0.6-mm leaded glasses, which have been shown to reduce the eye exposure six to eight times [117]. Unfortunately, the leaded glasses are generally heavy and uncomfortable if worn over extended periods. Further, the optical quality of leaded glasses is poor and they tend to be brittle and can break causing eye damage. Whether or not to wear eye protective devices during bronchoscopy is largely an individual decision. Movable leaded glass barriers, frequently used in radiology departments, are not practical for operators during bronchoscopy.

All personal protection devices such as lead aprons and thyroid collars should be readily available in any bronchoscopy suite that uses fluoroscopy. The bronchoscopist is responsible for making sure that no health-care worker enters the bronchoscopy suite without appropriate personal shielding measures. The Joint Commission on Accreditation of Health Organizations (JCAHO) requires health organizations to test the lead aprons under fluoroscopy for any defects every year and to keep a careful record of test results.

### Monitoring radiation exposure

Health-care workers who work with fluoroscopy must monitor their occupational radiation exposure. Film badges and thermoluminescent dosimeters (TLDs) are the most popular radiation dosage monitors for individual use. The film badge contains a piece of radiograph film that is exchanged and analyzed every month to measure the amount of radiation exposure. Filters in the badge holder provide information on radiation energy and direction. The TLD uses lithium crystals which absorb energy when exposed to radiation. When heated, the crystal emits the stored energy as light, the intensity of which is proportional to the amount of radiation absorbed. Film badges and TLDs each have advantages. Film badges may give erroneous readings if exposed to high temperature, but they are inexpensive and the pieces of used film may be stored so readings can be rechecked later. TLDs are stable at high ambient temperature but are relatively expensive. Also, the dosimetric information in these badges is erased each time they are read.

A new monitoring device introduced recently is the optically stimulated luminescence (OSL) dosimeter [118]. These monitors contain aluminum oxide to detect radiation. Instead of using heat, OSL dosimeters use a laser to monitor the radiation dose. OSL dosimeters are more sensitive to lower doses of radiation and are more stable than TLDs. Another type of dosimeter is photoluminescence glass (PLG) dosimeters which can give repeated readouts until reset to zero. Because these dosimeters are small and radiolucent, they are ideally suited for monitoring the radiation dose to the patients [119].

A variety of electronic dosimeters are also available [120]. Many of them are equipped with an alarm that beeps whenever predefined radiation exposure limits are exceeded. The electronic dosimeters provide immediate readouts, allowing case-by-case or daily assessment of radiation exposure. Unfortunately, they are unreliable in estimating cumulative radiation exposure, so they are not a suitable substitute for conventional monitoring devices. Nevertheless, the electronic dose monitors may be a useful adjunct to film badges or TLDs when close monitoring of radiation exposure is desired, such as for pregnant health-care workers.

Film badges are typically turned in for analysis on a monthly basis. A careful record of personal exposure is an absolute necessity. Because some health-care workers discount radiation risks, problems with compliance are occasionally encountered. Laxity in this matter is unacceptable and may place the person responsible for the radiation safety of the workers and the institution at legal risk.

The current recommendation is to wear the radiation badge outside the lead apron at the level of the collar. The effective dose is calculated by dividing the monthly radiation reading by 5.6 [121]. However, a single personal dosimeter is not sufficient for accurate assessment of radiation exposure to the entire body [122]. A monitoring badge worn outside the lead apron at collar level provides an accurate estimate of radiation exposure to the head, the lens of the eye, and the thyroid gland, but it overestimates ED by a factor of 5 to 20. In contrast, a single badge worn under the lead apron at waist level provides a more accurate estimate of ED but underestimates exposure to the head, neck, and hands. For these reasons, some authorities have advocated using two badges for radiation monitoring. However, this is not popular, except for the pregnant health-care workers.

A thorough investigation is in order whenever one person's exposure exceeds acceptable limits or when there is an unusual increase in the staff radiation exposure readings in a particular month. An appropriate investigation would include a careful review of the caseload, equipment performance, duration of fluoroscopy use, compliance with personal protection devices, and individual radiation safety practices. Removing an individual temporarily from the work force without carefully investigating the cause or causes of overexposure is inappropriate. In fact, every bronchoscopy suite should follow a standardized protocol to investigate the cause of an unexpected increase in radiation exposure, similar to that followed in radiology departments. Input from a radiation physicist is strongly recommended in this situation.

### Conclusion

Even though the occupational radiation exposure to physicians who frequently use fluoroscopy in their practice is within the acceptable limits, every possible precaution should be taken to minimize the low-level occupational radiation exposure. Input from a qualified radiation physicist during the initial set-up, periodic calibration, and quality control of the fluoroscopy equipment is very useful in this regard. In addition, radiation physicists should also be involved in monitoring radiation exposure to personnel, investigating the cause of overexposure, and in education of health-care workers. Bronchoscopists who frequently use fluoroscopy receive virtually no formal training in radiation use. We feel that it is time to change this trend and recommend that all health-care workers working in the bronchoscopy suite receive training in the principles of diagnostic radiation, health risks, and radiation protection.

# References

1 Srinivasan A, Wolfenden LL, Song X, *et al*. An outbreak of Pseudomonas aeruginosa infections associated with flexible bronchoscopes. *N Engl J Med* 2003; **348**: 221–7.

2 Kirschke DL, Jones TF, Craig AS, *et al*. Outbreak of Pseudomonas aeruginosa and Seratia marcescens associated with a manufacturing defect in bronchoscopes. *N Engl J Med* 2003; **348**: 214–20.

3 Mehta AC, Minai OA. Infection control in the bronchoscopy suite: a review. *Clin Chest Med* 1999; **20**: 19–32.

4 Prakash UBS. Does the bronchoscope propagate infection? *Chest* 1993; **104**: 552–9.

5 Harvey J, Yates M. Do you clean or contaminate your bronchoscope? *Respir Med* 1996; **90**: 63–7.

6 Mughal MM, Minai OA, Culver DA, Mehta AC. Reprocessing the bronchoscope: the challenges. *Semin Respir Crit Care Med* 2004; **25**: 443–9.

7 Culver DA, Gordon SM, Mehta AC. Infection control in the bronchoscopy suite. *Am J Respir Crit Care Med* 2003; **167**: 1050–6.

8 Gubler JG, Salfinger M, von Graevenitz A. Pseudoepidemic of nontuberculous mycobacteria due to a contaminated bronchoscope cleaning machine. *Chest* 1992; **101**: 1245–9.

9 Brown NM, Hellyar EA, Harvey JE, *et al*. Mycobacterial contamination of fibreoptic bronchoscopes. *Thorax* 1993; **48**: 1283–5.

10 Nye K, Chadha DK, Hodgkin P, *et al*. Mycobacterium chelonae isolation from broncho-alveolar lavage fluid and its practical implications. *J Hosp Infect* 1990; **16**: 257–61.

11 Centers for Disease Control and Prevention. Nosocomial infection and pseudoinfection from contaminated endoscopes and bronchoscopes-Wisconsin and Missouri. *MMWR Morb Mortal Wkly Rev* 1991; **40**: 675–8.

12 Fraser VJ, Jones M, Murray PR, *et al*. Contamination of flexible fiberoptic bronchoscopes with Mycobacterium chelonae linked to an automated bronchoscope disinfection machine. *Am Rev Respir Dis* 1992; **145**: 853–5.

13 Campagnaro RL, Teichtahl H, Dwyer B. A pseudoepidemic of Mycobacterium chelonae: contamination of a bronchoscope and autocleaner. *Aust N Z J Med* 1994; **24**: 693–5.

14 Wang HC, Liaw YS, Yang PC, *et al*. A pseudoepidemic of Mycobacterium chelonae infection caused by contamination of a fiberoptic bronchoscope suction channel. *Eur Respir J* 1995; **8**: 1259–62.

15 Cox R, deBorja K, Bach MC. A pseudo-outbreak of Mycobacterium chelonae infections related to bronchoscopy. *Infect Control Hosp Epidemiol* 1997; **18**: 136–7.

16 Wallace RJ, Brown BA, Griffith DE. Nosocomial outbreaks/pseudo-outbreaks caused by nontuberculous mycobacteria. *Annu Rev Microbiol* 1998; **52**: 453–90.

17 Ramsey AH, Oemig TV, Davis JP, *et al*. An outbreak of Bronchoscopy-related Mycobacterium tuberculosis infections due to lack of bronchoscope leak testing. *Chest* 2002; **121**: 976–81.

18 Pappas SA, Schaff DM, DiCostanzo MB, *et al*. Contamination of flexible fiberoptic bronchoscopes [letter]. *Am Rev Respir Dis* 1983; **127**: 391–2.

19 Wheeler PW, Lancaster D, Kaiser AB. Bronchopulmonary cross-colonization and infection related to mycobacterial contamination of suction valves of bronchoscopes. *J Infect Dis* 1989; **159**: 954–8.

20 Southwick KL, Hoffmann K, Ferree K, *et al*. Cluster of tuberculosis cases in North Carolina: possible association with atomizer reuse. *Am J Infect Control* 2001; **29**: 1–6.

21 Agerton T, Valway S, Gore B, *et al*. Transmission of a highly drug-resistant strain (strain W1) of Mycobacterium tuberculosis. *JAMA* 1997; **278**: 1073–7.

22 Michele TM, Cronin WA, Graham NMH, *et al*. Transmission of Mycobacterium tuberculosis by a fiberoptic bronchoscope. *JAMA* 1997; **278**: 1093–5.

23 Whitlock, WL Dietrich RA, Steimke EH, *et al*. Rhodotorula rubra contamination in fiberoptic bronchoscopy. *Chest* 1992; **102**: 1516–19.

24 Hoffmann KK, Weber DJ, Rutala WA. Pseudoepidemic of Rhodotorula rubra in patients undergoing fiberoptic bronchoscopy. *Infect Control Hosp Epidemiol* 1989; **10**: 511–14.

25 Hagan ME, Klotz SA, Bartholomew W, *et al*. A pseudoepidemic of Rhodotorula rubra: a marker for microbial contamination of the bronchoscope. *Infect Control Hosp Epidemiol* 1995; **16**: 727–8.

26 Hanson PJ, Gor D, Clarke JR, *et al*. Recovery of the human immunodeficiency virus from fibreoptic bronchoscopes. *Thorax* 1991; **46**: 410–12.

27 Rutala WA, Weber DJ. Disinfection of endoscope: review of new chemical sterilents used for high-level disinfection. *Infect Control Hosp Epidemiol* 1999; **20**: 69–76.

28 Spaulding EH. Chemical disinfection in the operating room. *Mil Med* 1958; **123**: 437–43.

29 Talsma SS. Biofilms on medical devices. *Home Health Nurse* 2007; **25**: 589–94.

30 Stewart PS, Costorton JW. Antibiotic resistance of bacteria in biofilms. *Lancet* 2001; **358**: 135–8.

31 Pajkos A, Vickery K, Cossart Y. Is biofilm accumulation on endoscope tubing a contributor to the failure of cleaning and decontamination? *J Hosp Infect* 2004; **58**: 224–9.

32 Vickery K, Pajkos A, Cossart Y. Removal of biofilm from endoscopes: evaluation of detergent efficiency. *Am J Infect Control* 2004; **32**: 170–6.

33 Marion K, Freney J, James G, *et al*. Using an efficient biofilm detaching agent: an essential step for the improvement of endoscope reprocessing protocols. *J Hosp Infect* 2006; **64**: 136–42.

34 Alvarado CJ, Stolz SM, Maki DG. Nosocomial infections from contaminated endoscopes: a flawed automated endoscope washer. An investigation using molecular epidemiology. *Am J Med* 1991; **91**(3B): 272S–80S.

35 Kressel AB, Kidd F. Pseudo-outbreak of Mycobacterium chelonae and Methylobacterium mesophilicum caused by contamination of an automated endoscopy washer. *Infect Control Hosp Epidemiol* 2001; **22**: 414–18 .

36 Alvarado CJ, Reichelderfer M. APIC guideline for infection prevention and control in flexible endoscopy. *Am J Infect Control* 2000; **28**: 138–55.

37 Honeybourne D, Babb J, Bowie P, *et al*. British Thoracic Society guidelines on diagnostic flexible bronchoscopy. *Thorax* 2001; **56**: I1–I21.

38 Mehta AC, Prakash UBS, Garland R, *et al*. American College of Chest Physicians and American Association of Bronchology consensus statement. *Chest* 2005; **128**: 1742–55.

39 Alfa MJ, Sitter DL. In-hospital evaluation of orthophthalaldehyde as a high level disinfectant for flexible endoscopes. *J Hosp Infect* 1994; **26**: 15–26.

40 Hanson, PJV, Chadwick, MV, Gaya, H, *et al*. A study of gluterladehyde disinfection of fiberoptic bronchoscope experimentally contaminated with Mycobacterium tuberculosis. *J Hosp Infect* 1992; **22**: 137–42.

41 Alfa MJ, Olson N, DeGagne P, Jackson M. A survey of reprocessing methods, residual viable bioburden, and soil levels in patient-ready endoscopic retrograde choliangiopancreatography duodenoscopes used in Canadian centers. *Infect Control Hosp Epidemiol* 2002; **23**: 198–206.

42 Alfa MJ, Olson N, DeGagne P. Automated washing with the Reliance Endoscope Processing System and its equivalence to optimal manual cleaning. *Am J Infect Control* 2006; **34**: 561–70.

43 Cêtre JC, Nicolle MC, Salord H, *et al*. Outbreaks of contaminated broncho-alveolar lavage related to intrinsically defective bronchoscopes. *J Hosp Infect* 2005; **61**: 39–45.

44 *FDA-Cleared Sterilants and High Level Disinfectants with General Claims for Processing Reusable Medical and Dental Devices.* March, 2009. Available at: http://www.fda.gov/cdrh/ODE/germlab.html. Accessed April 2011.

45 Wendt C, Kampf B. Evidence-based spectrum of antimicrobial activity for disinfection of bronchoscopes. *J Hosp Infect* 2008; **70** (Suppl. 1): 60–8.

46 Rutala WA, Weber DJ. Disinfection and sterilization in health care facilities: What clinicians need to know. *Clin Infect Dis* 2004; **39**: 702–9.

47 Nelson DB, Jarvis WR, Rutala WA, *et al*. Multi-society guideline for reprocessing flexible gastrointestinal endoscopes. *Infect Control Hosp Epidemiol* 2003; **24**: 532–7.

48 Fraser VJ, Zuckerman G, Clouse RE, *et al*. A prospective randomized trial comparing manual and automated endoscope disinfection methods. *Infect Control Hosp Epidemiol* 1993; **14**: 383–93.

49 Sorin M, Segal-Maurer S, Mariano N, *et al*. Nosocomial transmission of imipenem-resistant Pseudomonas aeruginosa following bronchoscopy associated with improper connection to the Steris System 1 processor. *Infect Control Hosp Epidemiol* 2001; **22**: 409–13.

50 Chroneou A, Zimmerman SK, Cook S, *et al*. Molecular typing of Mycobacterium chelonae isolates from a pseudo-outbreak involving an automated bronchoscope washer. *Infect Control Hosp Epidemiol* 2008; **29**: 1088–90.

51 Muscarella LF. Application of environmental sampling to flexible endoscope reprocessing: the importance of monitoring the rinse water. *Infect Control Hosp Epidemiol* 2002; **23**: 285–9.

52 Muscarella LF. The importance of bronchoscope reprocessing guidelines: raising the standard of care. *Chest* 2004; **126**: 1001–2.

53 Pang J, Perry P, Ross A, Forbes GM. Bacteria-free rinse water for endoscope disinfection. *Gastrointest Endosc* 2002; **56**: 402–6.

54 Muscarella LF. Inconsistencies in endoscope-reprocessing and infection control guidelines: the importance of endoscope drying. *Am J Gastroenterol* 2006; **101**: 2147–54.

55 Vandenbroucke-Grauls CM, Baars AC, Visser MR, *et al*. An outbreak of Serratia marcescens traced to a contaminated bronchoscope. *J Hosp Infect* 1993; **23**: 263–70.

56 Kruse A, Rey J-F. Guidelines on cleaning and disinfection in GI endoscopy. *Endoscopy* 2000; **32**: 77–83.

57 Corne P, Godreuil S, Jean-Pierre H, *et al*. Unusual implication of biopsy forceps in outbreaks of Pseudomonas aeruginosa infections and pseudo-infections related to bronchoscopy. *J Hosp Infect* 2005; **61**: 20–6.

58 Spraggs PD, Hanekom WH, Mochloulis G, *et al*. The assessment of risk of cross-contamination with a multi-use nasal atomizer. *J Hosp Infect* 1994; **28**: 315–21.

59 Wilson SJ, Everts RJ, Kirkland KB, Sexton DJ. A pseudo-outbreak of Aureobasidium species lower respiratory tract infections caused by reuse of single-use stopcocks during bronchoscopy. *Infect Control Hosp Epidemiol* 2000; **21**: 470–2.

60 Reynolds CD, Rhinehart E, Dreyer P, Goldmann DA. Variability in reprocessing policies and procedures for flexible fiberoptic endoscopes in Massachusetts hospitals. *Am J Infect Control* 1992; **20**: 283–90.

61 Rutala WA, Clontz EP, Weber DJ, Hoffmann KK. Disinfection practices for endoscopes and other semicritical items. *Infect Control Hosp Epidemiol* 1991; **12**: 282–8.

62 Honeybourne D, Neumann CS. An audit of bronchoscopy practice in the United Kingdom: a survey of adherence to national guidelines. *Thorax* 1997; **52**: 709–13.

63 Srinivasan A, Wolfenden LL, Song X, *et al*. Bronchoscope reprocessing and infection prevention and control: bronchoscopy-specific guidelines are needed. *Chest* 2004; **125**: 307–14.

64 Shimono N, Takuma T, Tsuchimochi N, *et al*. An outbreak of Pseudomonas aeruginosa infections following thoracic surgeries occurring via the contamination of bronchoscopes and an automatic endoscope reprocessor. *Infect Chemother* 2008; **14**: 418–23.

65 Silva CV, Magalhães VD, Pereira CR, *et al*. Pseudo-outbreak of Pseudomonas aeruginosa and Serratia marcescens related to bronchoscopes. *Infect Control Hosp Epidemiol* 2003; **24**: 195–7.

66 Singh A, Goering RV, Simjee S, *et al*. Application of molecular techniques to the study of hospital infection. *Clin Microbiol Rev* 2006; **19**: 512–30.

67 Bou R, Aguilar A, Perpiñán J, *et al*. Nosocomial outbreak of Pseudomonas aeruginosa infections related to a flexible bronchoscope. *J Hosp Infect* 2006; **64**: 129–35.

68 Chroneou A, Zimmerman SK, Cook S. Molecular typing of Mycobacterium chelonae isolates from a pseudo-outbreak involving an automated bronchoscope washer. *Infect Control Hosp Epidemiol* 2008; **29**: 1088–90.

69 Morice A. Hazard to bronchoscopists. [Letter]. *Lancet* 1989; **1**: 448.

70 Malasky C, Jordan T, Potulski F, Reichman LB. Occupational tuberculous infections among pulmonary physicians in training. *Am Rev Respir Dis* 1990; **142**: 505–7.

71 Jereb JA, Burwen DR, Dooley SW. Nosocomial outbreak of tuberculosis in a renal transplant unit: application of a new technique for restriction fragment length polymorphism analysis of Mycobacterium tuberculosis isolates. *Infect Dis* 1993; **168**: 1219–24.

72 Fennelly KP. Personal respiratory protection against mycobacterium tuberculosis. *Clin Chest Med* 1997; **18**: 1–17.

73 Birnie GG, Quigley EM, Clements GB, *et al.* Endoscopic transmission of hepatitis B virus. *Gut* 1983; **24**: 171–4.

74 Sawchuk WS, Weber PJ, Lowy DR, Dzubow LM. Infectious papillomavirus in the vapor of warts treated with carbon dioxide laseror electrocoagulation: detection and protection. *J Am Acad Dermatol* 1989; **21**: 41–9.

75 Hanson PJV, Chadwick MV, Gaya H, Collins JV. A study of glutaraldehyde insinfection of fiberoptic bronchoscopes experimentally contaminated with mycobacterium tuberculosis. *J Hosp Infect* 1992; **22**: 137–42.

76 Seballos RL, Walsh AL, Mehta AC. Clinical evaluation of a liquid chemical sterilization system for the flexible bronchoscopes. *J Bronchol* 1995; **2**: 192–9.

77 Hanson PJ, Gor D, Jeffries DJ, Collins JV. Elimination of high titer HIV from fibreoptic endoscopes. *Gut* 1990; **31**: 657–9.

78 American Association for Gastrointestinal Endoscopy. Infection control during GI endoscopy. *Gastrointest Endosc* 2008; **67**: 781–90.

79 Bronowicki JP, Venard V, Botté C, *et al.* Patient-to-patient transmission of hepatitis C virus during colonoscopy. *N Engl J Med* 1997; **337**: 237–40.

80 Rutala WA, Weber DJ. Creutzfeldt-Jakob disease: recommendations for disinfection and sterilization. *Clin Infect Dis* 2001; **32**: 1348–56.

81 Axon AT, Beilenhoff U, Brumble MG, *et al.* Variant Creutzfeldt-Jacob disease (vCJD) and gastrointestinal endoscopy. *Endoscopy* 2001; **33**: 1070–80.

82 Colt HG, Beamis JJ, Harrell JH, Mathur PM. Novel flexible bronchoscope and single-use disposable-sheath endoscope system. A preliminary technology evaluation. *Chest* 2000; **118**: 183–7.

83 Margery J, Vaylet F, Guigay J, *et al.* Bronchoscopy with the Vision Sciences BF100 disposable-sheath device: French experience after 328 procedures. *Respiration* 2004; **71**: 174–7.

84 Jain P, Fleming P, Mehta AC. Radiation safety for the health care workers in bronchoscopy suite. *Clin Chest Med* 1999; **20**: 33–8.

85 Harrison JD, Streffer C. The ICRP protection quantities, equivalent, and effective dose: their basis and application. *Radiat Prot Dosimetry* 2007; **127**: 12–18.

86 Huda W. Radiation dosimetry in diagnostic radiology. *Am J Roentgenol* 1997; **169**: 1487–8.

87 Wrixon AD. New recommendations from the International Commission on Radiological Protection- a review. *Phys Med Biol* 2008; **53**: 41–60.

88 Mettler FA, Koenig TR, Wagner LK, Kelsey CA. Radiation injuries after fluoroscopic procedures. *Semin Ultrasound CT MR* 2002; **23**: 428–42.

89 Wall BF, Kendall GM, Edwards AA, *et al.* What are the risks from medical x-rays and other low dose radiation? *Br J Radiol* 2006; **79**: 285–94.

90 Cohen BL. The cancer risk from low-level radiation. *Health Phys* 1980; **39**: 659–78.

91 Shimizu Y, Schull WJ, Kato H. Cancer risk among atomic bomb survivors: The RERF life span study. *JAMA* 1990; **264**: 601–4.

92 Evans JS, Wennberg JE, McNeil BJ. The influence of diagnostic radiography on the incidence of breast cancer and leukemia. *N Engl J Med* 1986; **315**: 810–15.

93 Brenner DJ, Doll R, Goodhead DT, *et al.* Cancer risk attributable to low dose ionizing radiation: assessing what we really know. *Proc Natl Acad Sci* 2003; **100**: 13761–6.

94 Committee on the Biological Effects of Ionizing Radiation (BEIR V). *Health Effects of Exposure to Low Levels of Ionizing Radiation.* National Academy of Science. Washington (DC): National Research Council, 1990.

95 Valentin J. Avoidance of radiation injuries from medical interventional procedures. *Ann ICRP* 2000; **30**: 7–67.

96 Niklason LT, Marx MV, Chan HP. Interventional radiologists: occupational radiation doses and risks. *Radiology* 1993; **187**: 729–33.

97 Johnson LW, Moore RJ, Balter S. Review of radiation safety in the cardiac catheterization laboratory. *Cathet Cardiovasc Diagn* 1992; **25**: 186–94.

98 Goldstone KE, Wright IH, Cohen B. Radiation exposure to the hands of orthopedic surgeons during procedures under fluoroscopic control. *Br J Radiol* 1993; **66**: 899–901.

99 Giblin JG, Rubenstein J, Taylor A, Pahira J. Radiation risk to the urologist during endourologic procedures, and a new shield that reduces exposure. *Urology* 1996; **48**: 624–7.

100 McGowan C, Heaton B, Stephenson RN. Occupational x-ray exposure of anesthetists. *Br J Anaesth* 1996; **76**: 868–9.

101 Wrixon AD. New ICRP recommendations. *J Radiol Prot* 2008; **28**: 161–8.

102 Dendy PP. Radiation risks in interventional radiology. *Br J Radiol* 2008; **81**: 1–7.

103 Rehani MM, Ortiz-Lopez P. Radiation effects in fluoroscopically guided cardiac interventions-keeping them under control. *Int J Cardiol* 2006; **109**: 147–51.

104 Wall BF. Radiation protection dosimetry for diagnostic radiology patients. *Radiat Prot Dosimetry* 2004; **109**: 409–19.

105 Ost D, Shah R, Anasco E, *et al.* A randomized trial of CT fluoroscopic-guided bronchoscopy vs conventional bronchoscopy in patients with suspected lung cancer. *Chest* 2008; **134**: 507–13.

106 National Council on Radiation Protection and Measurement. *Implementation of the Principle of as Low as Reasonably Achievable (ALARA) for Medical and Dental Personnel.* Bethesda (MD): NCRP, 1990; NCRP report No. 107.

107 Faulknar K, Moores BM. An assessment of the radiation dose received by staff using fluoroscopic equipment. *Br J Radiol* 1982; **55**: 272–6.

108 Mahesh M. Fluoroscopy: patient radiation exposure issues. *Radiographics* 2001; **21**: 1033–45.

109 Chaffins J. Radiation protection and procedures in OR. *Radiol Technol* 2008; **79**: 415–28.

110 Herman-Schulman M. Can fluoroscopic radiation dose be substantially reduced. *Radiology* 2006; **238**: 1–2.

111 Norris TG. Radiation safety in fluoroscopy. *Radiol Technol* 2002; **73**: 911–33.

112 Lakkireddy D, Nadzam G, Verma, *et al*. Impact of a comprehensive safety program on radiation exposure during catheter ablation of atrial fibrillation: a prospective study. *J Interv Card Electrophysiol* 2009; **24**: 105–12.

113 Ernst A, Smith L, Gryniuk L, *et al*. A simple teaching intervention significantly decreases radiation exposure during transbronchial biopsy. *J Bronchol* 2004; **11**: 109–11.

114 Brateman L. Radiation safety considerations for diagnostic radiology personnel. *Radiographics* 1999; **19**: 1037–55.

115 Hubbert TE, Vucich JJ, Armstrong MR. Light weight aprons for protection against scattered radiation during fluoroscopy. *AJR Am J Roentgenol* 1993; **161**: 1079–83.

116 Tse V, Lising J, Khadra M, *et al*. radiation exposure during fluoroscopy: should we be protecting our thyroids? *Aust NZ J Surg* 1999; **69**: 847–8.

117 Richman AH, Chan B, Katz M. Effectiveness of leaded glasses in reducing radiation exposure. *Radiology* 1976; **121**: 357–9.

118 Yukihara EG, McKeever SW. Optically stimulated luminescence (OSL) dosimetry in medicine. *Phys Med Biol* 2008; **53**: R351–79.

119 Moritake T, Matsumaru Y, Takigawa T, *et al*. Dose measurement on both patients and operators during neurointerventional procedures using photoluminescence glass dosimeters. *Am J Neuroradiol* 2008; **29**: 1910–17.

120 Luszig-Bhadra M, Perle S. Electronic personal dosimeters will replace passive dosimeters in the near future. *Radiat Prot Dosim* 2006; **123**: 546–53.

121 National Council on Radiation Protection and Measurement. *Use of Personal Monitors to Estimate Effective Dose Equivalent and Effective Dose to Workers for External Exposure to LOW-LET Radiation*. Bethesda (MD): NCRP, 1995; NCRP report No. 122.

122 Al-Shakhrah A, Abu-Kaled YS. Estimation of effective radiation dose for physicians and staff members in contrast angiocardiography. *Heart Lung* 2000; **29**: 417–23.

# 3

# Examination of the Larynx Through the Flexible Bronchoscope

## Navatha Kurugundla,[1] Adnan Majid,[2] Luis F. Riquelme,[3] and Arthur W. Sung[2]

[1] Division of Pulmonary and Critical Care Medicine, New York Methodist Hospital, Brooklyn, NY, USA

[2] Section of Interventional Pulmonology, Beth Israel Medical Center, New York, NY, USA

[3] Center for Swallowing and Speech-Language Pathology, New York Methodist Hospital, Brooklyn, and New York Medical College, Valhalla, NY, USA

## Introduction

The larynx is situated between the pharynx and the trachea as part of the upper airway. It contributes to phonation, respiration, and protection of the tracheobronchial tree from aspirations. Laryngeal anatomy and physiology is complex, hence pathologies in structure and function can lead to a broad spectrum of symptoms. Although an otolaryngologist usually performs evaluations of the larynx, and the speech–language pathologist evaluates function in the context of voice and swallow, the pulmonary physician will also encounter patients with respiratory symptoms due to laryngeal diseases. For a bronchoscopist, therefore, detailed surveillance should include descriptions of functional and anatomical findings. Prior to an endoscopic examination, pertinent information, including clinical history, pulmonary function test, and computed tomography images should be reviewed, as laryngeal pathologies can cause non-specific signs and symptoms. A heightened clinical suspicion, therefore, can assist in identifying abnormal findings that can otherwise be missed on casual surveillance. This chapter will focus on laryngeal anatomy and function from the perspectives of the bronchoscopist. Computed tomography imaging of the larynx will also be discussed.

## Endoscopy of the larynx

Ernest Krakowizer introduced laryngoscopy in 1858 [1] and Gustav Killian introduced suspension laryngoscopy in 1912 [2]. Today, rigid suspension laryngoscopy is still commonly performed. The instrument is introduced into the pharynx and suspended on a surgical tray (Mayo instrument stand), allowing the surgeon to operate with both hands. The patient is placed in the Jackson position with extension at the atlanto-occipital joint and flexion of the cervical spine [3]. Suspension laryngoscopy is also used in deploying airway stents with jet ventilation [4]. It is a well-recognized procedure, but requires specialized training in order to be performed.

In the modern era, endoscopy has grown into a multidisciplinary science. Otolaryngologists, pulmonologist, gastroenterologists, and speech–language pathologists visualize the larynx from their respective endoscopic armamentarium. While most instruments are much less intrusive than rigid laryngoscopy, such as flexible bronchoscopes and laryngoscopes, familiarity with laryngeal anatomy is crucial to improve testing performance and to avoid complications. Familiarity with laryngeal anatomy is also of great significance when differentially diagnosing a myriad of diseases.

## Laryngeal anatomy

Proficient knowledge of laryngeal anatomy is essential in detecting pathologies and normal variants. The laryngeal apparatus is composed of mucosal folds, cartilages, bony structures, muscles, and their respective neural innervations.

### Mucosal folds

The mucosa overlies the laryngeal apparatus and is lined with squamous epithelium [5]. Underneath, elastic and collagenous fibers form the vocal fold ligaments. The thyroarytenoid (vocalis) muscles form the muscularis layer and

*Flexible Bronchoscopy*, Third Edition. Edited by Ko-Pen Wang, Atul C. Mehta, J. Francis Turner.
© 2012 Blackwell Publishing Ltd. Published 2012 by Blackwell Publishing Ltd.

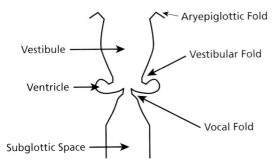

Aryepiglottic Fold

Vestibule

Vestibular Fold

Ventricle

Vocal Fold

Subglottic Space

**Fig. 3.1** Coronal view of mucosal folds of the larynx.

provide the predominant framework of the vocal folds [6]. The mucosal folds conform to the shape of the larynx. On coronal view (Fig. 3.1), there are two folds above the vocal folds; the paired aryepiglottic folds superiorly and the paired vestibular folds (structurally seen as false vocal folds) inferiorly. These supraglottic folds outline the vestibule. Below the vestibular folds are small cavities termed the ventricles, which are bounded inferiorly by the vocal folds.

### The cartilaginous framework of the larynx

The structural framework of the larynx is composed of nine cartilages, along with their connecting membranes and ligaments. Three are unpaired (thyroid, cricoid, epiglottis) and three are paired (arytenoids, corniculates, cuneiforms). The thyroid cartilage is the largest cartilage of the larynx, providing support for soft tissue structures. It is composed of two somewhat quadrilateral plates, called the thyroid laminae. They are fused with one another at midline anteriorly, and form the anterior and lateral walls of the larynx. The posterior margin of each thyroid lamina is prolonged upward and downward as two superior horns, which suspend the larynx from the hyoid bone, and two inferior horns that connect to the cricoid cartilage. On the lateral surface there are ridges connecting three extrinsic laryngeal muscles: the sternothyroid, thyrohyoid, and inferior pharyngeal constrictor.

The cricoid cartilage is situated below the thyroid cartilage and is the only complete cartilaginous ring. It supports the posterior laryngeal structure. The posterior aspect of the cricoid (i.e. the posterior quadrate lamina) is longer compared to its anterior dimension (i.e. anterior arch), with articulating surfaces for the arytenoid cartilages at the superior-lateral aspect. Laterally, the cricoid cartilage presents with small oval articular facets for articulation with the inferior horns of the thyroid cartilage.

The arytenoid cartilages are paired and are pyramidal in shape, thus each cartilage has a base, an apex, and three surfaces. The vocal folds attach to its medial surfaces via the muscular process and the vocal process. The cricoarytenoid muscles attach to its lateral aspects. The movement at the cricoarytenoid joint, which can be anteromedial or antero-lateral, allows the vocal folds to adduct during phonation and abduct during inspiration. The cricoarytenoid joint is an

occasional site of inflammation seen in rheumatoid arthritis where the synovial joint becomes fused [7]. Symptoms can include hoarseness or stridor in the most severe cases.

The two other pairs of small laryngeal cartilages include the corniculate and the cuineform cartilages [8]. The corniculate cartilages are paired and are located at the apices of arytenoid cartilages, assisting its rotation posteriorly and medially. Cuneiform cartilages are located within the aryepiglottic folds and tend to have a whitish discoloration.

### Muscles

The laryngeal muscles are divided into two groups: extrinsic and intrinsic muscles (Table 3.1). The extrinsic group includes the suprahyoid and infrahyoid muscles. These muscles are responsible for moving the larynx as a whole within the neck. The suprahyoid muscles, also known as the laryngeal elevators, elevate the larynx and include the stylohyoid, mylohyoid, digastric, geniohyoid, hyoglossus, stylopharyngeus, and the inferior pharyngeal constrictor. The infrahyoid muscles, also known as the laryngeal depressors, include the omohyoid, sternohyoid, and sternothyroid muscle. The exception is the thyrohyoid muscle, which elevates the thyroid and depresses the hyoid bone. Another description for the function of the extrinsic musculature is that they serve to support and fixate the larynx in position. The extrinsic muscles have at least one attachment to muscles outside the larynx.

The intrinsic musculature of the larynx may be categorized according the their effects on the shape of the glottis and on the vibratory behavior of the vocal folds. The "abductor muscles" separate the arytenoids and the vocal folds for respiration. The "adductor muscles" approximate the arytenoids and the vocal folds for phonation and for protective purposes. The "glottal tensors" are those that elongate and tighten the vocal folds; as opposed to the "relaxers" which shorten them. The intrinsic laryngeal muscles always act in pairs; one side does not contract independently from the muscles on the opposite side. The intrinsic muscles are responsible for the movement on the vocal folds and subtle tension adjustments needed during phonation. The intrinsic muscles are cricothyroid, posterior and lateral cricoarytenoids, transverse and oblique arytenoids, and thyroartenoids, which consist of thyromusuclaris (external thyroarytenoids) and thyrovocalis (internal thyroarytenoids, or vocalis) muscles. The cricothyroid is situated on the lateral aspect of the larynx; it tenses the vocal folds and is responsible for phonation. The posterior cricoarytenoids are responsible for vocal fold adduction, while the lateral cricoarytenoids cause vocal fold abduction (Fig. 3.2A). The arytenoids muscles act like sphincters bringing the arytenoids towards midline, assisting the posterior cricoarytenoids with adduction. External and internal thyroarytenoids relaxes, shortens vocal folds, and adducts vocal folds during speech. The vocalis muscles are primarily responsible

**Table 3.1** Muscles of the larynx and their function

| Muscles of the larynx | | | Function |
|---|---|---|---|
| Extrinsic muscles | Suprahyoid muscles | Stylohyoid | Elevates larynx |
| | | Digastric | Elevates larynx, depresses mandible |
| | | Geniohyoid | Depresses mandible |
| | | Mylohyoid | Elevates tongue and depress the mandibles |
| | | Stylopharyngeus | Elevates larynx |
| | Infrahyoid muscles | Omohyoid | Depresses larynx |
| | | Sternohyoid | Depresses larynx |
| | | Sternothyroid | Depresses larynx |
| | | Thyrohyoid | Depresses hyoid bone, elevates thyroid |
| Intrinsic muscles | | Cricothyroid | Stretches, tenses, and lengthens the vocal folds |
| | | Posterior cricoarytenoid | Abducts vocal folds |
| | | Lateral cricoarytenoid | Adducts vocal folds |
| | | Transverse arytenoid (interarytenoids) | Adducts focal folds |
| | | Oblique arytenoid (interarytenoids) | Narrows laryngeal inlet |
| | | External thyroarytenoid (thyromucularis) | Shortens and adducts vocal folds |
| | | Internal thyroarytenoid (thyrovocalis or vocalis muscle) | Shortens and adducts vocal folds |
| | | | Adjusts the tension in vocal folds |

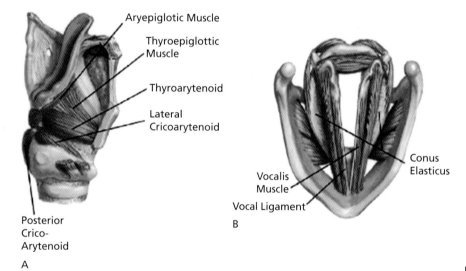

Aryepiglotic Muscle
Thyroepiglottic Muscle
Thyroarytenoid
Lateral Cricoarytenoid
Posterior Crico-Arytenoid
A

Conus Elasticus
Vocalis Muscle
Vocal Ligament
B

**Fig. 3.2** (A,B) Muscles of the larynx.

for adjusting the amount of tension of the vocal folds [5] (Fig. 3.2B).

### Nerve innervations

The vagus nerve (CN X) provides sensory and motor innervations to the laryngeal apparatus. The superior laryngeal nerve arises from the vagus nerve and divides into internal and external laryngeal nerve. The internal laryngeal nerve is responsible for sensory innervations to the larynx. The external laryngeal nerve is responsible for motor innervations to the cricothyroid muscle. The recurrent laryngeal nerve, which is also a branch of the vagus nerve, gives rise to inferior laryngeal nerve, which innervates all intrinsic laryngeal muscles except the cricothyroid. Superior and inferior laryngeal nerves both carry sympathetic and parasympathetic innervation. Injury to the external laryngeal nerve renders vocal folds flaccid, causing weak and breathy phonation. Damage to one of the recurrent laryngeal nerves can cause hoarseness, while bilateral damage can lead to glottic closure causing stridor and respiratory failure.

It is especially important when performing bronchoscopy that the patient is adequately anesthetized and sedated. Poor visualization is usually a result of excessive patient movements and coughing. Furthermore, trauma to the vocal folds

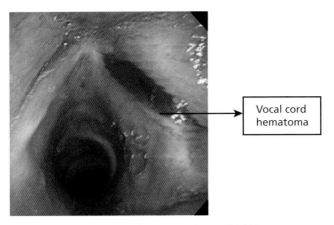

**Fig. 3.3** Trauma during bronchoscopy causing vocal fold hematoma.

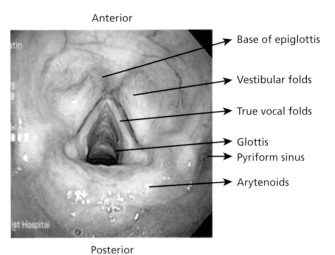

**Fig. 3.4** Bronchoscopic view of the larynx.

may occur when intubating the bronchoscope through the glottis. For example, real-time endobronchial ultrasound (EBUS) is commonly utilized (Chapter 13), where the visual field of the bronchoscope has a 30-degree forward oblique view; this may predispose to laryngeal injury when performed by amateur operators (Fig. 3.3). Hence it is crucial to be adept in moderate sedation protocols, topical anesthesia, as well as familiarity with bronchoscopic equipment.

It is advantageous for a bronchoscopist to become familiar with superior laryngeal nerve (SLN) block [9]. The procedure abolishes the gag reflex and reduces the need for sedatives. Superior laryngeal nerve pierces the thyrohyoid membrane and travels in the pyriform recesses (located at either side of the cricopharyngeus muscle, entering the cervical esophagus). When performing a SLN block, a syringe needle filled with lidocaine is inserted at the inferolateral portion of the hyoid bone, passing through the thyrohyoid membrane. Constant aspiration is maintained to ensure lack of blood return. When resistance is felt, 2–4 cc of 1% lidocaine is infiltrated to the region. This procedure should be performed on both sides.

## Bronchoscopic view of the larynx

The bronchoscope can be introduced either transnasally or orally and is directed towards the posterior pharynx. In a patient who has previously undergone a tracheotomy, the stoma site also provides direct access into the central airway, bypassing the larynx. However, the epiglottis is the first laryngeal structure examined when the bronchoscope is in the hypopharynx. It is important to recognize its anatomic variants. In some individuals, normal variants such as an omega-shaped epiglottis are seen [10]. The position of the epiglottis can be located posteriorly, resulting in enlarged valleculae. Additionally, certain medical conditions may predispose to mucosal edema and inflammation. For example, in patients with renal failure, the vocal folds and

epiglottis are often edematous, mimicking laryngopharyngeal reflux disease [11]. The epiglottis shape can also be significantly altered due to prior resection or as a result of radiation treatments to the area due to head and neck cancers [12].

Visualizing the larynx from the cephalic end of a supine patient (Fig. 3.4), it is bounded anteriorly by the free border of the epiglottis, laterally by aryepiglottic folds, and posteriorly by the corniculate tubercles of the arytenoid cartilages. The base of the tongue joins the anterior surface of the epiglottis and forms the medial and lateral glossoepiglottic folds. The space between the medial and lateral glossoepiglottic folds are called the valleculae. Lateral to the ariepiglottic folds are the pyriform sinuses (recesses) of the pharynx. Mucosal membrane over the epiglottis extends superiorly to the arytenoid cartilages forming aryepiglottic folds. Lateral to the folds, on either side of the cricopharyngeus (pharyngoesophageal segment) are the pyriform sinuses (recesses) of the pharynx. Inferior to the aryepiglottic folds are the false vocal folds, also known as ventricular folds. The true vocal folds lie below the false vocal folds (ventricular folds), extending from the anteroir surface of the arytenoid cartilage to the thyroid cartilage. The true vocal folds form an opening called the rima glotti, or glottis. The subglottic space begins at the inferior border of the true vocal folds and terminates at the level of the cricoid cartilage.

## Radiological imaging of laryngeal structures

Computed tomography (CT) and magnetic resonance imaging (MRI) assist in evaluating deep mucosal structures and laryngeal spaces [13]. CT images are acquired from the base of the skull to the upper trachea [14]. The patient is

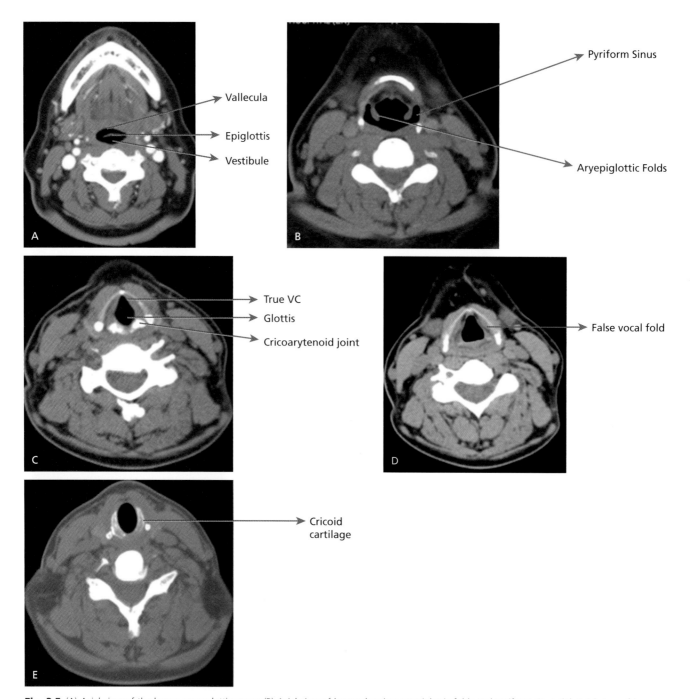

**Fig. 3.5** (A) Axial view of the larynx, supraglottic space. (B) Axial view of larynx showing aryepiglottic folds and pyriform sinus. (C) Axial view of larynx, glottic space. (D) Axial view of larynx showing false vocal folds. (E) Axial view of larynx showing cricoid cartilage.

placed in a supine position and is reminded to avoid swallowing or coughing.

Different views are used to delineate the structures of the larynx. On axial view of CT of the larynx, the epiglottis is seen at the level of the hyoid cartilage and it separates the vallecula from the laryngeal vestibule (Fig. 3.5A). The valleculae are separated from one another by the glossoepiglottic ligament. Aryepiglottic folds appear at the anterolateral aspect of the larynx, and are triangular in shape. They form a border between the laryngeal airway anteriorly and the pyriform sinuses posteriorly [15] (Fig. 3.5B). Supraglottic larynx consists of epiglottis, false/ ventricular folds, aryepiglottic folds, and the arytenoids. Beneath this level is the glottis, which consists of the true vocal folds, including the anterior commissure (Fig. 3.5C). Anterior commissure is the mucosa reflected from the anterior aspect of the true vocal folds, covering the posterior aspect of the thyroid cartilage in the glottis [16]. Superiorly, the glottis is bound by the vocal fold epithelium, which turns upward to form the lateral wall of the vestibules. The distinguishing feature between true and false vocal folds is the presence of fat in the false vocal folds [17] (Fig. 3.5D). True vocal folds appear thin and elliptical in shape and are bounded by the thyroid cartilage anteriorly and thyroarytenoid muscles laterally.

Beneath the glottis is the subglottic region. It is the narrowest part of the airway and is situated between the vocal folds and the upper trachea. The subglottic space is circular in shape and is bounded posteriorly by the cricoid cartilage (Fig. 3.5E).

## Laryngeal function

Direct visualization of the larynx can identify its various functions and related pathologies. The ability to recognize laryngeal dysfunction depends on the knowledge of normal physiology and the respective structural movements. Certainly, analysis of subtle movements that cause phonatory conditions will requirement more advance studies, such as videostroboscopy [18]. It is also important to bear in mind that surrounding structures such as the esophagus, for example, may present with pathologies such as acid reflux that can affect laryngeal function. This section will highlight important laryngeal functions, and how endoscopic examination can assist in identifying pathologies.

### Swallowing

Otolaryngologists and speech–language pathologists perform fiberoptic endoscopic evaluation of swallowing (FEES), for objective assessment in patients with suspected oropharyngeal dysphagia [19]. It is an important diagnostic test particularly in patients who are not candidates for a videofluoroscopic evaluation, or modified barium swallow, as in pregnant patients or patients with difficulties with transport to the radiology suite (i.e. intensive care unit). The FEES procedure also allows the examiner to assess the status of oral secretions, which cannot be observed fluoroscopically. Abnormal findings during a FEES procedure may include: aspiration of a bolus before/ during/ after the swallow, premature spilling into the hypopharynx prior to swallowing, bolus residue seen after the swallow, and a sluggish laryngeal closing maneuver. Reflecting a delayed initiation of swallowing process, reflux of esophageal contents after swallowing (esophagopharyngeal reflux) may also be observed during the exam [20]. Certainly, without formal training in FEES, the administration of the test and interpretation of results should remain with the otolaryngologist or speech–language pathologist. The scope of the swallowing mechanism is far too complex to be discussed thoroughly for the purpose of this chapter. The reader is referred to a more dedicated text for focused reading on oropharyngeal dysphagia [21]. However, the bronchoscopist should be able to identify some basic findings, if present, during endoscopic view of the hypopharynx and the larynx. Referral to an otolaryngologist or a speech–language pathologist is recommended if findings are suggestive of increased risks of aspiration or oropharyngeal dysphagia.

Of importance to the bronchoscopist is the pharyngeal stage of swallowing, which involves velopharyngeal closure to prevent nasal regurgitation, pharyngeal contraction to propel the bolus inferiorly and towards the esophagus, base of tongue excursion (to help push the bolus inferiorly), airway protection, and upper esophageal sphincter (UES) relaxation.

The airway protective component of swallowing involves the adduction of the vocal folds, the upward and anterior movement of the hyolaryngeal complex, and downward excursion of the epiglottis. Laryngeal and hyoid elevation is the first sign seen on video fluoroscopy indicating the initiation of swallowing. Endoscopically, medialization of the vocal folds marks the beginning of swallowing: the thyroarytenoid muscles rotate inwardly, bringing in the vocal folds and narrowing the rima glottis [22]. The arytenoids can be seen displaced anteriorly and in close apposition to the base of the epiglottis. The patient can be prompted to mimic swallowing before advancing the bronchoscope through the glottis to visualize potential issues.

The contour of the epiglottis guides food boluses into the esophagus and away from the glottis. During endoscopic examination, certain anatomical variants may identify increased risks for aspiration. These include narrow pharyngeal anteroposterior diameter, low-lying aryepiglottic folds, and incomplete laryngeal closure [21]. Pooling of secretions around the aryepiglottic folds, valleculae, or pyriform sinuses is also predictive of high risk of laryngeal aspiration (Fig. 3.6) [20,23].

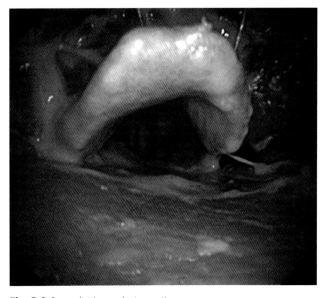

**Fig. 3.6** Supraglottic purulent secretions.

Cough reflex is a protective mechanism of the glottis and should be seen when stimulation of the larynx is performed [24]. For a bronchoscopist, this is usually seen in the initial topical anesthesia preparation of the patient undergoing bronchoscopy when lidocaine is instilled onto the larynx under endoscopic view. If this reflex is absent during the initial administration in a mildly sedated patient, sensory deficits of the larynx should be suspected.

## Phonation

Phonation is a process that transforms aerodynamic energy into acoustic sound, by means of oscillating sound waves, induced by the membranous portion of true vocal folds as air passes through. This process is precise, as vibration is manipulated by fine movements of the upper and lower lips of the true vocal folds in a semicyclical fashion, or the vibratory cycle [25]. Complex muscular adjustments result in pitch inflections and intensity changes. Vocal folds tension, or the stretch, controls the pitch of sound; while infraglottic pressure modulates the volume. The cricothyroid muscles, as part of the intrinsic laryngeal muscles, reduce the distance between the cricoid and thyroid cartilage, thus causing downward tilt of the thyroid process and increasing the tension of the vocal folds. In essence, vocal fold vibration encompasses the constant adduction and abduction created by air pressure changes. What is heard as voicing, or phonation, is the product of repeated opening and closing of the vocal folds. The motion of tissue and airflow disturb the molecules of air, causing the phenomenon called sound.

During bronchoscopic surveillance, phonatory lesions of the vocal folds (discussed later) may be identified in patients with voice change or respiratory symptoms. In general, lesions that are located in close proximity to the anterior commisure and the vocal folds have profound impact to both the pitch and strength of voice, while larger lesions in the posterior aspects, for example, laryngeal webs, may have little or no impact on voice production [26].

In presbylarynx, caused by age-related atrophy of soft tissues, there will be weak voice production [27]. It is important to pay close attention to laryngeal lesions as well as the overall condition of the patient when performing a bronchoscopic examination. For example, in a patients with myasthenia gravis, the structures of the larynx are normal, but diffuse neuromuscular weakness can involve its muscular content as well, causing voice and respiratory symptoms [28,29]. Having the patient produce multisyllabic words or single vowels, and observing vocal fold movement, symmetry, and overall structure are an important part of the examination. Further evaluation by experts in voice disorders, that is otolaryngologists and speech–language pathologist may be warranted. These may include phonatory function studies (acoustic and perceptual analyses), or videostroboscopy, for example.

## Respiration

During quiet breathing, there is minimal excursion of the vocal folds as they are positioned slightly adducted, that is in the paramedian fashion [5]. The expansion of the thoracic cage and downward movement of the laryngeal complex by infrahyoid muscles counteracted by attachments to the cricoid above, results in slight abduction during quiet inspiration. During more forceful inspiratory effort, the intrinsic respiratory muscles, including the thyromuscularis and the thyrovocalis muscles, act in concert to facilitate active glottic opening. During quiet expiration, the combined effects of the superior movement of the laryngeal complex and Bernoulli's effect of airflow against the closely apposed vocal folds, causes them to adduct [5]. During more active inspiration and expiration, the intrinsic muscles of the larynx participate in abduction and adduction, respectively.

Simultaneous adduction of vocal folds is a function of the posterior cricoarytenoid and transverse arytenoid muscles. Active inspiratory abduction by phasic muscular contraction of the lateral cricoarytenoid appears to be an essential component of respiration. Bilateral damage to posterior cricoarytenoid muscle causes inability to keep the vocal folds apart and causes difficulty in breathing [30].

## Vocal fold dysfunction

### Spasmodic dysphonia

Spasmodic dysphonia (or laryngeal dystonia) is classified as a neurological movement disorder but various types of classifications exist (early versus late onset; idiopathic versus secondary; and focal versus generalized or multifocal) [31]. There is inappropriate closure and opening of the vocal folds during speech. The pathophysiology stems from inappropriate contractions of adductor or abductor laryngeal muscles, and phonation may be abruptly cut off or breathy. There is no specific therapies for these entities, except with the option of injecting botulism toxin at regular intervals into respective musculatures [32]. Speech therapy can be employed but is usually met with variable results [31,33].

Various other neurological voice disorders affect voice quality, pitch, and volume. These include flaccid and spastic types, which are caused by lower and upper motor neuron pathologies, respectively. In Parkinson's disease, there is diffuse hypertonicity of the vocal folds causing reduced loudness and breathy, hoarse voice. Diagnosis of neurological vocal fold diseases cannot be established by endoscopy alone, and often requires a laryngologist who performs videostroboscopy, which allows slow-motion evaluation of vocal fold movements, symmetry, and structural integrity [18].

## Paradoxical vocal fold dysfunction

Vocal folds dysfunction, either functional (paradoxical movement and spasm) or fixed (edema), also can cause significant airway compromise. Normally, the true vocal folds abduct on inspiration and adduct during expiration, phonation, and swallowing. In contrast, paradoxical vocal fold motion (PVCM) is an inappropriate adduction of the true vocal folds throughout the respiratory cycle with the obliteration of glottic aperture except for a posterior diamond-shaped passage [34]. Patients with PVCM may exhibit signs of inability to speak, dyspnea, and stridor, which may progress to acute respiratory failure with the need for advanced airway management [35]. Speech pathology intervention can teach and train patients with milder degree of symptoms to recover from episodes of paradoxical vocal fold dysfunction [36].

## Vocal fold paralysis

Most often vocal fold palsies are due to peripheral lesions of recurrent laryngeal nerve or to disruption of vagal nerve [30]. Common causes are due to surgical manipulations after thyroidectomies, head and neck (such as carotid endarterectomies) or thoracic surgeries, malignancies such as primary lung cancers, trauma, or idiopathic causes [30]. In chronic vocal fold paralysis, the folds will atrophy (Fig. 3.7) and will be shortened in length. Left vocal fold paralysis is more common than the right as the left recurrent laryngeal nerve is longer and more convoluted, looping around the aortic arch and travels superiorly between the trachea and the esophagus [37]. The right recurrent laryngeal nerve travels via the right subclavian artery and is particularly susceptible to injury during thyroid surgeries. Vocal fold paralysis can either be unilateral or bilateral. Bilateral vocal fold paralysis presents with dyspnea, stridor, cyanosis, and apneic spells. Unilateral vocal fold paralysis may present with dysphonia [38].

The diagnosis is made by endoscopy with direct visualization of the folds and confirmed by absence of movement by videostroboscopy. They may be fixed in median or paramedian position. Patients with persistent dysphonia may respond to voice therapy, but sometimes require medialization procedures to prevent aspiration episodes [39]. Medialization procedure is performed for unilateral vocal fold paralysis to surgically displaced the paralyzed cord medially by injection with silicone, Teflon, or gelfoam [40]. This procedure improves vocal quality and swallowing. Other injectables include calcium hydroxyapatite, fat, or Bioplastique [41,42].

For patients with bilateral vocal fold paralysis presenting with stridor, tracheostomy is the most viable and safe option. Lateralization and reinnervation surgery can be performed in selected cases [43].

## Postintubation effects of vocal folds

Endotracheal intubation is an invasive but life-saving modality that requires significant expertise on oropharyngeal and laryngeal anatomy. Potential damage to laryngeal structures during intubation can occur but symptoms may manifest variably after extubation, with dysphagia, hoarseness, stridor, and even respiratory failure [44]. Prompt recognition and endoscopic examination can readily identify upper airway pathologies and stratify therapeutic management.

During intubation, dislocation of arytenoids can occur even under expert hands [45]. Post-extubation symptoms are often limited to hoarseness or odynophagia. In the setting of bilateral dislocations, vocal folds are closely approximated during inspiration, causing stridor and need for reintubation. Although complete recovery is the norm, temporary tracheostomy should be considered if symptoms are severe. Other side effects may include temporary oropharyngeal dysphagia, mostly in the form of reduced airway protection. This may be related to laryngeal edema or decreased laryngeal excursion for the swallow. Dysphagia management is important, so as to reduce the risk for aspiration, while airway protective mechanisms are regained.

## Anatomical/ structural abnormalities

### Benign conditions

*Vocal fold nodules and polyps* are also known as singer's nodule. They can occur in professionals who abuse or misuse their voices such as yelling or shouting [46]. Vocal fold nodules present as symmetrical lesions at the junction of anterior one-third of the vocal folds (Fig. 3.8) [47]. Symptoms include hoarseness, pain, reduced voice range, and loss of voice. Treatments include vocal rehabilitation, voice rest, or surgical removal.

Vocal fold polyps, on the other hand, are more commonly seen in men and are often unilateral and pedunculated (Fig. 3.9) [48]. During endoscopy blood vessels may be visible. They tend to occur in the middle third of the

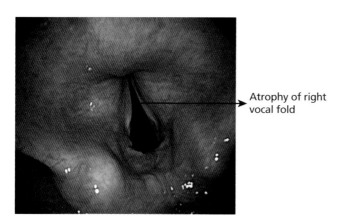

Atrophy of right vocal fold

**Fig. 3.7** Atrophy of right vocal fold.

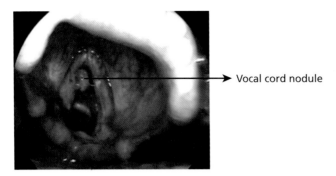

**Fig. 3.8** Left true vocal fold nodule.

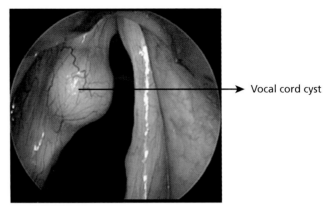

**Fig. 3.10** Left true vocal fold cyst.

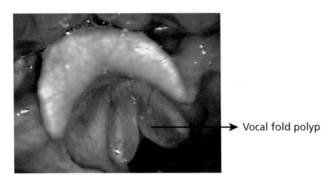

**Fig. 3.9** Bilateral true vocal fold polyp.

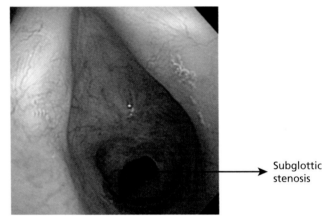

**Fig. 3.11** Subglottic stenosis.

membranous vocal folds. Common causes includes voice abuse and misuse, acid reflux, chronic inhalational irritants and allergies.

*Reinke's edema* is associated with cigarette smoking; it is a result of diffuse swelling of the lamina propria layer of the mucosa [49]. Due to the increase of the mass of the vocal folds, patients have a low-pitch voice. Endoscopically, the vocal folds are swollen lengthwise (sausage shape). Treatment is smoking cessation; but in cases that do not regress, surgery, or microlaryngoscopy may be required [50].

*Laryngeal cysts* are usually seen in the middle thirds of the vocal folds, and present with dysphonia and discomfort in the throat if they are located in the supraglottis (Fig. 3.10) [48].

*Laryngeal stenosis.* The incidence of subglottic stenosis is estimated to be 1–10% after endotracheal intubations [51]. The stenosis can be at the level of supraglottic or subglottic space. In some patients, the subglottic region is narrowed to a pinpoint diameter, causing stridor and respiratory failure.

Subglottic stenosis can be due to idiopathic or secondary causes. Acquired etiologies include prolonged intubation and tracheostomy cuff related injury with granulation tissue formation at the stoma site (Fig. 3.11). Additionally, over-

sized endotracheal tube or overzealous inflation of the balloon cuff can cause pressure necrosis, ulcer, and scar formation, which exacerbates the risk of stenosis [52]. Laryngotracheal reflux due to regurgitation of gastric acidic content may worsen stenosis and should be treated aggressively before surgical intervention [51,53].

*Laryngopharyngeal reflux (LPR).* LPR is a major cause of laryngeal inflammation and presents with different symptoms to those typically found in patients with gastroesophageal reflux disease (GERD) [54]. Koufman was the first to distinguish LPR from GERD, noting that in a combined reported series of 899 patients, throat clearing was a complaint of 87% of LPR patients versus 3% of those with GERD, while only 20% of LPR patients complained of heartburn versus 83% in the GERD group [55]. The laryngeal epithelium is particularly vulnerable to reflux of gastric content. Failure to recognize LPR in a symptomatic patient will delay prompt initiation of therapy, impairing patient global quality of life, and may place the patient at risk for developing complica-

Examination of the Larynx

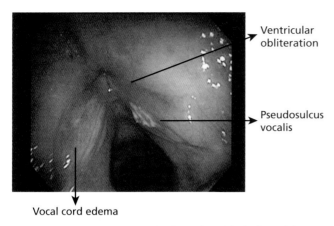

Fig. 3.12 Signs of laryngotracheal reflux: (1) vocal fold edema, (2) ventricular obliteration, and (3) pseudosulcus vocalis.

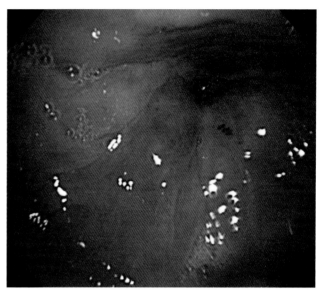

Fig. 3.13 Diffuse laryngeal edema.

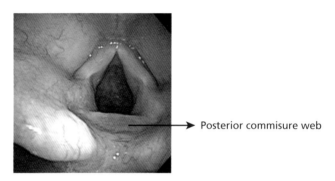

Fig. 3.14 Posterior commisure web.

tions such as ulcers, contact granulomas, subglottic stenosis, and lower airway disease [56,57].

Patients with LPR will typically present with symptoms such as throat clearing (98%), persistent cough (97%), globus sensation (95%), and hoarseness (95%). Only a few will have associated heartburn or regurgitation [58].

Although endoscopic evaluation of the laryngopharyngeal mucosa may suggest the presence of LPR, a definitive diagnosis requires demonstration of reflux events using a multichannel intraluminal impedance study and a dual pH probe monitor. LPR is confirmed when total acid exposure time (percentage of time during 24-hour monitoring when the sensor detects pH levels <4) is more than 1% [59].

Endoscopic evaluation usually reveals non-specific signs of laryngeal irritation and inflammation concentrated in the pharynx and posterior larynx. Since there are no pathognomonic LPR findings Belafsky *et al.*, developed an eight-item clinical severity scale for assessing laryngoscopic findings of LPR. The reflux finding score (RFS) is useful for the initial assessment and in the follow-up of LPR patients. There are eight LPR-associated findings with endoscopy that are graded in a 0–4 scale and include: (1) pseudosulcus vocalis (appearance of a groove lengthwise along the true vocal folds) (Fig. 3.12); (2) ventricular obliteration (edema of true and false vocal folds thus diminishing the space between the two structures) (Fig. 3.12); (3) diffuse erythema; (4) vocal fold edema (Fig. 3.12); (5) diffuse laryngeal edema (Fig. 3.13); (6) posterior commissure hypertrophy (Fig. 3.14); (7) granuloma; and (8) thick endolaryngeal mucus pooling (Fig. 3.6). The results could range from 0 (normal) to 26 (worst possible score). Based on their analysis, one can be 95% certain that a patient with a RFS of 7 or more will have LPR [60].

*Laryngeal papillomatosis,* in both pediatric and adult forms, are caused by human papillomavius (HPV) 6 and 11. There is an increased incidence of laryngeal papillomatosis in children born to mothers with genital warts via vertical transmission [61]. They present as multiple, warty lesion on both true and false vocal folds [61,62]. It is the most common benign neoplasm of the larynx. Papillomas can be found anywhere from the oral cavity to the lung parenchyma, but the most common site is the larynx. The first symptom is hoarseness, but can progress to dyspnea and stridor. Papillomas are characterized by multiple recurrences, requiring endoscopic removal every 2 to 3 months [63]. Endoscopically, they appear as pedunculated, exophytic, wart-like growths or cluster of grapes (Fig. 3.15A, B). Treatment options include microdebridement or direct injection of cidofovir [64]; however, lesions often recur with relapse of symptoms.

*Certain medical conditions* can involve the larynx and cause structural and functional abnormalities. They include inflammatory, infiltrative, and autoimmune diseases and are

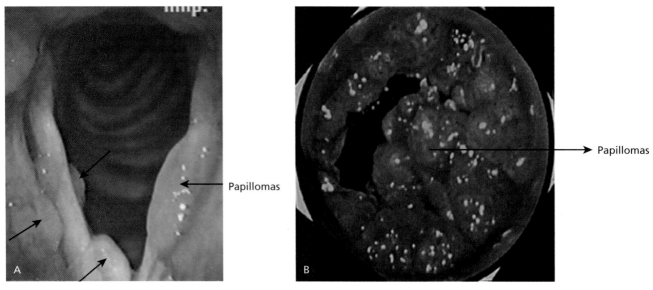

**Fig. 3.15** (A,B) Laryngeal papillomatosis.

**Table 3.2** Medical conditions affecting laryngeal structure and function

| Disease | Characteristics | Endoscopic findings |
|---|---|---|
| Sarcoidosis | Involves epiglottis, supraglottic, subglottic area and rarely true vocal folds | Pale edema, submucosal nodules, mass lesion [79] |
| Rheumatoid arthritis | Cricoarytenoid joint involvement | Edema, erythema, bowing of vocal folds |
| | | Normal in chronic rheumatoid arthritis [80] |
| Wegener's granulomatosis | Involves subglottis and upper trachea | Granulomas, crusting , ulceration, subglottic stenosis [65] |
| Amyloidosis | Involves larynx in the respiratory tract | Submucosal mass of vocal folds [81] |
| Relapsing polychondritis | Cartilagenous inflammation of the larynx | Vocal fold edema, subglottic stenosis, dynamic airway collapse [82] |
| Gout | Cricoarytenoid joint involvement | Fixed vocal folds, granular appearance of vocal fold mucosa, tophi |
| Laryngotracheal reflux | Involves whole larynx including the supraglottic to subglottic space | Granuloma, nodules, stenosis of subglottic and supraglottic area, erythema and edema of vocal folds, cobble stoning of interarytenoid area [60] |
| Myasthenia gravis | Involves laryngeal muscles [28,29] | Normal-appearing vocal folds |

listed in Table 3.2. For example, Wegener's granulomatosis can involve both the upper and lower respiratory tract. Necrotizing granulomas can be seen endoscopically (Fig. 3.16). Furthermore, repeated episodes of inflammatory response eventually lead to permanent airway injury, such as mucosal ulcerations. Vocal folds and subglottic involvements can present with hoarseness and shortness of breath in milder cases, but in more severe cases can present with stridor and respiratory failure [65].

*Laryngitis* can be acute or chronic. In acute laryngitis, there is inflammation and swelling of the larynx. It is caused by the common cold or by voice abuse. Chronic laryngitis is caused by exposure to smoke, dust, polluted air, and voice abuse.

*Vocal fold granulomas* are caused by direct irritation or chronic injury such as laryngotracheal reflux disease, postintubation trauma from endotracheal tube or rigid bronchoscopy, and hyperfunctional contact between the vocal folds (hence the name contact granuloma) [66–68]. Vocal fold granulomas can be either unilateral or bilateral; patients present with dysphonia, cough, and/or odynophagia. They are often located in close proximity to the posterior commisure, where closure of vocal folds occur, thus causing significant voice pathology (Fig. 3.17).

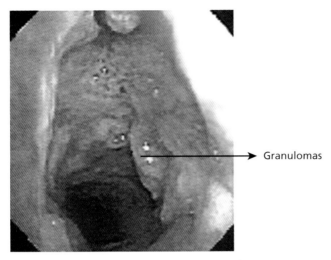

**Fig. 3.16** Granulomas secondary to Wegener's granulomatosis.

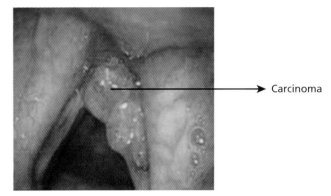

**Fig. 3.18** Squamous cell carcinoma of the larynx.

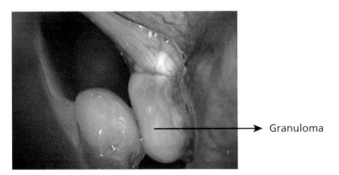

**Fig. 3.17** Laryngeal granuloma secondary to endotracheal intubation.

## Malignant lesions

*Squamous cell carcinoma of the larynx* is the most common malignancy of the larynx [69]. It is associated with smoking and alcohol abuse. Other risk factors are advanced age, male gender, radiation exposure, gastroesophageal reflux, and infection with human papilloma virus [70,71]. They can present as exophytic masses, ulcers or raised red patches called erythroplakia, or white lesions called leukoplakia (Fig. 3.18). They tend to be more aggressive and can metastasize to regional lymph nodes, with subsequent spread to the lungs [72]. Surgery and radiation therapy are possible treatment options [73].

*Verrucous carcinoma* is a variant of squamous cell carcinoma with minimal cellular atypia [74] associated with HPV16 [75]. It is an indolent tumor, commonly seen in the elderly. They present as warty and exophytic masses. However, they tend to have better prognosis with reduced incidence of metastasis [76]. Complete surgical excision is the treatment of choice.

Other malignant laryngeal tumors such as adenocarcinoma, chondrosarcoma, fibrosarcoma, rhabdomyosarcoma, lymphoma, and plasmacytoma are rare [77,78].

## Conclusion

Although pulmonary physicians do not typically manage laryngeal diseases, patients often present with respiratory symptoms. It behooves the bronchoscopist to gain proficient knowledge of laryngeal anatomy and physiology, because recognition of laryngeal pathologies during endoscopy can be significantly improved in addition to clinical history and imaging results. Close communication among other specialties, especially with otolaryngologists and speech–language therapists, helps to establish a multidisciplinary approach to the whole spectrum of laryngeal pathologies.

## Acknowledgement

The authors thank Lauren Stein MS, CCC-SLP for critical review of the manuscript.

## References

1 Garrison FG. *An Introduction to the History of Medicine*, 3rd edn. Philadelphia and London: W.B. Saunders; 1917: 649.

2 Zeitels SM, Burns JA, Dailey SH. Suspension laryngoscopy revisited. *Ann Otol Rhinol Laryngol* 2004; **113**: 16–22.

3 Klussman JP, Knoedgen R, Wittekindt C, *et al.* Complications of suspension laryngoscopy. *Ann Otol Rhinol Laryngol* 2002; **111**: 972–6.

4 Nouraei SAR, Kapoor KV. Results of endoscopic tracheoplasty for treating tracheostomy-related airway stenosis. *Clin Otolaryngol* 2007; **32**: 471–5.

5 Noordzij JP, Ossoff RH. Anatomy and physiology of the larynx. *Otolaryngol Clin N Am* 2006; **39**: 1–10.

6 Pretterklieber ML. Functional anatomy of the human intrinsic laryngeal muscles. *Eur Surg* 2003; **35**: 250–8.

7 Lofgren RH, Montgomery WW. Incidence of laryngeal involvement in rheumatoid arthritis. *N Engl J Med* 1962; **267**: 193–5.

8 Fried MP, Meller SM, Rinaldo A. Adult laryngeal anatomy. In: Fried MP, *et al.*, eds. *The Larynx*, 3rd edn. Plural Publishing; 2009.

9 Gotta AW, Sullivan CA. Anaesthesia of the upper airway using topical anaesthetic and superior laryngeal nerve block. *Br J Anaesth* 1981; **53**: 1055–8.

10 Petkar N, Georgalas C, Bhattacharyya A. High-rising epiglottis in children: should it cause concern? *J Am Board Fam Med* 2007; **20**: 495–6.

11 Ori Y, Sabo R, Binder Y. Effect of hemodialysis on the thickness of vocal folds: a possible explanation for postdialysis hoarseness. *Nephron Clin Pract* 2006; **103**: 144–8.

12 Yousefzadeh DK. Epiglottic enlargement following radiation treatment of head and neck tumors. *Pediatric Radiology* 1981; **10**: 165–8.

13 Yousem DM, Tufano RP. Laryngeal imaging. *Neuroimaging Clin N Am* 2004; **14**: 611–24.

14 Becker M, Burkhardt K, Dulguerov P, Alla A. Imaging of the larynx and hypopharynx. *Eur J Radiol* 2008; **66**: 460–79.

15 Lee JKT, Sagel SS, Stanley RJ, Heiken JP. *Computed Body Tomography with MRI Correlation*, 4th edn. Lippincott Williams and Watkins; 2005.

16 Kaflmes DF, Phillips CD. The normal anterior commissure of the glottis. *Am J Reontol* 1997; **168**: 1317–19.

17 Blitz AM, Aygun N. Radiologic evaluation of larynx cancer. *Otolaryngol Clin N Am* 2008; **41**: 697–713.

18 Bless DM, Hirano M, Feder RJ. Videostroboscopic evaluation of the larynx. *Ear Nose Throat J* 1987; **66**: 289–96.

19 Langmore SE, Schatz K, Olson N. Endoscopic and videofluoroscopic evaluations of swallowing and aspiration. *Ann Otol Rhinol Laryngol* 1991; **100**: 678–81.

20 Murray J, Langmore SE, Ginsburg S. The significance of oropharngeal secretions and swallowing frequency in predicting aspiration. *Dysphagia* 1996; **11**: 99–103.

21 Langmore S. *Endoscopic Evaluation and Treatment of Swallowing Disorders*, 1st edn. Georg Thieme Verlag; 2001: 37–60.

22 McCulloch TM, Perlman AL, Palmer PM, Van Daele DJ. Laryngeal activity during swallow, phonation, and the Valsalva maneuver: an electromyographic analysis. *Laryngoscope* 1996; **106**: 1351–8.

23 Hiss SG, Postma GN. Fiberoptic endoscopic evaluation of swallowing. *Laryngoscope* 2003; **113**: 1386–93.

24 Kidder TM. Esophago/ pharyngo/ laryngeal interrelationships: airway protection mechanisms. *Dysphagia* 1995; **10**: 228–31.

25 Kaszuba S, Garrett C. Strobovideolaryngoscopy and laboratory voice evaluation. *Otolaryngol Clin N Am* 2007; **40**: 991–1001.

26 Lalwani AK, ed. *Current Diagnosis and Treatment of Otolaryngology— Head and Neck Surgery*, 2nd edn. New York: McGraw-Hill; 2008.

27 Pontes P, Brasolotto A, Behlau M. Glottic characteristics and voice complaint in the elderly. *J Voice* 2005; **19**: 84–94.

28 Hara K, Mashima T, Matsuda A, *et al.* Vocal fold paralysis in myasthenia gravis with anti-MuSK antibodies. *Neurology* 2007; **68**: 621–2.

29 Mao VH, Abaza M, Spiegel JR, *et al.* Laryngeal myasthenia gravis: report of 40 cases. *J Voice* 2001; **15**: 122–30.

30 Woodson G. Evolving concepts of laryngeal paralysis. *J Laryngol Otol* 2008; **122**: 437–41.

31 Ludlow CL, Adler CH, Berke GS, *et al.* Research priorities in spasmodic dysphonia. *J Laryngol Otol* 2008; **122**: 437–41.

32 Grillone GA, Chan T. Laryngeal dystonia. *Otolaryngol Clin N Am* 2006; **39**: 87–100.

33 Ruotsalainen JH, Sellman J, Lehto L, *et al.* Interventions for treating functional dysphonia in adults. *Cochrane Database Syst Rev* 2007; **3**: CD006373.

34 Hicks M, Brugman SM, Katial R. Vocal fold dysfunction/ paradoxical vocal fold motion. *Prim Care* 2008; **35**: 81–103.

35 Altman KW, Mirza N, Ruiz C. Paradoxical vocal fold motion: presentation and treatment options. *J Voice* 2000; **14**: 99–103.

36 Goldman J, Muers M. Vocal fold dysfunction and wheezing. *Thorax* 1991; **46**: 401.

37 Aydin K, Ulug T. Bilateral vocal fold paralysis caused by cervical spinal osteophytes. *Br J Radiol* 2002; **75**: 990–3.

38 Ollivere B, Duce K, Rowlands G. Swallowing dysfunction in patients with unilateral vocal fold paralysis: aetiology and outcomes. *J Laryngol Otol* 2006; **120**: 38–41.

39 Sipp JA, Kerschner JE, Braune N, Hartnick CJ. Vocal fold medialization in children: injection laryngoplasty, thyroplasty, or nerve reinnervation? *Arch Otolaryngol Head Neck Surg* 2007; **133**: 767–71.

40 Gardnera GM, Altman JS, Balakrishnan G. Pediatric vocal fold medialization with silastic implant: intraoperative airway management. *Int J Ped Otorhinolaryngol* 2000; **52**: 37–44.

41 Bergamini G, Alicandri-Ciufelli M, Molteni G, *et al.* Therapy of unilateral vocal fold paralysis with polydimethylsiloxane injection laryngoplasty: our experience. *J Voice* 2010; **24**: 119–25.

42 Morgan JE, Zraick RI, Griffin AW, *et al.* Injection versus medialization laryngoplasty for the treatment of unilateral vocal fold paralysis. *Laryngoscope* 2007; **117**: 2068–74.

43 Lichtenberger G. Reversible lateralization of the paralyzed vocal fold without tracheostomy. *Ann Otol Rhinol Laryngol* 2002; **111**: 21–6.

44 Stauffer J, Olson D, Petty T. Complications and consequences of endotracheal intubation and tracheostomy: a prospective study of 150 critically ill adult patients. *Am J Med* 1981; **70**: 65–76.

45 Rubin AD, Hawkshaw MJ, Moyer CA, *et al.* Arytenoid cartilage dislocation: a 20-year experience. *J Voice* 2005; **19**: 687–701.

46 Pedersen M, McGlashan J. Surgical versus non-surgical interventions for vocal fold nodules. *Cochrane Database Syst Rev* 2001, Issue 2.

47 Lalwani AK, ed. *Current Diagnosis and Treatment of Otolaryngology— Head and Neck Surgery*, 2nd edn. New York: McGraw-Hill; 2008.

48 Altman KW. Vocal fold masses. *Otolaryngol Clin North Am* 2007; **40**: 1091–108.

49 Dikkers FG, Nikkels PG. Benign lesions of the vocal folds: histopathology and phonotrauma. *Ann Otol Rhinol Laryngol* 1995; **104**: 698–703.

50 Dursun G, Ozgursoy OB, Kemal O, Coruh I. One year follow-up results of combined use of CO2 laser and cold instrumentation for Reinke's edema surgery in professional voice users. *Eur Arch Otorhinolaryngol* 2007; **264**: 1027–32.

51 Lorenz RR. Adult laryngotracheal stenosis: etiology and surgical management. *Curr Opin Otolaryngol Head Neck Surg* 2003; **11**: 467–72.

52 Sue RD, Susanto I. Long-term complications of artificial airways. *Clin Chest Med* 2003; **24**: 457–71.

53 Terra RM, de Medeiros IL, Minamoto H, *et al*. Idiopathic tracheal stenosis: successful outcome with antigastroesophageal reflux disease therapy. *Ann Thorac Surg* 2008; **85**: 1438–9.

54 Koufman J, Sataloff RT, Toohill R. Laryngopharyngeal reflux: consensus conference report. *J Voice* 1996; **10**: 215–16.

55 Koufman JA. The otolaryngologic manifestations of gastro-esophageal reflux disease (GERD): a clinical investigation of 225 patients using ambulatory 24-hour pH monitoring and an experimental investigation of the role of acid and pepsin in the development of laryngeal injury. *Laryngoscope* 1991; **101** (Suppl. 53): 1–78.

56 Murry T, Medrado R, Hogikyan ND, *et al*. The relationship between ratings of voice quality and quality of life measures. *J Voice* 2004; **18**: 183–92.

57 Ylitalo R, Lindestad PA, Ramel S. Symptoms, laryngeal findings, and 24-hour pH monitoring in patients with suspected gastroesophago-pharyngeal reflux. *Laryngoscope* 2001; **111**: 1735–41.

58 Book DT, Rhee JS, Toohill RJ, Smith TL. Perspectives in laryngopharyngeal reflux: an international survey. *Laryngoscope* 2002; **112**: 1399–406.

59 Kawamura O, Aslam M, Rittmann T, *et al*. Physical and pH properties of gastroesophagopharyngeal refluxate: a 24-hour simultaneous ambulatory impedance and pH monitoring study. *Am J Gastroenterol* 2004; **99**: 1000–10.

60 Belafsky PC, Postma GN, Koufman JA. The validity and reliability of the Reflux Finding Score (RFS). *Laryngoscope* 2001; **111**: 1313–17.

61 Derkay CS, Wiatrak B. Recurrent respiratory papillomatosis: a review. *Arch Otolaryngol Head Neck Surg* 2009; **135**: 198–201.

62 Quiney RE, Hall D, Croft CB. Laryngeal papillomatosis : analysis of 113 patients. *Clin Otolaryngol* 1989; **14**: 217.

63 Andrus JG, Shapshay SM. Contemporary management of laryngeal papilloma in adults and children. *Otolaryngol Clin North Am* 2006; **39**: 135–58.

64 Derkay C. Use of cidofovir for treatment of recurrent respiratory papillomatosis. *Arch Otolaryngol Head Neck Surg* 2009; **135**: 198–201.

65 Blaivas AJ, Strauss W, Yudd M. Subglottic stenosis as a complication of Wegener's granulomatosis. *Prim Care Respir J* 2008; **17**: 114–6.

66 Devaney KO, Rinaldo A, Ferlito A. Vocal process granuloma of the larynx-recognition, differential diagnosis and treatment. *Oral Oncol* 2005; **41**: 666–9.

67 Heller AJ, Wohl DL. Vocal fold granuloma induced by rigid bronchoscopy. *Ear Nose Throat J* 1999; **78**: 176–8, 180.

68 Shin T, Watanabe H, Oda M, *et al*. Contact granulomas of the larynx. *Eur Arch Otorhinolaryngol* 1994; **251**: 67–71.

69 Glanz HK. Carcinoma of the larynx. Growth, p-classification and grading of squamous cell carcinoma of the vocal folds. *Adv Otorhinolaryngol* 1984; **32**: 1–123.

70 Galli J, Cammarota G, Volante M, *et al*. Laryngeal carcinoma and laryngo-pharyngeal reflux disease. *Acta Otorhinolaryngol Ital* 2006; **26**: 260–3.

71 Qadeer MA, Colabianchi N, Strome M, Vaezi MF. Gastroesophageal reflux and laryngeal cancer: causation or association? A critical review. *Am J Otolaryngol* 2006; **27**: 119–28.

72 Ferlito A, Shaha AR, Silver CE, *et al*. Incidence and sites of distant metastases from head and neck cancer. *J Otorhinolaryngol Relat Spec* 2001; **63**: 202–7.

73 Agrawal N, Ha PK. Management of early-stage laryngeal cancer. *Otolaryngol Clin North Am* 2008; **41**: 757–69, vi–vii.

74 Thompson LD. Diagnostically challenging lesions in head and neck pathology. *Eur Arch Otorhinolaryngol* 1997; **254**: 357–66.

75 Hagen P, Lyons GD, Haindel C. Verrucous carcinoma of the larynx: role of human papillomavirus, radiation, and surgery. *Laryngoscope* 1993; **103**: 253.

76 Ferlito A. Diagnosis and treatment of verrucous squamous cell carcinoma of the larynx: a critical review. *Ann Otol Rhinol Laryngol* 1985; **94**: 575–9.

77 Bathala S, Berry S, Evans RA, *et al*. Chondrosarcoma of larynx: review of literature and clinical experience. *J Laryngol Otol* 2008; **122**: 1127–9.

78 Lin HW, Bhattacharyya N. Staging and survival analysis for nonsquamous cell carcinomas of the larynx. *Laryngoscope* 2008; **118**: 1003–13.

79 Benjamin B, Dalton C, Croxson G. Laryngoscopic diagnosis of laryngeal sarcoid. *Ann Otol Rhinol Laryngol* 1995; **104**: 529–31.

80 Chen JJ, Branstetter BF, Myers EN. Cricoarytenoid rheumatoid arthritis: an important consideration in aggressive lesions of the larynx. *Am J Neuroradiol* 2005; **26**: 970–2.

81 Lalwani AK, ed. *Current Diagnosis and Treatment in Otolaryngology—Head and Neck Surgery*, 2nd edn. New York: McGraw-Hill; 2008.

82 Trentham DE, Le CH, Relapsing polychondritis—clinical review. *Ann Intern Med* 1998; **129**: 114–22.

# 4

# Applied Anatomy of the Airways

## Mani S. Kavuru,[1] Atul C. Mehta,[2] and J. Francis Turner Jr[3]

[1]Division of Pulmonary and Critical Care Medicine, Jefferson Center for Critical Care, Thomas Jefferson University and Hospital Philadelphia, PA, USA

[2]Respiratory Institute, Cleveland Clinic, Cleveland, OH, USA

[3]Interventional Pulmonary and Critical Care Medicine, Nevada Cancer Institute and University of Nevada School of Medicine, Las Vegas, NV

## The pharynx and the larynx

Flexible bronchoscopy is usually performed via either the oral or nasal route. Familiarity with the normal anatomy of this region is important to gain access to the trachea as well as to recognize local pathology. Certainly, bronchoscopy performed for the evaluation of hemoptysis or wheezing should include a careful evaluation of the upper airway. The nose extends from the external nares through the nasal cavity and the nasal pharynx. Each nasal cavity is bounded medially by the nasal septum, laterally by the three bony projections called turbinates or conchae, and inferiorly by the hard palate that separates the nasal cavity from the mouth. The paranasal sinuses open into an area below each turbinate called a meatus. The blood supply to the nasal mucosa is via branches of the maxillary artery and the facial artery that anastomose to form the Kisselbach's plexus at the anterior medial wall of the nose, which is a common site of nasal bleeding [1].

The pharynx is 12–15 cm long; it communicates anteriorly with the nasal cavity (nasopharynx) and the oral cavity (oropharynx) and extends to the cricoid cartilage inferiorly to encompass the hypopharynx or larynx [1]. The pharyngeal muscles, including the cricopharyngeous muscle, act as a sphincter to the proximal esophagus and help to prevent the reflux of esophageal contents. The adenoids or nasopharyngeal tonsils lie on the posterior wall of the nasopharynx. The oropharynx is bounded laterally by the tonsillar pillars, superiorly by the soft palate, anteriorly and inferiorly by the tongue, and posteriorly by the C2 and C3 vertebrae. The oropharyngeal cavity is not rigid and is subject to collapse easily. The hypopharynx lies between the epiglottis and the inferior border of the cricoid cartilage. The larynx, which is 5–7 cm in length and lies at levels C4, C5, and C6, is a complex organ composed of cartilages, ligaments, and muscles [1]. An endoscopic view of the larynx demonstrates the epiglottis anteriorly and superiorly, aryepiglottic folds bilaterally, with the pyriform sinuses alongside. The glottis is bounded anteriorly and laterally by the vestibular folds (false cords) and vocal folds (true cords) and posteriorly by the arytenoid cartilage [2]. During inspiration, the vocal cords are abducted away from the midline, and the rima glottidis has a triangular appearance. On expiration, the vocal cords are adducted medially with a very small opening between them. During maximal abduction the distance between the vocal processes is 19 mm in men and 12 mm in women. In adults, unlike children, the glottic chink is the narrowest part of the larynx [2].

## The tracheobronchial tree

The normal adult trachea begins at the lower margin of the cricoid cartilage and extends 10–14 cm until the bifurcation into the left and right main stem bronchi at the level of T5. One-third of the trachea is "extrathoracic," above the level of the suprasternal notch, and two-thirds is "intrathoracic" or below the notch. The average tracheal diameter is 2.5 cm and is supported anteriorly by 18 to 24 incomplete C-shaped cartilaginous elements and posteriorly by the membranous trachealis muscle. In the normal adult, the diameter of the entire trachea is well maintained throughout the respiratory cycle by the rigid support of the tracheal elements. In patients with obstructive airways disease or older individuals, the tracheal lumen may be reduced dynamically with coughing or during expiration because of collapse of the posterior membranous wall anteriorly [3]. Normally, the aortic arch compresses the mid to distal left lateral wall of the trachea to the right. The adult tracheal width–depth ratio can vary from 0.6 (high-domed variant) to 3.0 (lunate variant). The main carina is normally quite sharp and is mobile during the respiratory cycle [4]. The right main stem bronchus normally bifurcates at an angle of 25° to 30° from the midline, with a luminal diameter of around 16 mm and an average length of 2 cm before the bifurcation of the right upper lobe bronchus from the right main stem bronchus. The right upper lobe orifice averages 10 mm and usually branches into the apical, posterior, and anterior segmental bronchi [5]. After the bifurcation of the right upper lobe bronchus, the right main stem bronchus continues as the bronchus intermedius. The anterior wall of the intermedius bronchus continues to become the right middle lobe, which divides into the medial and lateral subsegments. By virtue of its anterior location, foreign bodies have a propensity to continue from the trachea and fall into the right middle lobe. The right lower lobe bronchus represents the posterior continuation of the bronchus intermedius, further dividing into five subsegments with frequent variation [6]. The superior or apical subsegment usually arises posteriorly opposite to the origin of the middle lobe bronchus. Next, the medial basal subsegment arises on the medial wall and may subdivide further. The right lower lobe subsequently divides into the anterior, lateral, and posterior basal subsegments. These latter three subsegments are usually stacked one on top of the other proceeding from anterior to posterior configuration (A–L–P).

The left main stem bifurcates from the trachea at a sharp 45° angle from the midline. It is narrower and much longer than its counterpart with an average length of 5 cm. The distal left main stem bronchus primarily divides into the left upper and the left lower lobe. The upper divides into the lingular division (composed of the superior and inferior lingular subsegments) and the upper lobe division (composed of the apical posterior and anterior subsegments). The lower lobe initially gives rise to the superior or apical subsegment, which is posteriorly located. The left lower lobe subsequently divides into the anterior–medial, lateral, and posterior basal subsegments. There is again considerable variability in the basilar subsegments of the left lower lobe [6,7].

## The relationship of airways to lymph nodes and vessels

As important as a thorough understanding of the normal endobronchial anatomy and the frequent congenital variations is a thorough familiarity with normal structures that reside outside the airway in intimate juxtaposition to the airway [8]. This knowledge is mandatory with the increasing use of endobronchial diagnostic and therapeutic modalities, including transbronchial needle aspiration (TBNA), laser therapy, and endobronchial radiation therapy. This anatomic knowledge will help facilitate access to lymph nodes or extraluminal mass lesions that may be important in either diagnosis or staging [9,10]. This understanding will hopefully avoid inadvertent access of vascular structures that are intimately associated with the airways in several areas.

The posterior aspect of the trachea is closely associated with the esophagus. The aortic arch lies anterior and to the left of the distal one-third of the trachea and makes an easily recognizable pulsatile imprint on the anterolateral tracheal wall; this area should be avoided for obvious reasons [8]. The superior vena cava and the azygos vein lie anteriorly and to the right of the distal third of the trachea. The aortic arch and the inominate artery lie directly anterior to the trachea at the level of the main carina. The right pulmonary artery lies immediately anterior to the right main stem bronchus and the origin of the right upper lobe bronchus. There is significant variability of the relationship of vascular structures to the right middle lobe and lower lobe bronchi. The aortic arch and the left pulmonary artery are in close association to the left main stem bronchus and left upper lobe bronchus.

Lymph nodes lie in close association to the airway. The paratracheal lymph nodes lie on either side of the length of the trachea in a posterolateral distribution. The right paratracheal lymphatic drainage is most easily accessed at one or two tracheal rings above the main carina before the bifurcation on the right posterolateral aspect (Fig. 4.1). The subcarinal mediastinal lymph nodes normally lie immediately inferior to the main carina. This chain can be most easily sampled not by direct aspiration of the main carina itself, but by entry with a transbronchial needle 3–5 mm below on either side of the main carina with a lateral to inferomedial entry (Fig. 4.2). This minimizes having to pass through the cartilaginous element itself. Hilar lymph nodes may be sampled at either the secondary carina, where the right upper lobe bifurcates from the bronchus intermedius, or at the level of the secondary carina, where the left upper lobe bifurcates from the left main stem bronchus (Fig. 4.3). The right pulmonary artery is in close association with the anterior wall of the right upper lobe bronchus; therefore, TBNA and other procedures are not recommended at this site (Figs 4.4, 4.5).

The left paratracheal lymph nodes are located at the origin of the left main stem bronchus from the main trachea (Fig. 4.6). This chain is particularly difficult to sample; however, aspiration can be performed by using a transbronchial needle anchored to the lateral tracheal wall of the distal trachea at the level of the carina with a subsequent downward or inferior movement of the entire bronchoscope, hence facilitating entry of the needle laterally. Figure 4.7 illustrates the association of left upper lobe bronchus and the left pulmonary artery. Figure 4.8 illustrates the location of left hilar lymph nodes.

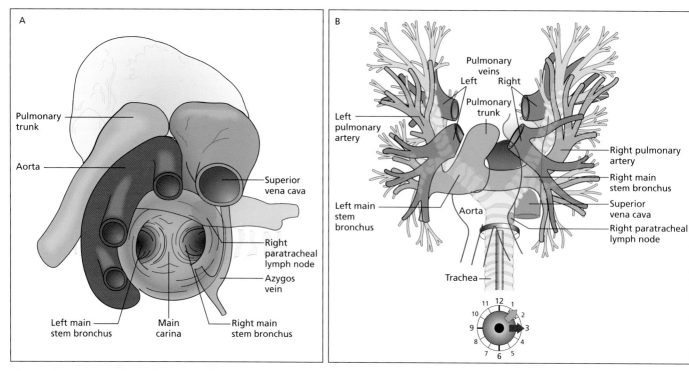

**Fig. 4.1** Representation of normal anatomic relationships at the level of the distal trachea. **(A)** The endoscopic view of the distal trachea, with adjacent vessels and lymph nodes superimposed. The right paratracheal lymph node is between the one and two o'clock position, whereas the azygos vein is located at the three o'clock position. **(B)** An endoscopic clock-face view. The arrow between one and two o'clock indicates the proper site for TBNA of the right paratracheal lymph node. The arrow at three o'clock indicates the unsafe location for aspiration (azygos vein).

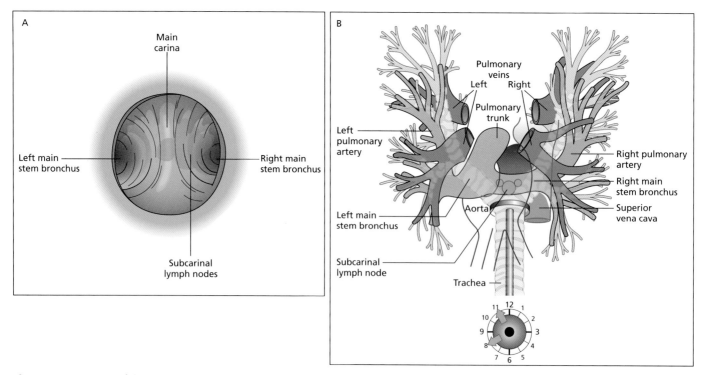

**Fig. 4.2** Representation of the normal anatomic relationships at the level of the main carina. **(A)** The endoscopic view of the main carina, with surrounding lymph nodes superimposed. **(B)** An endoscopic clock-face view at the right main stem bronchus orifice. The arrows at the eight and eleven o'clock positions indicate the proper site for TBNA of subcarinal lymph nodes.

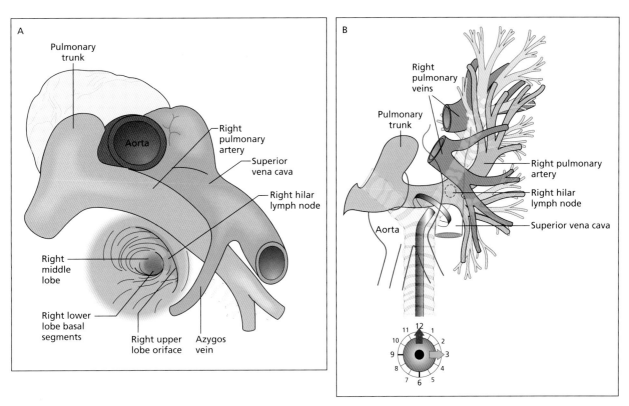

**Fig. 4.3** Representation of normal anatomic relationships at the level of the proximal bronchus intermedius. **(A)** The endoscopic view of the bronchus intermedius, with vessels and lymph nodes superimposed. **(B)** An endoscopic clock-face view. The arrow at three o'clock indicates the proper site for TBNA of the right hilar lymph node. The arrow at twelve o'clock indicates the unsafe location for TBNA (right pulmonary artery).

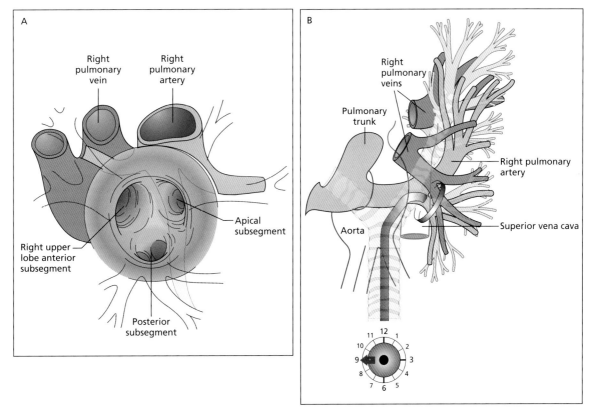

**Fig. 4.4** Representation of normal anatomic relationships at the level of the right upper lobe orifice. **(A)** The endoscopic view of the right upper lobe orifice, with surrounding vessels and lymph nodes superimposed. **(B)** An endoscopic clock-face view. The arrow indicates the location of the right pulmonary artery.

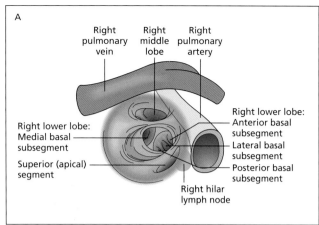

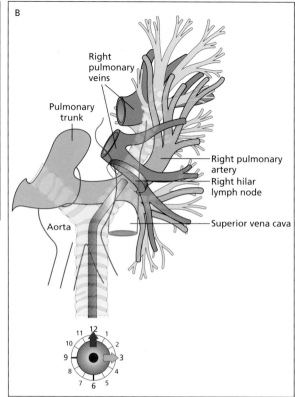

**Fig. 4.5** Representation of normal anatomic relationships at the level of the distal bronchus intermedius. Note the relationship of the right middle lobe bronchus with surrounding vascular structures. **(A)** The endoscopic view of the bronchus intermedius with hilar lymph node superimposed at the three o'clock position. **(B)** An endoscopic clock-face view. The arrow at three o'clock indicates the proper site for TBNA of right hilar lymph node. The arrow at twelve o'clock indicates the unsafe location (right pulmonary vein).

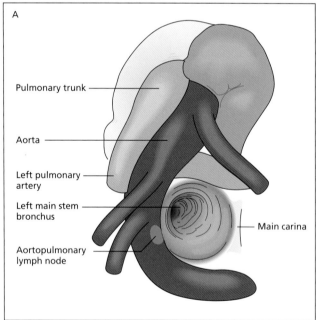

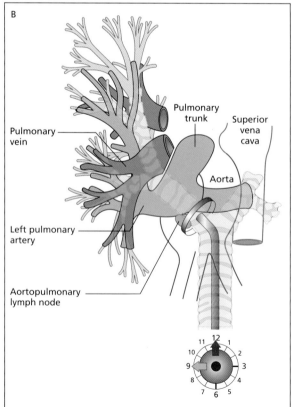

**Fig. 4.6** Representation of normal anatomic relationships at the level of the left main stem bronchus orifice. **(A)** The endoscopic view of the left main stem bronchus, with vessels and the aortopulmonary lymph node superimposed at the nine o'clock position. **(B)** An endoscopic clock-face view. The arrow at nine o'clock indicates the proper site for TBNA of aortopulmonary lymph node below the aortic knob. The arrow at twelve o'clock indicates the unsafe location (left pulmonary artery).

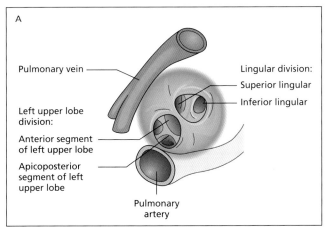

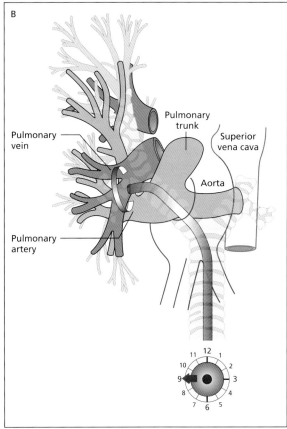

**Fig. 4.7** Representation of normal anatomic relationships at the level of the left upper lobe orifice. **(A)** The endoscopic view of the left upper lobe bronchus, with vessels superimposed. **(B)** An endoscopic clock-face view. The arrow at nine o'clock indicates the location of the left pulmonary artery.

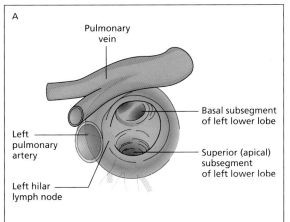

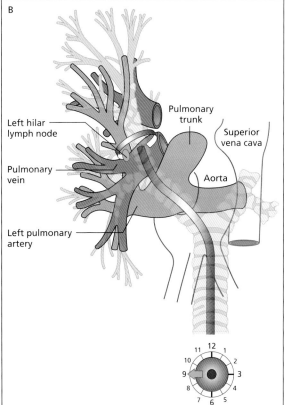

**Fig. 4.8** Representation of normal anatomic relationships at the level of the left lower lobe orifice. **(A)** The endoscopic view of the distal left main stem bronchus, with the left hilar lymph node at the nine o'clock position and vessels superimposed. **(B)** An endoscopic clock-face view. The arrow indicates the proper site for TBNA of the left hilar lymph node.

## References

1 Ovassapian A. Anatomy of the airway. In: Ovassapian A, ed. *Fiberoptic Airway Endoscopy in Anesthesia and Critical Care.* New York: Raven Press; 1990: 15–25.

2 Peter LG, Sasaki CT. Laryngeal anatomy and physiology. In: Heffuer JE, ed. *Clinics in Chest Medicine: Airway Management in the Critically Ill Patient.* Philadelphia: W. B. Saunders; 1991: 415–23.

3 Stradling P. *Diagnostic Bronchoscopy,* 4th edn. Edinburgh: Churchill Livingstone; 1981: 34–59.

4 Ikeda S. *Atlas of Flexible Bronchofiberscopy.* Baltimore and London: University Park Press; 1974.

5 Zavala DC. *Flexible Fiberoptic Bronchoscopy: A Training Handbook.* Iowa City: Iowa University Press; 1978.

6 Boyden EA. Developmental anomalies of the lung. *Am J Surg* 1955; **89**: 78–89.

7 Mehta AC, Ahmad M, Golish JA, Buonocore E. Congenital anomalies of the lung in the adult. *Cleve Clin Q* 1983; **50**: 401–16.

8 Durnon JF, Merlc B. *Handbook of Endobronchial Laser Surgery.* Marseilles, France: Salvator Hospital Publication; 1983: 7–22.

9 Mehta AC, Kavuru MS, Meeker DP, *et al.* Transbronchial needle aspiration for histology specimens. *Chest* 1989; **96**: 1228–32.

10 Mountain CF. Revisions in international system for staging lung cancer. *Chest* 1997; **111**: 1710–17.

# 5

# Anesthesia for Flexible Fiberoptic Bronchoscopy

## Mario Gomez[1] and Gerard A. Silvestri[2]

[1]Pulmonary and Sleep Center, West Laco, Texas, TX, USA
[2]Department of Internal Medicine, Medical University of South Carolina, Charleston, SC, USA

## Introduction

Flexible fiberoptic bronchoscopy is a technique that allows direct visualization of the tracheobronchial tree for diagnostic and therapeutic purposes. In the United States, over 500,000 flexible bronchoscopies are performed each year [1]. Although some authors [2–6] have suggested that sedation is not required for bronchoscopy, most guidelines in the United States [7] and Europe [8] endorse the use of sedation and topical anesthesia during flexible bronchoscopy. Sedative medications decrease patient anxiety, pain, oropharyngeal irritation, cough, and chest discomfort, thus increasing patients' ability to tolerate the procedure [9]. Several studies have demonstrated that sedation increases patient comfort and willingness to undergo future bronchoscopies [10–13]. In addition, with the increasing complexity and duration of bronchoscopic techniques (stenting, electrosurgery, balloon dilatation, endobronchial ultrasound), sedation improves the ability to obtain diagnostic and therapeutic results without interruption. The choice and dose of a sedative agent depends on patient characteristics that include age, medical comorbidities, concomitant medications, drug allergies; and the preference of the bronchoscopist. This chapter will review the pharmacologic properties of the most frequently used and newer agents that are under investigation or have recently become available for use, and will summarize the evidence supporting their use in flexible bronchoscopy.

## Patient evaluation and preparation

Prior to undergoing flexible bronchoscopy, the bronchoscopist should evaluate the patient and review the medical record, including current medications and drug allergies. Medical conditions such as chronic obstructive pulmonary disease, obstructive sleep apnea, congestive heart failure (CHF), renal insufficiency, liver cirrhosis, stroke, or neuromuscular disease may impact the optimal type and depth of sedation to be provided. A physical examination with emphasis on the airway, including assessment of the Mallampati score (Fig. 5.1), cardiac, pulmonary, and central nervous system should be performed. In addition, the physician should inquire about previous adverse experience with sedation-analgesia as well as regional and general anesthesia. Also, the physician must confirm that the patient has had an appropriate fasting period prior to sedation. The American Society of Anesthesiologists (ASA) Guidelines [14] recommend a fasting period of 2 hours for clear liquids (water, fruit juice without pulp, tea, or coffee), 4 hours for human breast milk, 6 hours for formula, non-human milk, or a light meal (toast and clear liquids), and 8 hours for a full meal (fried or fatty food or meat). Patients with a full stomach are at risk for vomiting and aspiration. If inadequate fasting is identified the procedure should be delayed; however, if bronchoscopy is deemed to be an emergency, the patient should be intubated for airway protection.

## Sedation for flexible fiberoptic bronchoscopy

Sedation and analgesia comprise a continuum of states ranging from minimal sedation (anxiolysis) through general anesthesia. Definitions of levels of sedation-analgesia, as developed and adopted by the ASA, are provided in Table 5.1 [15]. Because flexible bronchoscopy generally takes place in a procedure room and not an operating theater, moderate sedation (frequently called "conscious sedation"), is the goal level of sedation most frequently desired. However, staff should be aware that at times patients can slip into deep sedation.

*Flexible Bronchoscopy*, Third Edition. Edited by Ko-Pen Wang, Atul C. Mehta, J. Francis Turner.
© 2012 Blackwell Publishing Ltd. Published 2012 by Blackwell Publishing Ltd.

**Table 5.1** Continuum of depth of sedation: definition of general anesthesia and levels of sedation and analgesia

|  | Minimal sedation (anxiolysis) | Moderate sedation/ analgesia (conscious sedation) | Deep sedation/ analgesia | General anesthesia |
|---|---|---|---|---|
| Responsiveness | Normal response to verbal stimulation | Purposeful response to verbal or tactile stimulation | Purposeful response following repeated or painful stimulation | Unarousable even with painful stimulus |
| Airway | Unaffected | No intervention required | Intervention may be required | Intervention often required |
| Spontaneous ventilation | Unaffected | Adequate | May be inadequate | Frequently inadequate |
| Cardiovascular function | Unaffected | Usually maintained | Usually maintained | May be impaired |

Extracted from: *Continuum of Depth of Sedation Definition of General Anesthesia and Levels of Sedation and Analgesia*, American Society of Anesthesiologists, 1999. Reprinted with permission of the American Society of Anesthesiologists, 520 N Northwest Highway, Park Ridge, IL 60068-2573.

**Table 5.2** Pharmacokinetic properties of midazolam, lorazepam, fentanyl, meperidine, and propofol

| Parameter | Midazolam | Lorazepam | Fentanyl | Meperidine | Propofol |
|---|---|---|---|---|---|
| Onset of action (intravenous) | 1–2.5 min | 15–20 min | 1–2 min | 5 min | <2 min |
| Duration of action | 30–80 min | 20–30 min | 1–2 hour | 2–4 hour | 10–15 min |
| Protein binding (%) | 95–97 | 85–91 | 80–86 | 60–80 | 97–99 |
| Metabolism | Hepatic (oxidation, conjugation) | Hepatic (conjugation) | Hepatic (oxidative N-dealkylation) | Hepatic (demethylation, hydroxylation) | Hepatic (hydroxylation, conjugation) |
| Volume of distribution (L/kg) | 1–3.1 | 0.8–2.0 | 2.9–8 | 3.7–4.6 | 4.5 (±2.1) |
| Total body clearance (L/h/kg) | 0.25–0.54 | 0.0046–0.0055 | 0.72–0.78 | 0.41–0.66 | 1.1–2.11 |
| Renal excretion (%) | 45–57 | 88 | <5 | <5 | >1 |

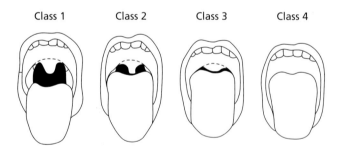

Class 1    Class 2    Class 3    Class 4

**Fig. 5.1** Mallampati score. Class 1, faucial pillars, soft palate and uvula visualized. Class 2, faucial pillars and soft palate visualized, but uvula masked by the base of the tongue. Class 3, only soft palate visualized. Class 4, soft palate not seen.

Moderate sedation is defined as a drug-induced depression of consciousness during which patients remain able to respond purposefully to verbal commands either alone or when accompanied by light tactile stimulation. It is important to note that spontaneous ventilation remains adequate and the patient requires no interventions to maintain a patent airway. In addition, the patient's cardiovascular status remains stable.

An ideal sedation agent should be easy to use and have a rapid onset, short duration of action, and quick recovery with a rapid return of cognition. The drug should also have a predictable pharmacokinetic and pharmacodynamic profile, analgesic and amnestic properties, and lack of respiratory depressant effects. The most commonly used agents include benzodiazepines [16,17], opioids, and to a lesser degree propofol. These sedatives have some of these ideal properties, but each has limitations which will be reviewed in this chapter. A summary of the pharmacokinetic properties of the most frequently used sedatives is provided in Table 5.2.

### Benzodiazepines

Benzodiazepines are frequently used to provide anterograde amnesia, relieve patient anxiety, and induce sedation. Their effect is mediated by the modulation of the gamma-aminobutyric acid (GABA) receptor. The two most commonly used benzodiazepines are midazolam and lorazepam.

Midazolam is water-soluble, highly lipophilic, and has a rapid distribution into the central nervous system (CNS) and adipose tissue, resulting in rapid onset of action (1–2.5 minutes) with an elimination half-life of 1 hour [18]. It is reported to be two to six times as potent as diazepam and it more reliably provides amnesia. In addition, the rapid redistribution of the drug from the brain to peripheral tissues produces a rapid recovery [19]. However, in patients with decreased renal clearance and/or when drug accumulates in adipose tissue prolonged sedation may occur. In adults, incremental doses of midazolam to a total of 1–3 mg are generally adequate to achieve patient comfort, amnesia, and tranquility. Large doses (0.15 mg/kg) may cause alveolar hypoventilation secondary to central respiratory depression and to a decrease in hypoxic respiratory drive.

On the other hand, lorazepam has lower lipophilicity and a slower onset of action (15–20 minutes) and a longer elimination half-life (10–20 hours) [18]. Additionally, intravenous diazepam provides a rapid onset of action but has a prolonged elimination half time (21–37 hours). Because diazepam is not soluble in water (it is dissolved in propylene glycol), it is associated with pain and inflammation at the injection site. For these reasons, it is less frequently used for sedation in bronchoscopy.

## Opioids

Opioids have sedative and analgesic properties. The most frequently used agents are fentanyl and meperidine. Morphine sulfate is the least commonly used opioid. Because of a synergistic effect, these agents are often used in combination with a benzodiazepine for sedation.

Fentanyl is a semisynthetic μ-opioid receptor antagonist that is 80 to 100 times as potent as morphine and highly lipid soluble. It has a rapid onset (1–2 minutes) and a short duration of action (1–2 hours). It produces dose-dependent analgesia, coupled with dose-dependent respiratory depression and sedation [18]. Furthermore, during bronchoscopy, fentanyl helps blunt airway reflexes and suppress coughing. Additionally, fentanyl is not associated with histamine release, an effect seen with meperidine or morphine, that may produce itching, hypotension, or bronchospasm [20]. Compared with fentanyl, meperidine is less potent, has a slower onset of action (5 minutes) and a longer duration of action (2–4 hours). Morphine sulfate has an onset of action similar to fentanyl (2–3 minutes) but a longer half-life (2–4 hours). Drug and metabolite accumulation can occur in patients with hepatic and renal insufficiency.

## Propofol

Propofol is a phenolic derivative structurally unrelated to other sedatives. It is a highly lipophilic compound that is formulated in a soybean, egg phosphatide, and glycerol emulsion. Propofol possesses sedative, amnestic, and analgesic effects. It exerts its anesthetic activity through GABA-mediated interactions. Because of its high lipophilicity it penetrates rapidly into the CNS, producing a rapid onset of action (<2 minutes), followed by a rapid redistribution and metabolic clearance from plasma, giving a rapid recovery time (10–15 minutes) [21].

## Clinical studies

Studies of benzodiazepines in patients undergoing flexible bronchoscopy have shown improved patient satisfaction [11] with minor side effects. The anterograde amnestic effect of benzodiazepines was demonstrated in a double-blind, placebo-controlled trial of oral lorazepam as premedication for bronchoscopy [12]. In the immediate postprocedure period, there was no difference in patient perception between the groups treated with lorazepam versus placebo. However, 24 hours after, those treated with lorazepam reported with lower frequency that the technique was difficult, and that they would be less reluctant to undergo a repeated bronchoscopy.

Comparative trials evaluating recovery time among patients receiving short-acting versus long-acting benzodiazepines have produced conflicting results. Driessen et al. [22] randomized patients between diazepam 10 mg and midazolam 15 mg orally prior flexible bronchoscopy. Patients receiving midazolam performed significantly better than those receiving diazepam on a psychomotor test performed 4 hours postprocedure. However, Korttila and colleagues [23] found that high-dose midazolam was associated with a longer time to recovery as assessed by the ability to stand steadily and walk along a straight line. Interestingly, they found no difference in psychomotor assessments, suggesting that midazolam offers no advantage over diazepam in terms of speed of recovery of psychomotor function.

Benzodiazepines are often combined with opioids for bronchoscopy given the sedative and amnestic properties of benzodiazepines, and the analgesic and antitussive properties of opioids. Despite this common practice, there are few studies comparing this approach to single-agent regimens. Greig et al [24] conducted a randomized, double-blind trial of 103 patients undergoing flexible bronchoscopy, evaluating sedation with midazolam versus alfentanyl versus the combination of the two. The study found less cough in the alfentanyl group and fewer supplemental lidocaine requirements in the alfentanyl and combination groups. No differences in discomfort scores were noted between the groups. More oxyhemoglobin desaturations were noted in the combination group. Another randomized, double-blind trial [25] compared sedation with the combination of midazolam and intravenous hydrocodone to midazolam and placebo. The perception of cough by the bronchoscopist and nursing staff was less in the midazolam and hydrocodone groups. Patient-rated discomfort was lower in the combination group. No differences in oxyhemoglobin desaturation were observed. A non-statistically significant trend toward a decrease in the requirement for supplemental lidocaine was seen in the combination group. In a randomized, double-blind trial of 69 patients undergoing bronchoscopy, there was no difference between midazolam and alfentanyl in postprocedure patient tolerance or discomfort, ease of procedure, or oxygen saturation [26]. Alfentanyl was associated with less cough, while patients given midazolam reported less discomfort when asked about the test 24 hours later [26].

Propofol is an effective sedative in patients undergoing flexible bronchoscopy [27–30]. In a randomized study comparing propofol with midazolam in 41 asthmatics undergoing outpatient flexible bronchoscopy, time to induction of sedation was significantly shorter in the propofol group (125 seconds versus 179 seconds; $P < 0.001$), as well as recovery time assessed by time to recall name and date of birth (2.3 minutes versus 6.3 minutes; $P < 0.0045$) and by Digital Symbol Substitution Test (DSST) scores. However, requirements for local anesthesia and investigator-rated patient tolerance were similar between groups [27]. In another study, computer-controlled infusion of propofol was compared with incremental doses of intravenous midazolam in 42 patients undergoing bronchoscopy [28]. Time to sedation and procedure duration were not significantly different, and both regimens produced similar patient and investigator satisfaction [28]. However, time to recovery was significantly shorter in patients receiving propofol compared with those in the midazolam group (5 minutes versus 10 minutes; $P < 0.01$), as assessed by psychomotor tests [28].

A summary of the randomized trials evaluating sedative regimens in patients undergoing flexible bronchoscopy is presented in Table 5.3.

**Table 5.3** Summary of randomized trials evaluating sedative regimens in patients undergoing bronchoscopy

| Study | No. of patients | Study design | Regimen | Patient assessment | Investigator assessment | Recovery | Cardiopulmonary safety |
|---|---|---|---|---|---|---|---|
| *Single-agent studies* | | | | | | | |
| Benzodiazepines | | | | | | | |
| Maltais *et al.* 1996 [12] | 100 | r, db, pc | LOR 1–2 mg po vs. PLA | LOR > PLA | NS | NR | NS |
| Driessen *et al.* 1982 [22] | 40 | r, db | MID 10 mg po vs. DZ 15 mg po | MID > DIAZ | NS | MID > DZ | NR |
| Korttila *et al.* 1985 [23] | 76 | r, db | MID 0.05 mg/kg iv vs. MID 0.1 mg/kg iv vs DZ 0.3 mg/kg iv | NS | NR | DZ > MID 0.1 mg/kg | NS |
| Opioids | | | | | | | |
| Houghton *et al.* 2005 [26] | 69 | r, db | ALF 0.5–1.0 mg iv titrated vs. MID 2.5–5 mg titrated | MID > ALF (at 24 h) | NS | NR | NS |
| Watts *et al.* 2005 [33] | 50 (elderly) | r, db, pc | ALF 250–500 μg iv vs. TEM 10 mg po + neb LIDO | TEM/ LIDO > ALF | NR | NR | NS |
| Propofol | | | | | | | |
| Randell *et al.* 1992 [30] | 30 | r, sb | PRO 1 mg/kg/h iv vs. FEN 1 μg/kg iv + DZ 0.05 mg/kg iv | NR | NR | NS | FEN/DZ: respiratory frequency ↓ vs. PRO |
| Clarkson *et al.* 1993 [27] | 41 | r, sb | PRO iv titrated vs. MID iv titrated | NR | NS | PRO > MID | NS |
| Crawford *et al.* 1993 [28] | 42 | r, db | PRO TCI vs. MID iv titrated | NS | NS | PRO > MID | NS |

*Continued*

**Table 5.3** *Continued*

| Study | No. of patients | Study design | Regimen | Patient assessment | Investigator assessment | Recovery | Cardiopulmonary safety |
|---|---|---|---|---|---|---|---|
| Fospropofol | | | | | | | |
| Silvestri *et al.* 2009 [39] | 252 | r, db | FOS 6.5 mg/kg iv vs. FOS 2.5 mg/kg iv | FOS 6.5 mg/ kg > 2.5 mg/kg | FOS 6.5 mg/ kg > 2.5 mg/ kg | FOS 6.5 mg/ kg > 2.5 mg/ kg | FOS 6.5 mg/kg: more desaturation vs. 2.5 mg/kg |
| *Combination studies* | | | | | | | |
| Benzodiazepine-based combinations | | | | | | | |
| Greig *et al.* 1995 [24] | 103 | r, db, pc | MID iv titrated vs. ALF iv titrated vs. MID + ALF titrated | NS | NS | NS | MID + ALF: more desaturation vs. ALF |
| Stolz *et al.* 2004 [25] | 120 | r, db, pc | MID iv titrated + HC 5 mg iv vs. MID iv titrated | MID/ HC > MID* | MID/ HC > MIC* | NR | NS |
| Propofol-based combinations | | | | | | | |
| Kestin *et al.* 1989 [34] | 46 | r, db | PRO 6–10 mg/kg/h iv + ALF 10 µg/kg vs. PRO 6–10 mg/kg/h iv + PLA | NR | NR | NS | PRO/ALF: ABP ↓ *vs* PRO/PLA |
| Voyagis *et al.* 2000 [68] | 40 | r | PRO 2 mg/kg iv + REMI 1 µg/kg vs. PRO 2 mg/ kg + FEN 3 µg/kg | NR | NR | NR | PRO/REMI: ABP ↓ vs. PRO/FEN |
| Hwang *et al.* 2005 [69] | 276 | r, db | PRO/ALF PCI vs. PRO/ KET PCI | PRO/ KET > PRO/ALF | NS | NS | PRO/ALF: SBP ↓ vs. PRO/KET |

>indicates a statistically significantly superior effect; ABP, arterial blood pressure; ALF, alfentanyl; db, double-blind; DZ, diazepam; FEN, fentanyl; FOS, fospropofol; HC, hydrocodone; iv, intravenous; KET, ketamine; LIDO, lidocaine; LOR, lorazepam; MID, midazolam; neb, nebulized; NR, not reported; NS, no significant difference; pc, placebo-controlled; PCI, patient-controlled infusion; PLA, placebo; po, oral; PRO, propofol; r, randomized; REMI, remifentanil; sb, single-blind; SBP, systolic arterial pressure; TCI, target-controlled infusion; TEM, temazepam.

*As assessed for perception of cough.

Adapted and updated from Vincent BD, *et al.* An update on sedation and analgesia during flexible bronchoscopy. *J Bronchol* 2007; **14**: 173–80, with permission [70].

## Safety and limitations

Benzodiazepines can produce cardiopulmonary depression. Though low to moderate doses of midazolam (i.e. <5 mg) do not appear to increase the risk of hypoxemia during flexible bronchoscopy, hypoxemia can occur with or without sedation [31]. Another potential disadvantage of benzodiazepines is a prolonged effect with repeat dosing due to drug accumulation in adipose tissue [18].

Opioids may cause respiratory depression, however, most comparisons of single-agent regimens have not demonstrated a significant difference in hypoxemia between opioids and benzodiazepines [24,26,32,33]. The risk of hypoxemia is increased when opioids are combined with

other sedatives. Also, opioids blunt cardiovascular responses of hypertension and tachycardia during mechanical stimulation of laryngeal and tracheal tissues and may cause hypotension [34].

Propofol may produce cardiopulmonary depression, leading to hypoxemia and hypotension, as well as injection site pain, and the risk of microbial contamination of the emulsion formulation [21,35]. The cardiopulmonary effects of propofol are generally dose dependent and are enhanced when combined with opioids [21,34,36]. Clinical studies comparing propofol and midazolam in bronchoscopy found no differences in either oxyhemoglobin desaturation or hemodynamic parameters [27,28]. Furthermore, one study showed that propofol was associated with less respiratory depression compared with a combination of fentanyl and diazepam, however, there was no significant difference between groups for oxyhemoglobin desaturation [30].

## New sedative agents

Fospropofol is a new agent with a promising therapeutic profile which may become available for use during bronchoscopy. It is a water-soluble prodrug of propofol with pharmacokinetic and pharmacodynamic properties that are different from the propofol emulsion. After intravenous administration, propofol is released from fospropofol by tissue alkaline phosphatases with a predictable rise and decline in plasma concentrations of propofol, and resultant lower peak concentrations and a more gradual decline in propofol concentrations compared to standard propofol injection [37,38].

Silvestri and colleagues [39] conducted a double-blind, randomized control trial evaluating the use of fospropofol in 252 patients undergoing flexible bronchoscopy. Patients were randomized to receive either 2 mg/kg or 6.5 mg/kg of fosfopropofol in addition to 50 μg of fentanyl and topical lidocaine. The primary end point was sedation success defined as three consecutive Modified Observer's Assessment of Alertness/ Sedation scores of equal to or less than 4, plus procedure completion without alternative sedative medication and/or mechanical/ manual ventilation. Sedation success rates were higher in the 6.5 mg/kg group than in the 2 mg/kg group (88.7 versus 27.5%, respectively; $P < 0.0001$). Fospropofol sedation at a dose of 6.5 mg/kg was associated with a higher frequency of hypoxemia compared to 2 mg/kg (15.4 versus 12.6%, respectively). Hypotension occurred in eight patients in the 6.5 mg/kg group. Other adverse events seen were transient and self-limited paresthesias and pruritus of mild-to-moderate severity. This study demonstrates that fospropofol provides safe and effective sedation for patients undergoing flexible bronchoscopy. Nevertheless, no trials comparing fospropofol and the combination of midazolam and fentanyl have been conducted yet.

A second new agent, dexmedetomidine, is a lipophilic α-2 agonist which causes sedation as a result of its action on the locus caeruleus. This produces a unique profile, as patients remain arousable despite being sedated with minimal respiratory depression. This profile makes the drug appealing for sedation of patients with pulmonary compromise undergoing bronchoscopy. In 2007, Abouzgheib et al. [40] conducted a prospective pilot study of the use of dexmedetomidine in 10 patients with severe COPD undergoing bronchoscopy. No patient exhibited marked hemodynamic changes, apnea, or oxygen desaturation during the procedure or recovery. More study is needed in a larger population of patients to confirm these findings. Furthermore, randomized trials comparing dexmedetomidine with conventional conscious sedation have not been conducted.

Other short-acting sedative agents that have been studied in flexible bronchoscopy but are not frequently used in clinical practice include ketamine [41] and chloral hydrate [42].

## Local anesthesia

Flexible bronchoscopy induces stimulation of the cough reflex, which may not be well tolerated by patients, who frequently try to expel the bronchoscope from the airways. Sedative agents alone will not produce blunting of the cough and other airway reflexes. For this reason, efficacious local anesthesia of the airway is necessary for an adequate examination.

Topical anesthetics are classified into two groups, the amides (lidocaine, prilocaine, mepivacaine, and bupivacaine) and the esters (tetracaine, benzocaine, and procaine). These agents inhibit the transfer of sensory signals from the periphery to the CNS by inhibiting sodium channels in the nerve membrane.

Topical lidocaine is the most commonly used topical anesthetic agent in flexible bronchoscopy. The drug can be delivered to the upper airway by several methods and in various preparations. Nasal anesthesia may be achieved with the application of 2% viscous lidocaine for the nasal mucosa. Oropharyngeal and laryngeal anesthesia may be obtained with nebulized 4% topical lidocaine, or injecting 1% lidocaine solution through the bronchoscopy channel directly onto the vocal cords. Lower airway anesthesia can also be induced by injecting 1% lidocaine onto the airway mucosa with the "spray as you go" technique.

Lidocaine is absorbed into the airways after topical application and metabolized by the liver into its active metabolites. The rate of lidocaine absorption varies, depending on the area of the respiratory tract and method of application. Application of lidocaine to the upper airway results in much lower blood concentrations compared with application to the lower airway, as the upper respiratory tract has a smaller surface area and less extensive vascularization than the lower tract. The effect is usually seen 2 to 5 minutes after application to the mucous membranes. The peak plasma concentration is reached 40 to 90 minutes after nasopharyngeal application and 5 to 30 minutes when applied to the larynx or trachea. The expected duration of action is 1 hour. The drug's elimination half-life is 90 minutes. A direct correlation exists between lidocaine's blood concentration and pharmacologic effect or toxicity. As lidocaine is almost exclusively metabolized by the liver, chronic liver disease patients can have an increase in the half-life of the drug to 300 minutes. In addition, clearance is decreased in patients with CHF because of decreased cardiac output, and empiric dosage reductions may be necessary in these patients.

The majority of lidocaine-related adverse effects involve the CNS and the cardiovascular system [43]. At low blood concentrations from 1 to 5 μg/mL the most common symptoms include drowsiness, euphoria, tingling of lips, ringing in the ears, a bitter taste in the mouth, and chills. Blood concentrations from 8 to 12 μg/mL may be associated with low speech, jerky tremors, and hallucinations, which may be followed by seizures. With very high blood concentrations from 20 to 25 μg/mL, toxic cardiorespiratory arrest may occur [44,45].

The efficacy of nebulized lidocaine to achieve airway anesthesia has come into question. Stolz and colleagues [46] randomized 150 patients to receive lidocaine or placebo via nebulization. There was no significant difference between the two groups in terms of cough score, hemodynamic parameters, discomfort, midazolam dose for additional sedation, or amount of supplemental lidocaine used. Further, the mean total lidocaine dose required in the lidocaine group was significantly higher compared to the placebo group. The authors concluded that the addition of nebulized lidocaine for airway anesthesia before initiating flexible bronchoscopy offered no benefit when bronchoscopy is performed using combined sedation with midazolam and hydrocodone.

The optimal concentration of topical lidocaine to achieve an acceptable level of satisfaction to the patient and the bronchoscopist has not been established. Mainland *et al.* [47] used various concentrations (1, 1.5, and 2%) and volumes of lidocaine to anesthetize the airways during bronchoscopy to determine the lowest dosage for effective airway anesthesia; however, it was found that all dosages compared in the study were equally effective in producing airway anesthesia. The effectiveness of anesthesia was measured by the number of patients with sustained coughing lasting longer than 5 seconds during bronchoscopy. Hasmoni and colleagues [48] conducted a prospective, double-blind, randomized-control trial, where patients were randomized to receive either lidocaine 1 or 2% for local anesthesia. They reported no difference in the mean number of coughs and perceived satisfaction for patients and bronchoscopists between the two groups. Not surprisingly, the authors found that the median total dose of lidocaine received in the 1% group was nearly half of that in the 2% group.

The maximum amount of topical lidocaine used for airway anesthesia during flexible bronchoscopy remains an ongoing question [49]. The National Institutes of Health (NIH) published guidelines in 1985 recommending a maximum cumulative lidocaine dose of 400 mg for asthmatic patients undergoing bronchoscopy [50]. Subsequent guidelines published in 1991 only indicated minimizing the dose to avoid potential toxicity [51]. Despite this published guidelines, apprehension was justifiably raised in 1996 when a 19-year-old healthy volunteer died from lidocaine toxicity after undergoing a research flexible bronchoscopy [52]. In 2000, Langmack *et al.* [45] reported that an average total dose of 600 mg (8.2 mg/kg) of lidocaine seems to be safe in mild-to-moderate asthmatics undergoing research bron-

choscopy. In 2001, the British Thoracic Society recommended a maximum dosage of 8.2 mg/kg in their guidelines (approximately 29 mL of a 2% solution and 58 mL of a 1% solution for a 70-kg patient) based primarily in this study [53]. Nevertheless, other studies have demonstrated the safety of lidocaine in much higher doses. In 2008, Frey and colleagues [49] evaluated serum lidocaine and methemoglobin levels in 154 patients who received airway anesthesia with 4% nebulized lidocaine, 2% viscous lidocaine for the nares, and as needed 1% lidocaine during bronchoscopy. The authors found a mean topical lidocaine dose of 15.4 mg/kg and a mean serum lidocaine levels of 1.55 ± 0.67 μg/mL without evidence of elevated methemoglobin levels or clinical toxicity. These results confirmed previous findings from smaller studies concluding higher topical lidocaine doses did not commonly lead to elevated serum lidocaine levels or clinical toxicity [54–58]. Although the recommended dose of lidocaine has been increasing, the patient should be monitored carefully for toxic signs such as CNS toxicity and cardiorespiratory toxicity. In Frey's study, there were no patients with significant CHF or chronic liver disease. As a result, mean serum lidocaine levels were lower than the toxic level. In patients with normal hepatic and cardiac function toxicity is rare, even if their total administered lidocaine doses were higher than 600 mg. However, in patients with CHF and liver disease, a lower dose of lidocaine is recommended. Until clear guidelines are established for doses in patients who require flexible bronchoscopy, precise monitoring is essential to assess and prevent lidocaine toxicity.

## Monitoring and equipment

Although the mortality and morbidity associated with bronchoscopy is low [59] (0.01–0.5%, 0.08–5%, respectively), several deaths and up to half of the major life-threatening complications have been related to the sedative regimen used. The safety of sedation during bronchoscopy depends not only on the agents used but also on the way their effects are monitored and on the facilities and personnel available.

The ASA has published guidelines for sedation and analgesia by non-anesthesiologists [60]. Recommendations include respiratory, hemodynamic, and neurological monitoring. Patient monitoring should be performed by a separate health care professional designated to administer medications and to monitor the patient.

The response of patients to commands serves as a guide to their level of consciousness. Spoken responses also provide an indication that patients are breathing. Patients whose only response is withdrawal from painful stimuli are deeply sedated, approaching a state of general anesthesia, and should be treated accordingly (Table 5.1).

Primary causes of morbidity associated with sedation-analgesia are drug-induced respiratory depression and airway obstruction. Monitoring of ventilatory function by observation and auscultation reduces the risk of adverse outcomes. The use of end-tidal carbon dioxide monitoring during procedural sedation in the emergency department has been shown to be a quicker, more sensitive detector of hypoventilation than pulse oximetry or emergency physician observer assessment [61]. In addition, this technique has been studied in children undergoing flexible bronchoscopy, showing a decrease in end-tidal carbon dioxide and oxygen saturation during the procedure that may be related to airway obstruction by the instrument [62,63]. Further study of end-tidal carbon dioxide monitoring needs to be conducted in adults prior to recommending its routine use.

Pulse oximetry should be employed to monitor oxygenation, as it effectively detects oxyhemoglobin desaturation and hypoxemia. Early detection of hypoxemia during bronchoscopy decreases the likelihood of adverse outcomes such as cardiac arrest and death. The use of supplemental oxygen during moderate sedation reduce the frequency of hypoxemia.

Sedation and analgesia agents can blunt the appropriate autonomic compensation for hypovolemia or procedure-related stress. On the other hand, if sedation and analgesia are inadequate, patients may develop potentially harmful autonomic stress responses such as hypertension or tachycardia. For this reason, heart rate and blood pressure should be measured and recorded every 5 minutes. Additionally, continuous electrocardiography is recommended in patients with heart disease or dysrhythmias.

Appropriately trained personnel should be immediately available for complications such as oversedation and loss of the airway. Resuscitative drugs and equipment must be immediately available, including a backup oxygen tank, airway equipment for bag-mask ventilation and endotracheal intubation, a suction setup, and resuscitative drugs including naloxone or flumazemil when narcotics or benzodiazepines are used. Furthermore, when moderate sedation is administered to patients with cardiovascular disease, a defibrillator should be available. Practitioners are cautioned that acute reversal of opioid- induced analgesia may result in pain, hypertension, tachycardia, or pulmonary edema.

## Sedation in special populations

Pregnant patients and their fetus are at risk of gas exchange impairment, severe cough, and barotrauma (e.g. pneumothorax, pneumomediastinum), during flexible bronchoscopy [64]. Furthermore, sedation agents per se may be teratogenic, or cause deleterious hemodynamic changes on the mother. There are no formal guidelines for bronchoscopy sedation in pregnancy, however, agents with an FDA pregnancy category D or X (e.g. midazolam, diazepam) should be avoided. Continuous cardiac monitoring, pulse oximetry, and blood pressure monitoring during bronchoscopy, with fetal monitoring, if available, should be performed.

Patients with asthma may experience bronchoscopy-induced bronchospasm and temporary decline in lung function and oxyhemoglobin saturation depending on the severity of asthma. However, studies have demonstrated that bronchoscopy with midazolam sedation can be performed safely [65,66]. Nevertheless, continuous and rigorous monitoring is advocated in patients with severe asthma undergoing bronchoscopy.

Elderly patients tend to have age-related decrease in lung function, increased sensitivity to sedatives, and an increase in sedation-related adverse events. They generally require smaller doses of sedative agents because of delayed or decreased drug metabolism, as well as attenuated airway reflexes associated with increasing age [67]. The increased risk should not be a contraindication for bronchoscopy in older persons.

## Conclusions

Sedation during flexible bronchoscopy improves patient comfort, tolerability of the procedure, the ability to obtain adequate specimens, and willingness to undergo future bronchoscopies. Adequate preprocedural evaluation of the patient with a special focus on cardiopulmonary reserve and airway anatomy is a must. Benzodiazepines and opioids are the most frequently used sedation agents. Topical anesthesia with lidocaine may blunt cough and airway reflexes, further improving procedure tolerance. As all sedation agents (alone or in combination) may produce cardiorespiratory depression, patient monitoring is advocated to ensure a safe outcome.

## References

1 Mehta AC, Prakash UB, Garland R, *et al.* American College of Chest Physicians and American Association for Bronchology [corrected] consensus statement: prevention of flexible bronchoscopy-associated infection. *Chest* 2005; **128**: 1742–55.

2 Banerjee A, Banerjee SN, Nachiappan M. Premedication for fibreoptic bronchoscopy (is sedation a must?) *Indian J Chest Dis Allied Sci* 1986; **28**: 76–80.

3 Colt HG, Morris JF. Fiberoptic bronchoscopy without premedication. A retrospective study. *Chest* 1990; **98**: 1327–30.

4 Hatton MQ, Allen MB, Vathenen AS, *et al.* Does sedation help in fibreoptic bronchoscopy? *Br Med J* 1994; **309**: 1206–7.

5 Pearce SJ. Fibreoptic bronchoscopy: is sedation necessary? *Br Med J* 1980; **281**: 779–80.

6 Sutherland FW. Sedation in fibreoptic bronchoscopy. Intravenous sedation is inappropriate in most minor procedures. *Br Med J* 1995; **310**: 872.

7 Green CG, Eisenberg J, Leong A, *et al.* Flexible endoscopy of the pediatric airway. *Am Rev Respir Dis* 1992; **145**: 233–5.

8 Honeybourne D, Babb J, Bowie P, *et al.* British Thoracic Society guidelines on diagnostic flexible bronchoscopy. *Thorax* 2001; **56**: i1–i21.

9 Poi PJ, Chuah SY, Srinivas P, *et al.* Common fears of patients undergoing bronchoscopy. *Eur Respir J* 1998; **11**: 1147–9.

10 Gonzalez R, De-La-Rosa-Ramirez I, Maldonado-Hernandez A, *et al.* Should patients undergoing a bronchoscopy be sedated? *Acta Anaesthesiol Scand* 2003; **47**: 411–15.

11 Maguire GP, Rubinfeld AR, Trembath PW, *et al.* Patients prefer sedation for fibreoptic bronchoscopy. *Respirology* 1998; **3**: 81–5.

12 Maltais F, Laberge F, Laviolette M. A randomized, double-blind, placebo-controlled study of lorazepam as premedication for bronchoscopy. *Chest* 1996; **109**: 1195–8.

13 Putinati S, Ballerin L, Corbetta L, *et al.* Patient satisfaction with conscious sedation for bronchoscopy. *Chest* 1999; **115**: 1437–40.

14 American Society of Anesthesiologists. Practice guidelines for preoperative fasting and the use of pharmacologic agents to reduce the risk of pulmonary aspiration: application to healthy patients undergoing elective procedures: a report by the American Society of Anesthesiologist Task Force on Preoperative Fasting. *Anesthesiology* 1999; **90**: 896–905.

15 American Society of Anesthesiologists. *Continuum of Depth of Sedation: Definition of General Anesthesia and Levels of Sedation/ Analgesia*, 1999.

16 Pickles J, Jeffrey M, Datta A, *et al.* Is preparation for bronchoscopy optimal? *Eur Respir J* 2003; **22**: 203–6.

17 Prakash UB, Offord KP, Stubbs SE. Bronchoscopy in North America: the ACCP survey. *Chest* 1991; **100**: 1668–75.

18 Horn E, Nesbit SA. Pharmacology and pharmacokinetics of sedatives and analgesics. *Gastrointest Endosc Clin N Am* 2004; **14**: 247–68.

19 Fragen RJ. Pharmacokinetics and pharmacodynamics of midazolam given via continuous intravenous infusion in intensive care units. *Clin Ther* 1997; **19**: 405–19; discussion 367–408.

20 Soifer BE. Procedural anesthesia at the bedside. *Crit Care Clin* 2000; **16**: 7–28.

21 Gan TJ. Pharmacokinetic and pharmacodynamic characteristics of medications used for moderate sedation. *Clin Pharmacokinet* 2006; **45**: 855–69.

22 Driessen JJ, Smets MJ, Goey LS, *et al.* Comparison of diazepam and midazolam as oral premedicants for bronchoscopy under local anesthesia. *Acta Anaesthesiol Belg* 1982; **33**: 99–105.

23 Korttila K, Tarkkanen J. Comparison of diazepam and midazolam for sedation during local anaesthesia for bronchoscopy. *Br J Anaesth* 1985; **57**: 581–6.

24 Greig JH, Cooper SM, Kasimbazi HJ, *et al.* Sedation for fibre optic bronchoscopy. *Respir Med* 1995; **89**: 53–6.

25 Stolz D, Chhajed PN, Leuppi JD, *et al.* Cough suppression during flexible bronchoscopy using combined sedation with midazolam and hydrocodone: a randomised, double blind, placebo controlled trial. *Thorax* 2004; **59**: 773–6.

26 Houghton CM, Raghuram A, Sullivan PJ, *et al.* Pre-medication for bronchoscopy: a randomised double blind trial comparing alfentanil with midazolam. *Respir Med* 2004; **98**: 1102–7.

27 Clarkson K, Power CK, O'Connell F, *et al.* A comparative evaluation of propofol and midazolam as sedative agents in fiberoptic bronchoscopy. *Chest* 1993; **104**: 1029–31.

28 Crawford M, Pollock J, Anderson K, *et al.* Comparison of midazolam with propofol for sedation in outpatient bronchoscopy. *Br J Anaesth* 1993; **70**: 419–22.

29 Erb T, Hammer J, Rutishauser M, *et al.* Fibreoptic bronchoscopy in sedated infants facilitated by an airway endoscopy mask. *Paediatr Anaesth* 1999; **9**: 47–52.

30 Randell T. Sedation for bronchofiberoscopy: comparison between propofol infusion and intravenous boluses of fentanyl and diazepam. *Acta Anaesthesiol Scand* 1992; **36**: 221–5.

31 Jones AM, O'Driscoll R. Do all patients require supplemental oxygen during flexible bronchoscopy? *Chest* 2001; **119**: 1906–9.

32 Papagiannis A, Smith AP. Fentanyl versus midazolam as premedication for fibre optic bronchoscopy. *Respir Med* 1994; **88**: 797–8.

33 Watts MR, Geraghty R, Moore A, *et al.* Premedication for bronchoscopy in older patients: a double-blind comparison of two regimens. *Respir Med* 2005; **99**: 220–6.

34 Kestin IG, Chapman JM, Coates MB. Alfentanil used to supplement propofol infusions for oesophagoscopy and bronchoscopy. *Anaesthesia* 1989; **44**: 994–6.

35 Kanto J, Gepts E. Pharmacokinetic implications for the clinical use of propofol. *Clin Pharmacokinet* 1989; **17**: 308–26.

36 Moerman AT, Struys MM, Vereecke HE, *et al.* Remifentanil used to supplement propofol does not improve quality of sedation during spontaneous respiration. *J Clin Anesth* 2004; **16**: 237–43.

37 Gibiansky E, Struys MM, Gibiansky L, *et al.* AQUAVAN injection, a water-soluble prodrug of propofol, as a bolus injection: a phase I dose-escalation comparison with DIPRIVAN (part 1): pharmacokinetics. *Anesthesiology* 2005; **103**: 718–29.

38 Struys MM, Vanluchene AL, Gibiansky E, *et al.* AQUAVAN injection, a water-soluble prodrug of propofol, as a bolus injection: a phase I dose-escalation comparison with DIPRIVAN (part 2): pharmacodynamics and safety. *Anesthesiology* 2005; **103**: 730–43.

39 Silvestri GA, Vincent BD, Wahidi MM, *et al.* A phase 3, randomized, double-blind study to assess the efficacy and safety of fospropofol disodium injection for moderate sedation in patients undergoing flexible bronchoscopy. *Chest* 2009; **135**: 41–7.

40 Abouzgheib WB, Littman J, Pratter M, Bartter T. Efficacy and safety of dexmedetomidine during bronchoscopy in patients with moderate to severe COPD or emphysema. *J Bronchol* 2007; **14**: 233–6.

41 Berkenbosch JW, Graff GR, Stark JM. Safety and efficacy of ketamine sedation for infant flexible fiberoptic bronchoscopy. *Chest* 2004; **125**: 1132–7.

42 Callahan CW. Chloral hydrate and sleep deprivation for sedation during flexible fiberoptic bronchoscopy. *Pediatr Pulmonol* 1997; **24**: 302.

43 Rademaker AW, Kellen J, Tam YK, *et al.* Character of adverse effects of prophylactic lidocaine in the coronary care unit. *Clin Pharmacol Ther* 1986; **40**: 71–80.

44 DiFazio CA. Local anesthetics: action, metabolism, and toxicity. *Otolaryngol Clin North Am* 1981; **14**: 515–19.

45 Langmack EL, Martin RJ, Pak J, *et al.* Serum lidocaine concentrations in asthmatics undergoing research bronchoscopy. *Chest* 2000; **117**: 1055–60.

46 Stolz D, Chhajed PN, Leuppi J, *et al.* Nebulized lidocaine for flexible bronchoscopy: a randomized, double-blind, placebo-controlled trial. *Chest* 2005; **128**: 1756–60.

47 Mainland PA, Kong AS, Chung DC, *et al.* Absorption of lidocaine during aspiration anesthesia of the airway. *J Clin Anesth* 2001; **13**: 440–6.

48 Hasmoni MH, Abdul M, Harun R, *et al.* Randomized-controlled trial to study the equivalence of 1% versus 2% lignocaine in cough supression and satisfaction during bronchoscopy. *J Bronchol* 2008; **15**: 78–82.

49 Frey WC, Emmons EE, Morris MJ. Safety of high dose lidocaine in flexible bronchoscopy. *J Bronchol* 2008; **15**: 33–7.

50 Anon. National Institutes of Health workshop summary. Summary and recommendations of a workshop on the investigative use of fiberoptic bronchoscopy and bronchoalveolar lavage in individuals with asthma. *J Allergy Clin Immunol* 1985; **76**: 145–7.

51 Anon. Workshop summary and guidelines: investigative use of bronchoscopy, lavage, and bronchial biopsies in asthma and other airway diseases. *J Allergy Clin Immunol* 1991; **88**: 808–14.

52 Day RO, Chalmers DR, Williams KM, *et al.* The death of a healthy volunteer in a human research project: implications for Australian clinical research. *Med J Aust* 1998; **168**: 449–51.

53 British Thoracic Society guidelines on diagnostic flexible bronchoscopy. *Thorax* 2001; **56** (Suppl. 1): i1–21.

54 Ameer B, Burlingame MB, Harman EM. Systemic absorption of topical lidocaine in elderly and young adults undergoing bronchoscopy. *Pharmacotherapy* 1989; **9**: 74–81.

55 Berger R, McConnell JW, Phillips B, *et al.* Safety and efficacy of using high-dose topical and nebulized anesthesia to obtain endobronchial cultures. *Chest* 1989; **95**: 299–303.

56 Efthimiou J, Higenbottam T, Holt D, *et al.* Plasma concentrations of lignocaine during fibreoptic bronchoscopy. *Thorax* 1982; **37**: 68–71.

57 Loukides S, Katsoulis K, Tsarpalis K, *et al.* Serum concentrations of lignocaine before, during and after fiberoptic bronchoscopy. *Respiration* 2000; **67**: 13–17.

58 Sucena M, Cachapuz I, Lombardia E, *et al.* [Plasma concentration of lidocaine during bronchoscopy]. *Rev Port Pneumol* 2004; **10**: 287–96.

59 Shelley MP, Wilson P, Norman J. Sedation for fibreoptic bronchoscopy. *Thorax* 1989; **44**: 769–75.

60 American Society of Anesthesiologists Task Force on Sedation and Analgesia by Non-Anesthesiologists. Practice guidelines for sedation and analgesia by non-anesthesiologists. *Anesthesiology* 2002; **96**: 1004–17.

61 Miner JR, Heegaard W, Plummer D. End-tidal carbon dioxide monitoring during procedural sedation. *Acad Emerg Med* 2002; **9**: 275–80.

62 Franchi LM, Maggi JC, Nussbaum E. Continuous end-tidal CO2 in pediatric bronchoscopy. *Pediatr Pulmonol* 1993; **16**: 153–7.

63 Taher MA, Kamash FA, Al-Momani JA. End-tidal carbon dioxide monitoring during flexible fiberoptic bronchoscopy. *Pak J Med Sci* 2006; **22**: 149–53.

64 Bahhady IJ, Ernst A. Risks of and recommendations for flexible bronchoscopy in pregnancy: a review. *Chest* 2004; **126**: 1974–81.

65 Djukanovic R, Wilson JW, Lai CK, *et al.* The safety aspects of fiberoptic bronchoscopy, bronchoalveolar lavage, and endobronchial biopsy in asthma. *Am Rev Respir Dis* 1991; **143**: 772–7.

66 Humbert M, Robinson DS, Assoufi B, *et al.* Safety of fibreoptic bronchoscopy in asthmatic and control subjects and effect on asthma control over two weeks. *Thorax* 1996; **51**: 664–9.

67 Hehn BT, Haponik E, Rubin HR, *et al.* The relationship between age and process of care and patient tolerance of bronchoscopy. *J Am Geriatr Soc* 2003; **51**: 917–22.

68 Voyagis GS, Dimitriou V. Remifentanil vs. fentanyl during rigid bronchoscopy under general anaesthesia with controlled ventilation. *Eur J Anaesthesiol* 2000; **17**: 404–5.

69 Hwang J, Jeon Y, Park HP, *et al.* Comparison of alfetanil and ketamine in combination with propofol for patient-controlled sedation during fiberoptic bronchoscopy. *Acta Anaesthesiol Scand* 2005; **49**: 1334–8.

70 Vincent BD, Silvestri GA. An update on sedation and analgesia during flexible bronchoscopy. *J Bronchol* 2007; **14**: 173–80.

# 6 Flexible Bronchoscopy Training

**Momen M. Wahidi,[1] Navreet Sandhu Sindhwani,[1] Scott L. Shofer,[1] and Ali I. Musani[2]**

[1] Department of Internal Medicine, Duke University Medical Center, Durham, NC, USA
[2] National Jewish Health Center, Denver, CO, USA

## Introduction

Learning medical procedures is a complex process that relies on the student's ability, teacher's effectiveness, teacher–learner interactions, and the context in which the procedure is performed. In addition to the skills component, learners need to acquire other essential aspects of procedural training including an understanding of indications and contraindications, knowledge of risk and benefit, and appreciation of one's own abilities and limitations. Once proficiency is obtained, continued practice and knowledge update are necessary to ensure mastery of the procedure.

Bronchoscopy is a common procedure with an estimated 500 000 bronchoscopies performed annually in the United States [1]. The majority of these bronchoscopic procedures are performed by pulmonologists, but bronchoscopies are also performed by surgeons, anesthesiologists, and intensivists.

Flexible bronchoscopy training for pulmonologists takes place during a 2 to 3-year fellowship following internal medicine residency. The current method of learning bronchoscopy relies on the traditional apprenticeship model, the so-called "see one, do one, teach one" philosophy.

Graduate medical education has undergone a profound revolution since the initial change brought about by the Flexner report in the late nineteenth century [2]. The Flexner report advocated education that integrated patient care and research, but as research and the acquisition of research funding has gained momentum in academic medical centers and the pressure on educators to produce clinical revenues has grown, education of trainees has suffered due to the "publish or perish" mentality, the long hours spent on patients' care, and, more recently, the limitations imposed by duty hours.

In this chapter, we will discuss the current methods in bronchoscopy education and competency measurement and explore the emerging data on the role of simulation technology in the learning of bronchoscopy.

## Current bronchoscopy training model

There are currently no published guidelines for bronchoscopy training. At present, training is based upon the apprenticeship model where the student learns from the mentor by passive observation, the so-called "see one, do one, teach one" philosophy. In this model, it is assumed that learners can acquire some basic understanding of the procedure by simple observation, then hone their skills by practicing on patients under faculty supervision. No preceding training or assessment of the learners is usually carried out prior to performing the procedures on patients. The advantage of this teaching model is the opportunity for the learner to learn directly from a skilled operator with one-on-one mentoring; however, the disadvantages are abundant, including the lack of consistency in teaching methodology across training centers, subjective evaluation of skill acquisition, and unnecessary and taxing practice on individual patients.

A few studies over the last decade have shed some light on the state of bronchoscopy education. Haponik *et al.* conducted a survey during a "hands-on" bronchoscopy symposium at the 1998 annual meeting of the American College of Chest Physicians in order to obtain a fellows' perspective on bronchoscopy training, and found that the majority of bronchoscopy learning was obtained via individualized instruction by faculty [3].

A more recent survey of 87 pulmonary fellowships program directors showed that all programs had an orientation for fellows that included bronchoscopy, as well as some form of wet labs for bronchoscopy and ventilator management; however, only 31 programs used simulators for bronchoscopy education [4]. This study confirmed that even though an orientation exists, at most programs, procedural training is done "on the job."

In a similar study, Pastis and his colleagues surveyed pulmonary fellowships on the types and number of advanced diagnostic and therapeutic pulmonary procedures offered to trainees and found a large variation in the spectrum of pulmonary procedures available in each program [5]. The majority of these training programs met the targeted number-based competency recommend by professional societies in only three out of 17 surveyed procedures [1].

Establishment of competency in bronchoscopy of trainees is currently based on the number of procedures and a global subjective assessment by faculty observers. Pulmonary fellowship training programs require the performance of at least 50 bronchoscopies for pulmonary trainees to achieve competency [6]. Although this number may be adequate for some learners, it may fall short for others. Moreover, a number-based competency metric does not test the cognitive component of procedural learning.

## Evolving tools for bronchoscopy education

Several training tools for bronchoscopy have been utilized with success, including inanimate airway models, extracted and preserved animal lungs, live animals, and airway simulation software [7–14]. However, none of them have been widely adopted.

Simulation offers an effective method of teaching which avoids using animals and offers a scenario-based interaction that imitates real-life situations. Other disciplines, such as the aviation industry, where errors can have serious consequences, rely heavily on simulation learning (http://www.faa.gov/education_research/training/).

Simulation technology in bronchoscopy is available in two forms: low-fidelity, inanimate mechanical airway models and high-fidelity, computer-based electronic simulation [10].

Low-fidelity models consist of molded tracheobronchial trees that offer realistic tubular-shaped, airway-like structures with accurate anatomy to the first subsegmental bronchial level (Fig. 6.1). This is an excellent tool for novice operators to build muscle memory and enhance hand–eye coordination.

High-fidelity simulators are computer-based and rely on the same technology as video games. The bronchoscopy simulator consists of a proxy bronchoscope, a robotic interface device, and a personal computer with a monitor (Fig. 6.2). The proxy bronchoscope is inserted into a plastic face and is maneuvered on the computer screen into a three-dimensional image recreation of the airways. The robotic interface device tracks the motions of the bronchoscope and reproduces the force felt during an actual bronchoscopy. The "virtual" patient on the screen breathes and coughs and the

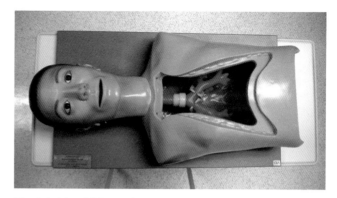

**Fig. 6.1** A low-fidelity mechanical airway model for bronchoscopy teaching.

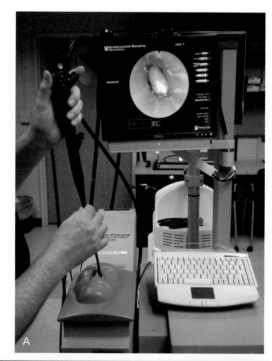

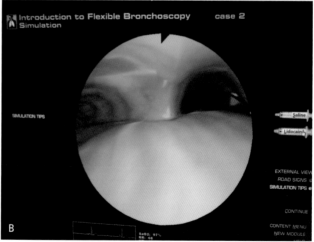

**Fig. 6.2** (A,B) A high-fidelity, computer-based simulator for bronchoscopy teaching.

vital signs are monitored in real time. Various scenarios are offered and the learner can choose to examine normal airways, intubate difficult airways, perform brushing or biopsy on an endobronchial tumor, or sample an enlarged lymph node with transbronchial needle aspiration (TBNA). The software tracks performance metrics such as time of procedure, amount of lidocaine used, incidence of wall collision, percentage of segments entered, and success in obtaining a sample from a targeted lymph node.

The data for simulation in the learning of various medical and surgical procedures are abundant; there have been numerous publications showing the efficacy, cost-effectiveness, and increase in patients' comfort and safety when simulation-based training is undertaken by trainees [15–18].

The first report of a high-fidelity bronchoscopy simulator was published in 1999 when Bro-Nielsen introduced the "Pre-Op Endoscopic Simulator" which integrated three-dimensional graphic simulation with force feedback technology to give a realistic bronchoscopy experience [19]. The first reports of the efficacy of the bronchoscopy high-fidelity simulator were published in 2001. Colt and colleagues reported the outcomes of five novice bronchoscopists who received 4 hours of training on a bronchoscopy simulator and then spent 4 hours practicing on their own without supervision; bronchoscopy skill sets obtained by the novices (dexterity, speed, and accuracy) reached those of a control group of skilled bronchoscopists (who had performed at least 200 bronchoscopies) after only 8 hours of training [9]. Ost *et al.* validated the bronchoscopy simulator as an assessment tool and demonstrated its ability to discriminate among bronchoscopists with varying levels of bronchoscopy; the study found that expert bronchoscopists (>500 bronchoscopies) performed better than intermediates (25–500) who in turn performed better than novices [13].

Most recently, the author of this chapter (MMW) reported the first prospective, multicenter study of performance-based metrics and educational interventions in the learning of bronchoscopy among starting pulmonary fellows [20]. In this study, two successive cohorts of pulmonary fellows, starting training between July 5, 2006 and June 30, 2008, were enrolled in the study. At prespecified milestones, validated tools were used to test their bronchoscopy skill and knowledge: the Bronchoscopy Skills and Tasks Assessment Tool (BSTAT), an objective validated evaluation of bronchoscopy skills with scores ranging from 0–24, and written multiple-choice question examinations.

The first cohort of fellows received training in bronchoscopy as per the standards set by each institution, while the second cohort received training in simulation bronchoscopy and was provided an on-line bronchoscopy curriculum. There was significant variation among study participants in bronchoscopy skills at their 50th bronchoscopy, the number previously set to achieve competency in bronchoscopy. An educational intervention, incorporating simulation bronchoscopy, enhanced the acquisition of bronchoscopy skills, as shown by the statistically significant improvement in mean BSTAT scores for seven of the eight milestone bronchoscopies ($P < 0.05$). The on-line curriculum did not improve the performance on the written tests; however, compliance of the learners with the curriculum was low.

In summary, simulation-based training in bronchoscopy can greatly enhance the speed of skills acquisition and is a great vehicle for individualized learning, repetition, correction of errors, and feedback, performed in a non-threatening environment and without the presence of an instructor. Simulation technology can help standardize the training of bronchoscopy across training programs and provide a tool for performance-based evaluation of competency.

## Preparation before live patient bronchoscopy

A core curriculum for bronchoscopy should be available to the bronchoscopy student. This may include bronchoscopy text books, selected review articles or landmark studies, atlases of still photographs, and case discussions. An invaluable educational resource for bronchoscopy knowledge is the Essential Bronchoscopist, a web-based open access bronchoscopy curriculum developed by a non-profit organization (www.bronchoscopy.org). It is organized in six modules, each covering an area of bronchoscopy knowledge presented in an interactive questions–answer format.

The student should gain a full understanding of bronchoscopy indications and contraindications, prevention and management of complications, safety to the operator and equipment, pharmacology and adverse events of medications used for topical anesthesia and sedation during bronchoscopy, and resuscitation methods and equipment.

Prior to the performance of bronchoscopy, the learners should familiarize themselves with the various components of the bronchoscope, including the proximal lever, suction port, working channel, light source, and optic. Equally important is to learn how to clean and sterilize the bronchoscope and protect it from damage. Although physicians may never perform the actual cleaning in their future practice, this knowledge is paramount to prevent infection complications. The American College of Chest Physicians and American Association for Bronchology consensus statement on prevention of flexible bronchoscopy-associated infection is a good resource on this topic [21].

Three motions are important in the manipulation of the bronchoscope and should be practiced repeatedly by the novice bronchoscopist:

**1** Advancing or retracting the bronchoscope using one hand
**2** Using the lever to flex or extend the tip of the bronchoscope

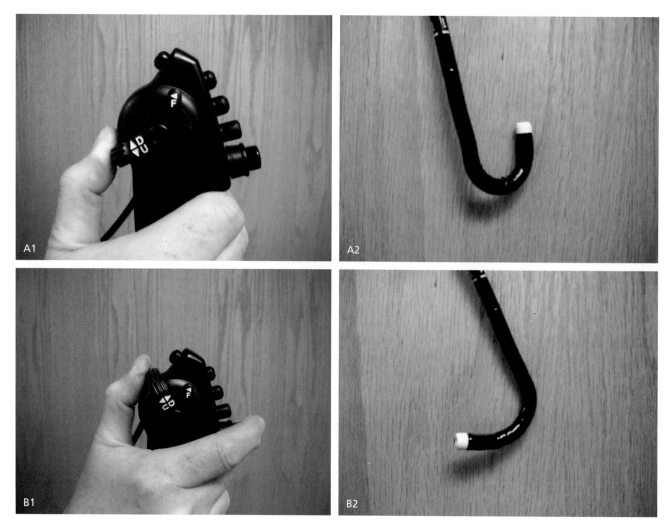

**Fig. 6.3** The bronchoscope's lever is moved in the opposite direction of the desired action at the tip of the bronchoscope (A) Lifting the lever results in downward motion. (B) Pressing the lever down results in upward motion.

**3** Rotating the tip of the flexible bronchoscope to the right or left direction via corresponding wrist movements

The first motion is intuitive and does not require much preparation. The second motion requires practice to grasp the concept that the lever is moved in the opposite direction to the desired action at the tip of the bronchoscope (lifting the lever results in downward motion and pressing the lever down results in upward motion) (Fig. 6.3). The third motion is the most commonly performed incorrectly, especially among novice operators. A bronchoscopist should turn the bronchoscope right and left by turning the wrist holding the proximal end of the scope and never by manipulating the shaft of the bronchoscope near the nose (or mouth) of the patient. The latter can cause twisting damage to the bronchoscope.

The Step-by-Step Bronchoscopy exercises, available on the Essential Bronchoscopist web site are highly recommended to enhance the hand-eye coordination of bronchoscopy skills (Fig. 6.4). These are a set of exercises that are designed to build muscle memory and facilitate laddered learning, and can be performed on low- or high-fidelity bronchoscopy simulators. The learners practice eight graded training maneuvers that direct them through incrementally more difficult moves of bronchoscopy; it begins with practicing passage through the oral or nasal orifice to the larynx, followed by navigating central, lobar, and segmental airways.

As confirmed by our recent study findings and discussed above, bronchoscopy simulation prior to human bronchoscopy is highly recommended to enhance the speed of acquisition of bronchoscopy skills.

## Training with live patients

After adequate preparation as outlined in the previous section, the learner is now ready to perform bronchoscopy

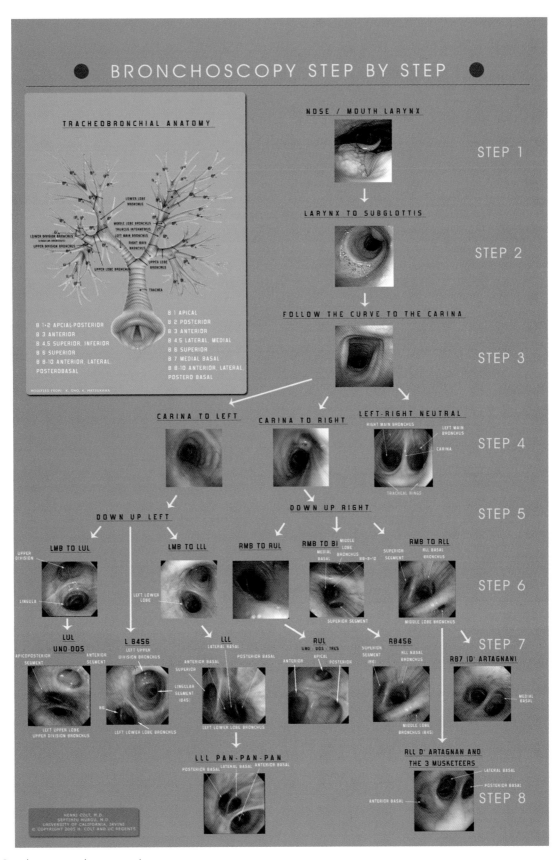

**Fig. 6.4** Bronchoscopy step-by-step exercises.

on a patient. This process starts with a full understanding of the indication of the planned procedure, careful analysis of the relative and absolute contradictions, and knowledge of adverse events and alternative approaches (observation, radiologically-guided procedures, or surgery). The learner should be able to discuss all these issues with the patient, as part of the informed consent, using simplified terminology that is easily understood by the lay person.

The learner should carefully review the radiographic studies prior to bronchoscopy to create a road map to the targeted lesion and decide on the best sampling modality. A useful tip is to invert the CT images horizontally to align the right and left lung views with the "bronchoscopist view" and aid with orientation. This is particularly helpful when the learner is trying to follow the bronchial branches to the target lesion.

The bronchoscope can be held in the right or left hand but it is estimated that there are far more left than right hand bronchoscopists. Some argue that this is mainly because Dr Shigeto Ikeda, the inventor of the flexible bronchoscope, was a left-handed person while others maintain that the right hand, the dominant hand for 90% of the population, is more suited to the fine operation of forceps and other accessory equipment through the bronchoscope [22]. It is ideal for the bronchoscopist to be comfortable operating the bronchoscope in either hand and make a choice based on the planned task.

Similarly, the best position of the bronchoscopist relative to the patient is debatable. Some prefer to stand behind the supine patient while others face the semirecumbent patient. The former provides better access to the anterior walls of the bronchial tree and the anterior segments of the lobar bronchi while the latter provides an easier access to the posterior walls and segments. Once again, it is best for the bronchoscopist to master both approaches and use the one most suited for the specific patient.

With respect to learning the various procedural aspects, we believe that the learner should concentrate on maneuvering the bronchoscope and learning anatomy during the early phase of the learning process. The learner should focus on keeping the bronchoscope centered, avoiding wall trauma, and accessing and inspecting all reachable bronchial segments and subsegments. The bronchoscopist should become extremely proficient with the anatomy of the bronchial segments and subsegments as this is really what defines an experienced bronchoscopist compared to a casual one, who merely performs a "suction" bronchoscopy where all bronchi are equal and mucous plugs are the target. An experienced bronchoscopist will apply knowledge gained from the radiographic studies of the bronchial tree to the precise subsegmental bronchial level. In our institution, we ask the fellows (even the advanced ones) to recite in order the name of every bronchial segment they enter with the bronchoscope so their teachers can correct any mistakes.

Once scope maneuverability and anatomy are learned, the student can progress to more complex sampling techniques such as endobronchial biopsy, transbronchial lung biopsy, and transbronchial needle aspiration.

At the end of the procedure, the learner should learn how to correctly label the specimens and document the procedure to produce a record of all findings and samplings that can be used to communicate with the referring physician and as a reference in future medical care.

## Maintenance and acquisition of skills for practicing physicians

Most of that has been discussed up to the point relates to bronchoscopy training for novice learners. However, practicing physicians often encounter important training issues relating to the need to get hospital credentialing, maintain learned skills on an annual basis, and learn new procedures.

The Credentialing process is the responsibility of each health care facility in the United States; professional societies usually issue consensus-based general recommendations that aid hospitals in this process. An example is the privileging and credentialing criteria for endoscopy and colonoscopy issued by the gastroenterology and surgical societies [23]. In 2003, The American College of Chest Physicians (ACCP) published guidelines for minimal numbers for interventional pulmonary procedures. For example, 25 procedures were needed to establish competency in TBNA and 10 annual procedures were recommended to maintain competency [1].These guidelines are based on experts opinions and not on scientific data evaluating variations in individual performance or patients' outcomes.

A more challenging issue is the learning of a new medical procedure once out of training [24]. A telling example is the recent introduction of endobronchial ultrasound, a technology that allows the real-time guidance of mediastinal lymph nodes sampling with sensitivity and specificity of 93 and 100%, respectively [25]. Physicians can acquire basic skills through focused courses with didactic and hands-on sessions which can provide the foundation of knowledge and basic skills for such a new procedure. Afterward, physicians can further enhance their skills by taking short sabbaticals in centers performing a high volume of the procedure, seeking proctorship from physicians who perform the procedure or a variation of it (gastroenterologists who perform esophageal ultrasound), or inviting experienced operators to supervise their performance. Clearly, none of these choices are easy to pursue and there are numerous legal and administrative obstacles that prevent physicians from pursing supervised training in other medical institutions. The ultimate goals of a credentialing process are proper procedure utilization and the delivery of high-quality patient care. More studies are needed to validate the effectiveness of simulation technology in establishing performance metrics and aiding in the certification process, especially for more complex procedures, which may facilitate learning of new medical procedures.

## Conclusions

Bronchoscopy is a procedure central to the pulmonogist's armamentarium to diagnose and treat respiratory diseases.

The apprenticeship model remains the major teaching method for bronchoscopy. Though, clearly, individual interaction with faculty represents a valuable experience in bronchoscopy and procedural education in general, innovative methods are necessary to assure clinical competency for trainees and delivery of high-quality medical care.

There is a mounting body of evidence that simulation-based training can enhance the speed of acquisition of bronchoscopy skills and provide a safe environment for structured training that is acquired away from patients and transferred to the bedside.

## References

1 Ernst A, Silvestri GA, Johnstone D. Interventional pulmonary procedures: Guidelines from the American College of Chest Physicians. *Chest* 2003; **123**: 1693–717.

2 Cooke M, Irby DM, Sullivan W, Ludmerer KM. American medical education 100 years after the Flexner report. *N Engl J Med* 2006; **355**: 1339–44.

3 Haponik EF, Russell GB, Beamis JF, *et al.* Bronchoscopy training: current fellows' experiences and some concerns for the future. *Chest* 2000; **118**: 625–30.

4 Lucarelli MR, Lucey CR, Mastronarde JG. Survey of current practices in fellowship orientation. *Respiration* 2007; **74**: 382–6.

5 Pastis NJ, Nietert PJ, Silvestri GA, Variation in training for interventional pulmonary procedures among US pulmonary/critical care fellowships: a survey of fellowship directors. *Chest* 2005; **127**: 1614–21.

6 Torrington KG. Bronchoscopy training and competency: how many are enough? *Chest* 2000; **118**: 572–3.

7 Blum MG, Powers TW, Sundaresan S. Bronchoscopy simulator effectively prepares junior residents to competently perform basic clinical bronchoscopy. *Ann Thorac Surg* 2004; **78**: 287–91.

8 Chen JS, Hsu HH, Lai IR, *et al.* Validation of a computer-based bronchoscopy simulator developed in Taiwan. *J Formos Med Assoc* 2006; **105**: 569–76.

9 Colt HG, Crawford SW, Galbraith O, 3rd. Virtual reality bronchoscopy simulation: a revolution in procedural training. *Chest* 2001; **120**: 1333–9.

10 Davoudi M, Colt HG. Bronchoscopy simulation: a brief review. *Adv Health Sci Educ Theory Pract* 2009; **14**: 287–96.

11 Di Domenico S, Simonassi C, Chessa L. Inexpensive anatomical trainer for bronchoscopy. *Interact Cardiovasc Thorac Surg* 2007; **6**: 567–9.

12 Moorthy K, Smith S, Brown T, *et al.* Evaluation of virtual reality bronchoscopy as a learning and assessment tool. *Respiration* 2003; **70**: 195–9.

13 Ost D, DeRosiers A, Britt EJ, *et al.* Assessment of a bronchoscopy simulator. *Am J Respir Crit Care Med* 2001; **164**: 2248–55.

14 Rowe R, Cohen RA. An evaluation of a virtual reality airway simulator. *Anesth Analg* 2002; **95**: 62–6.

15 Martin M, Vashisht B, Frezza E, *et al.* Competency-based instruction in critical invasive skills improves both resident performance and patient safety. *Surgery* 1998; **124**: 313–7.

16 Scott DJ, Bergen PC, Rege RV, *et al.* Laparoscopic training on bench models: better and more cost effective than operating room experience? *J Am Coll Surg* 2000; **191**: 272–83.

17 Sedlack RE, Kolars JC, Alexander JA. Computer simulation training enhances patient comfort during endoscopy. *Clin Gastroenterol Hepatol* 2004; **2**: 348–52.

18 Seymour NE, Gallagher AG, Roman SA, *et al.* Virtual reality training improves operating room performance: results of a randomized, double-blinded study. *Ann Surg* 2002; **236**: 458–63; discussion 463–4.

19 Bro-Nielsen M, Tasto JL, Cunningham R, Merril GL. PreOp endoscopic simulator: a PC-based immersive training system for bronchoscopy. *Stud Health Technol Inform* 1999; **62**: 76–82.

20 Wahidi MM, Silvestri GA, Coakley RD, *et al.* A prospective multicenter study of competency metrics and educational interventions in the learning of bronchoscopy among starting pulmonary fellows. *Chest* 2010; **137**: 1040–9.

21 Mehta AC, Prakash UB, Garland R, *et al.* American College of Chest Physicians and American Association for Bronchology [corrected] consensus statement: prevention of flexible bronchoscopy-associated infection. *Chest* 2005; **128**: 1742–55.

22 Gildea TR, Mehta AC, The flexible bronchoscope: which hand should hold it? Pro: right hand. *J Bronchol* 2003; **10**: 315–19.

23 Wexner SD, Eisen GM, Simmang C. Principles of privileging and credentialing for endoscopy and colonoscopy. *Surg Endosc* 2002; **16**: 367–9.

24 Ost D, Eapen GA, Jimenez CA, Morice RC. Improving procedural training and certification in pulmonary medicine. *Chest* 2010; **137**: 6–8.

25 Gomez M, Silvestri GA. Endobronchial ultrasound for the diagnosis and staging of lung cancer. *Proc Am Thorac Soc* 2009; **6**: 180–6.

# Indications and Contraindications in Flexible Bronchoscopy

## Robert F. Browning Jr,[1] J. Francis Turner Jr,[2] and Ko-Pen Wang[3]

[1] Division of Interventional Pulmonology, National Naval Medical Center and Uniformed Services University of Health Sciences, Bethesda, MD, USA
[2] Interventional Pulmonary and Critical Care Medicine, Nevada Cancer Institute and University of Nevada School of Medicine, Las Vegas, NV, USA
[3] Chest Diagnostic Center, Harbor Hospital, Baltimore, MD, USA

## Introduction

Since its introduction in 1897 by Killian, the role of the bronchoscope has been expanding with each new technical development resulting in yet another application [1]. Rigid bronchoscope was initially performed for visual examination of the trachea and proximal bronchi, with the therapeutic utility of being able to remove foreign bodies [2]. In 1964, Professor Shigeto Ikeda sought production of the prototype that was to become what is now known and utilized throughout the world as the flexible fiberoptic bronchoscope. With continued success of the prototypes produced by Machida and Olympus Corporation, the seventh model of the bronchofiberscope, and the first available in clinical practice, was completed in 1966 [3,4]. With Professor Ikeda's continued direction and technological improvements, this represented a tremendous advance in the field of bronchoscopy from the time of Killian. These new instruments first allowed the bronchoscopist better visualization of the upper lobes as well as the distil segments of the lower lobes. While allowing improved visualization, the new fiberscopes also were better tolerated by the patient, obviating the need for general anesthesia and facilitating the routine performance of this procedure in the outpatient department.

The subsequent development of instruments to be utilized with the flexible bronchoscope allowed sampling of endobronchial lesions [5,6]. The introduction of the Wang transbronchial needle allowed biopsies for cytology and histology specimens from outside the visualized tracheal bronchial tree [7,8].

With the rapidly expanding diagnostic use of flexible bronchoscopy we must not forget that one of the fathers of medicine, Hippocrates (460–370 BC), advised as to how a reed introduced into the windpipe could aid a suffocating patient. Thus the roots of endoscopy have long been in the active treatment of patients with respiratory compromise and, as such, there has now been a rapid expansion in the therapeutic application of the flexible bronchoscope. This chapter seeks to review the current indications and contraindications for the use of the flexible bronchoscope from a practical view and as first determined by the symptoms, signs, and imaging studies for which the patient will first present to the bronchoscopist (Table 7.1).

## Cough

Cough is an important symptom in the evaluation of patients who may have underlying lung disease. Although the frequency with which bronchoscopy is performed for cough and its low yield indicate that this is an overutilized procedure, we recommend a directed pulmonary evaluation in the context of the individual patient's presentation [9,10]. Acute cough in a non-immunocompromised patient with a normal chest X ray is most often fleeting and rarely requires bronchoscopy. However, in an immunocompromised patient with a low CD4 count (<200 cells/mm$^3$), bronchoscopy should be considered even in the context of a normal chest X ray if induced sputa is unrevealing [11]. Subacute and chronic cough, however, is defined as that symptom which persists for greater than 3 to 8 weeks and greater than 8 weeks duration, respectively [12]. The further evaluation of this symptom is then dependent upon the age, family history, risk factors, and additional symptoms with cough being a harbinger of more serious disease. In the immunocompromised patient, bronchoscopy for subacute or chronic cough should be considered to evaluate

*Flexible Bronchoscopy*, Third Edition. Edited by Ko-Pen Wang, Atul C. Mehta, J. Francis Turner.
© 2012 Blackwell Publishing Ltd. Published 2012 by Blackwell Publishing Ltd.

**Table 7.1** Indications for diagnostic bronchoscopy

Malignancy
  Diagnosis of bronchogenic carcinoma
  Staging of bronchogenic carcinoma
  Restaging after therapy and/or initial mediastinoscopy
  Abnormal sputum cytology
  Follow-up after treatment of carcinoma
  Evaluation of patients with head and neck malignancy
  Evaluation of patients with esophageal malignancy
  Metastatic carcinoma
  Mediastinal mass

Infection
  Recurrent or unresolved pneumonia
  Infiltrate in an immunocompromised patient
  Cavitary lesion

Unexplained lung collapse

Interstitial lung disease

Hemoptysis

Unexplained chronic cough

Localized wheezing

Stridor

Foreign body aspiration

Chest trauma
  Blunt or penetrating
  Chemical
  Thermal

Unexplained pleural effusion

Evaluation of the patient after lung transplantation

Endotracheal intubation
  Confirm tube position
  Evaluate for tube-related injury
  Confirm position of transtracheal oxygen catheter

Tracheobronchial stricture and stenosis

Hoarseness or vocal cord paralysis

Superior vena cava syndrome

Fistula
  Bronchopleural
  Tracheo- or bronchoesophageal
  Tracheo- or bronchoaortic

Persistent pneumothorax

Postoperative assessment of tracheal, tracheobronchial, bronchial, or stump anastomosis

Bronchography

for uncommon conditions after empiric treatment for the most common causes: upper airway cough syndrome, asthma, non-asthmatic eosinophilic bronchitis, and gastro-esophageal reflux syndrome (GERD) [12]. Chronic cough in the immunocompetent patient may still represent the initial presentation of a more serious disease. Bronchogenic carcinoma will have cough as an initial presenting symptom in 21–87% and occur sometime during the course in 70–90% of patients [13]. Algorithms evaluating chronic cough that include bronchoscopy after initial evaluation or unresponsiveness to treatment for postnasal drip, asthma, and GERD have been shown to be successful in determining an etiology for a significant number of unexplained cases of chronic cough [14].

We therefore we recommend early bronchoscopy be performed for acute cough only if the cough is associated with localizing lesion on chest X ray, hemoptysis, localized wheezing, or in an immunocompromised patient requiring a diagnosis. In patients with a chronic cough or whose cough has changed character, unresponsive to stopping smoking, or evaluation for the most common etiologies, we recommend performance of sputum cytology, white light bronchoscopy, and the addition of autofluorescence bronchoscopy if available [15–17].

## Wheezing

Although wheezing is frequently associated with asthma, the differential diagnosis is varied and large. The evaluation of wheezing in the non-asthmatic patient or patient poorly responsive to bronchodilator therapy requires a thorough examination including visual inspection of the upper and lower airways with bronchoscopy. "All that wheezes is not asthma" remains a sometimes hard-learned lesson. The differential diagnosis in these instances may include foreign bodies, tracheomalacia, extrinsic or intrinsic obstruction due to mass lesions, vascular abnormalities, or tracheobronchial stenotic lesions [18–22].

A chest X ray and pulmonary function testing with flow volume loops can provide important diagnostic clues [23]. However, if diagnosis remains elusive, fiberoptic bronchoscopy (FOB) offers direct airway examination in search of an obstructing airway lesion. Along with localized wheezing, an obstructing lesion may produce evidence of air trapping on X ray, the evaluation of which may require bronchoscopy. Additionally, bronchoscopy may be an important therapeutic tool for removing the offending lesion.

## Stridor

Stridor is an important sign of life-threatening upper airway obstruction. The etiology must be rapidly elucidated.

The causes are varied and can be grouped by age of presentation [24]. In infants and children the differential diagnosis should include epiglottis, croup, laryngomalacia, laryngeal papillomas, laryngotracheal clefts, subglottic hemangioma, pulmonary artery sling, anomalous inominate artery, and tracheal foreign bodies [25,26]. In adults the diagnostic considerations include acute bilateral vocal cord paralysis, rapidly growing tracheal lesions, extrinsic compression of the trachea by mediastinal or esophageal lesions, cricoarytenoid joint disease due to a rheumatologic disorder, Wegener's granulomatosis, infection, or acute laryngeal edema [25,27]. The radiographic studies should include evaluation of the neck as well as the chest. Soft tissue X rays or CT of the neck may be diagnostic of epiglottis or retropharyngeal abscess. Correct visualization of the upper airway can be diagnostic and occasionally therapeutic if the offending lesion or foreign body can be removed. Prior to starting the endoscopy, the bronchoscopist should ensure that equipment and the expertise to perform endobronchial intubation or emergent tracheostomy are immediately available.

## Hoarseness and vocal cord paralysis

Most patients with hoarseness and vocal cord paralysis tend to present to otolaryngologists rather than chest physicians. The etiologies of vocal cord paralysis are many and the offending lesion may be located in the chest, necessitating a referral to the chest physician [28]. In a review of 20 years of literature on the etiologies of vocal cord paralysis, Terris and associates noted that 36% were the result of a neoplastic process [29]. Of these, 55% were due to lung cancer. When history, physical examination, and imaging are non-diagnostic, endoscopy should be used because it can provide diagnosis in 20% of the patients [29]. The left recurrent laryngeal nerve, because of its circuitous path into the chest, can be involved with diseases in the area of the left hilum. Lesions in this area can be biopsied via transbronchial needles. The right laryngeal nerve is involved only if the lesion extends into the right side of the neck.

## Inhalational injury

Inhalation injury may be the result of thermal injury due to steam or super-heated air, smoke inhalation, or toxin exposure, and can be devastating, with a mortality rate of 30–90% when patients have combined cutaneous burns and inhalation injury [30]. Reliance on clinical criteria, such as facial or oral pharyngeal burns, production of carbonaceous sputum, wheezing, hoarseness, or singed nasal hairs, fails to diagnose a number of patients with burn injury [31,32]. Thermal injury may present as stridor with associated hoarseness and dysphagia. Facial burns, oropharyngeal edema, or carbonaceous sputa all may serve as warning signs that a significant thermal injury or smoke inhalation has occurred and the need for critical assessment of the airway should occur. Early radiographic diagnosis is difficult and not sensitive enough to diagnose mucosal damage in the airways. CT virtual bronchoscopy has been reported in a series of 10 burn patients as accurately identifying inhalational injury, but has yet to be shown equivalent or superior to bronchoscopy [33]. Bronchoscopy, should be performed as part of the initial assessment with identification of inflammation and mucosal edema. In patients with acute smoke inhalation, FOB should be performed promptly to identify early inflammation, ulceration, or swelling of the laryngeal area [34]. Patients may require concurrent intubation and use of the fiberoptic bronchoscope may facilitate intubations [35]. Use of fiberoptic bronchoscopy has also been shown to correlate with histologic findings and aids in outcome predictions [36,37]. Acute injury may produce severe airway edema, erythema, and mucosal sloughing. Subacute injury may cause mucosal necrosis and hemorrhagic tracheobronchitis, whereas chronic injury leads to scarring and stenosis, bronchiectasis, and formation of granulation tissue. Transbronchial biopsy in the chronic phase may demonstrate bronchiolitis obliterans [25]. The use of the bronchoscope, therefore, allows evaluation of airway injury for earlier diagnosis, with resultant rapid institution of treatment, including corticosteroids, humidified air, antibiotics, and assistance in clearing airway plugs.

Toxic exposure to carboxyhemoglobin, ammonia, nitrogen and sulfur dioxide, and chlorine gas also occurs as a product of incineration and may also precipitate airway injury [38]. Chemicals released during industrial accidents and during war also pose a substantial risk of injury to the lungs. Freitag and colleagues reported their experience in managing 21 Iranian soldiers who suffered lung injury following inhalation of mustard gas (dichlorodiethyl sulfide) and other poisonous gases during the Iran–Iraq War in the 1980s [39]. In the acute stage of injury bronchoscopy is used to assess the extent of damage and remove charred, necrotic debris from the airways. These patients produced large amounts of purulent, thick mucus that could not be expectorated by the patients in their weakened state. Later sequelae, including tracheobronchial stenosis and granulation tissue, may necessitate the use of the bronchoscope in a more aggressive therapeutic role [39].

## Hemoptysis

Hemoptysis is a frequent pulmonary symptom and may present as minimal blood streaked sputum to massive with quantities from 100 mL to 600 mL per day [40]. The most common causes are bronchitis, bronchiectasis, and carcinoma, and hemoptysis is the second most common reason for bronchoscopy [9,41–43]. Distinction between gastrointestinal, pharyngeal, nasal, and pulmonary sources is critical [44]. Flexible bronchoscopy should be reserved for those having persistent bleeding, bleeding that is brisk or of large volume, or those at increased risk for malignancy. The search for the source of bleeding must be meticulous. Applied appropriately, the bronchoscope can successfully localize the bleeding site in 75% to 93% of the cases [45]. A small-caliber bronchoscope may be needed to conduct a thorough examination of the distal bronchial tree [46]. If the initial examination is non-diagnostic, a repeat bronchoscopy following subsequent episodes of hemoptysis may be necessary. Although early bronchoscopy (within 48 hours) has a higher diagnostic yield than late bronchoscopy, the impact of timing of the procedure on overall patient management has not been shown [47–49]. Currently, CT scan to characterize the bleeding is often the first step. This approach can quickly demonstrate localized sources if limited abnormalities exist on the scan. Unfortunately, if diffuse bleeding is shown on the CT scan, there is no way of differentiating diffuse alveolar hemorrhage (DAH) from blood spilling over from a localized source. Despite the lack of any formal study, it is our impression that knowledge of the cause of hemoptysis and its location is critical in the patient's management, and thus we favor early evaluation with bronchoscopy for initial evaluation.

In the case of massive hemoptysis the role of rigid versus the flexible bronchoscope has been debated, but not studied in a head-to-head comparison. Most often, the greatest threat in massive hemoptysis is clot formation acutely obstructing the airways. The rigid instrument offers greater suction capacity, the ability to use larger instruments, and may afford the ability to directly tamponade the bleeding site, while intubation of the patient with a flexible and cuffed endotracheal tube offers the most control of the airway for ventilation and the flexible scope offers greater visibility to the smaller airways [50]. The flexible bronchoscope may also be utilized in the management of hemoptysis with the installation of epinephrine, thrombin solutions, or Fogarty balloons in an attempt to quell the bleeding [51,52]. Additionally new instruments have been used, such as the argon plasma coagulator, to provide for hemoptysis control and simultaneous treatment of malignant airway obstruction [53]. Ultimately, management will depend on the bronchoscopist's training and comfort level with the given instrument and the amount of bleeding.

In addition to the many symptoms outlined, patients often will be referred to the bronchoscopist with physical signs or diagnostic imaging that indicate bronchoscopy needs to be performed.

## Superior vena cava syndrome

Mediastinal lesions can compromise venous return, producing the superior vena cava syndrome. The bronchoscope may be used to perform transtracheal or transbronchial needle aspiration (TBNA) and biopsy on masses or enlarged lymph nodes in these areas. Knowledge of the location of the great vessels is of critical importance when sampling these areas. When patients with superior vena cava syndrome are being evaluated, vascular anomalies should be excluded prior to any invasive procedure. Superior vena cava syndrome in the era of antibiotic therapy is predominantly related to malignancy [54]. However, benign causes must also be kept in mind. Pathologic confirmation of the cause is needed before definitive treatment can be initiated. Bronchoscopic biopsy can establish the diagnosis in 60 to 70% of the cases [55,56]. This is particularly important in avoiding unnecessary thoracotomy under general anesthesia, which may be associated with prolonged intubation in patients with large mediastinal masses [57].

## Mediastinal mass

In the evaluation of mediastinal masses, bronchoscopy can often spare the patient a more aggressive mediastinoscopy. Conventional and ultrasound-guided transbronchial biopsies can often reach and diagnose mediastinal masses [8,58]. Because it can be safely performed in the outpatient setting, cost is reduced. The flexible bronchoscope is also seen as an important tool for anesthesiologists, allowing for intubation under topical anesthesia for patients that may have a compromised airway owing to an anterior mediastinal mass [59]. Previous guidance for the performance of upright and recumbent flow volume loops prior to procedures requiring anesthesia in patients with mediastinal mass has been shown to be unhelpful in risk stratification or operative planning [60].

## Interstitial lung disease

Interstitial lung disease encompasses a wide range of diagnoses [61]. Similarly, the role of bronchoscopy in the evaluation of these diseases is varied. Bronchoalveolar lavage (BAL) has been useful in studying the cells causing the inflammatory response in interstitial pulmonary fibrosis (IPF) [62,63] and to help determine the contribution of surfactant protein abnormalities to the development of chronic lung injury in a familial form of interstitial lung disease [64].

Bronchoscopy with BAL and biopsy can be diagnostic in diseases such as sarcoidosis, lymphangitic carcinomatosis, eosinophilic pneumonia, and pulmonary alveolar proteinosis. BAL, when demonstrating the presence of materials or cells not typically found in the lung, can lead to the diagnosis of diseases such as histiocytosis X, pulmonary alveolar proteinosis, asbestos exposure, and berylliosis [65–68]. In addition, the differential cell count of inflammatory cells identified may be helpful in narrowing the differential diagnosis of fibrosing interstitial pneumonias but is not diagnostic of IPF. In sarcoidosis, berylliosis, hypersensitivity pneumonitis, tuberculosis, and fungal infections, the T helper/T suppressor ratio is altered [69,70]. It should be noted that at present the T helper/T suppressor ratio is not commonly used in the clinical setting. Elevation of polymorphonuclear cells is noted in idiopathic pulmonary fibrosis, collagen vascular diseases, pneumoconiosis, and bronchiolitis obliterans organizing pneumonia [71,72]. Eosinophils are increased in chronic eosinophilic pneumonia and Churg–Strauss syndrome [73,74]. Lipid-laden macrophages provide clues to amiodarone exposure, whereas the hemorrhagic syndromes produce hemosiderin-laden macrophages [61]. It should be noted that although much is written about the use of BAL in interstitial lung disease, no clear role has been established for its use in prognosis or therapy [75,76]. Bronchoscopic transbronchial lung biopsies should be considered the diagnosis of interstitial lung diseases, especially in patients with contraindications to surgical lung biopsy. By the nature of the relatively small size of the transbronchial lung biopsy, they are not usually able to establish the diagnosis but may often reveal an alternative diagnosis, so surgical lung biopsy remains the gold standard [77–79].

## Infection

Pneumonia is a frequent disease encountered by the chest physician and such infections may be treated empirically or by microbiologic evaluation of sputum. The rate of radiographic resolution of community-acquired pneumonia depends on the patient's age and occurrence of underlying structural lung disease. Overall, 73% of patients have resolution within 6 weeks [80]. However, when pneumonia is recurrent or fails to resolve, bronchoscopy may be necessary [81]. Feinsilver and colleagues, in a review of 35 patients, reported on the role of the flexible fiberoptic bronchoscope in non-resolving pneumonia [82]. When a specific diagnosis other than community-acquired pneumonia was present, flexible FOB was able to yield the correct diagnosis in 12 of 14 patients. Of the 23 patients with non-diagnostic bronchoscopy, 21 had no other explanation for their infiltrate except community-acquired pneumonia, suggesting a high negative predictive value of a non-diagnostic bronchoscopy. Bronchoscopy is more likely to yield a specific diagnosis when the infiltrate has been present for more than 30 days and is multilobar rather than lobar or segmental, and when

the patient is less than 55 years old [82]. Patients who are older or those with impaired immune systems (e.g. those with chronic obstructive pulmonary disease, alcohol abuse, and diabetes) have slower resolution of their pneumonia [82]. Thus, bronchoscopy may be delayed in these patients.

Immunocompromised patients are particularly prone to opportunistic pulmonary infection by a variety of organisms. Huang et al. reviewed the diagnostic yield of bronchoscopy in patients with non-diagnostic induced sputa. In their study a diagnosis was established in 50.5% of evaluations with bronchoscopy providing the only or an early diagnosis of tuberculosis in 64% of cases [83]. Bronchoscopy with BAL offers a safe and relatively rapid means of sampling the lower respiratory tract. In patients with acquired immunodeficiency syndrome, *Pneumocystis jiroveci* is a major concern, and obtaining both BAL and transbronchial biopsy provides nearly 100% sensitivity [84]. In a study of 100 immunocompromised patients, Martin and associates were able to demonstrate opportunistic infection in 33%, obviating the need for open lung biopsy [85]. Through the use of smear, stains, and monoclonal antibody detection methods, the lavage fluid can be rapidly screened. If the preliminary results are negative and an open lung biopsy is deemed necessary, it can be done within a few hours. Thus, even a negative BAL need not cause significant delay in proceeding with the more definitive open lung biopsy.

Fiberoptic bronchoscopy is an important addition in the evaluation of critically ill patients with fever and infiltrates suggestive of pneumonia [35,86,87]. Pneumonia is the most common infection seen in patients admitted to an ICU and the risk for developing pneumonia in patients on mechanical ventilation at 1 month may be up to 60% [88,89]. Ventilator associated pneumonia (VAP) has become a significant threat to ventilated ICU patients and accurate and timely diagnosis is imperative to decrease mortality. National guidelines recommend lower respiratory tract samples be taken as soon as the infection is suspected and empiric antibiotic treatment given until Gram stain and culture data from the samples are available [87]. Fiberoptic bronchoscopy with BAL is a commonly used method for collecting these samples and also allows for visual inspection of the airways and removal of any retained secretions. In critically ill cancer patients, bronchoscopy with BAL, and sometimes transbronchial biopsy, is often essential for establishing a diagnosis, especially in the neutropenic patient [87,90,91]. Bronchoalveolar lavage may be safely undertaken in patients on positive pressure ventilation, with coagulopathy or thrombocytopenia [92].

Cavitary lung lesions represent a special diagnostic challenge for the chest physician. Although many are of an infectious origin, the incidence of associated carcinoma has been reported to be 7.6 to 17% [93]. Thus, bronchoscopic examination may be necessary to evaluate the possibility of cancer in patients presenting with cavitary lesions. In evaluating which patients are more likely to have underlying cancer, Sosenka and Glassroth noted that the cavitary lesion is more likely to be benign in patients with higher fevers, greater leukocytosis, and greater prevalence of systemic symptoms and who have risk factors for aspiration [93]. In patients with bronchogenic carcinoma, bronchoscopy was diagnostic of cancer in 58% and precipitated additional studies leading to diagnosis in another 16%. In addition to assessing for malignancy, bronchoscopy offers an opportunity to collect specimens for microbiologic studies. There are also reports of successful drainage of abscess via transbronchial catheters [94–96].

## Lobar collapse

Of all of the abnormal radiographic patterns, the diagnostic yield of bronchoscopy is highest when lobar collapse is being evaluated [97]. Persistent atelectasis may be a manifestation of an endobronchial lesion with post obstructive consolidation. Such a process requires endoscopic evaluation and appropriate treatment. Of the 54 patients undergoing bronchoscopy for lobar collapse, Su and coworkers noted that 35 (65%) had an endobronchial mass, eight (15%) had abnormal bronchial mucosa, and four (7%) had narrowed, compressed, or stenosed airway [97].

Fiberoptic bronchoscopy has also been used therapeutically in critically ill patients with lobar collapse or atelectasis. Hasegawa and coworkers noted that 27% of emergent bronchoscopy was performed for atelectasis and mucus plugging [98]. Patients with underlying neuromuscular disease, such as those with spinal cord injuries or Guillain–Barré syndrome, may especially benefit from removal of retained secretions [99]. Overall, improvement from performance of fiberoptic bronchoscopy may allow for weaning from mechanical ventilation, improvement in oxygenation (44%), X-ray improvement (58%), and significant clinical improvement in 41% of cases performed [100–102]. Thus the proposed indications for FOB in lobar collapse or atelectasis are for those patients with lobar or greater atelectasis not responding to chest physiotherapy or life-threatening whole lung atelectasis [35].

## Pleural effusions

Pleural effusions are generally evaluated by thoracentesis, closed pleural biopsy, pleuroscopy, or video assisted thorascopy (VATS) [103]. The recent widespread use of thoracoscopically guided pleural biopsies may serve as an alternative to bronchoscopy. The development of a semiflexible thoracofiberscope (Olympus™ LTF) in comparison to an Abram's biopsy needle demonstrated an improved sensitivity (81 versus 62%) and excellent views of the pleura and may aid

in the search for the elusive causes of perplexing pleural effusions [104]. The majority of effusions that remain undiagnosed have a high incidence of malignancy [105]. In such situations, FOB may play a role, particularly in the presence of cough or hemoptysis or if the chest X ray shows a concurrent pulmonary lesion. Chang and Perng performed thoracentesis, closed pleural biopsy, and bronchoscopy on 140 patients with pleural effusions [106]. The combination of these procedures resulted in a diagnosis in 100 (71%) of the patients. Sixty-eight patients were diagnosed by thoracentesis, or pleural biopsy, or both. Bronchoscopy provided diagnosis in an additional 32 patients. Bronchoscopy was more likely to be positive if the patient had hemoptysis or if the chest X ray demonstrated a parenchymal lesion in addition to the pleural effusion. In fact in the latter case, bronchoscopy was diagnostic more often than the pleural examination [106].

## Chest trauma

The chest is frequently subjected to various types of trauma. Physical trauma injuries may be due to either blunt or penetrating insult. Bronchoscopy is frequently necessary following major thoracic trauma, both blunt and penetrating, to assess for airway damage [107,108]. Hara and Prakash, in a retrospective review, noted bronchoscopy was of diagnostic value in 28 (53%) of 53 patients admitted with trauma [109]. High tracheal lesions have been overlooked, with resultant patient death in some cases, and some authors have suggested that all cases of major thoracic trauma be evaluated by bronchoscopy [110–112]. Fiberoptic bronchoscopy in trauma situations is able to provide both therapeutic and diagnostic benefit. Intubation with the fiberoptic scope can provide direct visualization of the airway and vocal cords while permitting simultaneous intubation, particularly in those with severe neck injury. In the evaluation of the multitrauma patient the occurrence of cervical or sternal fractures, pneumomediastinum, and persistent chest tube air leak are all markers of possible significant airway injury and the performance of FOB should be considered.

In addition to the initial evaluation of the trauma victim, bronchoscopy may also be necessary to diagnose and manage post-trauma complications, including aspiration and mucous plugging.

## Lung transplantation

With improved operative survival of patients undergoing lung transplant, the postoperative management of such patients presents a special challenge to the chest physician. The transplant patient is susceptible to complications related to the bronchial anastomosis, rejection, infection, and bronchiolitis obliterans. Bronchoscopy is of critical importance in the evaluation and management of airway complications and in the differentiation of rejection versus infection [113–115]. Although surgical advances have decreased the incidence of anastomotic dehiscence, bronchoscopy should be performed in patients with persistent chest tube air leak to assess the anastomotic site. The lung transplant patient may also develop suture granuloma with compromise of the airway. Bronchoscopy is used to evaluate these patients and may also serve a therapeutic role (e.g. stent placement or laser resection of the granulomas and offending suture material) [116]. In the lung transplant patient, infection and rejection can present with similar clinical and radiographic findings. Because the treatment for either is different, bronchoscopy with transbronchial biopsy must be performed to differentiate between the two entities [113–115,117]. The development of bronchiolitis obliterans remains a major obstacle to long-term survival of the lung transplant patient. Its manifestation includes the presence of new or increasing airway obstruction or restriction on pulmonary function testing. However, histologic confirmation requires tissue sampling via transbronchial biopsy [118].

## Bronchography

Prior to the advent of the bronchoscope and CT, bronchography was frequently used to define the airway anatomy. Now, three-dimensional reconstruction of CT images and virtual bronchoscopy have essentially replaced bronchography for defining airway anatomy. Still, the use of real-time endobronchial bronchography can aid in navigating the airways to locate cavities and lesions. This technique has been described by Ono and associates with mapping of the location of the peripheral lung lesion by selective peripheral bronchograms, performed through the flexible bronchoscope [119]. Combining this mapping technique with a double-hinged curet, Ono was able to establish diagnosis of peripheral lesions in 41 of 46 patients (89%) on the first bronchoscopy and 45 of 46 patients (98%) within two bronchoscopies [119].

## Pulmonary nodules

Peripheral lesions are those that cannot be directly viewed through the bronchoscope. The location, size, and technique used in the attempted bronchoscopic diagnosis of these lesions also play a significant role in the diagnostic yield. Lesions less than 2 cm historically have a diagnostic yield of 30%, compared with 80% in those over 4 cm [120–124]. With the use of advanced imaging techniques, such as endobronchial ultrasound, yield for pulmonary nodules less than 2 cm has been reported as high as 69% in lesions able to be reached by the ultrasound probe [125]. Distance from

the hilum has also been suggested to play a factor in diagnostic yield with nodules in the peripheral third of the lung having significantly lower yield than more central lesions [126]. Intuitively, this makes sense although most experienced bronchoscopists will agree that it is really dependent on the nodule's proximity to the airway and the angle and number of turns it takes to reach the lesion. Lesions in the apical segments and superior basal segments are often very difficult to reach with biopsy and diagnostic instruments. More peripheral lesions may also present a higher risk for pneumothorax complication, especially when using the ultrasound probe. Typically the radial ultrasound probe, electromagnetic navigation bronchoscopy (ENB) probe, catheters, and transbronchial needles have difficulty making sharp turns in the airway. Biplanar or C-arm fluoroscopy assisted transbronchial biopsy has been the standard for peripheral lesions, but in the past decade, additional techniques, such as radial ultrasound probe, CT fluoroscopy, CT guidance, virtual bronchoscopy (VB), electromagnetic navigation bronchoscopy (ENB), or some combination of these modalities, have become increasingly more common in practice and research and appear to demonstrate increased yield over fluoroscopy alone [125,127–129].

The type of biopsy instrument may also have a significant impact on diagnostic yield. There are a wide variety of instruments to use for biopsy including forceps, brush, needle, needle brush, and curette. Various other less-standard techniques have been described such suction catheter biopsy [130]. If a cytology brush is to be used to sample a peripheral lesion, it should be used before the transbronchial biopsy is performed, so as not to contaminate the airway with blood that may later cover the brush [121]. Some have suggested that BAL with 100 to 200 mL normal saline increases the yield for peripheral lesions as compared to brushings [131,132]. The needle brush, which combines the advantages of the brush and a needle, offers the highest yield of any technique used to sample a lesion [133]. Ultrathin FOB has been proposed to increase the yield of transbronchial biopsies. This involves passage of a 1.8- to 2.2-mm scope through a standard bronchoscope, allowing viewing of 10 to 12 generations of bronchi [134]. Although specimens cannot be collected through the ultrathin bronchoscope, preliminary visualization may result in increased success of biopsy. TBNA biopsy of the peripheral nodule produces a higher yield as compared to standard transbronchial forceps biopsy [135,136]. The addition of TBNA to transbronchial forceps biopsies, washings, and brushings increases a yield from 48 to 69% [135].

## Lung masses and mediastinal adenopathy

Lung cancer is the most common fatal malignancy in the United States. Its prevalence would explain why, in a recent survey of North American bronchoscopists, the presence of a mass on a chest radiograph was the most frequent indication for bronchoscopy [9]. From the bronchoscopist's viewpoint, masses can be divided into those centrally and those peripherally located [137]. Central masses or their effects on the central airways, such as extrinsic obstruction, may often be directly visualized through the bronchoscope. Endobronchial lesions may be easily biopsied using forceps with three to four biopsies being considered sufficient for sampling [138,139]. The diagnostic yield of forceps biopsy of central lesions ranges from 55 to 85%, depending on the cell type [137]. Flat lesions located on the wall of the bronchus may be also be sampled using the spear forceps [137]. Cytologic analysis of central lesions can be conducted through the collection of washings and cytology brushes. The yield of bronchial washings for cytologic evaluation ranges from 62 to 79% [140–142]. If washings are to be collected, it is generally recommended that the collection be performed after the lesion has been biopsied to increase the number of cells within the washings [140]. The reported diagnostic yield of washings ranges from 62 to 79% [140–144]. Collection of cytology specimens with a cytology brush appears to be effective as well, especially when used in combination with biopsies. Diagnostic yield of brushings ranges from 62 to 78% [140,141,145–148]. TBNA is felt to be useful with submucosal lesions or lesions that cause extrinsic compression of the bronchus [149–152]. TBNA is also recommended for use in those lesions that are necrotic or likely to bleed [153,154]. The diagnostic yield for TBNA is increased with proper, immediate preparation of the specimen. The most important role of TBNA is in the staging of lung cancer, as discussed below, where it can be used to aspirate hilar or mediastinal lymph nodes [151,155,156].

Shure and Fedullo utilized TBNA plus wash, forceps, and brush to help diagnose patient with central endobronchial lesions with a diagnostic yield of 97% [157]. Dasgupta *et al.* preformed a prospective study of 55 patients with submucosal or peribronchial disease. They compared the diagnostic yield of TBNA versus combined diagnostic procedures of wash plus brush plus forceps biopsy. The diagnostic yield for TBNA plus the combined procedures was 96%, with that of TBNA alone being 95.6%, in patients with submucosal or peribronchial disease [158]. The diagnostic yield of transthoracic needle aspiration is twice that of transbronchial biopsies without regard for the size of the lesions [124,137]. However, FOB allows direct examination of the airway where an incidental endobronchial malignancy is found in 3.5% of the cases of lung cancer [48]. FOB also offers a significantly lower rate of complications versus that of thoracic needle aspiration (0.01 versus 32 to 36%) [129,132,159].

The use of TBNA versus TTNA (transthoracic needle aspiration) in the diagnosis of patients with central and peripheral lesions was evaluated by Wang *et al.* in a prospective study of 329 patients [160]. TBNA established the diagnosis of malignant or benign disease in 68.1% of patients overall. The yield for patients with mediastinal lesions was 89.3%, with that of peripheral lesions without mediastinal abnormality being 45.6%. TTNA established the diagnostic in 83.3% of those with mediastinal lesions versus 66.7% of those with lung lesions. This study concluded that TBNA should be the invasive procedure of choice in patients with central chest lesions. In patients without mediastinal of hilar involvement, TBNA should be considered first owing to the reasonable percentage of obtaining a diagnosis, ability to visualize the central airways to rule out synchronous lesion, and the low complication rate compared to that of TTNA.

The evaluation of patients who present with suspicious or malignant cells in the sputum is another important area for diagnostic bronchoscopy. While screening for lung cancer with sputum cytology is not currently recommended on a population scale, it is still a non-invasive and cost effective initial diagnostic technique for evaluating lung abnormalities, including lung masses [161]. The bronchoscopic evaluation of a patient with positive sputum cytology and a normal chest X ray is less well defined [162]. The stepwise approach starts with a thorough examination of the mouth, pharynx, and larynx. If negative, bronchoscopy is performed. If no endobronchial lesion is noted, a detailed analysis of each segment and subsegmental bronchi is conducted, including collecting separate cytology specimens from each area. Lam *et al.* performed autofluorescence bronchoscopy (AFB) in 82 patients with an exposure history to asbestos or diesel demonstrating a sensitivity for moderate to severe dysplasia and carcinoma in situ of 52% for white light bronchoscopy (WLB) and 86% autofluorescence bronchoscopy (AFB) with specificity of 81 and 79%, respectively [163]. Nakhosteen and Khanavkar show autofluorescence bronchoscopy to be 2.6 times more sensitive in the diagnosis of dysplasia and carcinoma *in situ* when compared with WLB [164].

In addition to the diagnosis of bronchogenic carcinoma, the application of flexible bronchoscopy plus the utilization of TBNA represents a powerful combination giving the bronchoscopist the ability to stage and diagnose the patient. If surgical resection of a suspected bronchogenic carcinoma is anticipated, staging should be performed even before the diagnosis is firmly established. This is most important in situations where a parenchymal mass is clinically suspected to be malignant and there is mediastinal or hilar adenopathy. In such situations, transtracheal or transbronchial needle aspiration and transbronchial needle biopsies could be used to sample the enlarged lymph nodes. This should be done before the parenchymal lesion is disturbed because of the risk of contaminating the bronchoscope with malignant cells. If the parenchymal lesion is disturbed, the malignant cells could then be mixed with the specimen from the lymph nodes. The patient would then be considered to have inoperable disease, eliminating the option of potentially curative surgery for the patient. Shure and Fedullo studied the role of TBNA of subcarinal lymph nodes in patients with clinical stage I lung cancer [152]. The transbronchial needle aspirate provided the only evidence of non-resectability in 69% of these patients, thus saving the patient a staging surgical procedure [152]. Overall, TBNA can preclude the need for staging surgery in one-half of the patients whose tumors are unresectable because of mediastinal invasion [165]. TBNA has a sensitivity of 50%, with a specificity of 96% and an accuracy of 78% [165]. Additional imaging guidance techniques such as endobronchial ultrasound (EBUS), CT, fluoroscopy, virtual bronchoscopy, and electromagnetic navigation bronchoscopy have all been used as an adjunct to TBNA to increase diagnostic yields. Convex probe (CP) or linear EBUS TBNA has reported up to 95% sensitivity, 100% specificity, and 97% accuracy [166,167]. Despite these recent advances, it is still standard practice to proceed to a mediastinoscopy or mediastinotomy if the transbronchial needle aspirate is negative.

Restaging bronchoscopy is particularly important in patients already undergoing cancer therapy and response may be best assessed with the use of combined evaluation. Imaging procedures such as CT and PET scans are now regularly used in the follow up of bronchogenic carcinoma. However, among patients having an endobronchial lesion, prior to initiation of treatment, a bronchoscopy tempers the degree of response as determined by the CT scan. Parrat and colleagues were able to assess tumor response in 86% of patients with a bronchoscope as compared to 99% with CT scan [168]. However, the same study noted that in 33 of 88 patients (39%), CT scan either over or under evaluated tumor response as compared to direct visualization and biopsy assessment via bronchoscopy. Thus, FOB and CT scan should be viewed as complementary studies in evaluating the response to chemotherapy. Patients who initially received a mediastinoscopy or mediastinotomy often require diagnosis of mediastinal abnormalities or growths during or after therapy. Since repeat mediastinoscopy is technically difficult, especially if radiation therapy was also used, TBNA is often the best procedure to restage the mediastinum.

Because of common risk factors, patients with head and neck cancer frequently have multiple synchronous or metachronous tumors of the aerodigestive system [169,170]. It is recommended that all patients with head and neck cancer undergo screening endoscopy at the time of diagnosis of the index lesion and at 2 years after diagnosis [171]. Screening panendoscopy, including head and neck examination, esophagoscopy, and bronchoscopy, results in a 2.5-fold increase in the diagnosis of synchronous tumors [171].

Esophageal cancer, because of its close proximity, frequently involves the respiratory tract. The degree of involvement has an impact on resectability. In a review of 525 bronchoscopies on patients with esophageal cancer, Choi and associates noted 91 (17.3%) had impingement of the

airway, whereas 87 (16.6%) had direct invasion through the respiratory mucosa [172,173]. Although the surgical implications of the latter group are obvious, bronchoscopy has its shortcomings in patients found to have a normal airway or simple compression without obvious invasion. Seven percent of the "normal" and 20% of the "compression" patients have frank invasion at the time of surgery (62%).

The lung is frequently involved with metastatic carcinoma. Bronchoscopy plays an important role in the evaluation of these patients. In a report of 111 patients with metastatic disease, Argyros and Torrington noted that 44 patients (39.6%) had abnormal bronchoscopic findings [174]. Patients who present with cough, hemoptysis, and chest pain and those with localized wheeze or rhonchi are more likely to have abnormal findings on bronchoscopy [174,175]. Additionally, abnormality is more likely to occur if atelectasis is present on chest X ray [174]. Malignancies most likely to have endobronchial metastases include renal cell carcinoma, the adenocarcinomas, melanoma, sarcoma, Kaposi's sarcoma, and lymphoma [174].

## Therapeutic bronchoscopy

The roots of endoscopy as noted previously by Hippocrates is in the treatment of patients suffering. This ability markedly expanded in 1897, when Gustov Kilian reported the inspection of the tracheobronchial tree with a report of extraction of foreign bodies, most notably a chicken bone [1]. In the new millennium, we have seen the emphasis on bronchology come full circle. The introduction of the flexible bronchoscope has greatly expanded the role of the bronchoscope in clinical practice. The therapeutic applications of the bronchoscope are listed in Table 7.2. Frequently, the diagnostic and therapeutic applications of the bronchoscope occur simultaneously. The therapeutic applications of the flexible bronchoscope will be further detailed in later chapters in this text, but are briefly outlined in the following sections.

### Foreign body aspiration and removal
Aspiration of a foreign body served as the impetus for the first bronchoscopy [1]. The bronchoscope continues to play a major role in this entity, avoiding the need for major surgical procedures. Older children and adults can often provide a reliable history of foreign body aspiration. However, in younger children, and occasionally in adults, a clear history of aspiration may not be available. Pasaoglu and colleagues noted that 48% of 822 children gave a clear statement of aspiration [176]. Although radio-opaque objects can be detected by X-ray examination, radiolucent objects present with normal chest X ray or with focal hyperinflation, infiltrate, or atelectasis [176]. Traditionally, the rigid bronchoscope has been preferred, with successful removal in 85%

**Table 7.2** Indications for therapeutic bronchoscopy

Pulmonary toilet
Removal of foreign bodies
Removal of obstructive endobronchial tissue
   Malignant
      Brachytherapy
      Laser
      Cryotherapy
      Electrosurgery/ argon plasma coagulation
      Photodynamic therapy
   Non-malignant
Stent placement
Bronchoalveolar lavage
Aspiration of cysts
   Mediastinal
   Bronchogenic cysts
Drainage of abscesses
Lobar collapse
Intralesional injection
Thoracic trauma
Bronchoscopic bronchopleural fistula closure techniques
Airway maintenance (tamponade for bleeding)
Research indications
   Bronchoscopic lung volume reduction
   Gene therapy
   Bronchial thermoplasty

of the cases [177]. However, similar success has been reported with the FOB with lower morbidity and mortality [178,179]. As training of new pulmonologists offers increasingly less experience in the use of the rigid scope, the flexible scope will be used more and more to remove foreign bodies. The flexible scope offers the advantage of greater access to the periphery. It can also be used in patients with an unstable neck or those on mechanical ventilation. Various instruments for extraction are available for the flexible bronchoscope. Basket retrieval devices, three-pronged foreign-body forceps, endobronchial balloons, and cryoprobes have all been used successfully with the flexible bronchoscope for foreign body extraction. If sufficient time has passed since the aspiration, the foreign body may be completely surrounded by granulation tissue. The granuloma should be removed and dissected carefully to find the foreign body.

## Pulmonary toilet

Pulmonary toilet is probably the most common therapeutic application of the bronchoscope. This is commonly required in patients who have an impaired cough mechanism from a variety of causes or excessive sloughing of the endobronchial mucosa, as seen in airway burn patients [180]. Generally, the scope with the largest working channel is preferred to enhance removal of the secretions. Caution should always be exercised when the procedure is per-

formed to ensure that the risk of nosocomial infection is outweighed by the benefit of clearing the secretions and mucus.

## Electrosurgery and argon plasma coagulation

In addition to serving as a vehicle for the delivery of laser light and radiation catheters, the bronchoscope can also be used to deliver electricity for electrocautery. This is performed by the application of heat generated by an electrical current. This may be applied in either a contact or non-contact mode. Traditional contact electrosurgical modalities have been utilized for decades in surgery and now may be applied through various instruments developed for the flexible bronchoscope. A more recent addition to the performance of flexible bronchoscopy is the introduction of argon plasma coagulation (APC). APC utilizes ionized argon to produce an electrical current to the target site. This is applied in a non-contact technique and most frequently is used for endobronchial coagulation and debulking of friable or bleeding endobronchial lesions or tumors [181]. In comparison with laser photoresection, electrosurgery offers the advantage of a more superficial application of energy to the mucosal wall, lower startup cost, and shorter procedure time [182]. Despite the decreased risk for deeper penetration of the energy with the electrosurgical techniques, laser, electrocautery, and APC all have an inherent risk for endobronchial fire and oxygen levels must always be below 0.4 $F_1O_2$ prior to use of the thermal energy in the airways. Flammable material in the airway (i.e. endotracheal tube, silicone stents, covered stents, etc.) must be well removed from the area of electrocautery or APC use to avoid airway fires. As APC uses a jet of argon gas to carry the electrical charge to the endobronchial lesion, there have been reports of gas embolism as a result of APC use and perforation of the bronchial wall [183]. Animal studies indicate gas flow level to be proportional to the risk for gas embolism but further study to determine the optimal flow rate to minimize this risk is still needed [184].

## Cryosurgery

Although bronchoscopic cryosurgery has been available since the 1970s [185], its use has been rather limited. Its utility in comparison with laser and brachytherapy is a matter of some debate. Proponents argue that cryotherapy is safer because of the lack of risk of bronchial wall perforation and endobronchial ignition, no limitation of supplemental oxygen that may be used during the procedure, there is no danger to the operator's eyes, and a lower startup cost [186,187]. Additionally, cartilaginous, connective, and fibrous tissues are inherently resistant to the cryotherapy while mucous membranes, granulation tissue, and tumor are sensitive to its effects allowing for selective destruction of the abnormal tissue [188]. The pros are balanced by those who note that the cryotherapy may require several follow-up bronchoscopies to remove tissue slough and that there is a delay between application of the treatment and the establishment of maximal airway patency [189]. Mathur *et al.* studied the application of this technique with a cryoprobe through the flexible bronchoscope in 22 patients [190]. Twenty patients had malignant tracheobronchial obstruction and two had stenosis after lung transplantation. All therapy was carried out under conscious sedation in a bronchoscopy suite. Eighteen of the malignant endobronchial lesions were completely removed, with two patients experiencing easily treated bronchcospasm. Studies continue to demonstrate the effectiveness of cryosurgery for inoperable endobronchial tumors, including recanalization of the airway on the initial procedure with the cryoprobe [191]. As noted in the foreign body removal section above, a flexible cryoprobe can be extremely useful in removal of any porous object from the airway as well as large blood clots or mucus plugs.

## Laser photoresection

Indications and contraindications for the appropriate use of endoscopic laser therapy are dependent upon the anatomic characteristics of the obstructing lesion and clinical condition [192] (Table 7.3).

The application of laser to an obstructive lesion allows rapid re-establishment of airway patency, which in turn allows ventilation of the distal lung and drainage of postobstructive pneumonia. Coagulative effects of the laser energy can be used to palliate patients with hemorrhagic endobron-

chial tumors. Several reports have demonstrated improved airway patency in 79 to 92% of patients [193–195]. Laser light can only be applied to the visible endobronchial part of the lesion and a significant amount of extraluminal mass tumor in the case of malignancy may be left behind. This extraluminal tumor may be amenable to adjuvant radiotherapy, either via external beam or bronchoscopically administered brachytherapy. Once a lumen has been re-established, stent placement may delay reocclusion. Laser treatments may be used multiple times as the tumor grows back into the lumen. The complications of laser include hypoxemia, hemorrhage, perforation into adjacent structures, and endobronchial ignition of equipment [190,196]. The therapeutic role of laser is more apparent in the less commonly occurring benign airway obstructions. Its use in benign endobronchial tumor, such as endobronchial hamartoma, has been well described and can obviate the need for more aggressive surgical resection [193,194,197]. Other causes of benign airway obstruction treatable by laser photoresection include tracheal granulomas (e.g. suture granuloma), tracheal stenosis (e.g. postintubation injury), endobronchial amyloidosis, syphilis gumma, and osteoplastic tracheopathy [193,194,198], as well as closure of a bronchopleural fistula [199,200].

## Photodynamic therapy

This process requires the injection of a hematoporphyrin derivative, which serves as a photosensitizer. The subsequent delivery of laser light through the bronchoscope activates a hematoporphyrin derivative, resulting in tissue necrosis. Patients with inoperable carcinoma and needing definitive treatment of early lung cancer or palliation of unresectable bronchogenic carcinoma causing tracheobronchial obstruction are candidates [201,202]. Photodynamic therapy has also been seen to benefit control of tracheal papillomatosis [203]. Abramson has noted a reduction in the growth rate of endobronchial polyps in patients with juvenile laryngotracheobronchial papillomatosis [204] with preliminary analysis of a prospective trial of photodynamic therapy in patients with juvenile laryngotracheobronchial papillomatosis indicating that 50% have been disease free for at least 1 year [205]. Complications may include sunburn to skin exposed to bright light, hemoptysis, and production of necrotic tissue slough obstructing the airways. For over a decade, this technique has demonstrated potential for palliative treatment in patients with unresectable endobronchial tumor and more recently has shown some success in therapy for curative intent both alone or with external beam radiation in selected patients [206–210].

## Brachytherapy

The presence of an endobronchial obstruction, whether due to malignant cancer, benign tumor, or other benign lesion, often requires urgent medical attention. Bronchoscopy

**Table 7.3** Contraindications to laser bronchoscopy

| Anatomic contraindications | Clinical contraindications |
|---|---|
| Extrinsic obstruction without endobronchial lesion | Candidate for surgical resection |
| Lesion incursion into bordering major vascular structure (e.g. pulmonary artery) with potential for fistula formation | Unfavorable short-term prognosis without hope for palliation of symptoms |
| Lesion incursion into bordering esophagus with potential for fistula formation | Inability to undergo conscious sedation or general anesthesia |
| Lesion incursion into bordering mediastinum with potential for fistula formation | Coagulation disorder |
| | Total obstruction more than 4 to 6 weeks |

Table courtesy of: Turner JF, Wang KP. Endobronchial laser therapy. *Clin Chest Med* 1999; **20**: 107–22.

offers a unique means of delivering local treatment for these lesions. Large, malignant endobronchial tumors can be treated by a variety of methods depending on the characteristics of the tumor and previous treatment. Because the endobronchial tumor represents only "the tip of the iceberg", with substantial submucosal and parenchymal tumor load, external beam radiation is a preferred modality to attack the entire tumor burden. When external beam radiation cannot be provided because of the danger of exposure to adjacent structures, brachytherapy offers an alternative mode of radiation delivery. Both high does (>10 Gy/h) and low dose (<2 Gy/h) are utilized with a 60% response resulting in relief of symptoms, possibly for months [201]. Paradelo and coworkers, using a bronchoscopically positioned catheter to deliver radioactive seeds to the area of obstruction caused by tumor, noted symptomatic improvement in 30 of 34 patients (88%) [211]. Radiographic improvement or stability was noted in 22 of 24 patients (92%) [211]. Complications of brachytherapy include necrotic cavitation, fistula formation, and hemorrhage [212]. Implantation of radioactive seeds into inoperable lung tumor has also had some limited success in recent case series and may provide another modality for brachytherapy with a more precise delivery of the radiation dose and perhaps a decrease in the complication rate [213].

## Bronchoalveolar lavage

Bronchoalveolar lavage (BAL) has several well-known diagnostic applications, mostly in the diagnosis of infectious or diffuse lung disease. BAL does have a therapeutic role in bronchoscopy. In patients with pulmonary alveolar proteinosis, BAL plays a unique diagnostic and therapeutic role. The diagnosis by analysis of the lavage fluid can obviate the need for an open lung biopsy. Therapeutically, the lavage allows mechanical removal of intra-alveolar phospholipids [214,215]. Approximately two-thirds of patients will require lung washings. About 50% require only a single treatment, with multiple lavages necessary in other patients with pulmonary alveolar proteinosis [215,216]. There are few relative contraindications to BAL which include $FEV_1$ less than 1 liter, asthma with moderate airway obstruction, hypercapnia and hypoxemia which cannot be easily corrected, serious cardiac arrhythmia, hemodynamic instability, or bleeding diathesis [217].

## Aspiration of cysts

Bronchogenic cysts present a diagnostic and therapeutic dilemma, often in otherwise healthy, asymptomatic patients. Often surgery is required for histologic confirmation or to relieve compression on adjacent structures. However, there are several reports of successful diagnosis and therapeutic decompression of cysts using transbronchial needle aspiration [218,219].

## Drainage of lung abscesses

Lung abscesses are treated with antibiotics and adequate drainage. Drainage is usually attempted with chest physiotherapy and postural drainage. Surgical intervention is generally considered to be the next step in patients who do not respond to these drainage maneuvers [220,221]. However, the bronchoscope can be used not only to obtain culture material, but also to effectively drain the cavity [94,222]. Bronchoscopic placement of an indwelling drainage catheter has been attempted in a small number of patients with good results [95,223]. This technique not only allows avoidance of surgery, but also circumvents the problem of inadequate drainage that may occur when the catheter is removed at the end of the bronchoscopic session. The indwelling catheter not only maintains a patent route for drainage, but can also be used to irrigate the cavity when spontaneous drainage ceases [95]. Care must be exercised in using this technique to avoid spillage of the abscess fluid in the airway.

## Stents

Most of the above methods of removing airway obstruction are limited in their application to only endobronchial lesions. In situations where the airway is compromised by extrinsic compression or by loss of tracheal cartilaginous rings, placement of a prosthetic stent may be able to provide patency. Stents have also been used in patients with anastomotic stenosis following sleeve resection or lung transplant [116,224,225]. Stent placement may be performed by means of either the rigid or flexible scope [226,227] and is subsequently discussed more fully later in this book.

## Balloon dilation

Dilation of stenosis and coring out of central obstruction caused by benign or malignant disease of the airway has long been practiced with the rigid bronchoscope [201,228,229]. The flexible bronchoscope has also been demonstrated to allow effective balloon dilation. Hautmann *et al.* reported on 78 patients who underwent a total of 126 dilatation procedures for malignant tracheobronchial disease [230]. Indications included symptomatic stenosis of the tracheobronchial tree (dyspnea or stridor), retention pneumonia, atelectasis, retention of secretions, or lung abscess. The two lung abscess noted both resolved with improvement in atelectasis, pneumonia, and dyspnea in 62, 92, and 37% respectively. Complications consisted of one fatality due to hemoptysis and minor bleeding which did not require specific therapy. Balloon dilatation has also been used in successfully with flexible bronchoscopy and laser therapy in the treatment of benign laryngotracheostenosis (LTS) thus avoiding tracheal surgery and a significant proportion requiring only one dilation [231]. Balloon dilation has also played an integral role in the evolution of expandable metallic endobronchial stent deployment [232]. Dilation equipment typically includes a standard flexible bronchoscope with a balloon catheter ranging in sizes from 8 to 16 French and a balloon length of 2.5 to 4.0 cm [233].

## Fistula

Fistulas are known to occur between the airway and its surrounding structure. Bronchopleural fistulas are the most common and generally occur after surgery. Bronchopleural fistulas are also associated with tuberculosis, pneumonia, empyema, and lung abscess [234,235]. Proximally located fistulas may be directly visualized. However, localization of fistulas distal to the reach of the flexible bronchoscope are more challenging. In such situations an occluding balloon is systematically passed into each bronchial segment and inflated. When the correct segment is located, inflation of the balloon will result in a reduction in the air leak [234,236]. Once localized, the bronchoscope can also be used therapeutically to seal the leak with a variety of tissue sealants or endobronchial valves [234, 237–240].

Tracheoesophageal fistulas may be the result of a congenital defect or, more commonly in the adult, related to a malignancy of the aerodigestive system and its treatment. The most frequent symptom indicating the presence of a fistula is cough, especially triggered by swallowing or being in the decubitus position [241]. The overall yield of bronchoscopic detection of a tracheal esophageal fistula is 83% [241]. In addition to this diagnostic role, bronchoscopy performed in conjunction with esophagoscopy allows preoperative analysis and planning for surgical correction.

Aortobronchial fistula represents an uncommon but often lethal problem. The most common setting of aortobronchial fistula is prior surgical repair of the aorta [242]. Other causes include syphilitic and atherosclerotic aneurysms and tuberculous involvement of the aortic wall [242]. Aortograms frequently fail to demonstrate the fistula. Graeber and coworkers reported only one of five aortograms to be positive [242]. Bronchoscopy is diagnostic in 50% of cases (seven of 14 cases) [243]. The bronchoscopist must understand the inherent danger of performing bronchoscopy in the presence of an aortobronchial fistula. Manipulation of the fistula or its overlying clot, may precipitate massive hemorrhage [242]. Thus, one must be prepared to quickly isolate the hemorrhaging lung and proceed to immediate surgical repair.

## Endotracheal intubation

Traditionally, the laryngoscope is used to visualize the glottis for correct intubation of the airway. However, in difficult cases a fiberoptic bronchoscope offers an excellent alternative. Situations where the need for flexible bronchoscopy may be anticipated include patients with either fixed or unstable cervical spines, ankylosis of the temporal mandibular joint, and patients with large oral pharyngeal tumors [244]. Additionally, the fiberoptic bronchoscope may be emergently needed when the glottis is unexpectedly difficult

to visualize. Another role of the fiberoptic bronchoscope in the management of airways is confirmation of correct endotracheal tube position. Although a portable chest X ray is frequently adequate to confirm position, a few settings are better suited for the bronchoscope. These include the obese patient where radiographic penetration of the mediastinum is insufficient and in unstable patients where a delay is anticipated in obtaining a chest X ray. Some have also advocated the use of the bronchoscope to check endotracheal tube position in the pediatric patient to decrease the radiation dose from routine chest X ray [245].

Endobronchial intubation and tracheostomy are potential sources for iatrogenic airway injury [246]. Direct trauma to the vocal cords during passage of the endotracheal tube can lead to scarring of the anterior commissure. The pressure at the various contact points along the path of the endotracheal tube results in ischemic ulceration [247]. Frequently, these injuries heal properly. However, with prolonged injury, cricoarytenoid joint fixation and scarring of the posterior commissure can occur [248,249]. Overinflation of the cuff leads to circumferential ischemic necrosis of the trachea. The result may be loss of cartilaginous support and tracheomalacia or formation of fibrous stenosis during the repair process [250]. The transmission of cuff pressure through the tracheal wall may injure the recurrent laryngeal nerve, with a resultant vocal cord paresis [247]. Although tracheostomy eliminates the risk of glottic and subglottic injury, the stoma site is subject to stenosis by granulation, scarring, and contraction [247]. Bronchoscopy and laryngoscopy allow full anatomic assessment of these injuries and the institution of proper therapeutic maneuvers. Both the flexible and rigid scope can be used to assess the airway proximal to the narrow airway. However, in situations of tight stricture, examination distal to the lesion may not be possible with the flexible scope. In these situations a rigid bronchoscope, which is capable of delivering mechanical ventilation, may be used to complete the airway examination. The bronchoscopist should be aware that any manipulation of a critically narrowed stenosis may precipitate complete obstruction by increasing secretions, hemorrhage, or edema. Thus, one should be prepared to perform immediate dilation.

Bronchoscopy may be used to assess the proper length and placement of transtracheal oxygen catheters. Patients receiving transtracheal oxygen therapy may have a catheter that has retroflexed through the vocal cord or is too long, thus producing irritation and traumatizing the carina or bronchi. Although these conditions may be assessed by chest X ray, direct visualization with the bronchoscope may be needed. Irritation from the transtracheal oxygen catheter may also lead to granulation tissue formation along the cutaneotracheal tract, requiring bronchoscopic visualization and treatment. The transtracheal catheter also serves as a nidus for large mucous plug formation, which may require bronchoscopic evaluation and removal [251].

## Gene therapy

In 1996, the NIH evaluated the current development of gene therapy with the recommendation that additional bench research was required in the hope that future efficacy in human therapy could be developed [252]. Gene therapy is a technique whereby cells are modified outside or inside the target tissue by means of non-viral or viral vectors [253]. Although still a research tool in pulmonary medicine, the introduction into the target tumors of these agents may best be accomplished by flexible bronchoscopy [254,255].

## Bronchial thermoplasty

Recently, studies have been targeting therapy for medically refractory asthma by bronchoscopically administering radiofrequency (RF) energy to the bronchial walls and destroying the underlying smooth muscle that bronchoconstricts the airways in asthma [256,257]. While the initial Asthma Intervention Research trial (AIR) and Research in Severe Asthma trial (RISA) study results appeared to improve asthma control over a 6 to 12-month period, the more severe asthmatics had significantly more postprocedural complications and hospitalizations than the control group [256,257]. Further studies that include sham procedures are needed to minimize the influence of placebo affect in the results.

## Bronchoscopic lung volume reduction (BLVR)

Various bronchoscopic techniques are currently being studied in efforts to duplicate some of the positive outcomes that selected emphysema patients in the National Emphysema Treatment Trial (NETT) of 2003 experienced with surgical lung volume reduction surgery without the morbidity of a thoracic surgical procedure [258]. Currently, these techniques fall into three categories: endobronchial valves, airway bypass systems, and biological remodeling. The endobronchial valves are inserted into airways leading to overinflated and emphysematous lung with the intent to allow air and secretions to exit the distal portion of lung but not allow air to enter, thus reducing the volume of that area of lung or collapsing it completely [259,260]. The airway bypass technique essentially attempts to reduce lung volume by using a radiofrequency balloon catheter to create an "airway" passage from a central airway to the hyperinflated portion of lung and allow for exist of the trapped air into the larger airways [261]. The third main technique is biological remodeling, which attempts to collapse the areas of hyperinflated lung using a biological sealant that is administered through the bronchoscope into the target areas of lung [262]. The sealant collapses the lung section permanently at the parenchymal and alveolar level [262]. All of these techniques are still under evaluation, but the initial results from some of the earlier phase trials suggest that there will likely be a role for the bronchoscopic treatment of emphysema in the near future [263].

## Contraindications

Bronchoscopy has been shown to be a safe procedure since its early beginning [264,265]. The American Thoracic Society guidelines give only four contraindications to bronchoscopy [266]. Of these, three (absence of informed consent, inexperienced operator, and inadequate facilities) are applicable to any medical intervention. The fourth contraindication is the inability to adequately oxygenate the patient for the procedure. Additionally, when considering rigid bronchoscopy, the patient must not have an unstable neck, severely ankylosed cervical spine, or restricted temporomandibular joint [20]. For patients on mechanical ventilation, flexible FOB is preferred to rigid bronchoscopy [266].

Although generally a safe procedure, the risks of complications of bronchoscopy are increased in the presence of several conditions (Table 7.4). The risk is especially increased in the presence of malignant cardiac arrhythmia, severe refractory hypoxemia, or severe bleeding diathesis (if biopsy is anticipated) [266,267]. The safety of fiberoptic bronchoscopy in patient with underlying coronary artery disease has been reviewed by several authors. Matot *et al.* studied the incidence of myocardial ischemia in sedated patients undergoing fiberoptic bronchoscopy. In these 29 patients who

**Table 7.4** Contraindications to bronchoscopy

*Absolute contraindications*
  Inadequate oxygenation during the procedure
  For rigid bronchoscopy:
    Unstable neck
    Severely ankylosed cervical spine
    Restricted temporomandibular joint

*Relative contraindications*
  Malignant arrhythmia
  Unstable cardiac status
  Refractory hypoxemia
  Bleeding diathesis or severe thrombocytopenia (if biopsy is anticipated)

*Factors associated with increased risk of complications*
  Uncooperative patient
  Recent or unstable angina
  Unstable asthma
  Moderate to severe hypoxemia
  Hypercarbia
  Uremia
  Thrombocytopenia
  Pulmonary hypertension
  Lung abscess
  Immunosuppression
  Superior vena cava obstruction
  Debility, advanced age, or malnutrition
  Recent use of clopidogrel

were 50 years of age or older undergoing elective bronchoscopy [268], there was a significant rise in heart rate with 17% demonstrating myocardial ischemia. Of note is that only one of the five patients demonstrating ST segment changes had a history of myocardial infarction and angina pectoris. Subsequently, a study by Dunagan *et al.* in patients undergoing FOB within 10 days of a myocardial infarction showed no episodes of chest pain or ischemic events and no significant increase in major complications [269]. The implication of these and other studies indicate that while FOB remains an extremely safe procedure in patients with underlying coronary artery disease, the indications to perform bronchoscopy should be critically reviewed in all patients with cardiac risk factors [270–274].

The importance of bleeding diathesis depends on the bronchoscopic procedure. Airway examination and BAL can generally be performed safely. To decrease the risk of nasal hemorrhage, oral rather than nasal intubation is preferred. If biopsy or resection is anticipated, the coagulopathy should be corrected. Uncorrected thrombocytopenia (less than 50,000/dL) or platelet dysfunction in the setting of uremia, are considered to be relative contraindications to bronchoscopy [265,275]. Procedures that involve large biopsies using a shearing or tearing force without direct visualization of the biopsy site, such as transbronchial lung biopsy, involve the highest risk. Proximal airway biopsies also carry an increased risk for substantial bleeding, as they are closer to the larger vessels. In the setting of bleeding diathesis, if TBNA can be performed, instead of a transbronchial forceps biopsy, less bleeding can be expected [247]. However, when absolutely necessary, transbronchial biopsy can be successfully obtained with lower platelet counts. We have performed a number of transbronchial biopsies on immunocompromised bone marrow transplant recipients with platelet counts of less than 20,000/dL who were not candidates for open lung biopsy. All patients received platelet transfusion during the procedure and the flexible bronchoscope was firmly wedged into a segment before the biopsy was obtained. After the biopsy, suction was turned off and the scope was left in the wedged position to tamponade any bleeding for at least 5 minutes. Three to four biopsies were obtained from each patient without complication. Transbronchial lung biopsy in the setting of the commonly prescribed platelet inhibitor, clopidogrel, has been shown to significantly increase intraprocedure bleeding and patients are advised to discontinue this medication prior to biopsy [276]. Again, this is not an absolute contraindication but if time allows, stopping the clopidogrel approximately 5 to 7 days prior to the procedure should minimize the risk for bleeding.

In patients with baseline poor respiratory function, the risk for pneumothorax from biopsies or instrumentation during the procedure should be considered and may be a relative contraindication in selected patients. The use of fluoroscopy to visualize the distal end of instruments during the procedure is advised to limit proximity to the pleural surface. The incidence of pneumothorax varies among institutions, individual bronchoscopists, type of instruments used, biopsies performed, as well as imaging used for biopsy guidance. Overall, the incidence of iatrogenic pneumothorax from bronchoscopy is low and mortality from this complication, even in severe chronic obstructive pulmonary disease patients, is low [277,278].

## References

1 Nakhosten J. History of bronchoscopy: removal of tracheobronchial foreign body, Gustav Killian. *J Bronchology* 1994; **1**: 76.

2 Jackson C. Bronchoscopy; past, present and future. *N Engl J Med* 1928; **199**: 759–63.

3 Ikeda S, Yawai N, Ishikawa S. Flexible bronchofiberscope. *Keio J Med* 1968; **17**: 1–133.

4 Miyazawa T. History of the flexible bronchoscopy. In: Bollger CT, Mathur PN, eds. *Interventional Bronchoscopy. Progress in Respiratory Research*, vol. 30. Basel: Karger; 2000: 16–21.

5 Popavich J, Kvale PA, Ikanhornit L. Diagnostic accuracy of multiple biopsies from flexible fiberoptic bronchoscopy. A comparison of central vs. peripheral carcinoma. *Am Rev Respir Dis* 1982; **125**: 521–3.

6 Chur D, Asterita RW. Carcinoma presenting as endobronchial mass. Optimum number of biopsies specimens for diagnosis. *Chest* 1983; **83**: 865–7.

7 Wang KP, Terry PB, Marsh B. Bronchoscopic needle aspiration biopsy of paratracheal tumors. *Am Rev Respir Dis* 1978, **118**: 17–21.

8 Wang KP, Marsh B, Summer DR, *et al.* Transbronchial needle aspiration for diagnosis for lung cancer. *Chest* 1981; **80**: 48–50.

9 Prakash UBS, Stubbs SE. Bronchoscopy in North America: The ACCP survey. *Chest* 1991; **100**: 1660–75.

10 Poe RH, Israel RH, Utell MJ, Hall WJ. Chronic cough: bronchoscopy or pulmonary function testing? *Am Rev Respir Dis* 1982; **126**: 160–2.

11 Rosen MJ. Overview of pulmonary complications. *Clin Chest Med* 1996; **17**: 621–31.

12 Pratter MR, Brightling CE, Boulet, LP, Irwin RS. An empiric integrative approach to the management of cough. *Chest* 2006; **129**: 222–31S.

13 Hyde L, Hyde CI. Clinical manifestations of lung cancer. *Chest* 1974; **65**: 299–306.

14 Decalmer S, Woodcock A, Greaves M, *et al.* Airway abnormalities at flexible bronchoscopy in patients with chronic cough. *Eur Respir J* 2007; **30**: 1138–42.

15 Lam S, MacAulary C, Hung J, *et al.* Detection of dysplasia and carcinoma in situ using a lung imaging fluorescence endoscopy (LIFE) device. *J Thorac Cardiovasc Surg* 1993; **105**: 1035–40.

16 Kennedy TC, McWilliams A, Edell E, *et al.* Bronchial intraepithelial neoplasia/early central airways lung cancer: ACCP evidence-based clinical practice guidelines (2nd edition). *Chest* 2007; **132**: 221S–33S.

17 Lam B, Lam SY, Wong MP, *et al.* Sputum cytology examination followed by autofluorescence bronchoscopy: a practical way of

identifying early stage lung cancer in central airway. *Lung Cancer* 2009; **64**: 289–94.

18 Aslan AT, Kiper N, Dogru D, *et al.* Diagnostic value of flexible bronchoscopy in children with persistent and recurrent wheezing. *Allergy Asthma Proc* 2005; **26**: 483–6.

19 Schellhase DE, Fawcett DD, Schutze GE, *et al.* Clinical utility of flexible bronchoscopy and bronchoalveolar lavage in young children with recurrent wheezing. *J Pediatr* 1998; **132**: 312–18.

20 Wood RE. The emerging role of flexible bronchoscopy in pediatrics. *Clin Chest Med* 2001; **22**: 311–17.

21 Irwin RS. ACCP-SEEK board review question of the month. *Chest* 2000; **117**: 892–3.

22 Mehra PK, Woessner KM. Dyspnea, wheezing, and airways obstruction: is it asthma? *Allergy Asthma Proc* 2005; **26**: 319–22.

23 Kryger M, Bode F, Antic R, Anthonisen N. Diagnosis of obstruction of the upper and central airways. *Am J Med* 1976; **61**: 85–93.

24 O'Hollaren MT, Everts EC. Evaluating the patient with stridor. *Ann Allergy* 1991; **67**: 301–5.

25 Prakash UBS. Bronchoscopy. In: Bone RC, ed. *Pulmonary and Critical Care Medicine*. St. Louis: Mosby-Yearbook; 1993, F(5): 1–18.

26 Mancuso RF. Pediatric otolaryngology. Stridor in neonates. *Pediatr Clin North Am* 1996; **43**: 1339–55.

27 Langford CA, Van Waes C. Life-threatening complications of autoimmune disease. *Rheum Dis Clin North Am* 1997; **23**: 345–63.

28 Parnell FW, Brandenburg JH. Vocal cord paralysis: a review of 100 cases. *Laryngoscope* 1970; **80**: 1036–45.

29 Terris DJ, Arnstein DP, Nguyen HH. Contemporary evaluation of unilateral vocal cord paralysis. *Otolaryngol Head Neck Surg* 1992; **107**: 84–90.

30 Mlcak RP, Suman OE, Herndon DN. Respiratory management of inhalation injury. *Burns* 2007; **33**: 2–13.

31 Hunt JL, Agee RN, Pruitt BA. Fiberoptic bronchoscopy in acute inhalation injury. *J Trauma* 1975; **15**: 641.

32 Moylan JA. Smoke inhalation and burn injury. *Surg Clin North Am* 1980; **60**: 1533–40.

33 Gore MA, Joshi AR, Nagarajan G, *et al.* Virtual bronchoscopy for diagnosis of inhalation injury in burnt patients. *Burns* 2004; **30**: 165–8.

34 Marek K, Piotr W, Stanislaw S, *et al.* Fibreoptic bronchoscopy in routine clinical practice in confirming the diagnosis and treatment of inhalation burns. *Burns* 2007; **33**: 554–60.

35 Raoof S, Mehrishi S, Prakash UBS. Role of bronchoscopy in modern medical intensive care unit. *Clin Chest Med* 2001; **22**: 241–61.

36 Masanes MJ, Legendre C, Lioret N, *et al.* Fiberoptic bronchoscopy for the early diagnosis of subglottal inhalation injury. *J Trauma* 1994; **36**: 59–67.

37 Endorf FW, Gamelli RL. Inhalation injury, pulmonary perturbations, and fluid resuscitation. *J Burn Care Res* 2007; **28**: 80–3.

38 Moylan JA, Adib K, Birnbaum M. Fiberoptic bronchoscopy following thermal injury. *Surg Gynecol Obstet* 1975; **140**: 541–3.

39 Freitag L, Firusian N, Stamatis G, Greschuchuna D. Bronchoscopy: the role of bronchoscopy in pulmonary complications due to mustard gas inhalation. *Chest* 1991; **100**: 1436–41.

40 Thompson AB, Teschler H, Rennard SI. Pathogenesis, evaluation, and therapy for massive hemoptysis. *Clin Chest Med* 1992; **13**: 69.

41 Johnston H, Reisz G. Changing spectrum of hemoptysis. Underlying causes in 148 patients undergoing diagnostic flexible fiberoptic bronchoscopy. *Arch Intern Med* 1989; **149**: 1666.

42 Santiago S, Tobias J, Williams AJ. A reappraisal of the causes of hemoptysis. *Arch Intern Med* 1991; **151**: 2449.

43 Hirshberg B, Biran I, Glazer M, Kramer MR. Hemoptysis: Etiology, evaluation, and outcome in a tertiary referral hospital. *Chest* 1997; **112**: 440.

44 Lyons HA. Differential diagnosis of hemoptysis and its treatment. *Basics RD* 1976; **5**: 26–30.

45 Smiddy JF, Elliot RC. The evaluation of hemoptysis with fiberoptic bronchoscopy. *Chest* 1973; **92**: 77–82.

46 Prakash UBS. The use of the pediatric fiberoptic bronchoscope in adults. *Am Rev Respir Dis* 1985; **132**: 715–17.

47 Pursel SE, Lindskog GE. Hemoptysis: a clinical evaluation of 105 patients examined consecutively on a thoracic surgical service. *Am Rev Respir Dis* 1961; **84**: 329–36.

48 Gong H Jr, Salvatierra C. Clinical efficacy of early and delayed fiberoptic bronchoscopy in patients with hemoptysis. *Am Rev Respir Dis* 1981; **124**: 221–5.

49 Stoller JK. Diagnosis and management of massive hemoptysis: a review. *Respir Care* 1992; **37**: 564–81.

50 Jean-Baptiste E. Clinical assessment and management of massive hemoptysis. *Crit Care Med* 2000; **28**: 1642–6.

51 Freitag L. Development of a new balloon catheter for management of hemoptysis with bronchofiberscopes. *Chest* 1993; **103**: 593.

52 Saw E, Gottlieb L, Yokoyama T, *et al.* Flexible fiberoptic bronchoscopy and endobronchial tamponade in the management of massive hemoptysis. *Chest* 1976; **70**: 589–91.

53 Morice RC, Ece T, Ece F, *et al.* Endobronchial argon plasma coagulation for the treatment of hemoptysis and neoplastic airway obstruction. *Chest* 2001; **119**: 781–7.

54 Abner A. Approach to the patient who presents with superior vena cava obstruction. *Chest* 1993; **103**: 394S–7S.

55 Armstrong BA, Perez CA, Simpson JR, *et al.* Role of irradiation in the management of superior vena cava syndrome. *Int J Radiat Oncol Biol Phys* 1987; **13**: 531–9.

56 Chen JC, Bongard F, Klein SR. A contemporary perspective on superior vena cava syndrome. *Am J Surg* 1990; **160**: 207–11.

57 Ferrari LR, Bedford RF. General anesthesia prior to treatment of anterior mediastinal masses in pediatric cancer patients. *Anesthesiology* 1990; **72**: 991–5.

58 Yasufuku K, Chiyo M, Sekine Y, *et al.* Real-time endobronchial ultrasound-guided transbronchial needle aspiration of mediastinal and hilar lymph nodes. *Chest* 2004; **126**: 122–8.

59 Ovassapian A. The flexible bronchoscope: a tool of anesthesiologists. *Clin Chest Med* 2001; **22**: 281–99.

60 Hnatiuk OW, Corcoran PC, Sierra A. Spirometry in surgery for anterior mediastinal masses. *Chest* 2001; **120**: 1152–6.

61 Depaso WJ, Winterbauer RH. Interstitial lung disease. *Dis Mon* 1991; **37**: 61–133.

62 European Society of Pneumology Task Group on BAL. Clinical guidelines and indications for bronchoalveolar lavage (BAL): Report of the European Society of Pneumonology Task Group on BAL. *Eur Respir J* 1990; **3**: 937–76.

63 Goldstein RA, Rohatgi PK, Bergofsky EH, *et al.* Clinical role of bronchoalveolar lavage in adults with pulmonary disease. *Am Rev Respir Dis* 1990; **142**: 481–6.

64 Amin RS, Wert SE, Baughman RP, *et al.* Surfactant protein deficiency in familial interstitial lung disease. *J Pediatr* 2001; **139**: 85–92.

65 Chollet S, Soler P, Dournovo P, *et al.* The diagnosis of pulmonary histiocytosis X by immunodetection of Langerhan's cell in BALF. *Am J Pathol* 1984; **115**: 225–32.

66 Martin RJ, Coalsen JJ, Rogers RM, *et al.* Pulmonary alveolar proteinosis: the diagnosis by segmental lavage. *Am Rev Respir Dis* 1980; **121**: 819–25.

67 Helmers RA, Hunninghake GW. Broncho-alveolar lavage in the non-immunocompromised patient. *Chest* 1989; **96**: 1184–90.

68 Rossman MD, Kern JA, Elias JA, *et al.* Proliferative response of bronchoalveolar lymphocytes to beryllium, a test for chronic beryllium disease. *Ann Intern Med* 1988; **108**: 687–93.

69 Hunninghake GW, Crystal RG. Pulmonary sarcoidosis: a disorder mediated by excess helper T-lymphocyte activity at sites of disease activity. *N Engl J Med* 1981; **305**: 429–34.

70 Semenzato G. Current concepts on bronchoalveolar lavage cells in extrinsic allergic alveolitis. *Respiration* 1988; **54**: 59–65.

71 Studdy PR, Rudd RM, Gellert AR, *et al.* Bronchoalveolar lavage in the diagnosis of diffuse pulmonary shadowing. *Br J Dis Chest* 1984; **78**: 46–54.

72 Hunninghake GW, Kawanami O, Ferrans VJ, *et al.* Characterization of inflammatory and immune effector cells in the lung parenchyma of patients with interstitial lung disease. *Am Rev Respir Dis* 1981; **123**: 407.

73 Aguayo SM, Niccole SA, Martin RJ, *et al.* Is BAL eosinophilia clinically useful in the differential diagnosis of unexplained pulmonary infiltrates? *Am Rev Respir Dis* 1989; **139**: 385.

74 Pesci A, Bertorelli G, Manganelli P, *et al.* Bronchoalveolar lavage in chronic eosinophilic pneumonia: analysis of six cases in comparison with other interstitial lung diseases. *Respiration* 1988; **54**: 16–22.

75 Meyer KC. The role of bronchoalveolar lavage in interstitial lung disease. *Clin Chest Med* 2004; **25**: 637–49.

76 Nagai S, Izumi T. Bronchoalveolar lavage. Still useful in diagnosing sarcoidosis? *Clin Chest Med* 1997; **18**: 787–97.

77 Raghu G, Mageto YN, Lockhart D, *et al.* The accuracy of the clinical diagnosis of new-onset idiopathic pulmonary fibrosis and other interstitial lung disease: A prospective study. *Chest* 1999; **116**: 1168–74.

78 Romagnoli M, Bigliazzi C, Casoni G, *et al.* The role of transbronchial lung biopsy for the diagnosis of diffuse drug-induced lung disease: a case series of 44 patients. *Sarcoidosis Vasc Diffuse Lung Dis* 2008; **25**: 36–45.

79 Ryu JH, Daniels CE, Hartman TE, *et al.* Diagnosis of interstitial lung diseases. *Mayo Clin Proc* 2007; **82**: 976–86.

80 Mittle RL Jr, Schwab RJ, Duchin JS, *et al.* Radiographic resolution of community acquired pneumonia. *Am J Respir Crit Care Med* 1994; **149**: 630–5.

81 Kuru T, Lynch JP, 3rd. Nonresolving or slowly resolving pneumonia. *Clin Chest Med* 1999; **20**: 623–51.

82 Feinsilver SH, Fein AM, Niederman MS, *et al.* Utility of fiberoptic bronchoscopy in nonresolving pneumonia. *Chest* 1990; **98**: 1322–6.

83 Huang L, Hecht FM, Stansell JD, *et al.* Suspected *Pneumocystis carinii* pneumonia with a negative induced sputum examination. Is bronchoscopy useful? *AmJ Respir Crit Care Med* 1995; **151**: 1866–71.

84 Gal AA, Klatt EC, Koss MN, *et al.* The effectiveness of bronchoscopy in the diagnosis of *Pneumocystis carinii* and cytomegalovirus pulmonary infections in acquired immunodeficiency syndrome. *Arch Pathol Lab Med* 1987; **111**: 238–41.

85 Martin WJ II, Smith TF, Sanderson DR, *et al.* Role of bronchoalveolar lavage in the assessment of opportunistic pulmonary infections: utility and complications. *Mayo Clin Proc* 1987; **62**: 549–57.

86 Liebler JM, Markin CJ. Fiberoptic bronchoscopy for diagnosis and treatment. *Crit Care Med* 2000; **16**: 83–100.

87 O'Grady NP, Barie PS, Bartlett JG, *et al.* Guidelines for evaluation of new fever in critically ill adult patients: 2008 update from the American College of Critical Care Medicine and the Infectious Diseases Society of America. *Crit Care Med* 2008; **36**: 1330–49.

88 Allen R, Dunn W, Limper A. Diagnosing ventilator associated pneumonia: The role of bronchoscopy. *Mayo Clinic Proc* 1994; **69**: 962–8.

89 Langer M, Moscini P, Cigada M, *et al.* Long-term respiratory support and risk of pneumonia in critically ill patients. *Am Rev Respir Dis* 1989; **140**: 302–5.

90 White P. Evaluation of pulmonary infiltrates in critically ill patients with cancer and marrow transplant. *Crit Care Clin* 2001; **17**: 647–70.

91 Jain P, Sandur S, Meli Y, *et al.* Role of flexible bronchoscopy in immunocompromised patients with lung infiltrates. *Chest* 2004; **125**: 712–22.

92 Peikert T, Rana S, Edell ES. Safety, diagnostic yield, and therapeutic implications of flexible bronchoscopy in patients with febrile neutropenia and pulmonary infiltrates. *Mayo Clin Proc* 2005; **80**: 1414–20.

93 Sosenko A, Glassroth J. Fiberoptic bronchoscopy in the evaluation of lung abscesses. *Chest* 1985; **87**: 489–94.

94 Jeong MP, Kim WS, Han SK, *et al.* Transbronchial catheter drainage via fiberoptic bronchoscope in intractable lung abscess. *Korean J Int Med* 1989; **4**: 54–8.

95 Schmitt GS, Ohar JM, Kanter KR, Naunheim KS. Indwelling transbronchial catheter drainage of pulmonary abscess. *Ann Thorac Surg* 1988; **45**: 43–7.

96 Herth F, Ernst A, Becker HD. Endoscopic drainage of lung abscesses: technique and outcome. *Chest* 2005; **127**: 1378–81.

97 Su WJ, Lee PY, Perng RP. Chest roentgenographic guidelines in the selection of patients for fiberoptic bronchoscopy. *Chest* 1993; **103**: 1198–201.

98 Hasegawa S, Terada Y, Murakawa M, *et al.* Emergency bronchoscopy. *J Bronchol* 1998; **44**: 284–7.

99 Jolliet P, Chevrolet JC. Bronchoscopy in the intensive care unit. *Intensive Care Med* 1992; **18**: 160–9.

100 Djukanovic R, Wilson JW, Lai CKW, *et al.* The safety aspects of fiberoptic bronchoscopy, bronchoalveolar lavage, and endo-

bronchial biopsy in asthma. *Am Rev Respir Dis* 1991; **143**: 772–7.

101 Greally P. Human recombinant Dnase for mucus plugging in status asthmaticus. *Lancet* 1995; **346**: 1423–4.

102 Snow N, Lucas AE. Bronchoscopy in the critically ill surgical patient. *Am Surg* 1984; **50**: 441–5.

103 Frank W. [Current diagnostic approach to pleural effusion]. *Pneumologie* 2004; **58**: 777–90.

104 Lee P, Hsu A, Lo C, *et al.* Prospective evaluation of flex-rigid pleuroscopy for indeterminate pleural effusion: accuracy, safety and outcome. *Respirology* 2007; **12**: 881–6.

105 Gunnels JJ. Perplexing pleural effusion. *Chest* 1978; **74**: 390–3.

106 Chang SC, Perng RP. The role of fiberoptic bronchoscopy in evaluating the causes of pleural effusions. *Arch Intern Med* 1989; **149**: 855–7.

107 Balci AE, Eren N, Eren S, *et al.* Surgical treatment of post-traumatic tracheobronchial injuries: 14-year experience. *Eur J Cardiothorac Surg* 2002; **22**: 984–9.

108 Eckert MJ, Clagett C, Martin M, *et al.* Bronchoscopy in the blast injury patient. *Arch Surg* 2006; **141**: 806–9; discussion 810–11.

109 Hara KS, Prakash UBS. Fiberoptic bronchoscopy in the evaluation of acute chest and upper airway trauma. *Chest* 1989; **96**: 627–30.

110 Baumgartner F, Seppard B, de Virgilio C, *et al.* Tracheal and main bronchial disruptions after blunt chest trauma. *Ann Thorac Surg* 1990; **50**: 569–74.

111 Payne WS, DeRemee RA. Injuries of the trachea and major bronchi. *Postgrad Med* 1971; **49**: 152–8.

112 Travis SPL, Layer GT. Traumatic transection of the thoracic trachea. *Ann R Coll Surg Engl* 1983; **65**: 240–1.

113 Lehto JT, Koskinen PK, Anttila VJ, *et al.* Bronchoscopy in the diagnosis and surveillance of respiratory infections in lung and heart-lung transplant recipients. *Transpl Int* 2005; **18**: 562–71.

114 Glanville AR. The role of bronchoscopic surveillance monitoring in the care of lung transplant recipients. *Semin Respir Crit Care Med* 2006; **27**: 480–91.

115 Greene CL, Reemtsen B, Polimenakos A, *et al.* Role of clinically indicated transbronchial lung biopsies in the management of pediatric post-lung transplant patients. *Ann Thorac Surg* 2008; **86**: 198–203.

116 Seballos RJ, Mehta AC, McCarthy PM, Kirby TJ. The management of airway complications following lung transplantation [abstract]. *Am Rev Resp Dis* 1993; **147**: A602.

117 Sibley RK, Berry GJ, Tazelaar HD, *et al.* The role of transbronchial biopsies in the management of lung transplant recipients. *J Heart Lung Transplant* 1993; **12**: 308–24.

118 Paradis I, Yousem S, Griffith B. Airway obstruction and bronchiolitis obliterans after lung transplantation. *Clin Chest Med* 1993; **14**: 751–63.

119 Ono R, Loke J, Ikeda S. Bronchofiberscopy with curette biopsy bronchography in the evaluation of peripheral lung lesions. *Chest* 1981; **79**: 162–6.

120 Cortese DA, McDougall JC. Biopsy and brushing of peripheral lung cancer with fluoroscopic guidance. *Chest* 1979; **75**: 141–5.

121 Radke JR, Conway WA, Eyler WR, *et al.* Diagnostic accuracy in peripheral lung lesions. *Chest* 1979; **76**: 176–9.

122 Zavala DC. Diagnostic fiberoptic bronchoscopy: techniques and results of biopsy in 600 patients. *Chest* 1975; **68**: 12–19.

123 Stringfield JT, Markowitz DJ, Bentz RR, *et al.* The effect of tumor size and location on diagnosis by fiberoptic bronchoscopy. *Chest* 1977; **72**: 474–6.

124 Wallace JM, Deutsch AL. Flexible fiberoptic bronchoscopy and percutaneous needle lung aspiration for evaluating the solitary pulmonary nodule. *Chest* 1982; **81**: 665–71.

125 Eberhardt R, Ernst A, Herth FJ. Ultrasound-guided transbronchial biopsies of solitary pulmonary nodules less than 20 mm. *Eur Respir J* 2009; **34**: 1288–7.

126 Baaklini WA, Reinoso MA, Gorin AB, *et al.* Diagnostic yield of fiberoptic bronchoscopy in evaluating solitary pulmonary nodules. *Chest* 2000; **114**: 1049–54.

127 Okimasa S, Yoshioka S, Shibata S, *et al.* Endobronchial ultrasonography with a guide-sheath and virtual bronchoscopy navigation aids management of peripheral pulmonary nodules. *Hiroshima J Med Sci* 2007; **56**: 19–22.

128 Gibbs JD, Graham MW, Higgins WE. 3D MDCT-based system for planning peripheral bronchoscopic procedures. *Comput Biol Med* 2009; **39**: 266–79.

129 Steinfort DP, Finlay M, Irving LB. Diagnosis of peripheral pulmonary carcinoid tumor using endobronchial ultrasound. *Ann Thorac Med* 2008; **3**: 146–8.

130 Eberhardt R, Morgan RK, Ernst A, *et al.* Comparison of suction catheter versus forceps biopsy for sampling of solitary pulmonary nodules guided by electromagnetic navigational bronchoscopy. *Respiration* 2010; **79**: 54–60.

131 Pirozynski M. Bronchoalveolar lavage in the diagnosis of peripheral, primary lung cancer. *Chest* 1992; **102**: 372–4.

132 Shiner RJ, Rosenman J, Katz I, *et al.* Bronchoscopic evaluation of peripheral lung tumors. *Thorax* 1988; **43**: 887–9.

133 Arroliga AC, Matthay RA. The role of bronchoscopy in lung cancer. *Clin Chest Med* 1993; **14**: 87–98.

134 Ovchinikov A, Narizhny A. Value of ultra-thin bronchofibroscope in the diagnostics of peripheral cancer [abstract]. *Chest* 1991; 100: 89S.

135 Shure D, Fedullo PF. Transbronchial needle aspiration of peripheral masses. *Am Rev Respir Dis* 1983; **128**: 1090–2.

136 Wang KP, Haponik EF, Britt EJB, *et al.* Transbronchial needle aspiration of peripheral pulmonary nodules. *Chest* 1984; **86**: 819–23.

137 Mori K, Yanase N, Kaneko M, *et al.* Diagnosis of peripheral lung cancer in cases of tumors 2 cm or less in size. *Chest* 1989; **95**: 304–8.

138 Popovich J Jr, Kvale PA, Eichenhorn, *et al.* Diagnostic accuracy of multiple biopsies from flexible fiberoptic bronchoscopy: a comparison of central versus peripheral carcinoma. *Am Rev Respir Dis* 1982; **125**: 521–3.

139 Shure D, Astarita RW. Bronchoscopic carcinoma presenting as an endobronchial mass: optimal number of biopsy specimens for diagnosis. *Chest* 1983; **83**: 865–7.

140 Chaudhary BA, Yoneda K, Burki NK. Fiberoptic bronchoscopy: comparison of procedures used in the diagnosis of lung cancer. *J Thorac Cardiovasc Surg* 1978; **76**: 33–7.

141 Jay SJ, Wehr K, Nicholason DP, *et al.* Diagnostic sensitivity and specificity of pulmonary cytology: comparison of techniques used in conjunction with flexible fiberoptic bronchoscopy. *Acta Cytol* 1980; **24**: 304–12.

142 Payne CR, Hadfield JW, Stovin PG, *et al.* Diagnostic accuracy of cytology and biopsy in primary bronchial carcinoma. *J Clin Pathol* 1981; **34**: 773–8.

143 Bedrossian CWM, Rybka DL. Bronchial brushing during fiberoptic bronchoscopy for the cytodiagnosis of lung cancer: comparison with sputum and bronchial washings. *Acta Cytol* 1976; **20**: 446–53.

144 Castella J, del la Heras P, Puzo C, *et al.* Cytology of post bronchoscopically collected sputum samples and its diagnostic value. *Respiration* 1981; **42**: 116–21.

145 Kvale PA, Bode FR, Kini S. Diagnostic accuracy in lung cancer: comparison of techniques used in association with flexible fiberoptic bronchoscopy. *Chest* 1976; **69**: 752–7.

146 Buccheri G, Barberis P, Delfino MS. Diagnostic, morphologic and histopathologic correlates in bronchogenic carcinoma: a review of 1,045 bronchoscopic examinations. *Chest* 1991; **99**: 809–14.

147 Cummings CLM, Brooks IO, Stinson JM. Increases in diagnostic yield of fiberoptic bronchoscopy by fluoroscopy. *J Natl Med Assoc* 1982; **74**: 239–41.

148 Matsuda N, Horai T, Nakamura S, *et al.* Bronchial brushing and bronchial biopsy: comparison of diagnostic accuracy and cell typing reliability in lung cancer. *Thorax* 1986; **41**: 475–8.

149 Gay PC, Bruntinel WM. Transbronchial needle aspiration in the practice of bronchoscopy. *Mayo Clin Proc* 1989; **64**: 158–62.

150 Horsley JR, Miller RE, Amy RWM, *et al.* Bronchial submucosal needle aspiration performed through the fiberoptic bronchoscope. *Acta Cytol* 1984; **28**: 211–17.

151 Shure D. Transbronchial needle aspiration—current status [editorial]. *Mayo Clin Proc* 1989; **64**: 251–4.

152 Shure D, Fedullo PF. The role of transcarinal needle aspiration in the staging of bronchogenic carcinoma. *Chest* 1984; **86**: 693–6.

153 Schenk DA, Bryan CL, Bower JH, *et al.* Transbronchial needle aspiration in the diagnosis of bronchogenic carcinoma. *Chest* 1987; **92**: 83–5.

154 Shure D. Is transbronchial needle aspiration worthwhile? *Pulmonary Perspectives* 1991; **8**: 1–13.

155 Harrow E, Halbert M, Hardy S, *et al.* Bronchoscopic and roentgenographic correlates of a positive transbronchial needle aspiration in the staging of lung cancer. *Chest* 1991; **100**: 1592–6.

156 Wang KP, Gupta PK, Haponik EF, *et al.* Flexible transbronchial needle aspiration: technical considered. *Ann Otol Rhinol Laryngol* 1984; **93**: 233–6.

157 Shure D, Fedullo PF. Transbronchial needle aspiration in the diagnosis of submucosal and peribronchial bronchogenic carcinoma. *Chest* 1985; **88**: 49–51.

158 Dasgupta A, Jain P, Minai OA, *et al.* Utility of transbronchial needle aspiration in the diagnosis of endobronchial lesions. *Chest* 1999; **115**: 1237–41.

159 Swinburn CR, Veale D, Peel ET, *et al.* A prospective randomized comparison of fine needle aspiration biopsy and fiberoptic bronchoscopy in the investigation of peripheral pulmonary opacities. *Respir Med* 1989; **83**: 493–5.

160 Wang KP, Gonullu U, Baker R. Transbronchial needle aspiraiton versus transthorcic needle aspiration in the diagnosis of pulmonary lesions. *J Bronchol* 1994; **1**: 199–204.

161 Raab SS, Hornberger J, Raffin T. The importance of sputum cytology in the diagnosis of lung cancer a cost-effective analysis. *Chest* 1997; **112**: 937–45.

162 Martini N, Melamed MR. Occult carcinomas of the lung. *Ann Thorac Surg* 1980; **30**: 215–23.

163 Lam S, Hung J, Kennedy SM, *et al.* Detection of dysplasia and carcinoma in situ by ration fluorometry. *Am Rev Respir Dis* 1992; **146**: 1458–61.

164 Nakhosteen JA, Khanavkar B. Autofluorescence bronchoscopy: the laser imaging fluorescence endoscope. In: Bolliger CT, Mathur PN, eds. *Interventional Bronchosocopy. Progress in Respiratory Research*, vol. 30. Basel: Karger, 2000: 236–42.

165 Schenk DA, Bower JH, Bryan CL, *et al.* Transbronchial needle aspiration staging of bronchogenic carcinoma. *Am Rev Respir Dis* 1986; **134**: 146–8.

166 Yasufuku K, Chiyo M, Sekine Y, *et al.* Real-time endobronchial ultrasound-guided transbronchial needle aspiration of mediastinal and hilar lymph nodes. *Chest* 2004; **126**: 122–8.

167 Anantham D, Koh M, Ernst A. Endobronchial ultrasound. *Respir Med* 2009; **103**: 1406–14.

168 Parrat E, Pujol JL, Gautier V, *et al.* Chest tumor response during lung cancer chemotherapy: computed tomography vs fiberoptic bronchoscopy. *Chest* 1993; **103**: 1495–501.

169 Abemayor E, Moore DM, Hanson DG. Identification of synchronous esophageal tumors in patients with head and neck cancer. *J Surg Oncol* 1988; **38**: 94–6.

170 Leipzig B, Zellmer JE, Klug D. The role of endoscopy in evaluating patients with head and neck cancer: a multi-institutional prospective study. *Arch Otolaryngol* 1985; **111**: 589–94.

171 Haughey BH, Gates GA, Arfken CL, Harvey J. Meta-analysis of second malignant tumors in head and neck cancer: the case for an endoscopic screening protocol. *Ann Otol Rhinol Laryngol* 1992; **101**: 105–12.

172 Choi TK, Siu KF, Lam KH, Wong J. Bronchoscopy and carcinoma of the esophagus I: findings of bronchoscopy in carcinoma of the esophagus. *Am J Surg* 1984; **147**: 757–9.

173 Choi TK, Siu KF, Lam KH, Wong J. Bronchoscopy and carcinoma of the esophagus II: carcinoma of the esophagus with tracheobronchial involvement. *Am J Surg* 1984; **147**: 760–2.

174 Argyros GJ, Torrington KG. Fiberoptic bronchoscopy in the evaluation of carcinoma metastatic to the lung. *Chest* 1994; **105**: 454–7.

175 Poe RH, Ortiz C, Isreal RH, *et al.* Sensitivity, specificity, and predictive values of bronchoscopy in neoplasm metastatic to lung. *Chest* 1985; **88**: 84–8.

176 Pasaoglu I, Dogan R, Demircin M, *et al.* Bronchoscopic removal of foreign bodies in children: retrospective analysis of 822 cases. *Thorac Cardiovasc Surg* 1991; **39**: 95–8.

177 Weissberg D, Schwartz I. Foreign bodies in the tracheobronchial tree. *Chest* 1987; **91**: 730–73.

178 Cunanan OS. The flexible fiberoptic bronchoscope in foreign body removal: experience in 300 cases. *Chest* 1978; **73**: 725–6.

179 Lan RS, Lee CH, Chaing YC, Wang WJ. Use of fiberoptic bronchoscopy to retrieve bronchial foreign bodies in adults. *Am Rev Respir Dis* 1989; **140**: 1734–7.

180 Cha SI, Kim CH, Lee JH, *et al.* Isolated smoke inhalation injuries: acute respiratory dysfunction, clinical outcomes, and

short-term evolution of pulmonary functions with the effects of steroids. *Burns* 2007; **33**: 200–8.

181 Reichle G. Argon plasma coagulation in bronchology: a new method—alternative or complimentary? *Pneumologie* 2000; **54**: 508–16.

182 Gerasin VA, Shafrovsky BB. Endobronchial electrosurgery. *Chest* 1988; **93**: 270–4.

183 Reddy C, Majid A, Michaud G, *et al.* Gas embolism following bronchoscopic argon plasma coagulation: a case series. *Chest* 2008; **134**: 1066–9.

184 Feller-Kopman D, Lukanich JM, Shapira G, *et al.* Gas flow during bronchoscopic ablation therapy causes gas emboli to the heart: a comparative animal study. *Chest* 2008; **133**: 892–6.

185 Carpenter RJ, Neel HB, Sanderson DR. Cryosurgery of bronchopulmonary structures. *Chest* 1977; **72**: 279–84.

186 Marasso A, Gallo E, Massaglia GM, *et al.* Cryosurgery in bronchoscopic treatment of tracheobronchial stenosis: indications, limits, personal experience. *Chest* 1993; **103**: 472–4.

187 Walsh DA, Maiwand MO, Nath AR, *et al.* Bronchoscopic cryotherapy for advanced bronchial carcinoma. *Thorax* 1990; **45**: 509–13.

188 Gage AA, Baust JG. Cryosurgery for tumors. *J Am Coll Surg* 2007; **205**: 342–56.

189 George PJ, Rudd RM. Bronchoscopic cryotherapy for advanced bronchial carcinoma. *Thorax* 1991; **46**: 150.

190 Mathur PN, Wolf KM, Busk MF, *et al.* Fiberoptic bronchoscopic cryotherapy in the management of tracheobronchial obstruction. *Chest* 1996; **110**: 718–23.

191 Hetzel M, Hetzel J, Schumann C, *et al.* Cryorecanalization: a new approach for the immediate management of acute airway obstruction. *J Thorac Cardiovasc Surg* 2004; **127**: 1427–31.

192 Turner JF, Wang KP. Endobronchial laser therapy. *Clin Chest Med* 1999; **20**: 107–22.

193 Brutinel WM, Cortese DA, McDougall JC, *et al.* A two-year experience with the neodymium-YAG laser in endobronchial obstruction. *Chest* 1987; **91**: 159–65.

194 Cavaliere S, Foccoli P, Farina PL. Nd: YAG laser bronchoscopy: a five-year experience with 1,396 applications in 1,000 patients. *Chest* 1988; **94**: 15–21.

195 Unger M. Bronchoscopic utilization of the Nd: YAG laser for obstructing lesions of the trachea and bronchi. *Surg Clin North Am* 1984; **64**: 931–8.

196 Unger M. Lasers and their role in pulmonary medicine: present and future. In: Fishman AP, ed. *Update: Pulmonary Diseases and Disorders.* New York: McGraw Hill; 1992: 419–32.

197 Wang KP, Turner JF. Nd: YAG resection of hamartoma. *J Bronchol* 1196; **3**: 112–15.

198 Mehta AC. Laser applications in respiratory care. In: Kacmarek RM, Stoller JK, eds. *Current Respiratory Care.* Toronto: Mosby-Year Book; 1988: 100–6.

199 Wang KP, Turner JF. Closure of bronchopleural fistula with Nd-YAG Laser. *Am J Respir Care Crit Med* 1995; **151**: A847.

200 Wang KP, Schaeffer L, Heitmiller R, *et al.* Nd: YAG Laser closure of a bronchopleural fistula. *Monaldi Arch Chest Dis* 1993; **48**: 301–3.

201 Prakash UBS. Global theme issue: emerging technology in clinical medicine. Advances in bronchoscopic procedures. *Chest* 1999; **116**: 1403–8.

202 Ahmad M, Dweik RA. Future of flexible bronchoscopy. *Clin Chest Med* 1999; **20**: 1–17.

203 Dweik RA, Patel SR, Mehta AC. Tracheal papillomatosis. *J Bronchol* 1994; **1**: 226.

204 Abramson AL, Shikowitz MJ, Mullooly VM, *et al.* Clinical effects of photodynamic therapy on recurrent laryngeal papillomas. *Ann Otol Head Neck Surg* 1992; **118**: 25–9.

205 Patel SR, DeBoer G, Mehta AC. Role of photodynamic therapy in juvenile laryngotracheobronchial papillomatosis [abstract]. *Chest* 1993; **104**: 161S.

206 Imamura S, Kusunoki Y, Takifuji N, *et al.* Photodynamic therapy and/or external beam radiation therapy for roentgenological occult lung cancer. *Cancer* 1994; **73**: 1608–14.

207 Balchum O, Doiron DR. Photoradiation therapy of endobronchial lung cancer. *Clin Chest Med* 1985; **6**: 255–75.

208 McCaughan JS. Overview of experience with photodynamic therapy for malignancies in 192 patients. *Photochem Photobiol* 1987; **46**: 903–9.

209 Freitag L, Ernst A, Thomas M, *et al.* Sequential photodynamic therapy (PDT) and high dose brachytherapy for endobronchial tumour control in patients with limited bronchogenic carcinoma. *Thorax* 2004; **59**: 790–3.

210 Moghissi K, Dixon K, Thorpe JA, *et al.* Photodynamic therapy (PDT) in early central lung cancer: a treatment option for patients ineligible for surgical resection. *Thorax* 2007; **62**: 391–5.

211 Paradelo JC, Waxman MJ, Throne BJ, *et al.* Endobronchial irradiation with 192Ir in the treatment of malignant endobronchial obstruction. *Chest* 1992; **102**: 1072–4.

212 Khanavkar B, Stern P, Alberti W, Nakhosteen JA. Complications associated with brachytherapy alone or with laser in lung cancer. *Chest* 1991; **99**: 1062–5.

213 Lee W, Daly BD, DiPetrillo TA, *et al.* Limited resection for non-small cell lung cancer: observed local control with implantation of I-125 brachytherapy seeds. *Ann Thorac Surg* 2003; **75**: 237–42; discussion 242–3.

214 Goldstein RA, Rohatgi PK, Bergofsky EH, Block ER. Clinical role of bronchoalveolar lavage in adults with pulmonary disease. *Am Rev Respir Dis* 1990; **142**: 481–6.

215 Prakash UBS, Barham S, Carpenter HA, *et al.* Pulmonary alveolar phospholipoproteinosis: experience with 34 cases and a review. *Mayo Clin Proc* 1987; **62**: 499–518.

216 Murray MJ, DeRuyter ML, Harrison BA. "How I do it" Bilateral lung washings for pulmonary alveolar proteinosis. *J Bronchol* 1998; **5**: 324–6.

217 Colt HG. "How I do it" Bronchoalveolar lavage. *J Bronchol* 1995; **2**: 154–6.

218 Schwartz DB, Beals TF, Wimbish KJ, Hammersley JR. Transbronchial fine needle aspiration of bronchogenic cysts. *Chest* 1985; **88**: 573–5.

219 Schwartz AR, Fishman EK, Wang KP. Diagnosis and treatment of a bronchogenic cyst using transbronchial needle aspiration. *Thorax* 1986; **41**: 326–7.

220 Delarue NC, Pearson FG, Nelems JM, Cooper JD. Lung abscess: surgical implications. *Can J Surg* 1980; **23**: 297–302.

221 Estrera AS, Platt MR, Mills LJ, Shaw RR. Primary lung abscess. *J Thorac Cardiovasc Surg* 1980; **79**: 275–82.

222 Connors JP, Roper CL, Ferguson TB. Transbronchial catheterization of pulmonary abscesses. *Ann Thorac Surg* 1975; **19**: 254.

223 Herth F, Ernst A, Becker HD. Endoscopic drainage of lung abscesses: technique and outcome. *Chest* 2005; **127**: 1378–81.

224 Colt HG, Janssen JP, Dumon JF, Noirclerc MJ. Endoscopic management of bronchial stenosis after double lung ransplantation. *Chest* 1992; **102**: 10–16.

225 Tsang V, Goldstraw P. Endobronchial stenting for anastomotic stenosis after sleeve resection. *Ann Thorac Surg* 1989; **48**: 568–71.

226 Dumon JF. A dedicated tracheobronchial stent. *Chest* 1990; **97**: 328–32.

227 deCastro FR, Lopez L, Varela A, *et al.* Tracheobronchial stents and fiberoptic bronchoscopy [letter]. *Chest* 1991; **99**: 792.

228 Turner JF, Ernst A, Becker HD. "How I do it" Rigid bronchoscopy. *J Bronchol* 2000; **7**: 171–6.

229 Ayers ML, Beamis JF. Rigid bronchoscopy in the twenty-first century. *Clin Chest Med* 2001; **22**: 355–64.

230 Hautmann H, Gamarra F, Pfeifer KJ. Fiberoptic bronchoscopic balloon dilatation in malignant tracheobronchial disease. *Chest* 2001; **120**: 43–9.

231 Andrews BT, Graham SM, Ross AF, *et al.* Technique, utility, and safety of awake tracheoplasty using combined laser and balloon dilation. *Laryngoscope* 2007; **117**: 2159–62.

232 Susanto I, Peters JI, Levine SM, *et al.* Lung transplantation. Use of balloon-expandable metallic stents in the management of bronchial stenosis and bronchomalacia after lung transplantation. *Chest* 1998; **114**: 1330–5.

233 Sheski FD, Mathur PN. "How I do it" Balloon bronchoplast using the flexible bronchoscope. *J Bronchol* 1998; **5**: 242–6.

234 Baumann MH, Sahn SA. Medical management and therapy of bronchopleural fistulas in the mechanically ventilated patient. *Chest* 1990; **97**: 721–8.

235 Steiger Z, Wilson RF. Management of bronchopleural fistulas. *Surgery* 1984; **158**: 267–71.

236 Regal G, Sturm A, Neumann C, *et al.* Occlusion of bronchopleural fistula after lung injury: a new treatment by bronchoscopy. *J Trauma* 1989; **29**: 223–6.

237 Shah AM, Singhal P, Chhajed PN, *et al.* Bronchoscopic closure of bronchopleural fistula using gelfoam. *J Assoc Physicians India* 2004; **52**: 508–9.

238 Snell GI, Holsworth L, Fowler S, *et al.* Occlusion of a bronchocutaneous fistula with endobronchial one-way valves. *Ann Thorac Surg* 2005; **80**: 1930–2.

239 Ferguson JS, Sprenger K, Van Natta T. Closure of a bronchopleural fistula using bronchoscopic placement of an endobronchial valve designed for the treatment of emphysema. *Chest* 2006; **129**: 479–81.

240 Travaline JM, McKenna RJ Jr, De Giacomo T, *et al.* Treatment of persistent pulmonary air leaks using endobronchial valves. *Chest* 2009; **136**: 355–60.

241 Campion JP, Bourdelat D, Launois B. Surgical treatment of malignant esophagotracheal fistulas. *Am J Surg* 1983; **148**: 641–6.

242 Graeber GM, Farrell BG, Neville JF Jr, Parker FB Jr. Successful diagnosis and management of fistulas between the aorta and the tracheobronchial tree. *Ann Thorac Surg* 1980; **29**: 555–61.

243 Ishizaki Y, Tada Y, Takagi A, *et al.* Aortobronchial fistula after an aortic operation. *Ann Thorac Surg* 1990; **50**: 975–7.

244 Edens ET, Sia RL. Flexible fiberoptic endoscopy in difficult intubations. *Ann Otol* 1981; **90**: 307–9.

245 Dietrich KA, Strauss RH, Cabalka AK, *et al.* Use of flexible fiberoptic endoscopy for determination of endotracheal tube position in the pediatric patient. *Crit Care Med* 1988; **16**: 884–7.

246 Streitz JM, Shapshay SM. Airway injury after tracheotomy and endotracheal intubation. *Surg Clin North Am* 1991; **71**: 1211–31.

247 Bishop MJ. Mechanisms of laryngotracheal injury following prolonged tracheal intubation. *Chest* 1989; **96**: 185–6.

248 Colice GL, Stukel TA, Dain B. Laryngeal complications of prolonged intubation. *Chest* 1989; **96**: 877–84.

249 Whited RE. A prospective study of laryngotracheal sequelae on long term intubation. *Laryngoscope* 1984; **94**: 376–7.

250 Kastanos N, Estopa Miro R, Marin Perez A, *et al.* Laryngotracheal injury due to endotracheal intubation: incidence, evolution, and predisposing factors. A prospective long-term study. *Crit Care Med* 1983; **11**: 362–7.

251 Rai NS, Mehta AC, Meeker DP, Stoller JK. Transtracheal oxygen therapy—does practice make perfect? *J Bronchol* 1994; **1**: 205–12.

252 Orkin SH, Motulsky AG. *Report and Recommendations of the Panel to Assess the NIH Investment in Research on Gene Therapy.* NIH Panel Report, 1996.

253 Mastrangeli A, Harvey BG, Crystal RG. Gene therapy for lung disease. In: Crystal RG, West JB, Wibel ER, *et al.*, eds. *The Lung: Scientific Foundation*, 2nd edn. Philadelphia, Lippincott-Raven; 1997: 2795.

254 Rochlitz CF. Gene therapy for lung cancer. In: Bolliger CT, Mathur PN, eds. *Interventional Bronchoscopy. Progress in Respiratory Research*, vol. 30. Basel: Karger; 2000: 280–9.

255 Kruklitis RJ, Sterman DH. Endobronchial gene therapy. *Semin Respir Crit Care Med* 2004; **25**: 433–42.

256 Cox G, Thomson NC, Rubin AS, *et al.* Asthma control during the year after bronchial thermoplasty. *N Engl J Med* 2007; **356**: 1327–37.

257 Pavord ID, Cox G, Thomson NC, *et al.* Safety and efficacy of bronchial thermoplasty in symptomatic, severe asthma. *Am J Respir Crit Care Med* 2007; **176**: 1185–91.

258 Fishman A, Martinez F, Naunheim K, *et al.* A randomized trial comparing lung-volume-reduction surgery with medical therapy for severe emphysema. *N Engl J Med* 2003; **348**: 2059–73.

259 Strange C, Herth FJ, Kovitz KL, *et al.* Design of the endobronchial valve for emphysema palliation trial (VENT): a non-surgical method of lung volume reduction. *BMC Pulm Med* 2007; **7**: 10.

260 Wood DE, McKenna RJ Jr, Yusen RD, *et al.* A multicenter trial of an intrabronchial valve for treatment of severe emphysema. *J Thorac Cardiovasc Surg* 2007; **133**: 65–73

261 Choong CK, Cardoso PF, Sybrecht GW, *et al.* Airway bypass treatment of severe homogeneous emphysema: taking advantage of collateral ventilation. *Thorac Surg Clin* 2009; **19**: 239–45.

262 Reilly J, Washko G, Pinto-Plata V, *et al.* Biological lung volume reduction: a new bronchoscopic therapy for advanced emphysema. *Chest* 2007; **131**: 1108–13.

263 Ingenito EP, Wood DE, Utz JP. Bronchoscopic lung volume reduction in severe emphysema. *Proc Am Thorac Soc* 2008; **5**: 454–60.

264 Pereira W Jr, Kovnat DM, Snider GL. A prospective cooperative study of complications following flexible fiberoptic bronchoscopy. *Chest* 1978; **73**: 813–16.

265 Suratt PM, Smiddy JF, Gruber B. Deaths and complications associated with fiberoptic bronchoscopy. *Chest* 1976; **69**: 747–51.

266 Burgher LW, Jones FL, Patterson JR, Selecky PA. Guidelines for fiberoptic bronchoscopy in adults. *Am Rev Respir Dis* 1987; **136**: 1066.

267 Katz AS, Michelson EL, Stawicki J, Holford FD. Cardiac arrhythmias: frequency duringfiberoptic bronchoscopy and correlation withhypoxemia. *Arch Intern Med* 1981; **141**: 603–6.

268 Matot I, Kramer MR, Glantz L, *et al.* Myocardial Ischemia in Sedated Patients Undergoing Fiberoptic Bronchoscopy. *Chest* 1997; **112**: 1454–8.

269 Dunagan DP, Burke HL, Aquino SL. Fiberoptic bronchoscopy in coronary care unit patients. *Chest* 1998; **114**: 1660–7.

270 Kvale PA. Is it really safe to perform bronchsocpy after a recent myocardial infarction? *Chest* 1996; **110**: 592.

271 Liebler JM. Fiberotpic bronchoscopy for diagnosis and treatment. *Crit Care Clin* 2000; **16**: 83–100.

272 Dweik RA, Mehta AC, Meeker DP, Arroliga AC. Analysis of the safety of bronchosocpy after recent acute myocaridal infarction. *Chest* 1996; **110**: 825–8.

273 Matot I, Drenger B, Glantz L, *et al.* Coroanry spasm during outpatient fiberoptic laser bronchoscopy. *Chest* 1999; **115**: 1744–6.

274 Bein T, Pfeifer M. Fiberoptic bronchoscopy after recent acute myocarcial infarciton: stress for the heart? *Chest* 1997; **112**: 295–6.

275 Prakash UBS, Stubbs SE. The bronchoscopy survey: some reflections. *Chest* 1991; **100**: 1660–7.

276 Ernst A, Eberhardt R, Wahidi M, *et al.* Effect of routine clopidogrel use on bleeding complications after transbronchial biopsy in humans. *Chest* 2006; **129**: 734–7.

277 Sun SW, Zabaneh RN, Carrey Z, Incidence of pneumothorax after fiberoptic bronchoscopy (FOB) in community-based hospital; are routine post-procedure chest roentgenograms necessary? *Chest* 2003; **124**: 145.

278 Hattotuwa K, Gamble EA, O'Shaughnessy T, *et al.* Safety of bronchoscopy, biopsy, and BAL in research patients with COPD. *Chest* 2002; **122**: 1909–12.

# 2 Diagnostic Bronchoscopy

# 8 Bronchoscopy for Airway Lesions

## Heinrich D. Becker

Thoraxclinic-Heidelberg, Academic Teaching Hospital, University of Heidelberg, Heidelberg, Germany

After extensive examinations the experienced endoscopist knows how to add image upon image before his inner eye and combine different aspects of the same finding correctly. By the time the complete image becomes so clear, that the endoscopist lives like in a separate world of which a person outside has no imagination.

G. Killian, 1906 [1]

Everything we see hides another thing, we always want to see what is hidden by what we see. There is an interest in that which is hidden and which the visible doesn't show us.

Rene Magritte, Painter (1898–1967) [2]

## Introduction

On May 29, 1898, Gustav Killian of Freiburg University stated at the fifth annual meeting of the South German Laryngological Society at Heidelberg, in his first report on direct bronchoscopy, "The practical relevance of bronchoscopy cannot be assessed accurately at the moment. I hope that, apart from foreign bodies and bronchial diseases, it may also be applied to diagnosis and therapy of afflictions of the lung" [3]. Today, more than 100 years after Killian's invention of direct bronchoscopy in 1897, it has become one of the most important diagnostic and therapeutic tools in pulmonary medicine.

The possibility of direct visualization of the central airways through the rigid bronchoscope was further improved by the development of lens optics (Hopkins and Lumina optic), providing a far better field of view and visualization of details. The introduction of the fully flexible bronchofiberscope by Ikeda in 1967 made the peripheral bronchial system—even every part of the lung parenchyma—easily accessible for the endoscopist. Due to its comparative ease of handling and comfortable application for the patient, it has provided a strong impetus for the spread of bronchoscopic techniques to many institutions. Further, because of

improvements in technique and the pharmacology of general and local anesthesia, the risks of complications have become so few [4] that bronchoscopy, despite its invasive nature, today belongs to the basic procedures in pulmonary medicine, and is applied early in the diagnostic process.

This is all the more important for lesions of the central airways because these are located deep inside the thoracic cavity, surrounded by a complexity of mediastinal organs, and are poorly visualized by radiologic examination, despite profound technical revolutions such as the computed tomography (CT) scan and magnetic resonance imaging (MRI). Early consideration of endoscopy of the airways is further enhanced by the fact that most diseases involving the central airways produce uncharacteristic clinical symptoms, which are often not pathognomonic for the underlying process.

In this brief overview on bronchoscopy for airway lesions, I shall point out a few aspects of the technical approach and systematization of endoscopic findings in the airways that, in my experience, seem to be important.

## Technical considerations

The general technical considerations concerning instrumental equipment, operational approach, and anesthesiologic management are all dealt with elsewhere in this book. Here, special considerations on the approach in airway diseases are offered.

### Systematic inspection

The first consideration is the systematization of bronchoscopic examination. Because many diseases of the airways are not strictly localized to only one site, but rather frequently tend to be part of a more systemic spread, one should always strictly adhere to a scheme of systematic inspection of the entire airway tract during the procedure.

*Flexible Bronchoscopy*, Third Edition. Edited by Ko-Pen Wang, Atul C. Mehta, J. Francis Turner.
© 2012 Blackwell Publishing Ltd. Published 2012 by Blackwell Publishing Ltd.

This will frequently include the upper airways above the larynx as well.

The attention of the examiner is easily drawn toward obvious pathologies of the airways, so first examine those areas of the airways that do not appear to be involved in the pathologic process radiologically or endoscopically. Unexpected alterations may thus be discovered early during the diagnostic procedure and will not be missed after attention has been distracted by the exploration of the obviously pathologic process. This may occur easily if difficulties arise due to obscured vision caused by mucus, purulent secretions, and bleeding, or by technical problems in providing specimens for laboratory examinations [5].

## Documentation

All endoscopic findings must be meticulously documented by verbal and graphic description, together with the resultant diagnostic and therapeutic conclusions. Additional diagnostic, documentary, and therapeutic measures must be noted. Video documentation may be useful in longitudinal follow-up of diseases and information for colleagues. But one should always keep in mind that on the video only sequences that have been documented are seen; important additional information may be missed or lost. Direct communication among the physicians involved is still indispensable.

## Instrumentation

The second consideration involves the instrument and approach chosen by the examiner. The examination by flexible fiberscope under local anesthesia obviously needs less staff and instrumental equipment and seems to be comfortable for the patient. Further, a detailed functional analysis of the pharyngeal space, the vocal cords, and the stability of the tracheobronchial system under almost physiologic conditions is only possible under local anesthesia.

Visualization of details and management under conditions of poor compliance and obstruction of view by excessive secretions or bleeding are, however, not so easily managed under local anesthesia. Sometimes even under local anesthesia after inspection of the larynx and the upper trachea, it seems advisable to insert a tracheal tube if the instrument has to be withdrawn frequently for cleansing. This prevents excessive coughing due to repeated passage of the larynx.

Under these conditions, the rigid bronchoscope is still regarded as an ideal instrument because it provides an optimal overview and a much safer airway for ventilation in all circumstances. To obtain large and reliable biopsy specimens; for most therapeutic procedures such as removal of large foreign bodies, especially in children; for laser treatment; for dilatation of stenoses and stenting; and for optimal photographic and video documentation, the rigid bronchoscope is still used.

The rates of complications of flexible bronchoscopy under local anesthesia, when compared to rigid bronchoscopy under general anesthesia and high-frequency jet ventilation, according to major comparative studies and in our experience, seem to be almost equal. Whereas in rigid bronchoscopy traumatic lesions due to instrumentation and larger biopsies are more frequent, in flexible bronchoscopy side effects of local anesthetics and problems in ventilation are more common [6].

Because the general risk of bronchoscopy is higher when compared to gastroenterologic endoscopy, and the time for examination is limited due to the vanishing effect of anesthesia, meticulous planning and preparation for the procedure are necessary.

## Prerequisites

### History and physical examination

Because the amount of information from endoscopic examination is limited and frequently may also be ambiguous, some information before starting the procedure is essential. The history of symptoms and physical examination of the patient must be established. Frequently, signs of central airway disease are subtle but pathognomonic, and diagnosis may be suspected by careful examination. Anamnesis of smoking for decades, progressive dyspnea and coughing, hemoptysis or purulent secretions, acute persistent hoarseness, or a history of traumatic lesions of the airways such as prolonged intubation or tracheotomy may give the first hint of airways involvement.

On clinical examination, asymmetrical excursions of the thorax and one-sided "asthmatic" wheezing or reduction of breathing sounds are typical for obstruction of a main stem bronchus, especially if the onset of symptoms occurs in adults without a prior history of asthma. Signs of overinflation or of impaired ventilation of parts of the lungs can be pathognomonic for localized airway obstruction, rales, and signs of pleurisy for postobstructive infiltration.

### Laboratory tests and radiologic examination

These findings may be further quantified by lung function tests, giving an idea of the stability of the airways and especially of organic obstruction. A preoperative analysis of the blood gases will help in taking special precautions for safe ventilation during the procedure.

Laboratory blood tests do not usually afford much information about airway pathology. However, these are needed for assessment of risks prior to bronchoscopy.

Because during bronchoscopy, frequently, only indirect signs of central airway problems may be visualized, it is essential to establish an orienting survey on the thoracic organs. Therefore, radiologic exploration before bronchoscopy is essential. Plain frontal and lateral X rays are indispensable prerequisites. On these areas of impaired ventilation, malformations of respiratory organs and tumorous lesions of the lung, the bronchi, or neighboring organs may be suspected, if not already diagnosed.

Depending on these findings and according to the urgency of endoscopic examination, further investigations may be necessary for the exact localization of a pathologic process. Fluoroscopy with examination of the esophagus is helpful in assessing dynamic alterations of the great vessels, heart and lungs, and of the esophageal passage. Because even by CT scan and MRI, detailed visualization of the central airways and the hilar region is still unsatisfactory, hilar tomography with filters is frequently performed whenever a lesion of these structures is suspected.

## Safety measures

For early recognition and prevention of complications, safety precautions must be taken: safe intravenous access, oxygen insufflation, electrocardiographic and blood pressure monitoring, percutaneous pulse oximetry and sometimes transcutaneous $CO_2$ measurement. All instruments for intervention in the case of complications must be readily available and regularly tested for accuracy and performance.

## Anatomic considerations

Every textbook on pulmonary medicine and every bronchoscopy atlas contains ample information on the endoscopic appearance of the normal bronchial tree and nomenclature of its ramifications. Looking at the complexity of the bronchopulmonary system, one always marvels at the constancy of the basic anatomic structure that is found in most patients.

For example, there is a constant number of 22 tracheal cartilage rings and the well-known asymmetry of lobes on both sides with 19 segmental bronchi. The pulmonary vessels cross at definite regions so that inadvertent puncture during transbronchial needle biopsy of the regional lymph nodes and tumor masses can be avoided. The regional lymph nodes have been numbered according to their regular distribution along the bronchial tree, which is essential for the staging of involvement in bronchial carcinoma. The pulmonary fissures are a fairly safe guideline to assess the segmental localization of intrapulmonary lesions.

By these examples, without having mentioned the close anatomic relation of the tracheobronchial tree to neighboring organs of the mediastinum, the importance of a thorough knowledge of the anatomy is demonstrated. Table 8.1 lists five aspects that deserve further discussion [7].

**Table 8.1** Anatomic aspects in bronchology

| | |
|---|---|
| 1 | Anatomic orientation |
| 2 | Normal anatomy |
| 3 | Variations without clinical relevance |
| 4 | Pathologic malformations |
| 5 | Considerations regarding resectability |

## Anatomic orientation

To the beginner, the number and nomenclature of the bronchi will appear confusing. But once accustomed to it, orientation will become comparatively easy because the tracheobronchial system is not easily deformed and has no motility in itself, compared to the gastrointestinal tract.

An obstacle to orientation is its confinement, especially if vision is further impaired by mucus, blood, or tumor infiltration. This will be experienced more frequently in flexible bronchoscopy under local anesthesia than during rigid bronchoscopy under general anesthesia because the mucosa may be damaged easily due to forced maneuvers and coughing. Repeated withdrawal for cleansing of the lens of the fiberscope and reintroduction of the instrument will not be readily tolerated by the patient.

Once one has lost the anatomic orientation during the procedure one should withdraw the instrument to a distinct landmark, such as the main bifurcation of the trachea or into the trachea itself, and restart the examination from there. Many of the suspected "anatomic variations" will then clearly become misinterpretation of the actual inspected region.

## Normal anatomy

During development of the embryonic lung, the tracheobronchial system adopts its definitive structure by the sixteenth gestational week. In the newborn and child up to approximate age 4 to 6 years, the trachea has an almost round shape and the dorsal ends of the cartilages may almost meet, especially during forced breathing and coughing, which must not be mistaken for complete cartilage rings. It is only at about age 8 to 10 years that the typical horseshoe shape is completed. In children, the bifurcation of the trachea appears blunt and the angle wider than in the adult [8], in whom this would be a sign of displacement by extraluminal infracarinal masses.

Because the cartilages are still very soft at that age, total tracheal and bronchial collapse during coughing and forced breathing maneuvers in younger children is physiologic so long as the airways remain open in the resting or inspirating position. The diameter of the trachea varies according to the size and physical condition of the child. Rather than using tables as a guideline to choose the appropriate diameter of the bronchoscope, use the individual child's little finger, the caliber of which usually closely resembles that of the trachea ("rule of the little finger").

In the young adult, the trachea has grown in length and diameter, and has adopted the typical horseshoe form. Only during coughing does the paries membranaceus bulge toward the anterior wall; otherwise, the trachea is stable under physiologic conditions. The main carina is usually sharp and the angulation of the main bronchi is narrow.

Although the branching of the lobar and segmental bronchi is astonishingly consistent, some variations are so frequent that they may be considered as harmless. However, because severe pathologic malformations may be similar, some experience is required for their discrimination.

## Anatomic variations without clinical relevance

Many variations are seen in the branching of the segmental bronchi. Early branching of the subsegments may mimic additional segmentation. On the other hand, segmental bronchi that are normally separated may arise from a common stem. This should not be confused with agenesis of segments. These variations can cause difficulties in localization and access to peripheral lesions by transbronchial biopsy. Sometimes segmental or even lobar bronchi may be found as an "anlage" only; that is, bronchial buds, forming diverticulous excavations of the bronchial system. This will be most often be found with the paracardial segment in the lower lobe of the right side.

The most frequent surplus variation is an additional bronchus of the apical segments of both lower lobes, the so-called subapical segments. An additional, completely developed lobus cardiacus on the left side is comparatively rare. On the right side, the apicodorsal segments of the upper lobe may branch separately from the main bronchus, thus producing a double upper lobe carina. These segments or even the whole upper lobe bronchus may separate from the distal trachea as a so-called tracheal or "pig bronchus," as this is the normal anatomy in pigs, which are used as animal models in training (Fig. 8.1). This has been observed far more frequently on the right side than on the left. On the left side, sometimes there is no common upper lobe bronchus if the lingula arises directly from the main bronchus. A trifurcation may be formed or even a short intermediate bronchus if the branching occurs at the level of the apical segment of the lower lobe.

These branching variations cause clinical symptoms only if the bronchus is hypoplastic or shows some kinking due to its abnormal course, leading to impairment of ventilation or clearing of secretions of the corresponding part of the lungs.

In cartilage development, fusions of branchings or whole rings may be found as variations. A common variation is the finding of echondromas—harmless protrusions of normal cartilaginous tissue resembling compression by expansive extraluminal tumor growth. These may be distinguished easily due to their garland-like appearance, being restricted to the cartilages only and leaving the intercartilaginous spaces unharmed. At biopsy, the tissue will be very hard and, after removal of the mucosa, white cartilage will be laid bare.

This is not to be confused with the so-called tracheobronchopathia chondro- sive osteoplastica, a condition of excessive exophytic tumor-like growth of cartilaginous and mostly ossified tissue in the mucosa and submucosa without anatomic restriction to the cartilages. The inflammatory etiology of this disease is still debated; rarely is mechanical or laser removal used if it is obstructing the large airways.

## Pathologic malformations of the bronchial system

Many of the pathologic malformations can be explained as developmental disorders at different stages of fetal organ formation. They may be solitary lesions restricted to the bronchial tree only or they may be part of complex disorders of the bronchopulmonary system, which in themselves again may be part of a multiple organ malformation syndrome. Because the complex history of embryologic organ formation is still not completely understood, the classification of developmental malformations is arbitrary to some extent. Nevertheless, a systematic overview will help understanding [9], and because it will enhance orientation, the most important malformations will be discussed below in the order that they are encountered passing down the tracheobronchial tree.

### Larynx

By far the most frequent anomaly and cause of stridor in the newborn is laryngomalacia due to immature soft cartilages (85%), causing a "flabby larynx" with excess folding of the epiglottis and shortness with inward bending of the aryepiglottic folds. The larynx will most frequently stabilize spontaneously after some time of stabilization by a soft tracheal tube or, recently, by non-invasive continuous positive airway pressure (CPAP) ventilation. The diameter of the tube should be rather small so as not to cause further damage to the mucosal lining and to the cartilages by exertion of pressure.

Laryngeal stenoses due to supraglottic, glottic, or subglottic webs are far more frequently the sequelae to intubation trauma during neonatal intensive care than a congenital anomaly. These can be treated by endoscopic mechanical removal or laser resection.

Laryngotracheal clefts and fistulas are rare events caused by a defect in development of the tracheoesophageal septum. These require surgery because they cause symptoms of repeated aspiration. Endoscopic closure by fibrin application will rarely be successful and may only be considered in very small hair fistulas.

The involvement in hemangiomas or hamartomas, such as in familial neurofibromatosis, causes symptoms of upper airway obstruction due to submucosal tumors protruding

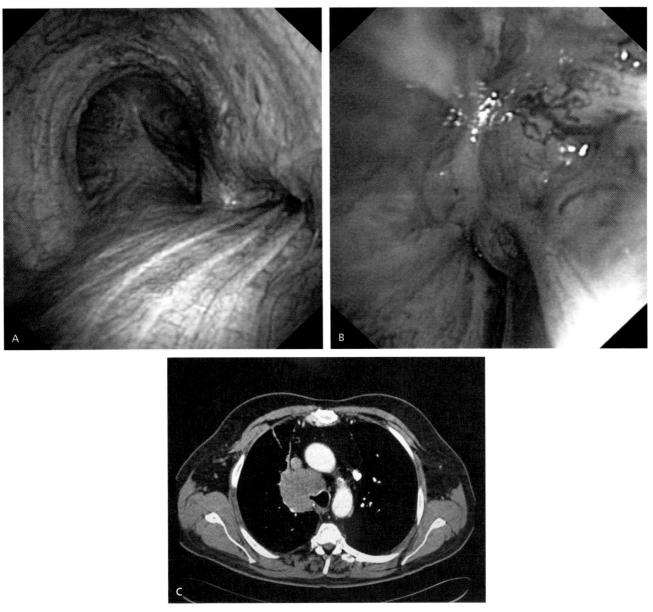

**Fig. 8.1** Anatomical variation. (A) An atypical bronchus is arising from the right tracheal wall in the distal third. It represents the apicodorsal segment of the right upper lobe and is regularly seen in pigs. (B) At closer inspection, it is occluded by a squamous cell cancer. (C) The corresponding CT shows the tracheal bronchus and the occluding tumor in the right upper lobe.

into the lumen of the larynx and the upper trachea. Hemangiomas may frequently be coagulated by neodymium:yttrium-aluminum garnet (Nd:YAG) laser if they do not resolve spontaneously. Recently there have been reports on successful systemic treatment by betablockers.

### Trachea

Mechanical instability of the trachea is so common in early childhood that it can be regarded as an almost normal finding, so long as the airways regain their normal diameter during the resting position. It takes several years for the cartilages to gain their definite stability. Complete rings and complete agenesis of the cartilages are rare malformations, causing life-threatening symptoms due to chronic obstruction and inflammation. Surgical management using grafts of cartilages or pericardium is still restricted and not always successful.

It is especially in combination with other developmental disorders of the vascular system, aberrant bronchi, or malformations of the esophagus that tracheal stenosis due to chondromalacia may become pathologic. In these instances, the cartilages can be softened due to chronic pressure or partially absent as fistulas, or aberrant bronchi may cause defects in the structures of the tracheal wall.

Congenital tracheobronchomegaly (Mounier–Kuhn) usually becomes symptomatic in adulthood only because the sequelae of chronic inflammation develop gradually over the years.

Tracheal diverticula will be formed either by rudimentary accessory bronchi or rudimentary tracheoesophageal fistulas. Sometimes these are found as the result of traction by scars from healed lymph nodes after specific inflammation or after perforation.

Esophagotracheal fistulas cause symptoms of aspiration in early infancy and are most frequently associated with esophageal atresia. Closure by endoscopic means, such as laser obliteration or application of fibrin glue, are frequently unsuccessful and surgical repair must be performed [10].

## Bronchi

Branching abnormalities of the bronchi cause symptoms only if they are associated with problems of ventilation or drainage of secretions from the parts of the lung parenchyma to which they lead. Accessory bronchi frequently have narrow ostia due to malformations of the corresponding cartilages, causing retention of secretions due to their instability. Abnormal cartilage spurs or complete rings at the branching levels lead to major stenoses of the large airways, which is especially common in aberrant tracheal bronchi.

Aberrant branching is most common in the right upper lobe, arising either from the main bronchus or from the trachea. Repeated inflammatory infiltration in the dependent lung tissue due to retention of secretions is not uncommon.

On the medial wall of the intermediate bronchus one occasionally sees a fistulous opening, which is the ostium of an accessory lobus cardiacus. This is also the most common location for bronchogenic cysts if the accessory lobe has not fully developed into a pulmonary segment.

Stenoses of the bronchi by webs are usually secondary, due to inflammation during early childhood. They are probably the most common cause of isolated bronchiectasis. Bronchiectasis due to agenesis of cartilages in the segmental bronchi, resulting in localized bronchial stenosis or due to complete malformation of the "anlage", is far less frequent.

Membranes or complete atresia of bronchi are rare events. I have found these in two cases of lobar sequestration. The hyperlucent lung tissue on the x-ray in these cases obviously was inflated via Kohn's pores from adjacent areas.

The syndromes associated with immotile cilia, specifically, Kartagener's disease or Young's syndrome, are always associated with diseases of the bronchi, mostly chronic inflammation or bronchiectasis.

Whether the syndrome of unilateral hyperlucency (Swyer–James or MacLeod's syndrome) is caused by primary hypoplasia of the pulmonary artery or is due to peripheral obliterative bronchiolitis of viral origin is still debated. Any malformations of the lung parenchyma, especially those associated with regional hypo- or hyperinflation, may lead to displacement or obstruction of the central bronchial system.

Pulmonary vascular disorders are visible only to the bronchoscopist if the bronchial circulatory system is involved or if they are part of systemic malformation syndromes; for diagnosis of these, endobronchial ultrasound has been found most useful. The latter are rarely found in arteriovenous fistulas (as, for example, in Osler's disease or as spider nevi in liver cirrhosis), the former in cardiac vitia that are causing redistribution of the intrathoracic blood flow to the bronchial vessels [11]. In these instances, I have found bronchial varicosis that resolved after surgical repair of the cardiac vitium.

## Anatomic considerations regarding resectability

Resectability is one of the most important anatomic aspects for the bronchoscopist in daily routine work. In the presurgical staging procedures, to assess the resectability of lesions of the central airways, accurate—to the millimeter—assessment of the structures involved is essential. The distances of lesions to structures marking crucial limitations for standard surgical procedures have to be watched closely, because involvement of central parts of the tracheobronchial system proximal to the pulmonary lesion will usually only be manageable by extensive surgical procedures. In these situations, bronchoplastic operations must be considered in favor of the conservation of healthy functioning lung tissue [12].

This is most important at the level of the right and left main bronchus for so-called sleeve lobectomy and at the level of the main carina and bifurcation for sleeve pneumonectomy, when resection of the bifurcation and reimplantation of the remaining main bronchus has to be planned. In a large prospective study for the evaluation of staging and therapeutic procedures in bronchogenic carcinoma, however, routine biopsy of macroscopically normal carinas proximal to the lesion hardly ever produced positive results.

Because the resectability of tracheal lesions is limited, it is essential that the bronchoscopist exactly measures not only the dimensions of the lesion itself but also its distances to crucial landmarks, especially the carina, the cricoid cartilage, and the vocal cords. Counting the number of cartilage rings involved may prove helpful.

The involvement of mediastinal structures surrounding the central airways—the mediastinal lymph nodes, the esophagus, or the major blood vessels—may be suspected due to displacement or direct involvement of the central airways at the corresponding level. In these cases the bronchoscopist can induce further investigational studies such as esophagoscopy, exploration by ultrasound and radiology, or even mediastinoscopy for the staging procedure.

## Semiotics

To establish a diagnosis by endoscopy of the airways, we have to consider the structures that can be seen and the changes due to pathologic processes when compared to the normal situation.

As in every kind of morphologic diagnosis in medicine, interpretation of bronchoscopic findings and establishment of a diagnosis is based on a synopsis of changes of the morphologic structures that is finally integrated into the clinical context. This procedure—the art of interpretation of appearances of diseases—is called semiotics (from Greek to semeion, "the sign") [13].

In contrast to the complex information that one obtains at the bedside, in endoscopy one has to rely mainly on visual information, rarely on additional indirect palpation. A diagnosis by bronchoscopic examination is achieved by interpreting the alterations of the visible structures of the tracheobronchial structures. Table 8.2 lists the structures that should be recognized in relation to their anatomy.

A detailed discussion of each of these items and how they may be set into a clinical context in establishing a diagnosis follows. Although the discussion covers the different aspects separately in an arbitrary arrangement, it must be stressed that in most instances various combinations of several components will be found, and only the complete mosaic will make the diagnosis. Obviously, some structures will be discussed under more than one category.

### Contents of the bronchi

Physiologically, in the normal subject the bronchi are filled mainly by air. The mucosal lining is covered by a thin layer of translucent fluid which is transported orally in a well-coordinated, mostly counterclockwise, spiral movement by the mucosal cilia. Recent observations, however, suggest that rather than by a spiral movement of the ciliary beat, this kind of transport is generated by the peculiar motion of the air inside the airways, as could also be seen in other reports [14]. In contrast to the general assumption that the flow is more or less laminar along the walls, during laser treatment in humans as well as in animals it has been

**Table 8.2** Structures as diagnostic guidelines in bronchoscopy

| 1 | Contents of bronchi |
|---|---|
| 2 | Coloration and surface of mucosa |
| 3 | Blood vessels |
| 4 | Lymph vessels |
| 5 | Integrity of the mucosa |
| 6 | Integrity of the bronchial wall |
| 7 | Involvement by surrounding structures |
| 8 | Clinical context |

repeatedly observed as a turbulent transport of smoke toward the larynx. Interestingly, this most efficient type of transportation for clearance of debris has been used in technical solutions such as sinks and sewers [15]. This kind of airflow also continues in the inbound direction right down to the alveolar spaces [16]. Probably, this is due to the turbulent or turbine-like motion of the sticky secretions with high concentration of eosinophils (first described as spirals in the sputum of asthmatics by Curschmann).

Pathologic changes in the bronchial mucous glands or of the alveolar fluid formation, may alter the composition of secretions in quantity and quality, consistency, and color.

Abundant clear liquid, and sometimes foamy fluid secretions, are pathognomonic for bronchioalveolar carcinoma. The abundant secretions in alveolar proteinosis and the not always copious secretions in *Pneumocystis carinii* pneumonia usually are more opaque due to their high protein content. In pulmonary edema, the foamy secretions are frequently stained by traces of blood.

The sticky, clear secretions in the asthmatic patient are well known and may even be so viscous that they form casts of the smaller bronchi, known as Curschmann's spirals. Larger agglomerations may form mucoid impactions, causing the obstruction of segmental or even larger bronchi. The resulting shadows on the plain X ray mimic obstructive pneumonia due to bronchial carcinoma.

The grayish-brown sticky secretions, which are full of macrophages loaded with condensed remnants of tobacco smoke at cytologic examination, are pathognomonic for the smoking patient suffering from chronic bronchitis. During episodes of bacterial infection, these may turn more yellowish.

Severely purulent secretions will be found in bacterial pneumonia—especially in its obstructive form—and in patients with abscess formation. The abundant, purulent secretions with "mouthful expectorations" are pathognomonic for bronchiectasis, which is found in its most extensive form in mucoviscidosis due to chronic infection by *Pseudomonas*. When recovered for bacteriologic examination, the secretions settle in three layers: foam on top, cloudy fluid in the middle, and sediments of leukocytes at the bottom of a vessel. The purulent secretions may also form thick plugs, causing bronchial obstruction by mucoid impactions, thereby further aggravating the distension of the peripheral bronchi. Tomography frequently shows "sausage-shaped" shadows that are suggestive of the diagnosis.

Superinfection of these plugs by *Aspergillus fumigatus* makes the secretions even more sticky, almost rubberlike, giving the clinical picture of allergic bronchopulmonary aspergillosis, a hypersensitivity reaction to the pathologic agent [17] (Fig. 8.2).

In all these diseases, cytologic and microbiologic examination of the bronchoscopically gained secretions will yield further information on the nature of the underlying

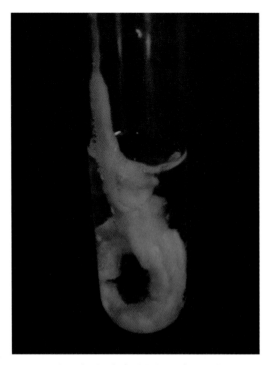

**Fig. 8.2** Mucus plug. This kind of solid plug is frequently seen in bronchiectasis. In this case it was colonized by *Aspergillus* species and associated with the clinical symptoms of allergic bronchopulmonary aspergillosis.

pathogenic cause. The samples may be obtained by special, sheathed catheters or microbiology brushes. Experience has demonstrated that asservation by simple suction through the biopsy channel of the fiberscope will yield reliable results for most routine clinical purposes [18]. Bronchoalveolar lavage (BAL) is the method of choice in the diagnosis of infections of the alveolar space, which have become the most important pneumologic problem in the immunocompromised patient, especially in acquired immunodeficiency syndrome (AIDS) [19].

Frequently, under varying conditions, blood staining of differing degrees will be mixed with the secretions. If these stains accompany clinical symptoms of chronic bronchitis with endoscopic findings of distended mucosal blood vessels, they are readily interpreted as benign. Unfortunately, the same patients—that is chronic smokers—also run a high risk of bronchial carcinoma. Therefore, one should always insist on visualizing the actual site of bleeding because this may be the early sign of an otherwise occult bronchial carcinoma.

In my opinion, every patient with hemoptysis, apart from the obvious clinical picture of pulmonary embolism, should undergo bronchoscopic examination immediately during the episode of bleeding. Thus, at least the site of bleeding may be assessed and further investigations (bron-chography, angiography, etc.) can be focused on the potential source of bleeding. Sometimes acribic sequential lavage of each lobar bronchus may be necessary for localization. In some cases of episodic hemoptysis the procedure has to be repeated. Every patient with an unexplained source of hemoptysis must be regarded as carrying an occult bronchogenic carcinoma and must be kept under close observation [20].

Malignant diseases make up 25% of the sources of bleeding in my patients. In 50%, chronic inflammatory processes are the source of bleeding, of which chronic bronchitis (15%), bronchiectasis (8%), and tuberculous caverns (8%) are the most frequent underlying causes. In about 70% of my cases the source of bleeding could be established by bronchoscopy. With the addition of positive results of conventional radiology, bronchography, and angiography, a definite diagnosis of the bleeding source was not established in only 10%. This has been especially true for catamenial hemoptysis, if the ectopic uterine mucosa is neither found endobronchially nor showing on the plain X-ray film in the lung parenchyma [21].

## Coloration and surface of the mucosa

The normal bronchial mucosa is a pink-colored, glistening layer smoothly covering all the structures of the bronchial wall. Only the cartilages are yellow-whitish in color. The nourishing capillary vessels are clearly seen as a delicate network. In the normal bronchial mucosa the lymph vessels are not seen, nor are the openings of the mucous glands visible. The submucosal longitudinal bundles of connective tissue may be somewhat prominent, giving a washboard-like appearance to the paries membranaceus, especially during forced breathing or coughing, but these cannot be observed through healthy mucosa.

Many of the factors causing changes in the secretions also influence the bronchial mucosa, thereby changing its color and the structures described above. Acute inflammatory reactions due to infectious or toxic agents frequently cause diffuse bright or dark reddening of the mucosa, according to the extent of vascular congestion. In this situation, the capillary network can no longer be discriminated.

By a concomitant edematous swelling, the mucosa may be thickened, leveling the contours of the bronchial wall. Especially in the asthmatic patient, edematous swelling is the main feature of mucosal alteration, whereas the vascular injection may be far less prominent. In these patients, the mucosa appears pale and has a cushion like swelling, which may cause mechanical bronchial obstruction on top of the functional bronchospasm.

In the most common form of chronic bronchitis, the mucosa appears thinned and rather pale. The underlying structures of the bronchial wall are prominent. This is conspicuous in the elastic layers of connective tissue on the dorsal parts of the larger airways. Longitudinal strands of white color, sometimes branching, can be seen lying directly beneath the thinned mucosa.

The mucosa and submucosal tissue may sag between the fiber bundles because the chronic inflammatory process and the continuous mechanical stress of coughing cause the elastica to be distended, as in the cutaneous striae due to pregnancy. In addition, the chronic liberation of polymorphonuclear leukocyte elastase leads to destruction of the elastic fibers. Typical changes in the mucous glands are found; because of the formation of viscous bronchial secretions, the ducts become distended by mucous retention and their normally invisible openings appear as small holes in the mucosa. All of these features make up the picture of chronic deforming and destructing bronchitis.

During episodes of acute inflammation due to viral or bacterial superinfection there may be some reddening. The blood vessels, however, will still be visible and even more prominent due to the congestion.

In the rarer form of chronic hypertrophic bronchitis there is marked swelling of the pale mucosa by an excessive lymphocytic infiltration of the submucosal layers, producing thickened folds that can even mimic amyloidosis of the bronchial wall or submucosal tumor infiltration. This also may cause mechanical obliteration of the bronchial lumina.

The transparent nodular lesions in sarcoidosis are easily recognized. Frequently in these lesions, as in discontinuous lymphangitic tumor spreading on close view, small capillary vessels may be seen extending into the nodular lesions. Sometimes patchy mucus collections may appear in a similar pattern but, in contrast, these can be removed easily by gentle suctioning.

## Blood vessels

The normal bronchial mucosa is nourished by a delicate network of arterial blood vessels, which can be seen clearly. In the trachea these vessels enter the mucosa in a segmental array between the cartilages, spreading like small trees upward and downward to the adjacent segment where they form scarce anastomoses. By compression due to a cuffed tube these anastomoses become easily obliterated, which then results in mucosal ulcerations and finally in chondromalacia due to malnutrition of the cartilages. It is only in the dorsal membranaceous wall that these take a longitudinal course, covering several segments.

In the larger bronchi the vascularization is arranged longitudinally, covering larger areas. Here anastomoses are scarce, so they have to be regarded as end arteries. The postcapillary venous blood is collected in an intra- and submucosal plexus from where it is carried directly to the pulmonary venous system [22]. In contrast to the blood vessels, the lymphatics are not seen in the normal bronchial mucosa.

In acute bacterial, and especially in viral, infections of the lower respiratory tract, the mucosa is frequently dark red so

that the capillary network is completely blurred. Although in these cases the discoloration is spread evenly over the entire mucosa, in localized types of inflammatory reactions, such as sarcoidosis, the reddening may be patchy, sometimes arranged around granulomas, leaving spaces of completely normal vascular structure in between.

It is especially in sarcoidosis that we see the phenomenon of vascular engorgement due to enhanced blood flow in the inflammatory process and impairment of venous drainage due to compression of the vessels by enlargement of the hilar lymph nodes adjacent to the bronchial wall.

Most frequently, vascular engorgement is due to swelling of the lymph nodes by malignant infiltration. Especially if a lymph node is penetrating the bronchial wall or if lymphangitic tumor is spreading submucosally, the blood vessels have an irregular, corkscrew-like appearance; the mucosal tumor nodules also show an irregular structure with a tendency to confluence (Fig. 8.3).

In chronic bronchitis, the mucosal blood vessels become more prominent as the inflammatory reddening of the mucosa is much less conspicuous than in acute bronchitis. The mucosa, due to chronic edema and scar formation, becomes pale. In chronic bronchitis, with a rise of pressure in the pulmonary circulation, marked distention of the bronchial blood vessels may develop because there are many

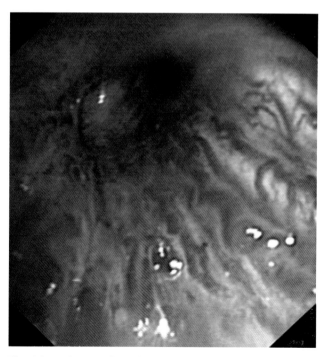

**Fig. 8.3** Ectatic mucosal vessels. The left upperlobe bronchus is narrowed by external compression from a bronchogenic cancer. The tumor is obstructing the veins in the deeper layers and adjacent to the bronchial wall. Therefore, the blood is transported via distended superficial mucosal varicosal vessels.

anastomoses between the bronchial and pulmonary circulation. This is also true for chronic congestive cardiovascular disease where, in severe cases, observed bleeding bronchial mucosal varices were treated by laser coagulation.

Acute bacterial infection in chronic bronchitis may cause further distention of blood vessels by an enhancement of blood flow; additional inflammatory damage to the mucosal lining can lead to hemoptysis. This is a most common complication of bronchiectatic lung disease and may even be life threatening because, in bronchiectasis, the source of bleeding is usually the bronchial artery with high systemic pressure, which may be distended to the caliber of a knitting needle due to the chronic inflammatory process.

The vascular pattern in chronic inflammation may also become fairly irregular, even forming small angiomatous structures. Rarely have true spider nevi of the bronchial mucosa in liver cirrhosis been seen. Hemangiomas in Osler's disease, in contrast, are smaller, more evenly distributed, and regular. True submucosal hemangiomas of the bronchial wall mostly show a cushion like appearance, and especially in children one will often find further lesions on the body surface.

### Lymphatic vessels

In contrast to the blood vessels, the lymphatics are mostly not seen in the normal bronchial mucosa. Sometimes these appear as whitish "tramlines" running parallel to the blood vessels in the major bronchi. Only if there is marked obstruction of the lymphatic drainage due to malignant invasion of lymph nodes, scar formation, or postoperative lymphedema after surgical interruption of lymph drainage are the mucosal lymphatic vessels prominent and visible. Due to the congestion by lymphatic edema, the mucosa may then be markedly swollen and show a cobblestone pattern on its surface. The distended lymph vessels are then seen as a fine, whitish network between the polyploidy formations. If enlarged lymph nodes adjacent to the bronchi are obstructing the lymphatic drainage, the distended larger mucosal lymph vessels may become visible as milky streaks, resembling "glass noodles," running parallel to the blood vessels.

Lymphatic cysts of the mucosa due to malignant occlusion of the lymph ducts in the mediastinum never occur in benign inflammatory disease.

Foreign material, such as anthracotic pigment that is inhaled into the alveolar space, may be carried by the intra- and interlobular lymphatics toward the hilar lymph nodes and to the bronchial mucosa, where it then is deposited and may become visible as black streaks, especially if the lymph vessels are further distended by lymphangitic tumor invasion.

### Integrity of the mucosa

Ordinary acute viral and bacterial infections leave the macroscopic structure of the mucosa intact, showing only the secondary reactions described above. The inflammatory process is seen only on the microscopic level. However, in some instances of non-specific viral and non-viral infections (*Mycoplasma pneumoniae* and some strains of streptococci among others), a granulomatous reaction can develop which may lead to polypoid and ulcerative formations. If this reaction is progressive and inflammatory destruction of the bronchial wall becomes invasive, severe scar formation may set in afterward during the process of healing with consecutive obliteration of the lumina. This may be one of the causes of bronchocentric granulomatosis. This kind of etiology, besides scar formation due to perforation of specific lymph nodes, is believed to be the most common cause of secondary isolated bronchiectasis in single lobes.

Rapid and extensive swelling and granuloma formation occurs after impaction of foreign bodies, especially due to oily substances contained in peanuts and the like. These swellings respond readily to corticosteroid medication. Thus, if given on the evening before a scheduled removal, frequently the foreign body has disappeared by the next day as the swelling has disappeared and the foreign body been coughed up and swallowed. If foreign bodies are not removed soon after accidental aspiration, inflammatory pseudotumors may develop with consecutive complete bronchial obstruction, resulting in chronic atelectasis or poststenotic bronchiectasis. The same can be true for penetrating lymph nodes in tuberculosis or anthracosilicosis.

Granulomatous inflammatory reaction is the typical form of bronchial involvement in sarcoidosis and tuberculosis. Whereas granulomata in sarcoidosis usually are clearly separated, pinhead-sized glassy nodules, in mycobacterial disease there is a tendency to confluence of the lesions and superficial necrosis of the mucosa, showing the picture of specific bronchitis. This is either due to bronchogenic propagation from the lung or specific lymph node invasion.

Beside tuberculous inflammation, ulcerative bronchitis may also be found in bronchial involvement of Wegener's granulomatosis and other forms of vasculitis. The same will happen if pulmonary granulomata invade the adjacent bronchial wall. Biopsy will show granulomatous destruction of the blood vessels by histologic examination. Chronic relapsing polychondritis may have the appearance of ulcerative bronchitis, most frequently involving proximal parts of the airways as well, especially the region of the cricoid cartilage, the arytenoids, and the cartilages of the nose [23].

The most common cause of ulcerative bronchitis is malignant infiltration of the bronchial wall. This must always be excluded by sufficient biopsies. The inflammatory process of common chronic bronchitis gradually affects the mucosa itself and the underlying structures of the bronchial wall. The recurrent infiltration by polymorphonuclear leukocytes, with the liberation of destructive substances such as elastase, causes atrophy of the mucosa and distention of the underlying layers of elastic connective tissue, leading to the morphologic changes described above. Due to the altered viscosity of the secretions, mucus is retained in the glands. This gradually leads to distension of orifices of the ducts that are seen as small holes in the mucosa, forming one of the distinctive features of chronic deforming bronchitis. Over years of duration the chronic inflammatory process also involves the deeper structures, thereby affecting the bronchial wall as a whole.

### Integrity of the bronchial wall

In chronic non-specific bronchitis the destruction of the elastic connective tissue of the bronchial wall is gradually followed by a loss of stability, leaving the larger airways even more susceptible to the damaging effects of excessive chronic recurring changes in pressure from attacks of coughing (Fig. 8.4). The result of these ongoing, combined destructive processes is a relaxation and prolapse of the paries membranaceus and chondromalacia of the larger airways. These cause further mechanical obstruction, thereby closing the vicious circle.

The most extensive kind of destruction in non-specific chronic inflammation is found in bronchiectasis. Here the destruction of the bronchial wall leads to saccular excavations between the cartilages and membranaceous scars in

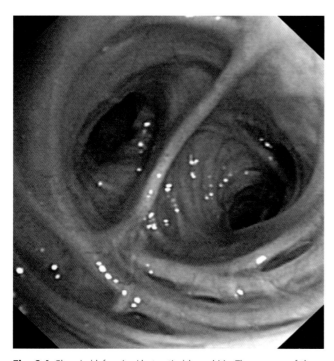

**Fig. 8.4** Chronic (deforming/destructive) bronchitis. The mucosa of the lingula bronchus is rough and shows several holes. Chronic inflammation by invasion of leukocytes that are liberating elastase has destroyed major parts of the submucosal connective tissue. Only the stronger supporting fibers are still present between the sagging mucosa. The holes are distended mucus gland openings, widened by the forced evacuation of sticky secretions.

between. The accumulation of the sticky secretions causes further distention. The most severe form of this disease can be seen in patients suffering from mucoviscidosis.

The deep-reaching destructive processes of chronic relapsing polychondritis have been mentioned above. Healing after immunosuppressive therapy may leave extensive scar formation and malacic stenosis after destruction of the supporting cartilages. Even more extensive scar formation is seen after inhalation injury due to toxic agents.

Cartilages are sensitive to pressure (intubation), heat (Nd : YAG laser) and irradiation. These reactions are especially observed in the long term after high-dose radiotherapy, especially after endobronchial brachytherapy. After this treatment, chondromalacia and chondroradionecrosis may develop with sequestration of the necrotic cartilages. After 6 months or longer, extensive scar formation may result in strictures that are difficult to treat.

The same may also be true for the destruction of the bronchial wall by invasion of inflammatory lymph nodes. Tumor invasion will be the most common reason for the destruction of the bronchial wall. One of the specific features in contrast, however, is the rare involvement of the cartilages. Even in extensive and deep malignant necrosis the cartilaginous structures may frequently be seen fairly intact. Currently, there is no satisfactory explanation for this.

Because of the tremendous progress in intensive-care procedures, many iatrogenic traumas are seen involving the tracheobronchial wall. Tracheomalacia and granulomatous inflammatory destruction at the site of mechanical alteration are the most serious sequelae of this kind of damage. In contrast to former expectations, these complex stenoses do not easily resolve and stabilize after internal support by stenting, but in 70 to 80% they recur after stent removal, which leads to new considerations with regard to long-term stability in these devices.

### Involvement by diseases of the surrounding structures

The central airways are surrounded by the complex anatomy of the organs in the mediastinum. A vast variety of pathologic processes of these organs may go along with involvement of the trachea and bronchi. In the newborn and young child, congenital malformations of the foregut and larger vessels are the most common causes of compression of the central airways. During later life, enlargement of the thymus, then the thyroid gland and the mediastinal lymph nodes due to their proximity to the central airways, is frequently followed by breathing impairment.

Lymph node invasion is never seen in ordinary sarcoidosis or in anthracosis (Fig. 8.5). Only if there is additional involvement in silicosis or tuberculosis will penetration or even perforation occur. If the lymph node is still covered by intact mucosa, the typical bronchial pseudotumor is formed that cannot be differentiated macroscopically from

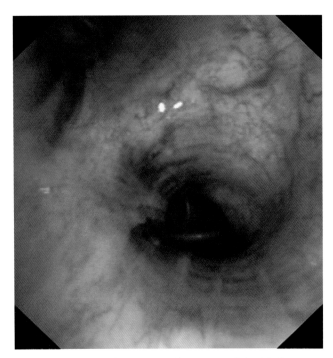

**Fig. 8.5** Anthracosis. The mucosa at the entrance of the right lower lobe shows a dark discoloration. This is due to anthracotic pigment deposition within the adjacent lymph node. There are no signs of lymph node penetration or perforation.

malignant disease. Calcified specific lymph nodes that are not evacuated after perforation will remain inside the bronchial lumen as broncholiths and cause postobstructive bronchiectasis [24].

The most frequent penetration of lymph nodes is caused by malignant infiltration. Endoscopically it can be difficult to assess the depth of penetration from the outer layers of the bronchial wall. Whether endobronchial sonography in this situation is helpful in guiding the needle for transbronchial needle biopsy is currently being investigated so that in the future it may become a routine procedure in staging of bronchial carcinoma (Fig. 8.6).

Deviation of the spinal column in severe kyphoscoliosis or Bechterew's disease as well as pectus excavatum can involve the trachea by compression or distortion. Differentiation from impression by aortic aneurysms is easy because, in the latter, pulsation of the mass is obvious. Only in small children are the airways still so soft that it may be difficult to discriminate intrinsic instability from extrinsic compression. Also in this situation, according to preliminary experience, endobronchial ultrasonography may be helpful.

All pathologic processes causing deviation or enlargement of the mediastinal organs, such as lymphomas, thymomas, cardial distention or pericardial effusions, esophageal diverticula and tumors, mesothelioma, or pleural effusions, may cause extrinsic compression of the central airways.

## Clinical context

Because the repertoire of reactions to different noxes is limited, the diagnosis is not always clear from the endoscopic aspect by itself. Before any final conclusions can be drawn, all the clinical and technical information achieved by anamnesis, physical examination, and technical investigations before and after the endoscopic examination must be considered. In context of this information as a whole the diagnosis is finally established.

## Findings in airway lesions

### Upper airways

Although the upper airways, nose, and nasopharynx, are not exactly considered the domain of bronchoscopy, one should always keep in mind that they are an integral part of the airway system. Because diseases of the airways are frequently systemic, involvement of the upper airways should always be considered. This especially applies to systemic diseases such as Wegener's granulomatosis, chronic relapsing polychondritis, and bronchiectasis in Kartagener's syndrome. Not uncommonly, malignant tumors of the upper and the lower airways are associated because the impact of noxes—especially cigarette smoke—affects both. Organic obstruction of the upper airways due to conchal hyperplasia or deformation, and functional obstruction such as airway collapse in sleep apnea, may cause secondary afflictions of the bronchial system such as chronic inflammation or aspiration pneumonia. A source of hemoptysis should always be excluded in the upper airways if it cannot be found in the tracheobronchial system or in the lung itself (Fig. 8.7).

### Larynx

The larynx is the most complicated and sensitive structure of the tracheobronchial system, and thorough knowledge of its anatomic and functional properties is essential for diagnosis [25].

The most frequent functional disorder to be diagnosed is paralysis of a vocal cord, which is mainly caused by compression or destruction of the recurrent laryngeal nerve due to malignancies of the thyroid gland or, more frequently, by bronchial carcinomas as a sign of tumor spreading to the aortopulmonary window beneath the aortic arch. Secondary paralysis after resection of goiter or bronchial carcinoma with extensive lymph node resection is not uncommon. For accurate assessment of laryngeal function, visualization under local anesthesia is required. In small children this can be performed easily under sedation, for example, by propofol, and additional local anesthesia while breathing spontaneously.

In early infancy, developmental malformations or delay of maturation are frequent causes of breathing problems.

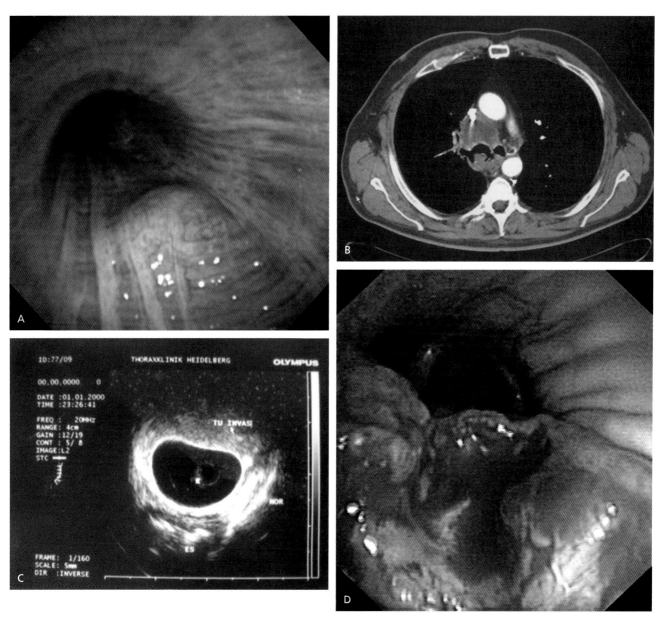

**Fig. 8.6** Mural tumor invasion. (A) A malignant lymph node, invaded by non-small-cell lung cancer (NSCLC) is bulging inward the dorsal wall of the left main bronchus. (B) From CT, invasion cannot not always be diagnosed. In contrast to the dorsal wall in this example, the lymph node anterior to the bifurcation might not be penetrating into the wall. (C) However, endobronchial ultrasound (EBUS, Olympus Co.) clearly shows the invasion (tu invas), seen by the loss of the layer structure of the anterior war of the trachea as compared to the normal wall (nor). Dorsally, the multilayer structure of the adjacent esophagus (ES) is visible. (D) In the case of invasion into the bronchial wall without perforation, a so called "button hole" biopsy is possible by removing the mucosa and penetrating with the forceps deep into the invading tumor.

Whereas instability of the cartilaginous support of the epiglottis and the cricoid are frequent (especially in the premature infant), laryngeal clefts or fistulas between the pharynx and esophagus are comparatively rare. Hemangiomatous obstructing lesions in the larynx may be found in children with cutaneous hemangiomas. Spontaneous resolution is seen frequently, but in severe cases laser destruction may give immediate relief.

In older children and in the adult, traumatic and inflammatory lesions are the most frequent laryngeal lesions besides neoplasias. Since diphtheria has become a rare disease, it is unspecific bacterial or viral infection causing even necrotic inflammation of the larynx that may result in membranes and synechiae after resolution. Specific tuberculous inflammation of the vocal cords with its typical nodular aspect has become extremely rare in my patients.

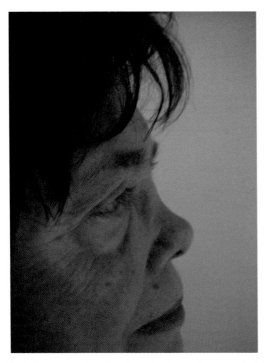

**Fig. 8.7** Deformation of nasal cartilage in Wegener's disease. In this patient the cartilage of the nose is severely damaged (so-called "saddle nose"), which is frequently seen in Wegener's granulomatosis. Clinical observation will guide the diagnosis in these cases with severe stenosis of the central airways and can be a sign for complications to be awaited after surgical procedures. Also, this patient had recurrent subglottic stenosis after surgical resection, which had to be treated by endoscopic insertion of a Montgomery T-stent.

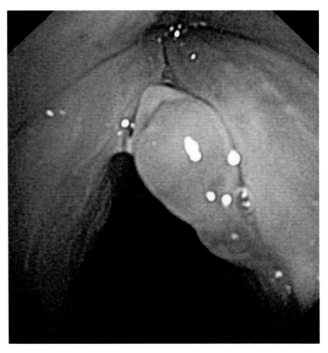

**Fig. 8.8** Vocal chord cyst. The right vocal cord shows a polypoid, shiny lesion close to the anterior commissure of the glottis. The smooth surface and the translucency at closer inspection are pathognomonic for a cyst. In case of doubt, EBUS can clearly differentiate it from solid structures.

Chronic inflammatory processes (such as relapsing polychondritis or Wegener's granulomatosis) involve the mucosa as well as the cartilages and result in severe stenotic scars if not treated aggressively from the beginning. Ankylosis of the arytenoid cartilages due to inflammatory processes at the joints may be diagnosed by gently moving the cartilages with a forceps.

In the larynx, the most frequent benign neoplasias are cysts of the epiglottis and the vocal cords. In the latter, differentiation from chronic Reinke's edema may be difficult and is only possible by biopsy (Fig. 8.8). Polyps due to strain or postintubational trauma have a smooth and shiny surface when compared to the more villous aspect of papillomas.

Primary malignant neoplasias of the larynx frequently arise from the vocal cords. If the lumen is compromised by extensive tumor growth, passage with the endoscope may result in severe swelling with imminent suffocation. Preparations for an emergency intubation should therefore always be made. Because treatment will usually be performed by a laryngologist, exact estimation of the extent of these tumors will not be necessary for the bronchoscopist. Synchronous tumors of the lower airways are not uncommon, so thorough examination of these should be performed.

Secondary malignancies mostly arise from direct invasion of hypopharyngeal carcinomas, of neoplasias of the thyroid gland, or of metastatic lymph node involvement.

The larynx is sensitive to trauma. Today, iatrogenic trauma during resuscitation and intensive care occurs far more frequently than lesions by accidents. Due to improved materials for intubation and improved methods of intensive care therapy, lesions are no longer induced as easily as formerly. But trauma due to intubation in an emergency situation is still common. Damage will mostly harm the subglottic area at the level of the cricoid cartilage because it is the narrowest part for intubation. Lesions or damage due to prolonged intubation are difficult to treat because these are combined lesions of endoluminal granulomata and invasive inflammatory reactions with chondromalacia.

### Trachea

Although the trachea and its bifurcation are part of the central airways, it assumes a special role in airway pathology. Owing to its position and structure, it is subject to major functional and organic changes under physiologic and pathologic conditions. Because it is a single organ and is vital to survival, severe impairment of air passage at this level will always be life threatening. The position of the trachea makes it especially prone to involvement in diseases of adjacent organs such as the esophagus, the great vessels, the heart, thymus, lymph nodes, and spinal column. Owing to both its intrathoracic and extrathoracic position, it is subject to considerable changes in pressure, up to 300 mm Hg, causing major changes in diameter. During forced respiratory maneuvers it may also undergo a change of several centimeters in length. These high functional demands are met by its intricate structure, combining rigid and flexible structures in the most delicate arrangement.

Functional impairment of the trachea is mostly due to loss of its stability. As the mechanical stability gradually develops during maturation in early infancy, comparative instability with nearly total collapse during coughing is almost physiologic in this age. Only if the collapse persists during normal ventilation does prolonged intubation using atraumatic material become necessary. In the adult, instability is most frequently caused by chronic inflammatory damage. Destruction of the collagen fibers by elastase of polymorphonuclear leukocytes, and weakening of the cartilages by chronic coughing, finally results in total collapse of the stabilizing tracheal structures.

Congenital malformations will usually become symptomatic during childhood. The most frequent is esophagotracheal fistula causing chronic aspiration. In my experience, tracheal stenosis due to complete rings of the tracheal cartilages is a rare event. Because in early childhood the cartilages are almost completely round in shape and the dorsal ends almost meet dorsally in the midline—especially during forced respiratory maneuvers and coughing—it may be easily misdiagnosed. Surgical repair by splinting and insertion of cartilaginous or pericardial flaps is a risky procedure; therefore, the diagnosis should be established by further radiologic studies before taking any such measures. Aberrant tracheal bronchi usually cause problems only if they are combined with malformations of the cartilages and additional tracheal stenosis or if narrowing of their ostia interferes with ventilation or drainage of the secretions.

Viral and bacterial inflammation is the most common disease of the airways and usually will not be an indication for bronchoscopy. Sometimes, however, staphylococci or other bacterial infections result in ulcerative lesions and, if unrecognized, may cause severe scar formation and tracheal stenosis. Chronic inflammatory processes caused by immunologic disorders such as Wegener's granulomatosis, chronic relapsing polychondritis, and rheumatoid arthritis involve the deeper structures, especially the cartilages, eventually resulting in strictures and instability. Diagnosis frequently can only be established by the clinical synopsis and not only by histologic examination of biopsy specimens. Inflammatory granulomatous reactions or invasion by specific lymph nodes may appear as pseudotumors and can only be proved benign by biopsy.

True benign neoplasias of the trachea are not frequent. Whether tracheopathia chondrosive osteoplastica is regarded as true neoplasia or an inflammatory reaction is still debated. By its typical macroscopic appearance and hard consistency, it may be diagnosed easily. As in the larynx, polypoid lesions such as fibrolipomas may be distinguished from papillomas due to viral infection by their smooth, shiny surface. The most common primary malignant neoplasias of the trachea are squamous cell carcinomas and adenoid cystic carcinomas. The latter are remarkable because they commonly grow slowly and metastasize only at late stages. There are two types of this tumor: one localized in a polypoid fashion, the other expanding submucosally over a large portion of the central airways so that its boundaries are not clear by macroscopic appearance.

Far more frequent is secondary neoplastic involvement of the trachea. Because the trachea is adjacent to many structures in the mediastinum, it may easily become involved in malignancies of the neighboring organs such as neoplasias of the thyroid gland, the esophagus, the thymus, or the mediastinal lymph nodes. Direct infiltration by bronchial carcinomas or invasion of lymph node metastases, as well as continuous lymphangitic tumor spreading, will usually represent a barrier to radical surgical therapy that only rarely can be overcome. Endotracheal metastasis in the mucosa from distal endobronchial carcinomas is an extremely rare event which, in my opinion, is an argument against the induction of metastatic tumor implantation by bronchoscopic biopsy, the theoretical risk of which is surely overcome by the advantage of establishing a definitive diagnosis for further treatment.

Frequently, patients with obstructing tracheal tumors present as emergency cases. Even high-grade stenosis of the trachea may remain unrecognized for a long time, or misinterpreted as "asthma" because the radiographic density of the surrounding structures of the mediastinum does not provide a good contrast of the trachea on routine chest radiograph, and tomography of the trachea may be obscured by sectional artifacts. Stenosis may be compensated down to a minimal lumen of 3–5 mm until acute obstruction is caused by retention of sticky secretions. For this reason, bronchoscopy is the principal diagnostic tool in this area of the airways and should always be considered in otherwise unexplained symptoms, as stated above [26].

Because the trachea is surrounded by many organs in its extrathoracic and intrathoracic course, and is not covered by protecting tissues, it is easily afflicted by pathologic processes of these surrounding structures. Processes causing an increase in volume or deviation will involve the trachea frequently because, due to the narrow space, it may not give way easily. In its cervical portion one of the most frequent causes is enlargement of the thyroid gland which, if not treated effectively, may eventually lead to almost total compression and asphyxia. And in long-standing compression simple surgical removal is no longer sufficient because tracheomalacia requires segmental tracheal resection as well. The compression by goiters may reach deep into the mediastinum, almost down to the carinal region.

In the upper and middle mediastinum the trachea may even more easily be compressed; its confinement between the spinal column and the sternum means giving way is more difficult. In contrast to displacement by deviations of the spinal column and pectus excavatum, which rarely cause problems of the central airways, abnormal vessels or enlargement of the heart are common causes of displacement and even obstruction. But the most frequent causes are tumors of the esophagus, the thymus gland, or the mediastinal lymph nodes. The most devastating affliction is esophagotracheal fistula due to necrotic invading tumors, the treatment of which is difficult.

Trauma is inflicted to the trachea as easily as to the larynx. The cartilages are extremely sensitive to mechanical (intubation trauma), thermal (laser treatment), or radiation trauma. Even if primarily only the mucosa is damaged, secondary inflammatory reactions frequently involve the deeper submucosal layers and the cartilages as well. This leads to chronification of the process, which eventually results in a combined stenosis due to malacia and strictures. The true extent of these lesions will always be larger than it appears by endoscopy.

For assessment of operability, exact measurement of the extent oaf tumor or traumatic lesion is essential. Distances to the main carina, the cricoid cartilage, and the vocal cords as well as total extent of the lesion must be measured exactly to calculate the possibility of segmental resection. The rigid or flexible endoscope is passed down to the carina and, during successive withdrawal, the respective distances may be measured easily by marking the level of the teeth (fiberscope) or the proximal end of the bronchoscope (on the rigid optic). Diameters of the airways may be calculated by the diameter of the bronchoscope that can be introduced through a stenosis or by placing an opened forceps close to the lesion and measuring the distance between the cups. For the exact intraoperative assessment of the tracheal segment to be resected, I find marking the proximal and distal end by needles under bronchoscopic control useful.

## Bronchi

Localized functional disorders of the bronchi obviously will cause less severe symptoms than is the case in the larynx or trachea. Bronchial collapse causes segmental or lobar symptoms of disturbances in ventilation such as atelectasis or overinflation.

Acute non-specific inflammation due to viral and bacterial agents is the most common affliction of the airways but will rarely be an indication for bronchoscopy. The mucosa is diffusely reddened, sometimes even hemorrhagic, and heavy more or less purulent secretions are seen. The most

frequent community-acquired bacterial agents found in probes are non-hemolytic streptococci, *Diplococcus pneumoniae*, *Hemophilus influenzae*, and in some populations also *Legionella* species; whereas in nosocomial infections staphylococci, *Pseudomonas* species, *Klebsiella*, and enterococci are the most frequent pathogens.

Several sampling devices have been proposed that are supposed to avoid contamination. Results of accuracy are inconclusive so fur. In a comparative study in 60 patients the authors were not able to demonstrate a significant difference in the results of bacteriologic sampling, whether different devices of protected microbiology brushes or simple suction through the biopsy channel of the fiberscope were used. The negative influence of some local anesthetics on bacterial growth, though, must be considered. In special cases, as in the immunocompromised host, the additional cost of these devices may be justified to establish a definite diagnosis. The value of special laboratory tests such as the polymerase chain reaction for the detection of *Mycobacteria tuberculosis* or cytomegalovirus has yet to be established.

Much more frequently, one will be confronted with a diagnosis of persistent or recurrent purulent infections due to resistant bacteria or to abnormalities such as localized bronchiectases or abscesses. In these cases, beside establishing a diagnosis of the pathologic agent, exact description of the anatomic cause and extent of the lesion is necessary. This is one of the comparatively rare cases, besides stenoses, cysts, or fistulas, where bronchography is still needed in addition to conventional radiologic analysis and CT scanning. In localized bronchiectasis or cavitational lesions the colonization by fungi, mostly *Aspergillus fumigatus*, must always be considered, which may cause asthmatic symptoms such as allergic bronchopulmonary aspergillosis.

The most common inflammatory finding is chronic bronchitis, mostly caused by chronic cigarette smoke inhalation. The macroscopic aspect and sequelae of this disease are described in some detail above.

The most common, specific form of inflammation of the bronchi today is sarcoidosis. Diagnosis is easy if the typical granulomas are seen, especially if further symptoms, such as enlargement of the parabronchial lymph nodes, are present and if the radiologic picture is consistent with the diagnosis. But positive endobronchial histology will also be achieved in 20 to 30% of the cases, even if no granulomas are visible at bronchoscopy. The most reliable histologic confirmation, however, will be found by transbronchial biopsy, the diagnostic yield of which, in my experience, is over 95%, even if granulomatous intrapulmonary lesions are not seen radiologically.

Regarding the technique of transbronchial biopsy in disseminated interstitial lung diseases, a significant improvement in diagnostic results was found if more than eight biopsies (usually 10–15) were performed from different parts of one lung and if damage to the biopsy specimens was avoided by not pulling the biopsy forceps through the biopsy channel of the fiberscope. Instead, the fiberscope is removed completely, leaving the tip of the forceps outside in front of the tip of the endoscope for recovery of the biopsy specimen. Irritation by frequent passage of the airways under local anesthesia can be avoided if a tube is inserted over the bronchoscope. Complications in our series are comparatively rare (2.5% of pneumothoraxes, and no severe bleeding), although in disseminated interstitial lung disease we normally do not apply fluoroscopy and we routinely use large forceps to obtain large biopsy specimens.

Primary specific tuberculous bronchitis due to bronchogenic spread has become comparatively rare. Specific ulcerating tuberculous bronchitis is mostly caused by penetration of lymph nodes. All stages, from invasion of the outer layers of the bronchial wall with still intact mucosal covering, to intramural penetration and finally ulceration and resulting scar formation, may be seen if the disease is taking its spontaneous course.

If calcified specific lymph nodes are penetrating into the bronchi, and if the masses are not evacuated due to bronchial stenosis, broncholiths will be seen. These frequently cause postobstructive atelectasis or bronchiectasis. Occlusion by specific lymph nodes has been the most frequent reason for the so-called middle lobe syndrome before the epidemic progress of bronchogenic carcinoma.

Immunologic inflammatory processes, such as vasculitis in Wegener's granulomatosis or in chronic relapsing polychondritis, are comparatively rare and may only be discerned by histology. Whether tumor-like bronchial amyloidosis is due to chronic inflammatory processes, or whether it is caused by the production and deposition of pathologic immunoglobulins in the bronchial mucosa, is still debated.

True benign neoplasias of the bronchi are rare compared to primary bronchial carcinoma. Metaplastic polyps and chondrofibrolipomas are the most frequent, whereas true benign adenomas are rare. Papillomas of the tracheobronchial tree may be due to chronic infection by papilloma viruses type 11 and 16, and there are descriptions of malignant transformation, as we have also seen ourselves. The so-called micropapillomatosis may be regarded as a precancerous lesion.

Counter to common opinion, carcinoid tumors have to be regarded and treated as true malignancies, because these show all signs of malignant growth: infiltration, recurrence after local treatment, and metastasis. We have seen metastatic lymph node skipping in very young adults, as well as late distant mucosal metastases and local recurrences after insufficient local treatment of these tumors.

The most common bronchial neoplasia is primary bronchial carcinoma. The prognosis of bronchial carcinomas is influenced by its histologic differentiation and by its extent, which are the main influences on therapeutic procedures.

**Table 8.3** TNM classification of the primary tumor in non-small-cell carcinoma using bronchoscopy

| T1 | The tumor is not visible endoscopically or has not yet extended beyond the respective lobar bronchus |
|----|----|
| T2 | The main bronchus is involved, but the lesion is still at least 2 cm distal to the main carina |
| T3 | The tumor is within 2 cm distance to, but has not yet involved, the main carina; or, there is altelectasis or obstructive inflammation of one entire lung |
| T4 | The main carina is involved, or the tumor has even infiltrated the trachea |

**Table 8.4** TNM classification of lymph node involvement and metastasis of non-small-cell carcinoma using bronchoscopy

| N1 | Involvement of the ipsilateral peribronchial and hilar nodes |
|----|----|
| N2 | Involvement of the ipsilateral mediastinal and/or subcarinal lymph nodes |
| N3 | Extension of tumor to the contralateral hilar or mediastinal lymph nodes |
| M1 | Intrabronchial or intrapulmonary metastasis or lymphangiosis carcinomatosa of the lung |

By bronchoscopy we are able to give the decisive answers to these questions in over 80% of all cases. In endobronchially visible tumors the accuracy of endoscopic staging is about 95%, which makes bronchoscopy the most important diagnostic procedure. For the bronchoscopist there exist clear definitions of the tumor, node, metastasis (TNM) classification (Tables 8.3, 8.4) regarding extension of the primary tumor, lymph node involvement, and metastases [21].

Endoscopists must be completely familiar with the TNM staging criteria and all macroscopic aspects of lung tumors, and with all conventional and surgical therapeutic options. They should be acquainted with the surgical resection procedures to ascertain bioptically that prospective lines of resection are free of tumor growth before operation. Routine biopsy from macroscopically unsuspected regions in a study at our institution did not yield enough positive results to advise it as a standard procedure.

Bronchoscopists must be familiar with the appearance of bronchial carcinoma from its earliest manifestations to its latest stages, and be aware of all the complications that may be caused by the primary tumor and its metastases. They must be familiar with indirect signs of spreading of the neoplasia and with routes of hematogenous and lymphogenous metastatic dissemination. They must know about typical surgical procedures and their endoscopic appearance to assess the postoperative result and to recognize and prevent imminent complications. Results and complications of conservative therapy must be distinguished from tumor relapse. Lastly, a large number of patients suffering from severe complications of advanced tumor growth may benefit from palliative therapeutic bronchoscopic procedures.

Secondary neoplasias involving the lung and bronchi have become a field of special interest in pulmonary medicine, because the therapeutic approach has changed tremendously over the past 10 years. It has been shown that surgical resection of isolated pulmonary metastases of tumors from other organs demonstrated an even better prognosis than many cases of primary lung carcinoma. This has been proved especially when these could be successfully treated in a multidisciplinary concept of preoperative chemotherapy, operation, and, if necessary, postoperative chemotherapeutic consolidation. In some tumors, such as metastasizing testicular tumors or osteosarcoma, 5-year survival rates of more than 50% could be achieved. Because involvement of the central bronchial system in these cases means a far more extensive resection of lung parenchyma, preoperative bronchoscopy is indispensable.

In metastases of a primary tumor of unknown localization and unknown histology, bronchoscopic biopsy may give the decisive histologic information for the original tumor. Involvement of the central airways or the lung itself in systemic malignancies, such as lymphomas, will have an enormous influence on staging and therapy. Every patient with suspected involvement of the airways or lung should undergo bronchoscopy.

Because the sensitivity of clinical assessment of hilar or mediastinal lymph node involvement in malignancies by conventional radiology, CT scan, or MRI still is no better than 60%, we developed endobronchial ultrasonography (EBUS), which proved superior to methods for conventional imaging and is discussed in more detail in a separate chapter.

As the bronchi are deep inside the thorax, they are better protected against traumatic lesions from internal iatrogenic or accidental external impact than are the larynx and trachea. Unrecognized damage to the central airways, such as bronchial rupture, can cause devastating secondary complications; therefore, early meticulous bronchoscopic examination should exclude such damage in every patient with severe thoracic trauma. This may be difficult because signs of bronchial rupture or perforation may be discreet, especially if the rupture has occurred submucosally and severe mucosal swelling with obliteration of vision has set in.

Aspiration of foreign bodies is still frequently unrecognized and extraction delayed for weeks and months when endoscopic removal is far more complicated than early after the accident. This is especially the case in small children who cannot relate their history. Early sequelae are marked mucosal swelling and reddening, with retention and bacterial infection of secretions. Later granuloma formation and in severe scar formation with postobstructive atelectasis, bronchiectasis, or abscess formation will result.

## New technologies

Since the first publication of *Flexible Bronchoscopy*, significant progress has been made in imaging technologies which have already become routine or are very close to clinical use. This applies to image quality as well as the range of resolution and penetration. By these techniques, structures down to the cellular level will become visible, and the bronchoscopist is now able to visualize structures within the bronchial wall and well into the parabronchial mediastinal structures. Because these new techniques will profoundly influence bronchoscopy and change the state of the art in the near future, the following descriptions of new technology are included [27].

### New imaging technologies

The gap of imaging technologies with regard to resolution, field of view, and penetration is continuously closing. Fiberoptic technology has been gradually introduced, and in our institution this is even being replaced by video chip technology. The rapid development of chip technology has had a tremendous impact on image quality and miniaturization of instruments. With the introduction of color chips the disadvantages of black-and-white chips (blurry images in fast movements and secretions or image breakdown by application of electrocautery or Nd-laser) are consigned to history. Also, for the first time, the quality of rigid instruments is equaled if not surpassed as the images can be electronically processed (Fig. 8.9). Thus, by structure enhancement, small lesions become easily visible that up to now needed intricate technologies such as autofluorescence for visualization (Fig. 8.10). Even autofluorescence systems have become handy instruments, far from the clumsy first-generation devices. Current chips in prototypes are hardly larger than $1\,mm^2$ with 50,000 pixels and prototypes of instruments of not much larger diameter are under investigation. These will provide access to regions currently still out of reach, with much superior image compared to conventional fiberscopes.

Miniaturization will enhance the incorporation of two objective lenses at the tip of one endoscope at a slightly different angles, providing a three-dimensional image. Computerized processing of the digital images will enhance endoscopic accuracy in objective measurement of vertical extent and square area of endobronchial lesions.

New laser probes will provide accurate measurement of diameter and length of stenoses for objective documentation

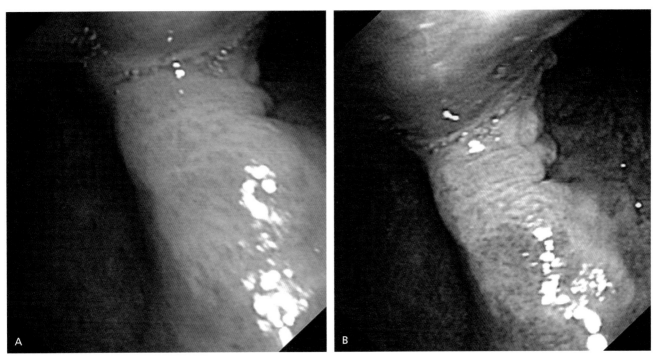

**Fig. 8.9** Dysplasia. (A) The mucosa at the carina of the right upper lobe in this patient is blunt and irregular. (B) Narrow band imaging (NBI, Olympus Co.) demonstrates irregularities in the vascular structure of the capillaries, namely atypical loops reaching under the surface of the mucosa, which is typical for precursor lesions for lung cancer. The patient had multifocal dysplastic lesions after laryngectomy for cancer.

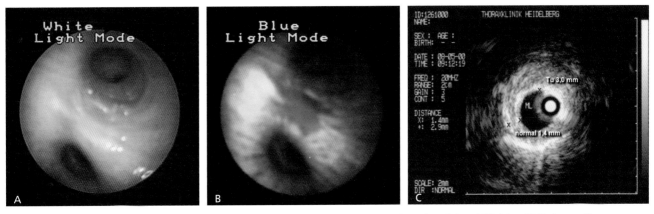

**Fig. 8.10** Early lung cancer. (A) In white light bronchoscopy a slight discoloration is seen at the carina of the middle lobe. (B) Under autofluorescence observation (D-light, Stortz Co.) the lesion and its extent become clearly visible. However, depth of penetration is not obvious. (C) Only EBUS is able to show the exact extent of the tumor (TU) within the bronchial wall as compared to the normal wall and is reliable to make a decision for bronchoscopic local treatment.

of results after treatment and as a basis for manufacturing individual stents.

Gaps in the current range of observation capabilities with regard to resolution, observation area, and depth of penetration will be closed by new imaging technologies, providing boundless imaging technology.

Chip endoscopes with an integrated microactuator of 2 mm outer diameter (by a piezo-electric device) will expand the view beyond the visible from normal to up to 100× magnification, adding zoom technology for endoscopic microscopy. Thus, the endoscopist will be able to predict the results of histopathological examinations and direct his or her diagnostic and therapeutic procedures more accurately.

Completely new imaging technologies will further close the gaps of optical imaging. One of these is endoscopic optical coherence tomography (EOCT). In this technology a low coherence laser light source is built into the tip of the endoscope, and a detector collects the images that are reflected by a reference mirror. The interference image is demodulated and processed by a computer. The spatial resolution of this new imaging technology is 10–20 mm, depth of penetration is up to 2–3 mm, and it allows visualization of tissue structures beyond the visibility of conventional fiber or chip endoscopes, and even high resolution ultrasound [28].

An additional technique that carries magnification even further is microconfocal scanning microscopy (μ COSM). This is achieved by an extremely miniaturized endoscopic laser scanning microscope. Two microscanning mirrors, driven by electrostatic actuators, are built into one chip at the tip of the endoscope. The laser light from the optical fiber is sent via a pinhole in a rotating scanning mirror and focused by a lens onto the tissue. The reflected light is collected by the optical fiber and reconstructed by computer software to an image of up to 800× magnification, allowing visualization of structures within individual cells [29]. Thus, in the not too distant future, the bronchoscopist will also become an *in vivo* pathologist.

The technology that has paved the road toward these new imaging techniques in a paradigmatic fashion is endobronchial ultrasonography (EBUS) . This technology was recently introduced after several obstacles were overcome by image processing and miniaturization of devices. It has opened a new dimension by expanding the bronchoscopist's view beyond the visible, closing the gap in penetration of optical technologies [30]. The resolution of current 20 MHz probes will be further enhanced by probes of 30 MHz and more, adding to the accuracy of diagnosis in small lesions. Electrical scanning systems and B-mode Doppler will open Doppler technology for the evaluation of small vessels in tumors and inflammatory lesions. Three-dimensional image reconstruction will improve assessment of tumor volume as a basis for dosimetry in photodynamic or brachytherapy. Image fusion technique with the endoscopic image will dramatically improve orientation in interdisciplinary planning for treatment. Endobronchial ultrasound is the ideal navigational tool to guide diagnostic biopsy and endotherapy devices. It will not only be useful for steering the instruments into deep organs but also for controlling the effect of therapeutic procedures such as radio-frequency waves or microwaves by change of impedance. Also, high intensity focused ultrasound (HIFU) itself will be an efficient tool for destruction of pathological tissues. By employing this technique, tissue is destroyed non-invasively at a distance from the probe by guiding the focus of the HIFU transducer to a limited portion of the tumor.

Another possible imaging technique is endoscopic magnetic resonance (MR) tomography. The reception antenna of the MR endoscope will receive signals of extremely high resolution and high S/N ratio of the mediastinal structures, far superior to conventional technology.

New procedures of *in vivo* imaging of the functional status such as ciliary beat, local bronchial and pulmonary interstitial inflammation, contraction of the bronchial muscles, bronchial and mediastinal blood flow, and tracheobronchial airflow, will generate new insights in pathomechanisms and also generate new technologies for non-invasive local treatment.

By these technologies, bronchology will become one of the most important tools for scientific research in pulmonary medicine and pulmonary oncology.

## New interactive technologies

*Steering mechanisms:* as new-generation instruments are more and more steered by remote control, new sensors will assist in guiding endoscopes through the sinuous pathways of the body with less discomfort.

*Optical sensors* computerize analysis of the endoscopic image. The computer verifies whether or not the endoscope can be advanced in the desired direction and redirects corrected automatic maneuvering by feeding in new data [31].

*Tactile sensors* will control the forces during introduction and assist in steering the endoscope. Tactile sensors function like the tentacles of a snail in activating the motion device. If they detect a particular level of resistance during insertion of the endoscope, the sensors will induce deflection of its tip by activating the sequential multichannel autoanalyzer (SMA) device or the remote control of the capsule endoscope [32,33].

*Force feedback systems* will be integrated into "intelligent" instruments such as forceps, needles, snares, baskets, and other probes, which will give an artificial impression of the forces to the operator who is no longer actually maneuvering these instruments directly by his or her hands but via a telemanipulator or even by a joystick.

*Integrated chip technology and neuronal structures* are directly connected to computers or computer-driven machines. Thus, manipulators will no longer be controlled by hand but by eye-trackers and brain-wave sensors. Brain and neurochips will be wired directly to the digital worlds and control devices [34]. This symbiosis between man and machine is a further step toward robotics.

*True robots* will no longer need human interface but will independently perform diagnostic and therapeutic procedures based on computerized feedback data. Humans will stand by to interfere only by trouble shooting [35].

### Energy transfer

Miniaturization of imaging instruments is making progress and so interventional systems will have to be redesigned. This applies especially to steering mechanisms. The diameters of instruments are becoming so slim that steering by conventional tendon-wire technology is no longer applicable because of the increasing friction in complicated airways and the lack of rigidity of these instruments [36].

*Miniaturized active bending catheter* is in development through which the miniaturized endoscope can be introduced. The bending mechanism is provided by shape memory alloy (SMA) technology. The crystals of "smart" alloys such as nitinol (nickel titanium) are arranged in complex folding patterns that change their internal structure according to force or temperature. Wires made from these materials bend and unbend to a preset geometric configuration when heated by electric current. This can be achieved by remote control. The wires can be extremely thin because they are actively bending and do not have to withstand stronger forces of traction. Thus, catheters of extremely thin external diameter, as small as 1.5 mm, can be produced with an internal lumen through which a 0.6 mm ultrathin endoscope can be inserted. Stabilization for insertion of these instruments is achieved by the mother–baby technique [37].

*Navigation instruments.* Remote-controlled instruments need advanced technologies for navigation. A technology that is currently under development is placing a patient on an examination table that is equipped with an electronic endoscope positioning system (BPS) (comparable to the GPS [Global Positioning System]). Coils generating magnetic fields are integrated into the examination table as well as into the endoscope. The fields generated by the source coils of endoscopes and instruments are detected by the sense coils and, by computer data processing, an exact virtual image of the endoscope position can be followed on the monitor, thus eliminating the necessity for fluoroscopy [38].

Automated navigation will be achieved by integrating the images of three-dimensional CT scanning and ultrasound. Lesions will be localized by virtual bronchoscopy on a computer monitor. The endoscope will then be guided down a virtual electronic track to approach the lesion.

Once the lesion has been localized and the probe brought into close contact, biopsies and interventional procedures, such as high-energy focused ultrasound. microwaves, or injection of cytotoxic agents or viral vectors, will be guided under ultrasonic control.

Training will become available on virtual mannequins in which all diagnostic techniques can be simulated by virtual imaging, and procedural instructions will be provided by integration of force feedback systems that impart the impression of "real touch" and transferring the movements of the surgeon's hand by transformation of its motions into electrical signals. Virtual scenarios can be constructed for the imitation of interventions such as lasering, stenting, or photodynamic therapy. Complications can be simulated for training in countermeasures.

## Summary

This concise overview on the aspects of bronchoscopy in airway lesions demonstrates the ever-growing potential and central diagnostic position of bronchoscopy in pulmonary medicine. Far from being at its limits, by continuous introduction of new methods and tools for applications, bronchoscopy seems to be just at the verge of a renaissance in its utility. This is clearly shown by the number of procedures being carried out throughout the world and also at our institution. We perform almost 5000 procedures annually and the numbers are increasing. This is especially due to the progress in diagnostic and therapeutic procedures introduced during the past 5 years. The growing interest shown by specialists of other disciplines, such as internists, anesthesiologists, surgeons, and pediatricians, is expressed in the growing number of participants in training courses and the growing demand for textbooks, and is encouraging enough to look for further applications of this over 100-year-old, but still young, procedure. The new technologies for imaging and steering, described here, will hopefully be available in the near future.

## References

1 Killian G. Die Grundlagen der modernen Rhino-Laryngologie. *Berliner Klin Wochenschr* 1906: 47, 6.

2 Magritte SD. *The Silence of the World*. New York: The Menil Foundation. Harry N. Abrams, Inc., 1992: 24.

3 Killian G. Ober directe Bronchoskopie. *MMW* 1898; **27**: 844–7.

4 Becker HD, Kayser K, Schulz V, *et al. Atlas of Bronchoscopy*. Philadelphia, Hamilton: BC Decker, 1991.

5 Prakash UBS, Cortese DA, Stubbs SE. Technical solutions to common problems in bronchoscopy. In: Prakash UBS, ed. *Bronchoscopy*. New York: Raven Press; 1994: 111–33.

6 Lukomsky Gr, Ovchinnikov AA, Bilal A. Complications of bronchoscopy: comparison of rigid bronchoscopy under general anesthesia and flexible fiberoptic bronchoscopy under topical anesthesia. *Chest* 1981; **79**: 316–21.

7 Becker HD, di Rienzo G. Anatomical considerations in bronchoscopy. *Atti 1. Corso Internationale di Bronchoscopia*. Editrice Roma; 1990: 13–18.

8 Thai W. *Kindetbrondwlogie*. Leipzig: J A Barth; 1972: 93–105.

9 Clements BS, Warner JO. Pulmonary sequestration and related congenital bronchopulmonary-vascular malformations: nomenclature and classification based on anatomical and embryonical considerations. *Thorax* 1987; **42**: 401–8.

10 Holder TM, Ashcraft KW, Sharp RJ, Armoury RA. Care of infants with esophageal atresia, tracheoesophageal fistula and associated anomalies. *J Thorac Cardiovasc Surg* 1987; **94**: 828–35.

11 Scwers HJ, Luhrner I, Oehlert H. Pulmonary venous obstruction following repair of total anomalous pulmonary venous drainage. *Ann Thorac Surg* 1987; **43**: 432–4.

12 Biilzebtuck H, Bopp R, Drings P, *et al.* New aspects in the staging of lung cancer. *Cancer* 1992; **70**: 1102–10.

13 Becker HD, di Rienzo G. On semiotics in bronchology: the interpretation of bronchoscopic findings by the example of inflammatory diseases. *Atti 1. Corso Internationale di Bronchoscopia.* Editrice Roma; 1990: 58–64.

14 Nilsson L. *Eine Reise in das Innere unseres Körpers.* Hamburg: Rasch und Rohrig Verlag; 1987: 138.

15 Barrois M. *Le Paris sous Paris.* Geneve: Hachette; 1964: 60–1.

16 Tsuda A, Rogers RA, Hydon PE, Butler JP. Chaotic mixing deep in the lung. *PNAS* 2002; **99**: 10173–8.

17 Katzenstein AA, Liebow A, Freidmann P. Bronchocentric granulomatosis, mucoid impaction and hypersensitivity reactions to fungi. *Am Rev Respir Dis* 1975; **11**: 497–537.

18 Torres A. Accuracy of diagnostic tools for the management of nosocomial respiratory infections in mechanically ventilated patients. *Eur Respir J* 1991; **4**: 1010–19.

19 Klech H, Hutter C, Costabel U, eds. Clinical guidelines and indications for bronchoalveolar lavage (BAL). *Eur Respir Rev* 1992; **2**: 8.

20 Cahill BC, Inghar DH. Massive hemoptysis. Assessment and management. *Clin Chest Med* 1994; **15**: 147–68.

21 Herth F, Ernst A, Becker HD. Long-term outcome and lung cancer incidence in patients with hemoptysis of unknown origin. *Chest* 2001; **120**: 1592–4.

22 Murata K, Ito H, Todo G, *et al.* Bronchial venous plexus and its communication with pulmonary circulation. *Invest Radiol* 1986; **21**: 24–30.

23 Dolan D, Lemmon GB Jr, Teitelhaum SL. Relapsing polychondritis: analytical literature review and studies of pathogenesis. *Am J Med* 1966; **41**: 285–98.

24 Igoe D, Lynch V, McNicholas WT. Broncholithiasis: bronchoscopic vs surgical management. *Respir Med* 1990; **84**: 163–5.

25 Hanafee WH, Ward PH. *The Larynx: Radiology, Surgery, Pathology.* New York: Thieme Medical Publishers; 1990.

26 Becker HD, Blersch E, Vogt-Moykopf I. Urgent treatment of tracheal obstruction. In: Grillo H, Eschapasse H, eds. *Major Challenges: International Trends in General Thoracic Surgery*, vol. 2. Philadelphia, London, Toronto: WB Saunders; 1987; **2**: 13–18.

27 Becker HD. Bronchoscopy, year 2001 and beyond. *Clin Chest Med* 2001; **22**: 225–39.

28 Huang D, Swanson EA, Lin CP, *et al.* Optical coherence tomography. *Science* 1991; **254**: 1178–81.

29 Dickensheets DL, Kino GS. Micromachined scanning confocal optical microscope. *Opt Lett* 1996; **10**: 764–6.

30 Becker HD, Herth PH. Endobronchial ultrasound. In: Braunwald E, Fauci AS, Isselhacher KJ *et al.*, eds. *Harrison's Principles of Internal Medicine* 1999. Available at: http://www.harrisonsonline. com.

31 Solomon SB, Acker DE, Polito AJ, *et al.* Real-time bronchoscope tip position technology displayed on previously acquired CT images to guide transbronchial needle aspiration (TBNA). *Cardiopulmonary Crit Care J* 1997; **112**: 3S.

32 Maezawa M, Imahashi T, Kuroda Y, *et al.* Tactile sensor using piezoelectric resonator. *Technical Digest of Transducers* 1997; **1**: 117–20.

33 Takizawa H, Tosaka H, Ohta R, *et al.* Development of a microfine active bending catheter equipped with MIF tactile sensors. *IEEE MEMS* 1999; 412–17.

34 Moravec H. *Robot: Mere Machine to Transcendent Mind.* New York: Oxford University Press; 2000.

35 Klein ST. Neuroprothetik. Handschlag mit der Zukunft. *GEO* 2000; **6**: 54–78.

36 Schulz S, Pylatiuk C, Brettauer G. A new class of flexible fluid actuators and their application in medical engineering. *At-Automatisierungstechnik* 1999; **47**: 390–95.

37 Mizuno H. Micromachines. *J Jap Soc Bronchoscopy* 2000; **22**: 590–5.

38 Forschungszentrum Karlsruhe Research Center. *Final Report: Steuerhares Flexibles Endoskop fur die Minimal Invasive Chirnrgie.* Forschungszentrum Karlsruhe, 2000.

# 9 Bronchoscopic Lung Biopsy

**Rajesh R. Patel and James P. Utz**
Mayo Clinic, Rochester, MN, USA

## Introduction

Bronchoscopic lung biopsy (BLB), also referred to as trans-bronchoscopic or transbronchial lung biopsy, is the technique by which biopsy of lung parenchyma can be obtained by using either the rigid or the flexible bronchoscope. Before BLB was described, lung biopsies were usually obtained by thoracotomy. Percutaneous needle biopsies using cutting needles and high-speed drills have largely been abandoned because of significant mortality and morbidity [1–6]. In 1965, Andersen and colleagues at the Mayo Clinic described the technique and results of BLB using a rigid bronchoscope in 13 patients [7]. This was followed by subsequent studies that support these results by Anderson *et al.* [8–11]. Among the first 450 cases of BLB performed via the rigid broncho-scope, lung tissue was obtained in 84% [8]. The introduction of the flexible bronchoscope in the late 1960s increased the popularity of the technique and demonstrated that BLB with the flexible instrument could be obtained with minimal mortality and morbidity [12–14]. The initial reports observed positive biopsies in 82% of cases [12]. BLB subsequently replaced thoracotomy lung biopsy in many instances. Currently, almost all the bronchoscopists exclusively use BLB with a flexible bronchoscope.

With several newer bronchoscopic techniques now available, there has been some confusion in the nomenclature used to describe various bronchoscopic procedures. The term BLB should be used to describe the procedure used to obtain specimens from abnormal lung parenchyma. Many bronchoscopists apply this term indiscriminately to describe bronchoscopic brushing and biopsy of peripheral nodules, masses, cavities, and other non- parenchymal lesions. For the current discussion, we will restrict the term BLB to the technique used for obtaining biopsies from lung parenchyma to diagnose diffuse parenchymal diseases. We find that the prefix trans- in transbronchoscopic lung biopsy does not add much to the description and therefore prefer the shorter term: bronchoscopic lung biopsy. We believe the word trans-bronchial should be reserved for bronchoscopic needle aspiration of paratracheal, subcarinal, or perihilar lesions.

## Indications

The roentgenologic presence of any diffuse lung disease without an obvious etiology is an indication for BLB. However, as with any diagnostic procedure, clinical correlation and consideration of other less-invasive diagnostic tests should be made before performing BLB. These may include studies of respiratory secretions, pleural effusions, blood, and other body fluids or tissues, as well as different imaging procedures. The development and application of newer non-bronchoscopic diagnostic tests and techniques has diminished the indications for BLB in recent years. The increasing clinical application of high-resolution computed tomography (HRCT) of the chest has contributed to the decreasing number of BLBs performed in diffuse lung disease. Typical HRCT findings in the presence of characteristic clinical features are highly indicative of the diagnosis of disease entities such as pulmonary Langerhan's cell granuloma, lymphangioleiomyomatosis, sarcoidosis, usual interstitial pneumonia (UIP), and lymphangitic pulmonary metastases [15–17]. Even though HRCT is a valuable tool in diagnosing the above listed entities, typical HRCT findings are not seen in all patients with these disorders [15–19]. Therefore, bronchoalveolar lavage (BAL) and BLB should both be considered when the results of HRCT are not definitive. The wide availability of BAL has decreased the need for BLB (and thoracotomy) in many patients with opportunistic infections, particularly those caused by *Pneumocystis jiroveci*, mycobacteria, and certain mycoses [20,21–23]. The role of BAL in the evaluation of non-infectious diffuse diseases such as sarcoidosis, idiopathic pulmonary fibrosis,

*Flexible Bronchoscopy*, Third Edition. Edited by Ko-Pen Wang, Atul C. Mehta, J. Francis Turner.
© 2012 Blackwell Publishing Ltd. Published 2012 by Blackwell Publishing Ltd.

**Table 9.1** Pulmonary diseases in which bronchoscopic lung biopsy provides a higher diagnostic yield

Sarcoidosis
Pulmonary Langerhan's cell histiocytosis (histiocytosis X)
Lymphangitic carcinomatosis
Pulmonary alveolar proteinosis
Diffuse lung infections caused by mycobacterium and mycoses
Diffuse pulmonary lymphoma
Diffuse alveolar cell carcinoma
Lymphagioleiomyomatosis
Silicosis

hypersensitivity pneumonitis, pneumoconioses, and others is less clear and often is confined to the research sphere. The clinical application of BAL to diagnose or monitor these diseases is not recommended. BAL does provide diagnostic information in certain non-infectious diffuse lung diseases such as pulmonary Langerhan's cell histiocytosis, pulmonary alveolar proteinosis, and lymphangitic pulmonary metastasis, though BLB provides a higher diagnostic yield in all these entities [24–27]. BAL and BLB may be complementary and increase the overall diagnostic yield under these circumstances [21,28,29]. More recently, video-assisted thoracoscopy (VAT) has contributed to the decreased utilization of BLB in diagnosing diffuse as well as focal interstitial lung diseases, as larger lung biopsies allow more complete and accurate histologic interpretation. This increased diagnostic utility is balanced against increased cost and morbidity of thoracoscopic biopsy compared to BLB. Nevertheless, BLB continues to be a valuable diagnostic tool in a variety of situations (Table 9.1).

## Contraindications

Even though there are very few absolute contraindications to routine bronchoscopy, there are several contraindications to BLB. BLB is absolutely contraindicated if a patient is unable to cooperate with the procedure [29]. Other absolute contraindications include an unstable cardiovascular status, status asthmaticus, severe hypoxemia during bronchoscopy despite maximal support, an inadequately trained bronchoscopist or bronchoscopy team, and inadequate instruments to perform the procedure properly. Relative contraindications include cough that is uncontrollable during the procedure, untreated hemorrhagic diatheses, advanced renal failure, significant hypoxemia in a patient with a single lung, extensive bullous changes in areas to be biopsied, and roentgenographic suggestion of vascular malformations adjacent to areas to be biopsied.

Pulmonary hypertension has been considered an absolute contraindication for BLB because of concern that the pul-

monary hypertension substantially increases the risk of bleeding associated with the procedure. Recent limited data suggest that that pulmonary hypertension may be less of a risk than previously anticipated. An experimental study of a sheep model with pulmonary hypertension reported no increase in the risk of hemorrhage when compared to control animals without pulmonary hypertension [30]. The same group of investigators extended their observation to 22 patients with interstitial lung disease and latent pulmonary hypertension to show that there was no significant difference in post-BLB bleeding between those with pulmonary hypertension when compared to patients with interstitial lung disease but without pulmonary hypertension [31]. Until more comprehensive experience is published, it seems reasonable to consider pulmonary hypertension a relative, rather than an absolute, contraindication in carefully selected patients. In recent years, the use of clopidogrel with coronary artery stents has been considered a contraindication for BLB. A small study in 16 healthy pigs with or without clopidogrel and aspirin showed no increased risk of bleeding with these medications [32]. The prospective study on humans by the same group was stopped early due to higher risk of bleeding in patients taking clopidogrel (89%) versus 3.4% in the control group, and almost 100% in patient on both aspirin and clopidogrel [33]. The 2007 and 2008, ACC guidelines recommended deferring non-urgent procedures while on clopidogrel or withholding the drug for 7–10 days to reduce the risk of bleeding [34,35]. If BLB is absolutely needed in patients on clopidogrel, we withhold the medication for at least 5 days prior to the procedure after discussion with the patient's cardiologist [34].

## Prerequisites

An informed consent should be obtained from all patients after details of the procedure, goals, and risks involved with bronchoscopy and BLB are explained. Table 9.2 indicates certain steps that are essential before bronchoscopy. It is essential that the patient undergo a thorough history and physical examination, with particular emphasis on conditions that might pose problems during or after bronchoscopy. In an otherwise healthy individual scheduled to undergo bronchoscopy with or without BLB, it is not essential to perform a complete blood count, blood chemistry, or urinalysis [36,37]. It is, however, particularly important to ask the patient about the presence of familial or acquired hemorrhagic diathesis. In the absence of a history of bleeding diathesis, it is not necessary to routinely perform coagulation studies before BLB. Further, no single test designed to examine the integrity of the coagulation system can predict bleeding during surgery [38,39]. Even combinations of coagulation tests will not predict the risk of bleeding following BLB [40]. Therefore, estimation of prothrombin time, acti-

**Table 9.2** Prebronchoscopy checklist

1  Is there an appropriate indication for bronchoscopy?

2  Has there been a previous bronchoscopy?

3  If the answer to the above question is "yes", then were there any complications?

4  Does the patient (and the close relative/s, if the patient is unable to communicate or consent) fully understand the risks, goal, benefit, and complications of bronchoscopy?

5  Does the patient's past medical history (allergy to medication and topical anesthesia) and present clinical condition pose special problems or predisposes to complications?

6  Are all the appropriate test completed and results available?

7  Are the premedications correct and the dosages available?

8  Does the patient require special consideration before (e.g. corticosteroids for asthma, insulin for diabetes mellitus, or prophylaxis against bacterial endocarditis) or during (supplemental oxygen or more sedation) the procedure?

9  Are the plans for the postbronchoscopy care appropriate?

10 Are all the appropriate instruments and personnel available to assist the procedure and to handle the potential complications?

Table reproduced with permission from Prakash UBS, Cortese DA, Stubbs SE. Technical Solutions to common problems in bronchoscopy In: Prakash UBS, ed. *Bronchoscopy*, New York: Raven Press, 1994: 111–133.

vated partial thromboplastin time, bleeding time, platelet count, and other parameters of coagulation are not warranted on a routine basis in the absence of known or suspected hemorrhagic diathesis. On the other hand, Zavala reported a 45% incidence of significant hemorrhage following BLB in uremic patients [41] and remarked "any biopsy procedure is avoided, if at all possible, on a uremic patient because of hemorrhage" [42]. Based on this observation, a serum creatinine level of 3 mg/dL or greater, or a serum urea level of 30 mg/dL or greater is considered a relative contraindication to BLB due to platelet dysfunction caused by renal failure leading to clinically significant post-BLB hemorrhage [36]. However, it should be noted that these criteria do not have a documented scientific basis. Yet, clinicians have continued to apply these criteria in their practice. Preparation of patients with coagulation disorders who are scheduled to undergo BLB is discussed below.

Many patients with diffuse lung disease who are referred for BLB have significant pulmonary dysfunction and are often hypoxemic. The presence of these abnormalities should not preclude BLB if supportive measures are employed. Routine pulmonary function testing and arterial blood gas analysis before BLB is unnecessary. If pulmonary function testing is otherwise planned, it should be performed before bronchoscopy because bronchoscopy can induce mucosal edema and spuriously alter lung function tests [43–45]. Special imaging procedures such as HRCT may be

helpful in identifying the abnormal areas to be biopsied. The identification of a particular roentgenologic pattern and its location by tomography or HRCT may optimize the application and diagnostic yield of BLB. Additionally, these imaging procedures may demonstrate areas that should be avoided by the biopsy forceps; namely, bullous lesions, vascular abnormalities, and pleural lesions.

## Technique

The preparation of the patient for BLB is similar to that for routine bronchoscopy and premedications and sedatives used are likewise identical. Most adult patients can undergo BLB under topical anesthesia. General anesthesia is indicated in patients who cannot cooperate under topical anesthesia and intravenous sedation or in cases of documented allergy to local anesthetics. Cough suppression is especially important during BLB and administration of optimal sedation or preoperative cough-suppressive therapy may be necessary. Before the administration of a sedative, the patient should be instructed to indicate by hand gestures or head-nod if pain is experienced during the procedure. If fluoroscopic guidance is used, metallic pads and wires to be placed on the patient's thoracic cage for electrocardiographic or other monitoring should be arranged in such a way that they do not interfere with the fluoroscopic image of the lesion to be biopsied.

Bronchoscopic examination is performed in the usual manner, and both bronchial trees are thoroughly examined prior to BLB. If other procedures, such as BAL, endobronchial brushings and biopsies, or bronchial washings, are required, they should be obtained before BLB. Performing BLB as the last procedure minimizes cough after BLB, avoiding subsequent instrumentation that may precipitate pneumothorax secondary to cough-induced barotrauma. Before starting BLB we tend to preanesthetize the area with topical lidocaine to avoid cough during the procedure. After positioning the fluoroscope to obtain an image of the area to be biopsied, the bronchoscope is advanced as far distally as possible. The bronchoscope is then maintained in this wedged position while the biopsy forceps are inserted into the working channel of the instrument. Once the distal end of the biopsy forceps exits the distal end of the bronchoscope, the forceps are further advanced distally until their tip is beyond bronchoscopic visualization. At this point, the fluoroscopic image is projected on the monitor and used to track the progress of the forceps to the lesion. If the lesion is localized, biplane fluoroscopy can be helpful in confirming that the biopsy has been taken from the lesion (Fig. 9.1). The biopsy forceps are opened 5–6 mm proximal to the area to be biopsied, advanced to the lesion, and then closed. At this point, the patient is asked if any pain is experienced. If the patient indicates pain (by prearranged signals), the forceps

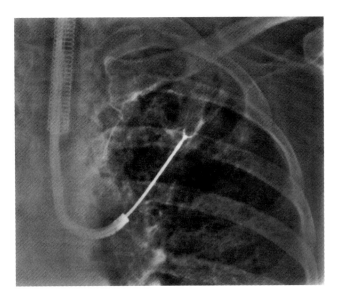

**Fig. 9.1** Fluoroscopic guidance used to obtain bronchoscopic lung biopsy from a localized parenchymal lesion in the left upper lobe. The use of biplane fluoroscopy enables the bronchoscopist to obtain lung specimens from selected areas.

are opened and withdrawn proximally without obtaining biopsy. The biopsy is then attempted from another area. If there is no indication of pain, the biopsy forceps are withdrawn. During the withdrawal of the forceps, the bronchoscope is maintained in the wedged position [41,42]. The advantage of this "wedge" technique is twofold: it maintains the tip of the bronchoscope in the optimal position so that more biopsies can be obtained without having to withdraw the bronchoscope to clean the objective lens; and, most importantly, if postbiopsy bleeding occurs, the wedged position limits the bleeding to the biopsied segment or subsegment. It is not necessary to apply prolonged suction to check for hemorrhage after each biopsy. In fact, applying suction at the biopsy can dislodge the clot and cause more bleeding. If a brief suctioning does not indicate serious hemorrhage, then the bronchoscopist can proceed to obtain more biopsies. The traditional teaching that carrying out BLB at the end of expiratory maneuvers will recruit more alveolar tissue into the biopsy forceps has been challenged by many bronchoscopists as there is no literature to support this notion [46,47].

If significant hemorrhage (more than 50 mL) is encountered immediately after BLB, the wedged position of the bronchoscope is maintained and suction applied as needed [41]. If bleeding persists or fails to diminish, the bronchoscopist can perform several maneuvers to minimize and control the hemorrhage. First, maintaining a wedge position for a more prolonged period to allow thrombus formation may be all that is required, particularly is wedging fully contains bleeding to the segment or subsegment to which the wedge is applied. If required, continuous or prolonged

intermittent suction may be used while the tip of the bronchoscope remains in the wedged position. Gentle instillation of 10–15 mL of iced saline through the bronchoscope into the bleeding area for several seconds can help stem bleeding. During the slow instillation of iced saline, the bronchoscopist should be able to visualize the distal bronchial tree through the saline. This "saline flooding" of the distal bronchus should be maintained for several seconds after completing the instillation of iced saline. A stream of blood coming from the distal bronchus and mixing with the just instilled saline usually indicates that bleeding from the biopsied site is persistent. If this is the case then bronchoscopic suction should be applied to remove the blood, and cold saline instillation as described above should be repeated. This technique can be repeated several times until bleeding stops. In many patients, this technique will diminish and eventually stop the bleeding caused by BLB [41]. Some advocate bronchoscopic instillation of epinephrine to help with vasoconstriction. This technique appears to have less efficacy in control of bleeding since the bleeding eliminates from distal areas and the small aliquot of epinephrine injected through the bronchoscope may not reach the bleeding site, particularly with more brisk bleeding. Other techniques to control BLB-induced hemorrhage include balloon tamponade, fibrin glue application, rigid bronchoscopic aspiration of blood and endobronchial packing of bleeding bronchus, isolation of bronchial trees by inserting double-lumen endotracheal tubes, and, lastly, surgical resection of the bleeding segment [48]. When the bleeding is brisk, the patient should be turned so that the bleeding side is dependent. This will keep the blood from spilling over to the nonbleeding side. It should be noted that the dead space volume is small (150–350 ml), so it does not require a large amount of blood to cause asphyxia from bleeding. Some of these techniques are described in other chapters in this volume. In our experience, these measures are seldom required to treat BLB-induced hemorrhage.

After the BLB is completed and lack of bleeding is confirmed, the bronchoscope is withdrawn from the airways. Routine chest X ray is unnecessary after BLB [49–51]. We usually perform fluoroscopic screening to exclude a pneumothorax. Chest X ray should be reserved for patients who, during BLB, cough excessively, repeatedly complain of pain, or after BLB in patients who develop other pulmonary symptoms (dyspnea, chest tightness, or chest pain). Clinical suspicion of post-BLB pneumothorax, presence of pneumothorax following BLB, serious hemorrhage following BLB, and development of unexplained dyspnea or other significant cardiorespiratory symptoms are indications for hospitalization. The patient should be instructed to contact the physician or report to the emergency department if new symptoms develop within the next 24 hours.

Processing of the lung specimens obtained by BLB is an important part of the procedure. Crush artifacts should be avoided by careful handling of specimens. Simply washing the specimen from the forceps into the formalin by swishing is preferred to manipulation with pick-up forceps, which may cause crush artifact. Appropriate preservatives and culture media should be selected before BLB. Touch preparations for identification of *P. jiroveci* is no longer used due to better sensitivity of BAL procedures. Crush artifact should be avoided so that histologic analysis of the tissue is not impaired. Communication with the pathologist regarding the clinical features and provisional diagnoses is also essential.

## Other considerations

### Coagulation disorders

In a 2001 survey involving 158 pulmonary physicians, bleeding secondary to anticoagulant medications was perceived as the major risk in the setting of lung biopsy and anticoagulant medications were held by most of the bronchoscopists in preparation for the procedure [52]. The limitation of the tests of coagulation to predict bleeding in BLB is discussed above. As noted, coagulation disorders are a relative contraindication to BLB. Thrombocytopenia is perhaps the most common disorder of coagulation encountered by the bronchoscopist. In one report, 25 BLBs were performed in 24 patients with a mean platelet count of 30,000/mm$^3$ (7000–60,000/mm$^3$); self-limited hemorrhage was noted in three patients and one developed fatal bleeding (this patient had a platelet count of 23,000/mm$^3$) [53]. Because of this increased risk of hemorrhage, documented thrombocytopenia is a relative contraindication to BLB. However, in the absence of known bleeding diathesis, routine measurement of platelet count is not warranted before BLB. Immunocompromised patients with bone marrow failure frequently require both fresh frozen plasma and platelet transfusions. Despite these measures, hemorrhage-associated morbidity and mortality may occur [53]. Failure of the platelet count to increase significantly 1 hour past platelet infusion indicates the presence of platelet antibodies [54]. BLB should be avoided in these patients although BAL can be safely performed [48]. In patients with thrombocytopenia (platelet count less than 50,000/mm$^3$), six to ten packs of platelets should be transfused 30 to 40 minutes before BLB [41,42,55,56]. It might be prudent to recheck the platelet count after transfusion and before BLB.

Platelet dysfunction (despite normal platelet count) in patients with renal failure is associated with increased risk of hemorrhage and may be manifested by prolonged bleeding time. If BLB is an absolute necessity in the presence of platelet dysfunction, then deamino-8D-arginine-vasopressin (DDAVP) can be administered before the procedure [57,58].

Iatrogenically induced (heparin and warfarin) abnormalities of coagulation should be corrected with discontinuation of the drug and monitoring of appropriate laboratory tests. BLB should be undertaken only after the bleeding tendency is reversed. Grouping and cross matching of blood type before BLB is unnecessary as blood transfusion is seldom required during the procedure or as a result of its complication. [37]. For patients on Coumadin we recommend adjusted international normalized ratio (INR) to be 1.5 or below to perform BLB. As discussed previously in this chapter, clopidogrel should be discontinued for at least 5 days before performing BLB [32,34,35]. This should be done only after weighing the risk and benefit of discontinuing clopidogrel, particularly in patients with a recent stent for a coronary event.

### Fluoroscopy

Fluoroscopic guidance is invaluable in obtaining optimal lung specimens. The main reason for using fluoroscopic guidance is to prevent pneumothorax secondary to BLB. Another important reason to employ fluoroscopic guidance is to guide the distal end of the bronchoscope and the biopsy forceps toward the localized abnormality seen on the fluoroscopy monitor. Some bronchoscopists, however, believe that fluoroscopy is not necessary to obtain BLB [59–61]. The 1989 survey of about 1800 North American bronchoscopists disclosed that more than 75% of the participants routinely used fluoroscopy for BLB [62]. However, the 1999 survey of 2500 bronchoscopists revealed that only 66% of the participants routinely used fluoroscopy for obtaining BLB [63,64]. Indeed, BLB can be performed without fluoroscopic guidance in the following situations: if the pulmonary parenchymal process involves an entire lung, if the infiltrate is localized to a lung apex, or if the infiltrate is roentgenographically well defined and involves an entire segment of any lobe [65]. Using tactile sensation (without fluoroscopy), a study analyzed the complications of BLB in 68 patients undergoing at least three BLBs; a single pneumothorax was reported and no significant hemorrhage ensued [60]. However, a mail survey of 231 British bronchoscopists reported that the incidence of pneumothorax following BLB was 1.8% when fluoroscopy was used and increased to 2.9% when fluoroscopy was not used [66]. For this reason, we recommend fluoroscopic guidance when performing BLBs. The cost of fluoroscopy equipment and the administrative control of the fluoroscopy equipment (usually by the radiologist) are the main impediments to the optimal utilization of fluoroscopy [38]. If fluoroscopy equipment is readily available, then it should be used to obtain maximal diagnostic yield. Fluoroscopy also provides an added advantage of post-BLB assessment of the thoracic cage to exclude pneumothorax and precludes routine post-BLB roentgenography [65]. The bronchoscopist should be trained in the appropriate use of fluoroscopic equipment or have a trained person available during the procedure. Every attempt must be made to minimize the exposure of the patient and bronchoscopy personnel to fluoroscopy-associated radiation.

## Localized peripheral lesions

These lesions include pulmonary parenchymal nodules, localized (segmental, subsegmental, or sub-subsegmental) infiltrates, and bronchoscopically invisible endobronchial lesions. The latter include distal carcinoma, carcinoid, hamartoma, or other lesions originating in the mucosa or wall of distal bronchi or bronchioles. The term BLB is a misnomer to describe biopsy of such lesions because the lung parenchyma is not biopsied. The lesions originating in the bronchoscopically invisible bronchi and very dense alveolar infiltrates (i.e. alveolar cell carcinoma and alveolar lymphoma) is less likely to result in pneumothorax following bronchoscopic biopsy because the biopsied area is either endobronchial or airless. In a study involving 205 localized lesion from 516 immunocompetent patients, the overall diagnostic yield from 530 consecutive BLBs performed was only 29% [67]. There are increasing numbers of reports of HRCT-guided transbronchial biopsy of peripheral lesions using virtual bronchoscopy [68]. A report of 25 patients with 26 peripheral lesions using this technique with a thin flexible bronchoscope (external diameter 2.8 mm) showed a success rate of 65.4% in reaching the target lesion and definitive diagnosis [69]. Increasing cost, time of the procedure, radiation involved, and availability of electromagnetic navigation has made this technique less favorable for small peripheral lesions.

## Rigid bronchoscopy

Although the first BLBs were obtained via the rigid bronchoscope with rigid bronchoscopy forceps [1,7,9], it is unlikely that many bronchoscopists currently use the rigid bronchoscope for this purpose. Nevertheless, BLB can be safely obtained using rigid bronchoscopic techniques. The technique is similar to that used with the flexible bronchoscope. Fluoroscopic guidance should be used to obtain BLB via the rigid bronchoscope. A disadvantage is the relative difficulty in introducing the rigid bronchoscope and biopsy forceps into upper lobe bronchi. The use of rigid bronchoscopy for routine BLB is no longer recommended.

## Biopsy forceps

No biopsy forceps are solely designed for the purpose of BLB. The forceps used to biopsy endobronchial lesions are usually used to obtain BLB. Among these, the two main types are the cup (without teeth) and alligator (toothed) forceps. There is no evidence that tooth forceps causes more hemorrhage due to its "tearing" action. We believe that either type of forceps can be used to obtain BLB. Although there have been no randomized controlled trials, cupped forceps have been used widely to obtain BLBs and the quality of the specimen is the same as with toothed forceps. Hence, the choice of type of forceps is a matter of personal preference and experience.

The small size (approximately 5–20 mm) of the tissue obtained by BLB may sometimes be inadequate to establish a histopathologic diagnosis [70]. The size of the specimen depends on the size of the cups in the biopsy forceps. Rigid bronchoscopic forceps are much larger than the flexible biopsy forceps. However, some authors observed that larger tissue pieces obtained by BLB do not provide additional diagnostic yield [71,72]. In a small study involving 27 patients, larger flexible biopsy forceps (cup size 3.0 × 2.0 × 0.9 mm) obtained significantly more tissue in 74% of the patients, contrary to small biopsy forceps (cup size 2.0 × 1.5 × 0.6 mm), which obtained more tissue in only 19% [73]. Large forceps also obtained more alveolar tissue in 73%, whereas small forceps obtained more alveolar tissue in only 27%. There was no difference in the post-BLB bleeding with either forceps. This may be clinically significant because another study demonstrated that the presence of a greater number of alveoli per individual tissue piece results in a statistically significant increase in the ability to make a diagnosis of infection [70]. Potential problems with the use of larger forceps are the inability to pass the forceps through the working channel of smaller adult flexible bronchoscopes and difficulty in getting the jaws to open in small peripheral airways [73]. To assess the adequacy of the biopsy specimens as soon as the biopsy is obtained, many bronchoscopists use the "float sign" [74]. If the biopsied lung tissue contains aerated alveoli, it should float when placed into the liquid fixative. This sign is not completely reliable because dense, non-aerated lesions may not float. A prospective, blinded, observational analysis of 43 patients who underwent 170 BLBs assessed the bronchoscopists' ability to predict specimen quality at the time of BLB. The results showed that the physician estimate of BLB specimen quality and float sign were not helpful in predicting that the biopsy specimens contained abnormal or diagnostic tissue. However, in 53% of cases the diagnosis was established by the first biopsy specimen and in 33.3% of the cases the second specimen was helpful in establishing the diagnosis. The authors concluded that a diagnostic BLB specimen will likely be obtained if the size of the specimen fills the forceps, two to four biopsies are performed, and toothed forceps are used [75].

## Number of biopsies

In addition to the size of the biopsy forceps, the number of biopsies also determines the diagnostic yield. However, it is intuitively obvious that the risk of pneumothorax is proportional to the number of BLBs obtained. Therefore, the least number of BLBs to establish the diagnosis is the optimal number, which in turn depends upon underlying pulmonary process and several other factors. The availability of frozen-section technique to immediately analyze the biopsy specimen also determines the number of biopsies obtained. For instance, if the first biopsy specimen is subjected to frozen-section examination and reveals a definitive diagnosis, an additional biopsy for permanent section may be all that is required. But the above scenario to limit the number of biopsies based on the results of the frozen section should be undertaken with caution as initial diagnostic impression may change upon further review and it prolongs the bronchoscopy time as well. Non-specific findings on frozen-section analysis may require a larger number of biopsies. Peribronchial or peribronchiolar disease processes (such as lymphangitic malignancy, sarcoidosis, or disseminated infections) are more likely to be diagnosed by BLB [76]. One study evaluated the diagnostic yield of BLB in 530 consecutive BLBs in 516 immunocompetent patients with chronic diffuse lung infiltrate, and observed that that there was a direct correlation between the number of samples obtained per BLB and the overall diagnostic yield (i.e. 38% with one to three tissue fragments versus 69% with six to ten, $P < 0.01$). Based on this result, the authors recommend that at least five to six BLB specimens should be taken [67].

The 1999, American Thoracic Society/ European Respiratory Society (ATS/ ERS) guidelines on sarcoidosis recommend BLB as the initial procedure to establish the diagnosis. This statement indicates that diagnostic yield from BLB depends largely on the experience of the operator, ranging from 40% to more than 90% when four to five lung biopsies are carried out [77]. In patients with stage II or stage III sarcoidosis, the diagnostic sensitivity is 95% when at least four biopsies are obtained [60,78–82]. However, patients with stage I sarcoidosis may need 10 BLBs to achieve similar diagnostic yield [83]. The overall diagnostic accuracy of BLB in all stages of sarcoidosis is 80 to 85% [84,85]. The size of the biopsy specimens may also influence the diagnostic utility of BLB [70]. Addition of endobronchial biopsy to BLB may slightly increase the diagnostic yield [86]. A positive endobronchial biopsy had a positive predictive value of 79% to diagnose sarcoidosis. The current use of endobronchial ultrasound guided aspiration of mediastinal lymph node can be helpful to establish a diagnosis of sarcoidosis as well. Some investigators recommend that the combination of bronchoscopic needle aspiration, endobronchial biopsy, and BLB in stages I and II, and of endobronchial biopsy and BLB in stage III, are safe and cost-effective as well as increase the diagnostic yield [87].

## Diagnostic accuracy

By definition, BLB denotes biopsy of lung or pathologic process occurring within the pulmonary parenchyma. As stated previously, biopsy of peripheral nodules originating in the bronchial wall does not represent BLB. Nevertheless, the term BLB is loosely used in clinical practice as well as the literature to describe biopsy of any bronchoscopically invisible lesion. As a result, the interpretation of diagnostic yield from "BLB" of a diffuse and localized lesion is difficult. The diagnostic accuracy also depends on the pathologist's understanding of the clinical features. Therefore, clear communication between the bronchoscopist and the pathologist may be helpful in difficult cases [88]. The diagnostic rates of BLB can be considered separately for diffuse and localized lesions.

## Diffuse lesion

Biopsy of uniformly diffuse lung infiltrates is more likely to provide diagnosis than a small (less than 1.0 cm) peripheral nodule. The rate of diagnostic accuracy from BLB depends also on the predetermined criteria for the diagnosis. For example, if non-specific fibrosis is accepted as a definitive diagnosis in the presence of typical clinical features, then the diagnostic yield can be considered high. One study evaluated the diagnostic yield of BLB in 530 consecutive BLBs in 516 immunocompetent patients with either a chronic diffuse lung infiltrates, a localized peripheral lung lesion, or hilar lymphadenopathy. In patients with chronic diffuse pulmonary infiltrates (n = 244), the overall diagnostic yield was 50%, but higher figures were obtained for hypersensitivity pneumonitis (92%), stage II and III sarcoidosis (75%), lymphangitic carcinomatosis (68%), and pneumoconiosis (54%). The diagnostic yield was lower in diffuse tuberculosis (38%) and interstitial pulmonary fibrosis (27%) [67]. A review of several series observes that the overall diagnostic yield from BLB was 72% [89]. However, when more specific diagnostic criteria were applied prospectively to 176 patients with interstitial lung disease, the diagnostic yield was substantially lower (37.7%) [89]. In addition, the acceptance of "specific" diagnoses based on non-specific histologic changes is tenuous and often that diagnosis is not confirmed when the patients are further subjected to surgical lung biopsy [90]. A retrospective analysis of 651 BLBs in 603 consecutive patients with diffuse lung disease showed results of BLB were "clinically helpful" in 75% of the cases (to prove or refute a diagnosis) and non-helpful in 25% of the cases. In patients with "non-helpful" data, 32% had no lung parenchyma on the BLB specimen [91]. The ATS statement on idiopathic pulmonary fibrosis concludes that surgical lung biopsy (open thoracotomy or video-assisted thoracoscopy) is recommended in most patients, especially those with suspected idiopathic pulmonary fibrosis who have clinical, physiological, or radiological features that are not typical for idiopathic pulmonary fibrosis and there are no contraindications to surgery [92]. This consensus statement recommended BLB in the absence of surgical biopsy, though many do not follow that recommendation when the diagnosis of idiopathic pulmonary fibrosis is otherwise secure based on a highly confident HRCT appearance and compatible clinical findings, given it is uncommon in that situation that the BLB suggests an alternative diagnosis. The ATS/ ERS International Multidisciplinary Consensus infers that BLB is not useful in the diagnosis of most idiopathic interstitial pneumonias, with the exception of diffuse alveolar damage/ acute interstitial pneumonias, and occasionally organizing pneumonia. The consensus also states that the primary role of BLB biopsies is to exclude sarcoidosis and certain infections [92,93]. Hence, BLB is not recommended in suspected usual interstitial pneumonia/idiopathic pulmonary fibrosis, except as an aid to exclude other processes in selected cases.

It may be prudent to avoid particular areas when performing BLB. In patients with diffuse disease, the lingula is often the site of chronic non-specific inflammation, hence the biopsy of the lingula might best be avoided [94,95], although this notion is challenged by some [96]. Areas of greatest involvement may seem to be the preferred sites of BLB, but it may be better to target areas of intermediate involvement, because the more severely involved areas may display only end-stage fibrosis, the final common pathway of innumerable diffuse lung diseases.

In immunocompromised patients with diffuse pulmonary infiltrates, BLB has been reported to provide diagnostic rates ranging from 28 to 68% [22,97]. A single-institution study of 104 immunocompromised patients with bilateral diffuse pulmonary infiltrates who underwent flexible bronchoscopy showed a diagnostic yield of 38% by BLB. The yield was increased to 70% when BLB was combined with BAL. The overall diagnostic yield was higher for infiltrates due to infectious etiology (80%) than non-infectious etiology (56%) [25]. In a study of renal transplant patients who developed lung infiltrates, BLB was felt to be diagnostic in 54% [98]. In patients with AIDS, BLB has been shown to provide a diagnostic yield of 88 to 97% in *P. jeroveci* infection [23,99,100]. The same data revealed a much lower diagnostic accuracy of BLB in those with cytomegalovirus pneumonia (22%), *Mycobacterium avium intracellulare* (MAI) infection (0 of 11 patients), and pulmonary Kaposi's sarcoma (0 of 11 patients) [100]. The diagnostic yield from BLB is lower, compared to bronchial washings or BAL, in pulmonary infection caused by MAI. Among 42 patients with this infection who had negative sputum smear on 3 consecutive days, bronchial washing was smear-positive for *Mycobacterium avium* complex (MAC) in 44%, and culture-positive in 85%. BLB specimens revealed specific findings (epithelioid cell granuloma and/or acid-fast bacilli) in 37%. Bronchial washing of all patients who showed specific histology in BLB grew MAC in culture. The authors of this study infer that to make a diagnosis of MAC, bronchial washing is superior to BLB, and should be done in the bronchus that drains the area demonstrating small nodular opacities around ectatic bronchi [101]. Others report a diagnostic yield of 67% for BLB in patients with AIDS and opportunistic infections caused by organisms other than *P. jiroveci* [102]. Currently, the BAL technique establishes the diagnosis in over 90% of patients with *P. jiroveci* pneumonia [103]. The addition of BAL related polymerase chain reaction (PCR) studies further increases the sensitivity [104]. Many major medical centers use a staged approach; that is, for patients in whom *P. jiroveci* pneumonia is a major diagnostic consideration but whose sputa are negative for *P. jiroveci* pneumonia, only a diagnostic BAL is performed initially; BLB is added to the initial BAL if other diagnostic possibilities are considered likely.

## Localized lesion

Because many bronchoscopists do not differentiate between the biopsy of a peripheral (bronchoscopically invisible) endobronchial lesion and a true BLB, we address this issue here. Bronchoscopic biopsy of a localized lesion should be performed under fluoroscopic guidance. The biopsy is reported to yield approximately a 60% diagnostic rate in primary lung cancer and a 50% diagnostic yield in metastatic cancer, when these tumors present as peripheral lung nodules [105]. Cytology brushing increases the diagnostic yield in both conditions. An important determinant of diagnostic yield is the size of the nodule. Biopsy of lesions larger than 2.0 cm may provide a greater than 60% diagnostic yield, whereas lesions less than 2.0 cm in diameter may yield a diagnosis in less than 25% of cases [105]. The use of ultrathin fiberoptic bronchoscopes, electromagnetic navigation and CT guided virtual bronchoscopy have improved diagnostic yield of peripheral nodules [87,106,107]. The details of the above procedures are discussed elsewhere in the book. The diagnostic rates are likely to be lower if non-malignant processes cause nodular or localized lesions. Bronchial washings, brushings, and BAL add to the diagnostic yield in both malignant and non-malignant processes.

## Mechanical ventilation

Mechanical ventilation is not an absolute contraindication to BLB although the incidence of pneumothorax is reported to increase [108,109]. The potential for a tension pneumothorax should be anticipated and appropriate planning for immediate treatment made. A review of BLB in 15 patients with diffuse lung disease on mechanical ventilation reported a 7% incidence of post-BLB tension pneumothorax [108]. But, the same study also observed a diagnostic yield of 47% and a significant alteration in management in 53% of the patients. Self-limiting hemorrhage occurred in 20% of the patients. The results may vary if the patients have had aggressive empiric therapy before BLB. The institution of positive end-expiratory pressure (PEEP) may increase the risk of pneumothorax. A retrospective analysis of 71 consecutive, mechanically ventilated patients who underwent 83 BLBs in the critical care unit reported that a specific histologic diagnosis was made in 29 (35%) patients; and the biopsy results changed management in 34 (41%) subjects. Several points should be recognized in this study: (1) the 71 patients selected in this report were in a group of 110 patients; 39 in the latter group was judged to be either at too great a risk for complications from BLB or the procedure was refused by the patient's attending physician or family; (2) pneumothorax occurred in 14%, nearly three times the risk in non-mechanically ventilated patients; (3) all patients who developed pneumothorax required thoracostomy tubes; (4) BLB can be performed in the patient's room; and (5) BLB did not cause patient deaths [110].

In the study described above, the $FiO_2$ was increased to 1.0 at least 10 minutes before the BLB, and the ventilator was changed to the assist-control mode. Attempts were made to decrease the level of PEEP to 5 cm of water before inserting the bronchoscope into the endotracheal tube. All patients received intravenous sedation, topical anesthesia, and in some, a short-acting neuromuscular-blocking agent was administered. BLB was performed under fluoroscopic guidance using a C-arm fluoroscope in the patient's room. The average number of biopsies per patient was 9.5 ± 4.5 (range 3 to 22). Lung transplant patients had significantly more biopsies compared to non-transplant patients (12.3 ± 3.4 versus 6.0 ± 2.9; $P < 0.001$) [110]. Hence, it is our suggestion to remove the PEEP and support ventilation with a hand-held Ambu-bag and continue ventilatory support without PEEP for 30–45 minutes to avoid PEEP induced barotrauma.

If BLB is planned in a mechanically ventilated patient, facilities should be immediately available to control the pleural space with thoracostomy tube if necessary [111]. As most of these patients on mechanical ventilation are critically ill, it may not be possible to easily move them to the bronchoscopy suite for BLB. If the procedure is to be performed in the critical care unit, every effort should be made to obtain a mobile fluoroscopy unit to facilitate optimal BLB.

## Lung transplant

Lung transplant recipients undergo BLB more frequently than any other group of patients. The main indications for bronchoscopy in this group include allograft rejection, opportunistic infections, and airway complications at tracheobronchial anastomosis site (wound dehiscence, fistula, stenosis, etc.). Lung transplant recipients may undergo surveillance bronchoscopy (SB) or clinically indicated bronchoscopy (CB). The role of SB has always been controversial in terms of sample adequacy, diagnosis of rejection, and clinical utility of the biopsy results.

An earlier prospective mail survey of 57 North American and eight international lung transplant programs observed that surveillance BLB after lung transplant is commonly performed. Of these 57 programs, 68% (39 of 57) performed surveillance BLBs; 92% of the programs performing surveillance BLBs did so within the first month, and 69% continued to do surveillance BLBs on a regular basis. Further, 69% (27 of 39) of programs performing surveillance BLBs continued to do so after 1 year. An overwhelming majority (86%) of respondents believed that surveillance BLB impacted on patient management at least 10% of the time

[112]. A retrospective study concluded that intensive induction and maintenance immunotherapy with surveillance BLBs and aggressive treatment of acute rejection is associated with a survival similar to that of patients without early acute rejection [113]. This study did not demonstrate decreased survival in those patients who were found to have acute rejection on surveillance BLB. A prospective study, from 2006, demonstrated that SB detects more clinically significant infections and rejections than CB. The diagnostic yield was higher in the first 12 months post transplant [114]. The diagnostic yield from BLB in this group of patients is high if the procedure is performed to diagnose acute rejection or infection. An earlier study observes that of 55 lung transplant recipients who underwent 203 BLBs (CB in 88, SB in 90, and follow-up of previous biopsy in 25), a specific histologic diagnosis was detected in 57% of surveillance procedures and 64% of the follow-up procedures [115]. The overall complication rate was 9%. In a report on a 5-year study of 99 patients who developed lung allograft rejection, follow-up BLB was used to monitor the pulmonary status. Bronchiolitis obliterans occurred in patients with persistent rejection on follow-up BLB at a median 2.0 years post-transplantation. The authors concluded that the practice of follow-up BLB after rejection within 2 years post-transplant is clinically useful, as it provides valuable diagnostic information [116]. A prospective analysis of 1235 BLBs (836 for SB and 399 for CB) in 230 post lung transplant patients concluded that an average of 6.4 biopsies per patient is required to get an adequate sample in 98% of their patients. The yield of SB for acute rejection was only 6.1% from 4 to 12 months post-transplant; hence the group did not favor SB. Obliterative bronchiolitis was diagnosed in 11 patients (0.84%) only [117]. Only 12% of the patients in the study showed acute rejection after 12 months post-transplant, concluding that BLBs after 12 months is done only if clinically indicated. The overall complication rate was 6.4% with no deaths. Currently, the role of SB versus CB is still not settled [118]. Multiple biopsies, usually six to eight separate biopsies, should be obtained to get adequate specimens but some pulmonologists prefer 10 to 12 biopsy specimens believing that the increased number of specimens increases diagnostic accuracy. The optimal site for BLB to document acute cellular rejection in the lung allograft was analyzed in a retrospective study of 73 patients and the results indicated that in absence of pulmonary infiltrates, biopsies of the lower lobes are more informative [116]. BLB is generally not helpful for diagnosing OB [114,117,119]. In the pediatric lung transplant patient population, SB was found to detect silent rejection in 4% of the patients [120], while a larger retrospective study found CB is equally efficacious in detecting infection and silent rejection in this population as well [121].

Complications from surveillance BLBs were minimal, with less than 5% rates of pneumothorax, requirement for chest tube placement, or significant bleeding [114,122]. The patient with a transplanted lung loses the ability to perceive pain and hence are not reliable when it comes to pain perception during BLB. This may increase the risk of pneumothorax if fluoroscopy is not used. The perception of pain by the patient may indicate that the biopsy forceps has come in contact with the parietal pleura and that a pneumothorax has occurred. Due to this uncertainty, we perform routine chest X ray after BLBs on post lung transplant patients. The loss of ability of the transplanted lung to react to stimulation of stretch receptors or tracheobronchial mucosa can be of procedural advantage, in that the patients do not cough as much. Brisk hemorrhage following BLB is uncommon as bronchial arterial blood supply is absent in the transplanted lung.

## Pediatric patients

Pediatric patients have undergone BLB [123,124], though the procedure is not used as often as in adults. BLB in pediatric patients has its greatest impact in detecting rejection in lung transplant recipients. High sensitivity and specificity (88 and 91%, respectively) have been reported in the diagnosis of rejection [124–126]. A study of 12 pediatric patients (median age 14.5 years) with diffuse pulmonary processes who underwent BLB reported a diagnostic yield of 50% [127]. The main impediment to obtaining BLB in children is the inability to insert a biopsy forceps through the narrow channel of a pediatric flexible bronchoscope. This can be overcome by using a rigid bronchoscope through which regular flexible biopsy forceps can be inserted to obtain BLB. The recent use of laryngeal mask with general anesthesia to perform bronchoscopy procedures in children is a great alternative [128,129]. The laryngeal mask airway is suitable in children with an endotracheal tube size of less than 6.5 mm [47]. This technique permits easy passage of a flexible bronchoscope with a biopsy channel in children as young as age 3, and hence can be employed to obtain BLB.

Another method is to use the pediatric (or ultrathin) flexible bronchoscope through an endotracheal tube and pass a flexible biopsy forceps alongside the bronchoscope. The tip of the bronchoscope can then be used to guide the biopsy forceps into the region of roentgenographic abnormality. Fluoroscopic guidance should be used to guide the bronchoscope as well as the forceps. The above technique permits introduction of larger flexible bronchoscopes into the airways of children so that biopsy forceps can be guided to the lung segment from where the biopsies are desired.

The major complication of BLB in children is pneumothorax. Earlier experience reported in a publication observed a rate of 8% among 92 procedures [124]. The same group, with increasing experience, particularly with the rigid bronchoscope, was able to reduce the rate of pneumothorax to 3% [47]. A study of 19 children who underwent 25 BLBs

(19 procedures using rigid bronchoscope) reported a 12.5% incidence of pneumothorax [127].

## Other issues

Many bronchoscopists recommend the use of an endotracheal tube to obtain BLB [30,34]. This enables the bronchoscopist to effectively control post-BLB hemorrhage. Others report that BLB can be safely performed using a transnasal or transoral approach without an endotracheal tube [130,131]. The use of an endotracheal tube is thus left to preferences and practice of the performing bronchoscopist.

The 2006 guidelines of the working party of the British Society for Antimicrobial Chemotherapy recommends against the use of prophylactic antibiotics for rigid as well as flexible bronchoscopy [132]. Many authors advise against endocarditis prophylaxis for BLB [133]. The 2007 American Heart Association guidelines recommend endocarditis prophylaxis for high-risk patients, as stated in Table 9.3 [134]. Hence, we recommend the use of endocarditis prophylaxis with bronchoscopic procedures in high-risk patients [49,135–137]. When in doubt it is advisable to consult the patients' cardiologist.

The inability to obtain optimal lung specimens is an occasional problem even when fluoroscopic guidance is used. Proper functioning of biopsy forceps and good technique will enhance the chance of collecting good biopsy specimens. Opening the biopsy forceps closer to the area of

**Table 9.3** Cardiac conditions associated with the highest risk of adverse outcome from endocarditis for which prophylaxis with dental procedures is reasonable

Prosthetic cardiac valve or prosthetic material used for cardiac valve repair

Previous IE

Congenital heart disease (CHD)*

Unrepaired cyanotic CHD, including palliative shunts and conduits

Completely repaired congenital heart defect with prosthetic material or device, whether placed by surgery or by catheter intervention, during the first 6 months after the procedure†

Repaired CHD with residual defects at the site or adjacent to the site of a prosthetic patch or prosthetic device (which inhibit endothelialization)

Cardiac transplantation recipients who develop cardiac valvulopathy

*Except for the conditions listed above, antibiotic prophylaxis is no longer recommended for any other form of CHD.

†Prophylaxis is reasonable because endothelialization of prosthetic material occurs within 6 months after the procedure.

Reprinted with Permission ©2007 American Heart Association Inc..

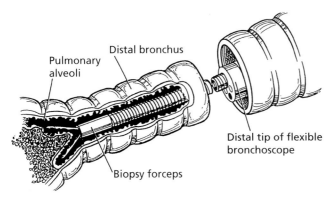

**Fig. 9.2** Diagrammatic representation of the technique of bronchoscopic lung biopsy. The biopsy forceps obtains lung tissue located between the two walls of branching terminal bronchioles. It is unclear if the biopsy forceps actually pierces the wall of the bronchioles to obtain lung specimen. Reproduced by permission from McDougall JC, Cortese DA. Bronchoscopic lung biopsy In: Prakash UBS, ed. *Bronchoscopy*. New York: Raven Press; 1994: 141–6.

parenchymal abnormality will help prevent biopsy of the bronchial wall [65]. If biopsy forceps fail to obtain adequate samples, a new or different forceps should be used or a new anatomic area should be selected for biopsy. It is also unclear whether the biopsy forceps pierces the bronchial wall to enter the lung parenchyma to obtain the biopsy or if the cups of the biopsy forceps pinch the lung tissue located between the two walls of the bronchioles, as shown in Fig. 9.2. The presence of bronchial tissue in a significant number of BLB specimens makes the latter hypothesis plausible.

BLB has a definite role in diagnosis of pulmonary parenchymal vasculitis, if the lesions are central and accessible via bronchoscope. A small retrospective study shows BLB to be less efficacious in patients with pulmonary vasculitis [138]. In an another retrospective report, bronchial biopsy was helpful to diagnose Wegener's granulomatosis in 50% of the cases with endobronchial abnormalities. Although BLB may increase the risk of significant hemorrhage [139], it is possible and has been performed in these patients if the benefit outweighs the risk. The finding of progressive hemorrhagic fluid return on BAL, and presence of hemosiderin-laden macrophages (>20%) in BAL fluid makes the diagnosis of pulmonary hemorrhage but cannot diagnose vasculitis. Current serological markers, with high sensitivity and specificity, help to diagnose vasculitides in the right clinical setting.

## Complications

Minor complications are the same as those associated with any bronchoscopic procedure. A report based on a postal survey of 231 British bronchoscopists notes that the overall complication rate from bronchoscopy increases from 0.12 to 2.7% and the mortality rate goes from 0.04 to 0.12% if BLB is included in the procedure [66]. Another study of 540 patients reported the rate of complication in those who did not undergo BLB was 0.18%, compared to 2.0% in those who underwent BLB [49].

The two major complications of BLB are hemorrhage and pneumothorax. An earlier study, based on a questionnaire survey of 5450 cases of BLB, reported a 1.2% incidence of post BLB hemorrhage (greater than 50 mL) and 13 (0.24%) deaths [140]. However, it is unclear if the deaths were directly related to BLB or other comorbid factors. A retrospective analysis of 3572 flexible bronchoscopy procedures performed at the Veterans Affairs Medical Center in Houston, Texas, by first and second year pulmonary/ critical care fellows (under the guidance of faculty), observed an overall complication rate of 1.58%. In this study, BLB was performed in 1408 patients, endobronchial biopsy in 926, BAL in 962, and bronchoscopic needle aspirations in 376 patients. BLB was the procedure most commonly associated with complications (n = 41) [141].

A study of 438 patients who underwent BLB observed mild to severe hemorrhage in 9% of patients, but the incidence was higher in immunocompromised patients (29%) and uremic patients (45%); with one death [41]. Andersen and colleagues reported a series of 939 patients who underwent BLB and less than 1% (six patients) had greater than 50 mL of BLB-associated bleeding [11]. In Gaensler's review of a series of studies comprising 1289 cases of BLB, only three (0.2%) deaths were recorded [94]. Prevention and treatment of BLB-induced hemorrhage is discussed above (see Technique section).

The incidence of post-BLB pneumothorax is between 1 and 4% [14,50,59,72,75,142–144]. The risk of pneumothorax can be decreased, as discussed above, by the use of fluoroscopic guidance [66], cough suppression, and proper biopsy techniques. Cerebral air embolism is a rare complication of BLB, and has been described in a patient who underwent this procedure [145].

## Current status of bronchoscopic lung biopsy

In a survey of 1800 North American bronchoscopists, nearly 70% reported that they performed BLB routinely in diffuse lung disease in non-immunocompromised patients [62]. An analysis of the registry on interstitial lung diseases from three countries in Europe (Belgium, Germany, and Italy) and Bernalillo County, New Mexico, USA, observed wide variations in the use of diagnostic techniques, such as HRCT, BAL, BLB, and open lung biopsy [146]. From our recent review of the literature and the experience at the Mayo Clinic, we infer that the number of BLB procedures performed in clinical practice is declining due to increased use of BAL, HRCT of the thorax, and video-assisted thoracoscopic lung biopsy in the diagnosis of diffuse lung disease. The decline in the need for BLB may continue with the introduction of newer, sophisticated imaging procedures. For now, BLB will remain an important diagnostic tool for the evaluation of a select group of diffuse lung diseases.

## References

1 Andersen HA, Miller WE, Bernatz PE. Lung biopsy: transbronchoscopic, percutaneous, open. *Surg Clin North Am* 1973; **53**: 785–93.

2 Vitums VC. Percutaneous needle biopsy of the lung with a new disposable needle. *Chest* 1972; **62**: 717–19.

3 Zavala DC, Bedell GN. Percutaneous lung biopsy with a cutting needle. An analysis of 40 cases and comparison with other biopsy techniques. *Am Rev Respir Dis* 1972; **106**: 186–93.

4 Mehnert JH, Brown MJ. Percutaneous needle core biopsy of peripheral pulmonary masses. *Am J Surg* 1978; **136**: 151–6.

5 Feist JH. Letter: Cutting needle biopsies. *Chest* 1976; **69**: 244–5.

6 Castellino RA. Percutaneous pulmonary needle diagnosis of *Pneumocystis carinii* pneumonitis. *Natl Cancer Inst Monogr* 1976; **43**: 137–40.

7 Andersen HA, Fontana RS, Harrison EG, Jr. Transbronchoscopic lung biopsy in diffuse pulmonary disease. *Dis Chest* 1965; **48**: 187–92.

8 Andersen HA, Fontana RS. Transbronchoscopic lung biopsy for diffuse pulmonary diseases: technique and results in 450 cases. *Chest* 1972; **62**: 125–8.

9 Palojoki A, Sutinen S. Transbronchoscopic lung biopsy as aid in pulmonary diagnostics. *Scand J Respir Dis* 1972; **53**: 120–4.

10 Andersen HA. Transbronchial lung biopsy in diffuse pulmonary disease. *Ann Thorac Surg* 1977; **24**: 1.

11 Andersen HA. Transbronchoscopic lung biopsy for diffuse pulmonary diseases. Results in 939 patients. *Chest* 1978; **73**: 734–6.

12 Levin DC, Wicks AB, Ellis JH, Jr. Transbronchial lung biopsy via the fiberoptic bronchoscope. *Am Rev Respir Dis* 1974; **110**: 4–12.

13 Scheinhorn DJ, Joyner LR, Whitcomb ME. Transbronchial forceps lung biopsy through the fiberoptic bronchoscope in *Pneumocystis carinii* pneumonia. *Chest* 1974; **66**: 294–5.

14 Hanson RR, Zavala DC, Rhodes ML, *et al.* Transbronchial biopsy via flexible fiberoptic bronchoscope; results in 164 patients. *Am Rev Respir Dis* 1976; **114**: 67–72.

15 Elliot TL, Lynch DA, Newell JD, Jr., *et al.* High-resolution computed tomography features of nonspecific interstitial pneumonia and usual interstitial pneumonia. *J Comput Assist Tomogr* 2005; **29**: 339–45.

16 Nishimura K, Izumi T, Kitaichi M, *et al.* The diagnostic accuracy of high-resolution computed tomography in diffuse infiltrative lung diseases. *Chest* 1993; **104**: 1149–55.

17 Sundaram B, Gross BH, Martinez FJ, *et al.* Accuracy of high-resolution CT in the diagnosis of diffuse lung disease: effect of predominance and distribution of findings. *AJR Am J Roentgenol* 2008; **191**: 1032–9.

18 Zompatori M, Sverzellati N, Poletti V, *et al.* High-resolution CT in diagnosis of diffuse infiltrative lung disease. *Semin Ultrasound CT MR* 2005; **26**: 332–47.

19 Halme M, Piilonen A, Taskinen E. Comparison of endobronchial and transbronchial biopsies with high-resolution CT (HRCIT) in the diagnosis of sarcoidosis. *APMIS* 2001; **109**: 289–94.

20 Peikert T, Rana S, Edell ES. Safety, diagnostic yield, and therapeutic implications of flexible bronchoscopy in patients with febrile neutropenia and pulmonary infiltrates. *Mayo Clin Proc* 2005; **80**: 1414–20.

21 Patel NR, Lee PS, Kim JH, *et al.* The influence of diagnostic bronchoscopy on clinical outcomes comparing adult autologous and allogeneic bone marrow transplant patients. *Chest* 2005; **127**: 1388–96.

22 Haponik EF, Summer WR, Terry PB, *et al.* Clinical decision making with transbronchial lung biopsies. The value of nonspecific histologic examination. *Am Rev Respir Dis* 1982; **125**: 524–9.

23 Broaddus C, Dake MD, Stulbarg MS, *et al.* Bronchoalveolar lavage and transbronchial biopsy for the diagnosis of pulmonary infections in the acquired immunodeficiency syndrome. *Ann Intern Med* 1985; **102**: 747–52.

24 Rennard SI, Spurzem JR. Bronchoalveolar lavage in the diagnosis of lung cancer. *Chest* 1992; **102**: 331–2.

25 Jain P, Sandur S, Meli Y, *et al.* Role of flexible bronchoscopy in immunocompromised patients with lung infiltrates. *Chest* 2004; **125**: 712–22.

26 Prakash UB, Barham SS, Carpenter HA, *et al.* Pulmonary alveolar phospholipoproteinosis: experience with 34 cases and a review. *Mayo Clin Proc* 1987; **62**: 499–518.

27 Linder J, Radio SJ, Robbins RA, *et al.* Bronchoalveolar lavage in the cytologic diagnosis of carcinoma of the lung. *Acta Cytol* 1987; **31**: 796–801.

28 Prakash U. Pulmonary eosinophilic granuloma In: III LJ, ed. *Immunologically Mediated Pulmonary Diseases.* Philadelphia: Lippincott; 1991.

29 McDougall JC CD. *Bronchscopic Lung Biopsy.* New York: Raven Press; 1994.

30 Morris MJ, Peacock PM, Lloyd WC III, Blanton HM. The effect of pulmonary hypertension upon bleeding in sheep undergoing bronchoscopic biopsy. *J Bronchol* 1996; **3**: 11–16.

31 Morris MJ, Peacock PM, Mego DM, *et al.* The risk of hemorrhage from bronchoscopic lung biopsy due to pulmonary hypertension in interstitial lung disease. *J Bronchol* 1998; **5**: 115–21.

32 Wahidi MM, Garland R, Feller-Kopman D, *et al.* Effect of clopidogrel with and without aspirin on bleeding following transbronchial lung biopsy. *Chest* 2005; **127**: 961–4.

33 Ernst A, Eberhardt R, Wahidi M, *et al.* Effect of routine clopidogrel use on bleeding complications after transbronchial biopsy in humans. *Chest* 2006; **129**: 734–7.

34 Fleisher LA, Beckman JA, Brown KA, *et al.* ACC/AHA 2007 Guidelines on perioperative cardiovascular evaluation and care for noncardiac surgery: Executive summary: A report of the American College of Cardiology/American Heart Association Task Force on Practice Guidelines (Writing Committee to Revise the 2002 Guidelines on Perioperative Cardiovascular Evaluation for Noncardiac Surgery) Developed in Collaboration

With the American Society of Echocardiography, American Society of Nuclear Cardiology, Heart Rhythm Society, Society of Cardiovascular Anesthesiologists, Society for Cardiovascular Angiography and Interventions, Society for Vascular Medicine and Biology, and Society for Vascular Surgery. *J Am Coll Cardiol* 2007; **50**: 1707–32.

35 Fleisher LA, Beckman JA, Brown KA, *et al*. ACC/AHA 2007 guidelines on perioperative cardiovascular evaluation and care for noncardiac surgery: executive summary: a report of the American College of Cardiology/American Heart Association Task Force on Practice Guidelines (Writing Committee to Revise the 2002 Guidelines on Perioperative Cardiovascular Evaluation for Noncardiac Surgery). *Anesth Analg* 2008; **106**: 685–712.

36 Prakash UB, Stubbs SE. The bronchoscopy survey. Some reflections. *Chest* 1991; **100**: 1660–7.

37 Prakash U. *Optimal Bronchoscopy*. New York: Raven Press; 1994.

38 Rodgers RP, Levin J. A critical reappraisal of the bleeding time. *Semin Thromb Hemost* 1990; **16**: 1–20.

39 Lind SE. The bleeding time does not predict surgical bleeding. *Blood* 1991; **77**: 2547–52.

40 Bjortuft O, Brosstad F, Boe J. Bronchoscopy with transbronchial biopsies: measurement of bleeding volume and evaluation of the predictive value of coagulation tests. *Eur Respir J* 1998; **12**: 1025–7.

41 Zavala DC. Pulmonary hemorrhage in fiberoptic transbronchial biopsy. *Chest* 1976; **70**: 584–8.

42 Zavala DC. Transbronchial biopsy in diffuse lung disease. *Chest* 1978; **73**: 727–33.

43 Matsushima Y, Jones RL, King EG, *et al*. Alterations in pulmonary mechanics and gas exchange during routine fiberoptic bronchoscopy. *Chest* 1984; **86**: 184–8.

44 Peacock AJ, Benson-Mitchell R, Godfrey R. Effect of fibreoptic bronchoscopy on pulmonary function. *Thorax* 1990; **45**: 38–41.

45 Belen J, Neuhaus A, Markowitz D, *et al*. Modification of the effect of fiberoptic bronchoscopy on pulmonary mechanics. *Chest* 1981; **79**: 516–19.

46 Kvale P. Bronchoscopic lung biopsy. *J Bronchol* 1994: 321–6.

47 Whitehead B. Bronchoscopic lung biopsy in pediatric patients. *J Bronchol Intervent Pulmonol* 1999; **6**: 48–54.

48 Prakash UBS FL. *Hemoptysis and Bronchoscopy-induced Hemorrhage*. New York: Raven Press; 1994.

49 Ahmad M, Livingston DR, Golish JA, *et al*. The safety of outpatient transbronchial biopsy. *Chest* 1986; **90**: 403–5.

50 Frazier WD, Pope TL, Jr., Findley LJ. Pneumothorax following transbronchial biopsy. Low diagnostic yield with routine chest roentgenograms. *Chest* 1990; **97**: 539–40.

51 Milam MG, Evins AE, Sahn SA. Immediate chest roentgenography following fiberoptic bronchoscopy. *Chest* 1989; **96**: 477–9.

52 Wahidi MM, Rocha AT, Hollingsworth JW, *et al*. Contraindications and safety of transbronchial lung biopsy via flexible bronchoscopy. A survey of pulmonologists and review of the literature. *Respiration* 2005; **72**: 285–95.

53 Papin TA, Lynch JP, 3rd, Weg JG. Transbronchial biopsy in the thrombocytopenic patient. *Chest* 1985; **88**: 549–52.

54 Cordasco EM, Jr., Mehta AC, Ahmad M. Bronchoscopically induced bleeding. A summary of nine years' Cleveland clinic experience and review of the literature. *Chest* 1991; **100**: 1141–7.

55 Cunningham JH, Zavala DC, Corry RJ, *et al*. Trephine air drill, bronchial brush, and fiberoptic transbronchial lung biopsies in immunosuppressed patients. *Am Rev Respir Dis* 1977; **115**: 213–20.

56 Schiffer CA, Anderson KC, Bennett CL, *et al*. Platelet transfusion for patients with cancer: clinical practice guidelines of the American Society of Clinical Oncology. *J Clin Oncol* 2001; **19**: 1519–38.

57 Mannucci PM, Remuzzi G, Pusineri F, *et al*. Deamino-8-D-arginine vasopressin shortens the bleeding time in uremia. *N Engl J Med* 1983; **308**: 8–12.

58 Mannucci PM, Vicente V, Vianello L, *et al*. Controlled trial of desmopressin in liver cirrhosis and other conditions associated with a prolonged bleeding time. *Blood* 1986; **67**: 1148–53.

59 de Fenoyl O CF, Lebeau B, Rochemaure J. Transbronchial biopsy without fluoroscopy: a five year experience in outpatients. *Thorax* 1989; **44**: 956–9.

60 Puar HS, Young RC, Jr., Armstrong EM. Bronchial and transbronchial lung biopsy without fluoroscopy in sarcoidosis. *Chest* 1985; **87**: 303–6.

61 Anders GT, Johnson JE, Bush BA, *et al*. Transbronchial biopsy without fluoroscopy. A seven-year perspective. *Chest* 1988; **94**: 557–60.

62 Prakash UB, Offord KP, Stubbs SE. Bronchoscopy in North America: the ACCP survey. *Chest* 1991; **100**: 1668–75.

63 Colt HG, Prakash UB, Offord KP. Bronchoscopy in North America: Survey by the American Association for Bronchology, 1999. *J Bronchol Intervent Pulmonol* 2000; **7**: 8–25.

64 Prakash UB, Colt HG. The AAB bronchoscopy survey: Does it reveal anything new? *J Bronchol Intervent Pulmonol* 2000; **7**: 1–3.

65 Prakash UBS, Cotese DA, Stubbs SE. *Technical Solutions to Common Problems in Bronchoscopy*. New York: Ravens Press; 1994.

66 Simpson FG, Arnold AG, Purvis A, *et al*. Postal survey of bronchoscopic practice by physicians in the United Kingdom. *Thorax* 1986; **41**: 311–17.

67 Descombes E, Gardiol D, Leuenberger P. Transbronchial lung biopsy: an analysis of 530 cases with reference to the number of samples. *Monaldi Arch Chest Dis* 1997; **52**: 324–9.

68 Asahina H, Yamazaki K, Onodera Y, *et al*. Transbronchial biopsy using endobronchial ultrasonography with a guide sheath and virtual bronchoscopic navigation. *Chest* 2005; **128**: 1761–5.

69 Shinagawa N, Yamazaki K, Onodera Y, *et al*. CT-guided transbronchial biopsy using an ultrathin bronchoscope with virtual bronchoscopic navigation. *Chest* 2004; **125**: 1138–43.

70 Fraire AE, Cooper SP, Greenberg SD, *et al*. Transbronchial lung biopsy. Histopathologic and morphometric assessment of diagnostic utility. *Chest* 1992; **102**: 748–52.

71 Shure D. Transbronchial biopsy and needle aspiration. *Chest* 1989; **95**: 1130–8.

72 Smith LS, Seaquist M, Schillaci RF. Comparison of forceps used for transbronchial lung biopsy. Bigger may NOT be better. *Chest* 1985; **87**: 574–6.

73 Loube DI, Johnson JE, Wiener D, *et al*. The effect of forceps size on the adequacy of specimens obtained by transbronchial biopsy. *Am Rev Respir Dis* 1993; **148**: 1411–13.

74 Anders GT, Linville KC, Johnson JE, *et al.* Evaluation of the float sign for determining adequacy of specimens obtained with transbronchial biopsy. *Am Rev Respir Dis* 1991; **144**: 1406–7.

75 Curley FJ, Johal JS, Burke ME, *et al.* Transbronchial lung biopsy: can specimen quality be predicted at the time of biopsy? *Chest* 1998; **113**: 1037–41.

76 Kvale PA. *Flexible Bronchoscopy with Brush and Forceps Biopsy.* New York: Raven Press; 1989.

77 Statement on sarcoidosis. Joint Statement of the American Thoracic Society (ATS), the European Respiratory Society (ERS) and the World Association of Sarcoidosis and Other Granulomatous Disorders (WASOG) adopted by the ATS Board of Directors and by the ERS Executive Committee, February 1999. *Am J Respir Crit Care Med* 1999; **160**: 736–55.

78 Gilman MJ, Wang KP. Transbronchial lung biopsy in sarcoidosis. An approach to determine the optimal number of biopsies. *Am Rev Respir Dis* 1980; **122**: 721–4.

79 Whitcomb ME, Hawley PC, Domby WR, *et al.* The role of fiberoptic bronchoscopy in the diagnosis of sarcoidosis. Clinical conference in pulmonary disease from Ohio State University, Columbus. *Chest* 1978; **74**: 205–8.

80 Koonitz CH, Joyner LR, Nelson RA. Transbronchial lung biopsy via the fiberoptic bronchoscope in sarcoidosis. *Ann Intern Med* 1976; **85**: 64–6.

81 Koerner SK, Sakowitz AJ, Appelman RI, *et al.* Transbronchinal lung biopsy for the diagnosis of sarcoidosis. *N Engl J Med* 1975; **293**: 268–70.

82 Poe RH, Israel RH, Utell MJ, *et al.* Probability of a positive transbronchial lung biopsy result in sarcoidosis. *Arch Intern Med* 1979; **139**: 761–3.

83 Roethe RA, Fuller PB, Byrd RB, *et al.* Transbronchoscopic lung biopsy in sarcoidosis. Optimal number and sites for diagnosis. *Chest* 1980; **77**: 400–2.

84 MacJannette R, Fiddes J, Kerr K, *et al.* Is bronchoscopic lung biopsy helpful in the management of patients with diffuse lung disease? *Eur Respir J* 2007; **29**: 1064.

85 Armstrong JR, Radke JR, Kvale PA, *et al.* Endoscopic findings in sarcoidosis. Characteristics and correlations with radiographic staging and bronchial mucosal biopsy yield. *Ann Otol Rhinol Laryngol* 1981; **90**: 339–43.

86 Shorr AF, Torrington KG, Hnatiuk OW. Endobronchial biopsy for sarcoidosis: a prospective study. *Chest* 2001; **120**: 109–14.

87 Bilaceroglu S, Perim K, Gunel O, *et al.* Combining transbronchial aspiration with endobronchial and transbronchial biopsy in sarcoidosis. *Monaldi Arch Chest Dis* 1999; **54**: 217–23.

88 Fechner RE, Greenberg SD, Wilson RK, *et al.* Evaluation of transbronchial biopsy of the lung. *Am J Clin Pathol* 1977; **68**: 17–20.

89 Wall CP, Gaensler EA, Carrington CB, *et al.* Comparison of transbronchial and open biopsies in chronic infiltrative lung diseases. *Am Rev Respir Dis* 1981; **123**: 280–5.

90 Nishio JN, Lynch JP, 3rd. Fiberoptic bronchoscopy in the immunocompromised host: the significance of a "nonspecific" transbronchial biopsy. *Am Rev Respir Dis* 1980; **121**: 307–12.

91 Ensminger SA, Prakash UB. Is bronchoscopic lung biopsy helpful in the management of patients with diffuse lung disease? *Eur Respir J* 2006; **28**: 1081–4.

92 American Thoracic Society. Idiopathic pulmonary fibrosis: diagnosis and treatment. International consensus statement. American Thoracic Society (ATS), and the European Respiratory Society (ERS). *Am J Respir Crit Care Med* 2000; **161**: 646–64.

93 American Thoracic Society/European Respiratory Society International Multidisciplinary Consensus Classification of the Idiopathic Interstitial Pneumonias. This joint statement of the American Thoracic Society (ATS), and the European Respiratory Society (ERS) was adopted by the ATS board of directors, June 2001 and by the ERS Executive Committee, June 2001. *Am J Respir Crit Care Med* 2002; **165**: 277–304.

94 Gaensler. *Open and Closed Lung Biopsy.* New York: Marcel Dekker; 1980.

95 Wilson RK, Fechner RE, Greenberg SD, *et al.* Clinical implications of a "nonspecific" transbronchial biopsy. *Am J Med* 1978; **65**: 252–6.

96 Newman SL, Michel RP, Wang NS. Lingular lung biopsy: is it representative? *Am Rev Respir Dis* 1985; **132**: 1084–6.

97 Matthay RA, Farmer WC, Odero D. Diagnostic fibreoptic bronchoscopy in the immunocompromised host with pulmonary infiltrates. *Thorax* 1977; **32**: 539–45.

98 Hedemark LL, Kronenberg RS, Rasp FL, *et al.* The value of bronchoscopy in establishing the etiology of pneumonia in renal transplant recipients. *Am Rev Respir Dis* 1982; **126**: 981–5.

99 Mones JM, Saldana MJ, Oldham SA. Diagnosis of *Pneumocystis carinii* pneumonia. Roentgenographic-pathologic correlates based on fiberoptic bronchoscopy specimens from patients with the acquired immunodeficiency syndrome. *Chest* 1986; **89**: 522–6.

100 Stover DE, White DA, Romano PA, *et al.* Diagnosis of pulmonary disease in acquired immune deficiency syndrome (AIDS). Role of bronchoscopy and bronchoalveolar lavage. *Am Rev Respir Dis* 1984; **130**: 659–62.

101 Ikedo Y. The significance of bronchoscopy for the diagnosis of *Mycobacterium avium* complex (MAC) pulmonary disease. *Kurume Med J* 2001; **48**: 15–19.

102 Chopra SK, Mohsenifar Z. Fiberoptic bronchoscopy in diagnosis of opportunistic lung infections: assessment of Sputa, Washings, Brushings and biopsy specimens. *West J Med* 1979; **131**: 4–7.

103 Kvale P. How much bronchoscopic sampling is enough (for HIV infected patients)? *J Bronchol* 1996; **3**: 83–4.

104 Ribes JA, Limper AH, Espy MJ, *et al.* PCR detection of *Pneumocystis carinii* in bronchoalveolar lavage specimens: analysis of sensitivity and specificity. *J Clin Microbiol* 1997; **35**: 830–5.

105 Cortese JM, McDougall JC. *Bronchoscopy in Peripheral and Central Lung Lesions.* New York: Raven Press; 1994.

106 Oki M, Saka H, Kitagawa C, *et al.* Novel thin bronchoscope with a 1.7-mm working channel for peripheral pulmonary lesions. *Eur Respir J* 2008; **32**: 465–71.

107 Eberhardt R, Anantham D, Ernst A, *et al.* Multimodality bronchoscopic diagnosis of peripheral lung lesions: a randomized controlled trial. *Am J Respir Crit Care Med* 2007; **176**: 36–41.

108 Papin TA, Grum CM, Weg JG. Transbronchial biopsy during mechanical ventilation. *Chest* 1986; **89**: 168–70.

109 Pincus PS, Kallenbach JM, Hurwitz MD, *et al.* Transbronchial biopsy during mechanical ventilation. *Crit Care Med* 1987; **15**: 1136–9.

110 O'Brien JD, Ettinger NA, Shevlin D, *et al.* Safety and yield of transbronchial biopsy in mechanically ventilated patients. *Crit Care Med* 1997; **25**: 440–6.

111 Stubbs SE. *Bronchoscopy*. New York: Raven Press; 1994.

112 Kukafka DS, O'Brien GM, Furukawa S, *et al.* Surveillance bronchoscopy in lung transplant recipients. *Chest* 1997; **111**: 377–81.

113 Swanson SJ, Mentzer SJ, Reilly JJ, *et al.* Surveillance transbronchial lung biopsies: implication for survival after lung transplantation. *J Thorac Cardiovasc Surg* 2000; **119**: 27–37.

114 McWilliams TJ, Williams TJ, Whitford HM, *et al.* Surveillance bronchoscopy in lung transplant recipients: risk versus benefit. *J Heart Lung Transplant* 2008; **27**: 1203–9.

115 Trulock EP, Ettinger NA, Brunt EM, *et al.* The role of transbronchial lung biopsy in the treatment of lung transplant recipients. An analysis of 200 consecutive procedures. *Chest* 1992; **102**: 1049–54.

116 Aboyoun CL, Tamm M, Chhajed PN, *et al.* Diagnostic value of follow-up transbronchial lung biopsy after lung rejection. *Am J Respir Crit Care Med* 2001; **164**: 460–3.

117 Hopkins PM, Aboyoun CL, Chhajed PN, *et al.* Prospective analysis of 1,235 transbronchial lung biopsies in lung transplant recipients. *J Heart Lung Transpl* 2002; **21**: 1062–7.

118 Valentine VG, Taylor DE, Dhillon GS, *et al.* Success of lung transplantation without surveillance bronchoscopy. *J Heart Lung Transpl* 2002; **21**: 319–26.

119 Glanville AR. The role of bronchoscopic surveillance monitoring in the care of lung transplant recipients. *Semin Respir Crit Care Med* 2006; **27**: 480–91.

120 Benden C, Harpur-Sinclair O, Ranasinghe AS, *et al.* Surveillance bronchoscopy in children during the first year after lung transplantation: Is it worth it? *Thorax* 2007; **62**: 57–61.

121 Greene CL, Reemtsen B, Polimenakos A, *et al.* Role of clinically indicated transbronchial lung biopsies in the management of pediatric post-lung transplant patients. *Ann Thorac Surg* 2008; **86**: 198–203.

122 Chhajed PN, Aboyoun C, Malouf MA, *et al.* Risk factors and management of bleeding associated with transbronchial lung biopsy in lung transplant recipients. *J Heart Lung Transpl* 2003; **22**: 195–7.

123 Levy M, Glick B, Springer C, *et al.* Bronchoscopy and bronchography in children. Experience with 110 investigations. *Am J Dis Child* 1983; **137**: 14–16.

124 Whitehead B, Scott JP, Helms P, *et al.* Technique and use of transbronchial biopsy in children and adolescents. *Peditric Pulmonol* 1992; **12**: 240–6.

125 Muntz HR, Wallace M, Lusk RP. Pediatric transbronchial lung biopsy. *Ann Otol Rhinol Laryngol* 1992; **101**: 135–7.

126 Scott JP, Higenbottam TW, Smyth RL, *et al.* Transbronchial biopsies in children after heart-lung transplantation. *Pediatrics* 1990; **86**: 698–702.

127 Fitzpatrick SB, Stokes DC, Marsh B, *et al.* Transbronchial lung biopsy in pediatric and adolescent patients. *Am J Dis Child* 1985; **139**: 46–9.

128 Smyth AR, Bowhay AR, Heaf LJ, *et al.* The laryngeal mask airway in fibreoptic bronchoscopy. *Arch Dis Child* 1996; **75**: 344–5.

129 Nussbaum E, Zagnoev M. Pediatric fiberoptic bronchoscopy with a laryngeal mask airway. *Chest* 2001; **120**: 614–16.

130 Kvale PA, Bode FR, Kini S. Diagnostic accuracy in lung cancer; comparison of techniques used in association with flexible fiberoptic bronchoscopy. *Chest* 1976; **69**: 752–7.

131 Feldman NT, Penningtonp JE, Ehrie MG. Transbronchial lung biopsy in the compromised host. *JAMA* 1977; **238**: 1377–9.

132 Gould FK, Elliott TS, Foweraker J, *et al.* Guidelines for the prevention of endocarditis: report of the Working Party of the British Society for Antimicrobial Chemotherapy. *J Antimicrob Chemother* 2006; **57**: 1035–42.

133 Witte MC, Opal SM, Gilbert JG, *et al.* Incidence of fever and bacteremia following transbronchial needle aspiration. *Chest* 1986; **89**: 85–7.

134 Wilson W, Taubert KA, Gewitz M, *et al.* Prevention of infective endocarditis: guidelines from the American Heart Association: a guideline from the American Heart Association Rheumatic Fever, Endocarditis, and Kawasaki Disease Committee, Council on Cardiovascular Disease in the Young, and the Council on Clinical Cardiology, Council on Cardiovascular Surgery and Anesthesia, and the Quality of Care and Outcomes Research Interdisciplinary Working Group. *Circulation* 2007; **116**: 1736–54.

135 Watts WJ, Green RA. Bacteremia following transbronchial fine needle aspiration. *Chest* 1984; **85**: 295.

136 Kane RC, Cohen MH, Fossieck BE, Jr., *et al.* Absence of bacteremia after fiberoptic bronchoscopy. *Am Rev Respir Dis* 1975; **111**: 102–4.

137 Pereira W, Kovnat DM, Khan MA, *et al.* Fever and pneumonia after flexible fiberoptic bronchoscopy. *Am Rev Respir Dis* 1975; **112**: 59–64.

138 Schnabel A, Holl-Ulrich K, Dalhoff K, *et al.* Efficacy of transbronchial biopsy in pulmonary vaculitides. *Eur Respir J* 1997; **10**: 2738–43.

139 Flick MR, Wasson K, Dunn LJ, *et al.* Fatal pulmonary hemorrhage after transbronchial lung biopsy through the fiberoptic bronchoscope. *Am Rev Respir Dis* 1975; **111**: 853–6.

140 Herf SM, Suratt PM, Arora NS. Deaths and complications associated with transbronchial lung biopsy. *Am Rev Respir Dis* 1977; **115**: 708–11.

141 Varon J, Fromme RE. Fiberoptic bronchoscopy: complications among physicians-in-training. *Internet J Emerg Intens Care Med* 1998; **2**: N1.

142 Joyner LR, Scheinhorn DJ. Transbronchial forceps lung biopsy through the fiberoptic bronchoscope. tdiagnosis of diffuse pulmonary disease. *Chest* 1975; **67**: 532–5.

143 Hernandez Blasco L, Sanchez Hernandez IM, Villena Garrido V, *et al.* Safety of the transbronchial biopsy in outpatients. *Chest* 1991; **99**: 562–5.

144 Zavala DC. Diagnostic fiberoptic bronchoscopy: Techniques and results of biopsy in 600 patients. *Chest* 1975; **68**: 12–19.

145 Shetty PG, Fatterpekar GM, Manohar S, *et al.* Fatal cerebral air embolism as a complication of transbronchoscopic lung biopsy: a case report. *Australas Radiol* 2001; **45**: 215–17.

146 Thomeer MJ, Costabe U, Rizzato G, *et al.* Comparison of registries of interstitial lung diseases in three European countries. *Eur Respir J* 2001; **32** (Suppl): 114s–8s.

# 10 Bronchoalveolar Lavage

**Brian Palen and Richard Helmers**

Mayo Clinic, Scottsdale, AZ, USA

Although the technique of washing the lung with physiologic saline to remove accumulated material and cells from the air space had been used therapeutically for many years, it was with the advent of widespread use of flexible fiberoptic bronchoscopy (FOB) in the 1970s that instillation of smaller quantities of saline directly into the distal airways and recovery of the aspirate for analysis—bronchoalveolar lavage (BAL)—became an important clinical and investigational tool [1,2]. BAL allows the recovery of both cellular and non-cellular components from the epithelial surface of the lower respiratory tract. BAL differs significantly from bronchial washings, which refer to aspiration of either secretions or small amounts of instilled saline from the large airways [3]. The conceptual basis of BAL is that cells and non-cellular components present on the epithelial surface of the alveoli are representative of the inflammatory and immune system of the entire lower respiratory tract. This has been confirmed by studies comparing cellular constituents obtained from open lung biopsy and BAL. BAL thus allows minimally invasive sampling of various components of the inflammatory and immune system at their site of action [1,4]. BAL is a widely used technique applied to virtually every area of pulmonary medicine.

## Technique

Historically, a lack of technique standardization from one institution to another created variability in reportable results from BAL. The European Respiratory Society (ERS) published consensus reports in 1989 and again in 1999, which contain thorough technical guidelines [5,6].

BAL is performed after routine inspection/ examination of the tracheobronchial tree and before biopsy or brushings to avoid contamination of the recovered fluid with excess blood, which would alter the concentrations of the cellular and non-cellular components. Using a clean suction channel, the tip of the bronchoscope is advanced distally until it is wedged (advanced to point of resistance and/or collapse of airway with gentle suction) into a subsegmental bronchus. The wedge position is usually at the level of the fourth to fifth branching. Care should be taken to avoid trauma and coughing because these may lead to excessive contamination of the recovered fluid with mucus and blood [7]. Passing the bronchoscope through a previously inserted endotracheal tube has been shown to reduce oropharyngeal contamination when BAL specimens are cultured [8].

In diffuse disease, segments of the lingula or the right middle lobe are routinely lavaged. Fluid recovery is typically greater in these lobes due to the effects of gravity in the supine position [1,2,9]. When localized disease is present radiographically, lavage should be carried out at the area of radiographic abnormalities, because the BAL results may be most abnormal from these areas [4,5,10]. Radiographic and clinical data will often dictate location and number of segments lavaged. It is important to specify the number of segments lavaged and whether the specimens were pooled or analyzed separately.

After the bronchoscope is wedged, sterile saline is infused with a syringe into the suction port of the bronchoscope. Mixed data are found regarding the use of warmed saline. Prewarming the lavage fluid to 37°C may help prevent coughing and bronchospasm, especially in patients with hyper-responsive airways, and may increase fluid recovery and cellular yield in comparison to instillations of fluid at room temperature [3,5,7]. Most institutions use aliquots of 20 to 60 mL. There are no significant data to support a specific aliquot size. The fluid is then removed from the lung by the use of negative pressure from a suction apparatus and collected into a specimen trap. The lavage procedure is then repeated to a total of at least 100 mL instilled volume.

The suction channel of the bronchoscope should be maintained in the center of the airway lumen. If an adequate

*Flexible Bronchoscopy*, Third Edition. Edited by Ko-Pen Wang, Atul C. Mehta, J. Francis Turner.
© 2012 Blackwell Publishing Ltd. Published 2012 by Blackwell Publishing Ltd.

"wedge" is maintained throughout the lavage, the patient should not experience cough because the lavage fluid should not "leak" proximal to the tip of the bronchoscope [4]. Gentle suction should be applied until free flow of return is diminished. The ERS recommends suction should be kept to less than 100 mm Hg; 50 mm Hg has been shown to easily cause airway collapse. Excess suction pressure can result in airway collapse and diminished return.

In an average-sized person at total lung capacity (TLC), the typical lavaged zone represents about 165 mL and the residual volume of this zone is approximately 45 mL [11]. It has been demonstrated that alveoli with pockets of residual gas yield higher total cell counts, but normal differentials [12]. The lavage of a normal adult with 100 mL of saline yields 40 to 60 mL of fluid containing 5 to $10 \times 10^6$ cells and 1 to 10 mg protein [1]. It has been estimated that a 100-mL lavage of a bronchial subsegment represents the sampling of about $10^6$ alveoli [2,11]. Lavage cellular counts are, in general, not considered valid if: the patient has purulent secretions in the airways, the bronchoscope is not maintained in the "wedge" position during the lavage procedure, or the volume of fluid recovered is less than 40% of the volume infused [4].

The volume of fluid infused is an important variable between institutions. Larger amounts of lavage fluid (up to 240 to 300 mL) have been used, particularly if a larger number of inflammatory cells are required; but it is generally agreed that increased patient morbidity may result, particularly local atelectasis and transient fevers [2,4,7]. Smaller amounts of BAL fluid, in contrast, may sample only small bronchi or relatively few alveoli. It has been demonstrated that a lavage volume of 60 mL sampled only proximal airways, but that a volume of 120 mL instilled into a single segment appeared to perfuse the entire segment (including distal airways and alveoli) and aspiration of this volume produced fluid movement from within the whole of the segment [13]. It is generally agreed that lavage should be terminated if the instilled volume exceeds recovery by more than 100 mL [14,15].

Several investigators have evaluated cell differential on sequential aliquots of recovered lavage fluid and have concluded that the initial aliquot (if the volume of the fluid is small, i.e. 20 mL) is different from subsequent aliquots in that the initial aliquot is likely to recover cells and proteins from distal bronchi and not alveoli [7,16–19]. For this reason, many institutions discard the initial 20 mL aliquot. Rennard and colleagues [19] found that pooling the initial 20 mL and subsequent aliquots resulted in a sample that was "mostly alveolar" and concluded it is unlikely that including the first aliquot, which represents 10% or less of the total recovered cells, will affect the cellular analysis in the absence of significant inflammation. If a patient does have obvious airway inflammation, the analysis may be heavily influenced by bronchial airway secretions.

In general, 40 to 60% of the infused volume is recovered and cell viability is generally greater than 80% [1,9,20]. In patients with loss of elastic recoil, the recovery of fluid is usually less since the bronchial walls collapse when suction is applied [1,2,7]. Obstructive lung disease is an established cause of decreased BAL fluid recovery. Patients with lower forced expiratory volume in one second ($FEV_1$) to forced vital capacity ($FVC$) ratios ($FEV_1/FVC$) have demonstrated a proportional decrease in lavage return. The volume of fluid recovered has also shown to be decreased with advancing age and with cigarette smoking [21].

The dynamic interaction of the alveolar and vascular space creates great difficulty in assessing true concentrations of alveolar materials. BAL fluid instilled into the alveoli mixes with existing alveolar fluid which is in constant exchange with the vascular space. This creates uncertainty in measurement of alveolar components. Endogenous dilutional markers such as urea and albumin have shown to be impacted by BAL itself, as well as disease states of altered epithelial permeability such as acute respiratory distress syndrome (ARDS). Exogenous markers such as methylene blue are prone to uptake by macrophages and thus may be altered in various disease states. An alternative is to express components of the lower respiratory tract as units per milliliter of lavage fluid. This remains an area of active debate [3,5,6,22].

## Safety and complications

Lavage is a relatively safe procedure that adds 5 to 15 minutes to a routine flexible fiberoptic bronchoscopic examination. There are no absolute contraindications to BAL, but one should be aware of high-risk situations and relative contraindications. These include an uncooperative patient, $FEV_1$ less than 800 mL, moderate to severe asthma, hypercapnia, hypoxia uncorrected to an oxygen saturation of 90% with supplemental oxygen, serious cardiac dysrhythmia, myocardial infarction within 6 weeks, uncorrected bleeding diathesis, and hemodynamic instability [3].

The most frequently seen complication is post-BAL fever [23,24]. Studies have demonstrated that a febrile response may occur in 10 to 50% of patients. The mechanism is a transient pyrogen effect due to the release of biologically active mediators such as cytokines [25]. Fever postprocedure is rarely associated with bacteremia [26] and may successfully be treated with antipyretics [27]. The incidence of post BAL fever has been shown to be proportional to the number of lobes lavaged and the total volume of fluid instilled into each lavage site. A recent study in children demonstrated that administration of intravenous dexamethasone prior to bronchoscopy significantly reduced subsequent fever. Further studies are needed prior to practice implementation [28].

Another commonly observed complication with BAL is transient decrease in $P_aO_2$. Cole and colleagues [29] noted an average fall in $P_aO_2$ of 22.7 mm Hg, which persisted for at least 2 hours. Degree of desaturation has been demonstrated to be proportional to the volume of fluid instilled [30]. Regardless of underlying pulmonary function, the patient should be administered supplemental oxygen throughout and immediately following the procedure [11].

Much debate in the literature has involved the safety of BAL in patients with asthma and COPD. Large-volume lavage (500 mL) has been associated with significant decrease in $FEV_1$, $FVC$, and peak expiratory flow rate ($PEFR$). In healthy subjects, small-volume (175 mL) lavage has not been shown to affect pulmonary function tests (PFTs) [31]. Recent literature reviews have confirmed safety in patients with compensated COPD and asthma by showing complication rates similar to those of control patients [32,33]. While reports have shown safety in asthmatic patients without use of bronchodilators, most institutions recommend the use of nebulized bronchodilators prior to procedure [34].

Multiple studies at different institutions have examined immunosuppressed and thrombocytopenic patients and have concluded that BAL has an acceptable morbidity as a diagnostic tool [35–39].

Post BAL, it has been shown that up to 90% of patients will display radiographic evidence of new or increased consolidation in the area lavaged. Resolution of these opacities is gradual, with 73% remaining at 240 minutes post lavage. Complete resolution is expected within 24 hours. The presence of these opacities correlates with the amount of retained saline solution, is limited to the area lavaged, and is not associated with clinical complications [40].

Pneumothorax is a rare complication with isolated case reports found in the literature. Elevations in intrathoracic pressure may be created by cough, and is of particular concern in patients with emphysematous bulla.

## Sample processing

Recovered fluid should be collected into traps made of material to which the cells are poorly adherent, such as polyethylene or polycarbonate; unsiliconized glass materials should not be used [5,7]. Macrophages, in particular, have shown to be adherent to glass. Specimens should be transported to a laboratory for evaluation within 1 hour. Cell counts have shown to preserve at 25°C for 4 hours [41,42] and 4°C for 24 hours [41]. Proteins are temperature sensitive and preservation is typically at −80°C [6].

Filtering of lavage fluid through sterile gauze or nylon mesh has traditionally been performed to remove excess mucus. This practice has subsequently been shown to affect cell count and sterility. It has also been noted to lead to a loss of potentially useful information such as ferruginous

bodies in patients with asbestos exposure as well as cells with increased adherence, such as activated neutrophils [7]. Current recommendations are to avoid filtering [43].

Differential cell counts are determined on slides prepared by cytocentrifugation or filtration. Cytocentrifugation is more commonly used and provides multiple advantages over filtering, including preserved lymphocyte concentration, limited cellular damage, and expense [44,45]. Prepared slides are then stained for interpretation. Wright–Giemsa stains are most commonly used for inflammatory cells. Papanicolaou staining is commonly used to analyze cells of infection or cancer. Cellular counting is performed using light microscopy to analyze stained slides. It has been proposed that a total of 300–500 nucleated cells should be counted to provide an adequate representation of the BAL [46]. Significant variability may be present in interpretation, and should be performed by designated laboratory personnel.

Lymphocyte subpopulations such as CD4 and CD8 are most commonly determined by flow cytometry [47]. An alternative method involves immunohistochemistry staining on slides prepared by cytocentrifugation [48]. Utility of immunofluorescent staining has also been shown in evaluation for infection and malignancy.

## Cellular analysis—normal values

Analysis of inflammatory cellular populations of bronchoalveolar lavage fluid was met with great enthusiasm for utility in disease diagnosis, prediction of clinical course, and measurement of response to therapy. Although not conclusive as a solitary tool, it has shown utility in the differentiation of interstitial disease processes as well as infectious evaluation.

BAL in healthy non-smokers produces 100,000 to 150,000 cells per mL of lavage fluid obtained [15]. BAL in a normal non-smoking adult will yield 80 to 95% macrophages, 5 to 15% lymphocytes, CD4/CD8 ratio of 1.5 to 1.8, less than 3% neutrophils, and less than 1% eosinophils, basophils, and mast cells [1,20,49,50].

The results of BAL cellular analysis should be expressed both as number/mL and as a percentage of the total cell population (plus an estimate of total cell numbers should be given). These numbers provide complementary information [1,21]. A normal cell differential does not always indicate that the lung is free of inflammation. Specifically, an abnormal percentage of one cell line may affect the relative percentages of others. It has been shown that a markedly increased number of cells with a normal differential may be associated with an inflammatory process in the lung [20]. Combining the differential count with the total cell count allows quantification of each cell type per set volume. The lack of standardized lavage volumes is a limiting factor in this practice.

Smoking, quantity of lavage return, lavage processing, and age are variables shown to affect the cellular profile.

Active smokers have been shown to have a four to tenfold increase in total cell count with proportional increase in macrophages and neutrophils as well as altered CD4/CD8 ratios. Former smokers should have cellular profiles similar to never smokers [21,51]. Advanced age has also been shown to increase percentages of lymphocytes and neutrophils [52].

The high normal percentage of lymphocytes in lavage fluid is considered to be in the 10 to 15% range, with most normal individuals falling under 10%. However, healthy non-smoking individuals have been shown to have transient levels greater than 20% [37]. The lymphocytes subtypes found within the alveolar structures of healthy individuals are similar to those of blood. The majority of alveolar lymphocytes are CD3$^+$ T cells, with B cells representing a minority at 4 to 7% [21]. T-helper (CD4$^+$) cells represent 39 to 48% of lymphocytes and T-suppressor (CD8$^+$) cells between 23 and 28%, so that the normal ratio of T-helper cells to T-suppressor cells (CD4/CD8) is 1.6 to 1.8.

The National Institute of Health (NIH) cooperative study showed lymphocyte phenotype variability consequent to age, gender, and smoking status [21]. These variables should be taken into consideration in data interpretation.

**1** The percentage of T-helper cells in individuals greater than 50 years old was, on the average, more than 10% higher than that in individuals under 37 years old.

**2** Total T cells, T-suppressor cells, and B cell percentages were significantly higher in men than in women and the CD4/CD8 ratio was significantly lower in men.

**3** T-helper cells were significantly lower (32.2%) in current smokers than in exsmokers (46%) and in never smokers (44.4%), and T-suppressor cells were higher in current smokers (29.2%) than in exsmokers (20.7%) and never smokers (20.7%). Thus, the CD4/CD8 ratio was significantly lower in current smokers than in either former smokers or never smokers.

Neutrophils typically represent less than 1% of the cell total. Causes of elevated neutrophils counts include blood contamination, active smoking, and inflammatory disease of the bronchi [1,4]. Elevated neutrophils levels have also shown to be present in advanced cases (containing fibrosis) of interstitial diseases. The presence of squamous epithelial cells suggests contamination from the upper airway.

### Acellular analysis—normal values

A multitude of proteins, enzymes, cytokines, chemokines, lipids, and electrolytes are present in bronchoalveolar fluid. The investigation of these non-cellular components has been overshadowed by efforts on cellular counterparts. Contributing factors include our evolving understanding or their function and limitations for quantification and analysis.

Quantifying non-cellular alveolar constituents is limited by a lack of a definitive dilution marker (see previous discussion). The dynamic interaction of the alveolar and vascular space especially impacts non-cellular components such as cytokines. Subsequently, samples obtained from BAL may reflect activity from the blood stream as well as the alveolar space. This creates great difficulty in assessing true concentrations of alveolar materials. Some have proposed simultaneous BAL fluid and serum measurements for interpretation [53].

## Clinical utility

In most situations, BAL, by itself, does not provide information to make specific diagnoses with absolute certainty. However, BAL has important diagnostic value when considered in conjunction with other information. If patients cannot safely undergo open lung biopsy, BAL can provide supportive evidence for a diagnosis, and if a patient has respiratory symptoms but near normal pulmonary functions and a normal chest X ray, an abnormal BAL result facilitates the decision to proceed with open lung biopsy [54].

### Sarcoidosis

BAL has served a pivotal role in the understanding of sarcoidosis. The discovery of intense alveolitis with elevated BAL lymphocyte populations refuted the prior doctrine that sarcoidosis was associated with a suppressed immune response [55,56]. Much debate has occurred in the literature regarding the utility of BAL in sarcoidosis patients as a diagnostic and prognostic tool. Current consensus is that BAL alone cannot be used to make a definitive diagnosis of sarcoidosis. However, analysis of BAL cellular profile can be of value in distinguishing sarcoidosis from other granulomatous and interstitial disease processes [57,58]. Current consensus also suggests a limited utility in use of BAL for prediction of disease course, duration, or response to therapy.

BAL cell differentials in sarcoidosis reflect current levels of alveolitis and can show great variability. Alveolitis may be present in patients without radiographic evidence of thoracic involvement. Takahashi and colleagues documented BAL lymphocytosis in patients with suspected ocular sarcoidosis and no evidence of pulmonary involvement [59]. Typically seen is a normal to slightly elevated total cell count, elevated lymphocytes, elevated CD4/CD8 ratio, and normal percentages of eosinophils and neutrophils. Notably absent are "foamy macrophages" and plasma cells [60,61].

BAL lymphocytosis in sarcoidosis is variable and may be normal in 10–15% of patients or reach values as high 80% of total cellular count [62,63]. Decreased lymphocyte counts are typically seen in active smokers. Significant variability of the CD4/CD8 ratio has also been shown in patients with sarcoidosis. Elevation of the CD4/CD8 ratio is found in approximately 60% of patients [64]. Various groups have published data showing a ratio greater than 3.5 to have sensitivity of 52–59% and specificity of 94–96% [48,61,65].

This has prompted in-depth discussion regarding the combination of elevated lymphocyte count (good sensitivity) and elevated CD4/CD8 ratio (good specificity) as a joint diagnostic tool. Costabel and colleagues proposed that in patients with a clinical presentation typical for sarcoidosis, an elevated CD4/CD8 ratio may confirm diagnosis without need for biopsy [66]. Lymphocytosis was initially anticipated to be predictive of disease activity and clinical response to steroids. This has been an active area of publication, and initial studies suggested a possible link. However, later studies did not find a correlation [48,62,67].

BAL neutrophil counts may be elevated in sarcoidosis patients with more advanced disease [68]. Ziegenhagen and colleagues demonstrated that values greater than 3% were associated with faster clinical decline and steroid resistance [69]. Another study showed that patients with advanced disease by PFT, radiographic findings, and functional impairment showed higher numbers of BAL neutrophils than those who responded spontaneously [68].

Evidence of increased macrophage activity has been demonstrated in the BAL of patients with sarcoidosis [70]. Cytokine release by alveolar macrophages has been shown to regulate granuloma formation and play a pivotal role in sarcoidosis. BAL measurement of cytokines has yet to show diagnostic or prognostic utility.

## Idiopathic interstitial pneumonias

Set diagnostic criteria and markers for disease prognosis have proven elusive with the idiopathic interstitial pneumonias. Publication of the American Thoracic Society/ European Respiratory Society Consensus Classification in 2002 provided a platform to apply previously existing data [71]. Seven types of idiopathic interstitial pneumonias (IIPs) were identified: idiopathic pulmonary fibrosis (IPF), non-specific interstitial pneumonia (NSIP) with cellular and non-cellular variants, cryptogenic organizing pneumonia (COP), acute interstitial pneumonia (AIP), desquamative interstitial pneumonia (DIP), respiratory bronchiolitis interstitial lung disease (RB-ILD), and lymphocytic interstitial pneumonia (LIP).

Cellular analysis of BAL fluid in IPF patients has shown low lymphocyte levels (5%) and elevated neutrophil levels (7%) [72,73]. The correlation between tissue and BAL lymphocyte subpopulations in IPF patients has been confirmed as well [74]. The diminished BAL lymphocyte counts may assist in distinguishing IPF from the other idiopathic interstitial pneumonias. Ryu and colleague showed particular use of BAL cell count in distinguishing IPF from NSIP [73]. Patients with pulmonary fibrosis (usual interstitial pneumonia (UIP) histologic pattern) secondary to collagen vascular disease have been shown to display elevated BAL cellularity [72,73,75]. This serves as a valuable tool in distinguishing idiopathic pulmonary fibrosis of non-idiopathic causes.

BAL analysis in NSIP of the cellular (non-fibrotic) variant typically shows elevated lymphocytes to 40%, slight increase of neutrophils, and a CD4/CD8 ratio less than 0.3 [76]. Normalization of the BAL lymphocytosis is typically seen in patients from this group who benefit from steroid therapy. NSIP of the non-cellular (fibrotic) variant shows a non-specific pattern with lymphocyte elevation to 33%, and neutrophils elevated to 14% [76]. These individuals are typically not responsive to steroids. BAL cell counts in either NSIP subtype of idiopathic origin are similar to those seen in patients with NSIP histologic pattern due to infection, CVD, drug reaction, or other non-idiopathic etiologies.

COP BAL cell counts typically show marked lymphocytosis (greater than 40%) with low CD4/CD8 ratio [76]. As with cellular NSIP, lymphoctyosis has shown the ability to normalize in steroid responsive individuals [77]. BAL cell counts in COP are not different from those seen in patients with organizing pneumonia histologic pattern of non-idiopathic etiology [76].

AIP cell count is typified by increased neutrophils with a mild lymphocyte elevation. Reactive pneumocytes and hyaline membrane fragments may be found, as seen with IPF exacerbation [71]. BAL cellular populations are similar in patients with exacerbation of underlying IPF.

Definitive diagnosis of idiopathic interstitial pneumonia requires elimination of other etiologies of interstitial disease. Analysis of BAL fluid has proven utility in the identification of materials and cultures specific to non-idiopathic causes of interstitial pneumonia such as asbestos bodies. In cases of established UIP histology without clear etiology, BAL cellular analysis may differentiate between idiopathic and non-idiopathic causes. Analysis of the BAL cellular profile can also be of use in differentiating between the seven idiopathic histologies. Particularly, it is of value in differentiating IPF from the other IIPs. BAL likely does not obviate need for definitive biopsy, but may provide assistance when biopsy is not feasible or histology is unclear. In summary, it is a useful adjunct tool for diagnostic challenges.

Utility of BAL as a prognostic tool in IIP is still actively debated. Despite initial hope, studies by authors such as Veeraraghavan showed limited efficacy [78]. A retrospective study by Ryu and colleagues suggested utility. In this study 122 patients with either UIP or NSIP underwent BAL and high resolution computed tomography (HRCT) prior to biopsy. Follow-up at 2 years suggested BAL lymphoctyosis to reflect non-UIP histologic pattern and better prognosis [73].

## Hypersensitivity pneumonitis

Hypersensitivity pneumonitis (HP) also known as extrinsic allergic alveolitis, is an inflammatory granulomatous response of the lungs to antigens from a wide range of inhaled organic dusts [79,80]. The characteristic feature of BAL cellular analysis in HP is an alveolitis shown by a two- to fivefold increased total cell count, significant lymphocytosis, and below normal CD4/CD8 ratio.

The percentage of lymphocytes may be strikingly increased (often above 50%) compared to normal controls [80,81]. Some of the lymphocytes have an atypical appearance suggestive of blast cells, having markedly indented multi-clefted nuclei and increased cytoplasmic area [79]. The CD4/CD8 ratio in this population has shown to be variable but typically is less than one. By the time of clinical presentation, patients with HP show increased BAL lymphocytes. These levels may remain elevated for months to years after removal of the antigen. Lymphocyte counts are commonly decreased with smoking. HP is more common in non-smokers, suggestive of an immunosuppressive effect from tobacco [80].

Macrophages account for a lower percentage of the total cells obtained by BAL in HP (often less than 40%), but the actual numbers are comparable to controls [81]. The macrophages may display a foamy cytoplasm.

Elevated neutrophil and eosinophil concentrations may also be present in the BAL in HP, especially if there has been a recent exposure to antigen. Fournier and colleagues [82] found a marked increase in neutrophils in BAL of patients with HP who underwent antigen inhalation in an experimental setting. Twenty-four hours after exposure, 41.2% of the BAL cells were neutrophils compared to 8.3% prior to antigen challenge. The increased numbers of neutrophils returned to baseline 5 to 8 days later. In this study, the presence of neutrophils in BAL was associated with clinical symptoms. There are also data showing neutrophil levels increased in HP patients who have progressed to fibrosis [83].

BAL samples from exposed patients with HP may also contain mast cells in increased numbers (as much as 10-fold higher) [79,84]. In most patients, the increase in mast cells occurs when individuals are currently or have been recently exposed, and fall soon after removal from exposure [79]. Mast cells and neutrophils may remain elevated with continued exposure and symptoms [79].

BAL cellular analysis is not diagnostic of HP as a solitary tool. A limitation of note is the presence of lymphocytosis in asymptomatic "sensitized" individuals without definitive HP. However, BAL fluid lacking the hypercellularity seen in alveolitis may rule out HP (or sensitization) as a cause of unknown interstitial disease. Increased lymphocytes and mast cells are thus neither a sign of lung disease nor a predictor of eventual development of HP [85]. Inhalation provocation tests have utilized BAL neutrophil counts as one of several measurable variables for diagnosis. However, these are cumbersome studies limited to designated facilities [86]. Much debate has occurred regarding utility of the BAL cell count as a prognostic tool in individu-

als with established HP. It has been demonstrated that BAL lymphocytes do not predict outcome or prognosis in these patients [87].

## Pneumoconioses

BAL cellular analysis in patients with pneumoconioses typically reflects alveolitis with a two- to threefold elevation in total cell count, lymphocytosis, and an elevated CD4/CD8 ratio. Neutrophil levels are variable but commonly elevated. Cellular analysis alone is an insufficient diagnostic tool. However, BAL retains utility in the documentation of specific exposures such as asbestos fibers, silica particles, and beryllium sensitized lymphocytes.

Asbestos is a commercial term for a group of naturally occurring fibers composed of hydrated magnesium silicates. Asbestos fibers are classified based on shape as serpentine or amphibole. Amphibole fibers are typically long and straight in shape. Amphibole fibers are considered more toxic and previously were associated with industrial use. Serpentine fibers are typically shorter and curved in shape. Serpentine fibers are associated with urban pollution and are generally considered less toxic. Asbestos exposure predisposes to fibrosis, lung cancers, and pleural diseases such as mesothelioma, fibrosis, effusion, and plaque formation [88].

Asbestos bodies (ABs) are inhaled asbestos fibril particles that are coated with iron-containing mucoprotein and embedded in lung tissue. AB formation is an intracellular process that occurs as one or more alveolar macrophages engulfs an asbestos fiber. The fiber then becomes incorporated into an intracytoplasmic vacuole and is coated with an acid mucopolysaccharide [89]. Iron accumulates in the coating initially as hemosiderin. Only a small portion of asbestos fibers in the lung become coated as ferruginous bodies [89,90]. Asbestos bodies rarely develop from serpentine fibers, and are formed primarily from amphibole fibers. The presence of ABs thus reflects primarily the burden of long amphibole fibers, which are most frequently associated with asbestosis and mesothelioma [91,92]. In the population without occupational asbestos exposure, but exposed to urban pollution, the bulk of the asbestos fibers are serpentine [93,94]. These small fibers do not form ABs, which explains why finding ABs in BAL usually correlates well with occupational exposure, implying inhalation of long industrial fibers. ABs represent only a fraction of the total asbestos burden in the lung and thus in BAL [89,91].

Measurement of ABs in lung parenchyma via biopsy remains the gold standard for detection of asbestos exposure. Parenchymal concentrations of greater than 1000 AB/g dried lung tissue is generally associated with past significant exposure to asbestos [93,94]. It has been demonstrated that a measured BAL concentration of one AB/mL is predictive of a parenchymal concentration between 1050 and 3010 AB/g [91]. Thus, BAL concentrations greater than one

AB/mL indicate significant asbestos exposure[93] and are associated with increased prevalence of radiographic abnormalities, respiratory symptoms, and reduced values on pulmonary function testing [95].

The finding of ABs on BAL fluid is an excellent objective measure of asbestos exposure but, in itself, is not a good marker for proof of disease [90,92,94]. The absence of ABs in a correctly performed BAL does not exclude asbestos-related pleural disease or significant AB parenchymal concentrations [94]. The concentration of ABs in BAL may positively correlate with length and intensity of exposure and may negatively correlate with time since last exposure. Use of ABs in induced sputum for screening purposes has shown to be less sensitive than BAL, and limited to use in settings of severe asbestos exposure [96,97].

Beryllium has found widespread application in modern industries such as ceramics, nuclear, electronics, and automotive. Inhaled beryllium metal dusts, beryllium oxide, or beryllium salts can cause either acute or chronic lung disease. The acute form appears to have a toxic and dose-related effect on the lungs, and has largely been eliminated by controls on environmental exposure. The chronic form develops over 1 to 20 years in 1 to 3% of exposed persons and is a granulomatous interstitial disease remarkably similar, histopathologically, radiographically, and clinically, to sarcoidosis. [20,98]. The diagnosis of chronic berylliosis is usually based on a history of beryllium exposure, typical clinical and histologic abnormalities, and elevated lung beryllium levels [20,98].

Bronchoalveolar lavage has shown value in the evaluation of a patient with suspected berylliosis. BAL cell counts from patients with berylliosis are similar to those from patients with sarcoidosis. The total numbers of macrophages and T cells are increased. The percentage of lymphocytes is increased, and most of these cells are helper T cells [20,98]. BAL in berylliosis has its greatest use in showing a local immunologic response to beryllium. Lymphocytes from the BAL of berylliosis patients proliferate when stimulated *in vitro* with soluble beryllium salts, with a sensitivity and specificity approaching 100% [20,98,99]. Beryllium lymphocyte proliferation tests are commonly performed on blood or BAL samples as an industry surveillance tool. Specimen mononuclear cells are incubated *in vitro* with beryllium salts at varying concentrations and intervals. Measurement of cell proliferation is laboratory dependant and universal standards are not defined. Patients with prior history of beryllium exposure and proof of lymphocyte proliferation, but lacking definitive granulomatous histology, may be considered as sensitized individuals. Sensitized patients have shown rates of progression to chronic beryllium disease as high as 6–8% per year [100].

### Eosinophilic lung disease

Normal BAL specimens from non-smokers typically show eosinophil concentrations less than 1% of the total cell count. The eosinophil concentration may be slightly elevated in current or former smokers [1,20]. Eosinophil counts greater than 5% should be considered significant [101]. A wide variety of disease processes, including infection, drug reaction, allergic response, and idiopathic mechanisms, can result in elevated eosinophil concentrations on blood and BAL cellular count. Moderate BAL eosinophil concentration elevations (5–20%) are typical in infection, allergic response, and drug reactions [101–105].

Eosinophilic pneumonia is classically defined as eosinophil predominance on histopathology from lung biopsy. It is accepted that in the appropriate clinical and radiographic context, BAL eosinophil elevation may obviate the need for lung biopsy. Costabel and colleagues proposed that normal cellular concentrations from a technically adequate BAL performed in an area of radiographic finding likely exclude an eosinophilic infiltrate [106]. BAL cellular counts in eosinophilic pneumonias may show eosinophil concentrations as high as 90% [106]. Although there are no universal diagnostic criteria for eosinophil concentrations, Lazor and colleagues have proposed minimum eosinophil concentrations of 25% as diagnostic criteria [107].

Idiopathic Acute Eosinophilic Pneumonia shows mean BAL cellular eosinophil concentrations from 37–54%, with slight elevation of Lymphocyte and neutrophil concentrations [108,109]. Pope–Harmon and colleagues have proposed a minimum eosinophil concentration of 25% as diagnostic criteria. BAL cellular counts in Idiopathic Chronic Eosinophilic Pneumonia have shown mean eosinophil concentrations of 58%, with mild elevation of lymphocyte and neutrophil populations [110,111]. Marchand and colleagues have proposed a minimum eosinophil concentration of 40% as a diagnostic criteria.

### Systemic sclerosis

BAL cellular counts in patients with systemic sclerosis typically reveal normal total cell counts with variable elevation of lymphocyte, neutrophil, and eosinophil populations. Elevated eosinophil levels are typically greater in patients with NSIP radiographic and histologic pattern than those with UIP histologic pattern. Lymphocyte populations are typically greater in cellular NSIP than in fibrotic NSIP (see prior discussion) [112]. This non-specific alveolitis limits the utility of BAL cellular count as a diagnostic tool in this population.

Much debate has occurred in the literature regarding the use of BAL alveolitis to predict disease course and monitor response to therapy. Initial studies suggested a possible correlation between alveolitis and worsening measurements on PFT, as well as response to treatment [113]. Subsequent studies demonstrated a correlation between neutrophil predominant alveolitis and severity of fibrotic disease on high resolution computed tomography scan (HRCT), as well as worsening measurements on PFT [114,115]. This suggested neutrophil predominant alveolitis to be indicative of patients with more advanced disease rather than a population of patients with early disease and poor prognosis. Goh and colleagues assessed 141 systemic sclerosis patients with BAL, HRCT, PFT, echocardiography at baseline and followed for 10 years. Their study demonstrated that a potential correlation between neutrophil predominant alveolitis and overall long term mortality was lost when baseline disease severity was taken into account. No correlation between lymphocyte predominant alveolitis and mortality was found [114]. This would suggest that clinical course is better predicted by disease severity at presentation, and that BAL cell count is of limited value in disease monitoring.

## Pulmonary Langerhans cell histiocytosis

Pulmonary Langerhans Cell Histiocytosis (PLCH) is a chronic granulomatous disorder that typically affects young adults with smoking history. Previous nomenclature has included Histiocytosis X and eosinophilic granuloma of the lung. Pathologically, there is an interstitial accumulation of antigen presenting cells known as Langerhans cells [20]. Langerhans cells are distinguished on electron microscopic examination by an indented nucleus and small (40 to 45 nm diameter) pentalaminar elongated bodies called Birbeck granules which are scattered throughout the cytoplasm [1,20,116]. They are further characterized by the presence of CD1 antigen on their cell surface and S100 protein in their cytoplasm on immunostaining. Low concentrations (less than 1%) of Langerhans cells may be detected in BAL of normal patients via immunostaining [117]. In PLCH, proliferation of Langerhans cells results in the formation of upper lobe reticulonodular infiltrates which progress to cystic changes and honeycombing.

BAL may be useful in the diagnosis of PLCH. Cellular counts typically show an increased total cell count, increased percentage of alveolar macrophages with smoker's inclusion bodies, slight elevation of neutrophil and eosinophil concentrations, and variable lymphocyte populations [4]. The distinguishing feature is the presence of CD1+ Langerhans cells. Langerhans cell concentrations less than 5% are commonly found in BAL of patients with other interstitial lung diseases, lung cancer, and healthy smokers [118]. Costabel and colleagues suggest that concentrations greater than 4% are diagnostic with good specificity, but poor sensitivity [106]. At this time, there is no established quantitative value of Langerhans cells to confirm diagnosis. Identification of Birbeck granules by electron microscopy is less practical secondary to time and expense [4].

## Diffuse alveolar hemorrhage

Diffuse alveolar hemorrhage (DAH) is a syndrome of alveolar vascular injury leading to the accumulation of red blood cells in the distal airways. The definition has traditionally included the triad of anemia, hypoxemia, and hemoptysis.

It should be noted that up to 33% of patients will not display hemoptysis despite significant alveolar accumulation [119]. DAH may be caused by a wide variety of disease mechanisms with vasculitis being the most common. Clinical and radiographic presentation is often confusing and may mimic infectious and other interstitial processes. A grossly bloody appearance to BAL is not always diagnostic because it may be secondary to bronchoscopy-induced trauma, infection, or other processes [4].

BAL performed in an area of radiographic finding can assist in diagnosis of DAH. Using appropriate BAL technique, sequential aliquots are instilled and retrieved. Retrieval of aliquots which are sequentially more hemorrhagic (increased red blood cell count) is consistent with diagnosis of DAH [120,121].

The presence of hemosiderin-laden macrophages via iron staining of cellular analysis has also shown great yield as a diagnostic tool. It has been proposed that a hemosiderin-laden macrophage population greater than 20% is diagnostic of DAH [122]. It is important to note that presence of macrophage hemosiderin uptake is relative to time of bleeding and is rarely detectable within 48 hours of bleeding onset [123,124]. Use of hemosiderin-laden macrophage population as a diagnostic tool has proven less cumbersome than the previously utilized Golde scoring system [122]. It should also be noted that hemosiderin-laden macrophages have been found in a variety of other lung diseases including IPF, cardiac disease, sarcoidosis, carcinoma, vasculitis, pulmonary alveolar proteinosis, and pulmonary Langerhans cell histiocytosis [4,20,125]. DAH has been shown to be safely and accurately diagnosed by BAL in immunocompromised, thrombocytopenic, and anticoagulated patients [125–128].

## Pulmonary alveolar proteinosis

Pulmonary alveolar proteinosis (PAP) involves the widespread filling of alveoli with a lipoprotein material that stains with a periodic acid-Schiff (PAS) reagent. The lipoprotein material is composed principally of surfactant phospholipid and protein debris. The presence of antigranulocyte–macrophage colony stimulating factor (GM-CSF) antibodies results in impaired macrophage clearance and subsequent alveolar accumulation of this material [129–131]. Congenital, acquired secondary, and acquired primary (idiopathic) variants of the disease are documented. This text will focus on the acquired primary variant.

Use of BAL as a research tool has proven instrumental in our understanding of this disease process [129–131]. Several characteristic findings of alveolar lavage fluid make BAL a significant tool in diagnosis of PAP. The gross appearance of the fluid is unique and frequently described as opaque, turbid, or milky. Typical findings on light microscopy include: "foamy" alveolar macrophages engorged with PAS-positive material; predominant PAS staining of proteinaceous materials and debris; acellular globules which are pink on PAS staining, and basophilic on May–Grunwald–Giemsa staining [7,132]. In addition, the lipoprotein material has been demonstrated to stain with specific antibodies to surfactant apoproteins confirming surfactant origin [20,133]. When performed, electron microscopic examination of the lipid material shows characteristic whorled lamellar bodies [20].

Characteristic BAL findings commonly obviate the need for biopsy in the appropriate radiographic and clinical setting [134–137]. Despite recent data supporting use of GM-CSF administration for treatment of PAP, whole lung lavage remains the most effective treatment. This procedure has shown to be safe when performed with use of double lumen endotracheal tube under general anesthesia [134].

## Drug-induced lung disease

Drug-induced pulmonary toxicity may be expressed in a wide range of clinical, histologic, and radiographic presentations. Hypersensitivity as well as cytotoxic findings may be noted at the level of the alveoli. BAL cellular changes may include alveolitis of eosinophil, neutrophil, or more commonly lymphocyte predominance. CD4/CD8 ratios are typically low, but elevated CD4 populations have been noted with methotrexate, nitrofurantoin, and ampicillin exposure. [138–141]. Drug reactions with specific underlying histologic pattern such as NSIP and COP have shown BAL cellular findings typical of that histology (see prior discussion) [139,142,143]. Certain drugs are linked to diffuse alveolar hemorrhage and patients display typical BAL findings such as hemosiderin-laden macrophages [139]. Although BAL cellular counts are not typically unique to drug-induced disease, BAL may be of use in the exclusion of other predisposed processes such as infection.

BAL has shown utility as an adjunctive test in the evaluation of suspected amiodarone lung toxicity [144]. Phospholipid accumulation in alveolar macrophages results in cytoplasmic lamellar body formations. These formations give the macrophages a "foamy" appearance [144]. This is relatively characteristic for drug effect secondary to amiodarone, and "foamy" inclusions are found in up to 50% of patients taking therapeutic levels. Their presence is thus, not exclusively diagnostic of toxicity. However, their absence makes the diagnosis of amiodarone pulmonary toxicity unlikely [144,145].

## Use of bronchoalveolar lavage in malignancy

Flexible bronchoscopy has shown significant utility in the diagnosis of malignancy involving the lung. Endoscopically visible lesions have reported diagnostic yield as high as 90% via endobronchial biopsy [146]. Non-endoscopically visible peripheral lesions have shown much lower diagnostic yield with transbronchial biopsy, brushing, and needle aspiration [146,147]. BAL has shown utility as an adjunctive tool in the diagnosis of these peripheral lesions.

BAL cellular counts typically reveal a non-specific alveolitis in patients with neoplastic processes [148]. Lymphocyte predominant alveolitis may be expected in patients with lung involvement of lymphoproliferative disorders [149]. Routine staining methods typically include May–Grunwald–Giemsa, Papanicolau, and Diff–Quik. Immunocytochemistry and histochemistry markers have been an active area of research involving pulmonary malignancy. The list of available markers is extensive and utility is variable with tumor type [150].

BAL has shown significant utility in the diagnosis of specific primary epithelial lung tumors. The greatest diagnostic yield has been found in diffuse processes which spread via lymphatic or lepidic growth. This includes tumors such as bronchioalveolar cell carcinoma (BAC) and adenocarcinoma. Wislez and colleagues showed diagnostic yield of adenocarcinoma as high as 66% in patients with consolidation on CT [151]. BAL smears alone may yield diagnostic neoplastic cells [152].

Utility of BAL in diagnosis of primary lung non-Hodgkin's lymphomas such as MALT (mucosa-associated lymphoid tissue), has been demonstrated [150,152]. Utility has also been shown in non-Hodgkin's lymphoma with secondary lung localization [150,152]. Yield of BAL in the diagnosis of non-Hodgkin's lymphoma has been reported as high as 67% [152]. Less commonly, Hodgkin's disease can be diagnosed by the identification of Reed–Sternberg cells in BAL cytology specimens [153,154].

Metastatic disease may also occasionally be detected by BAL cytology. Reported cases of diagnosis include metastatic breast cancer and melanoma [152,155,156].

In summary, BAL may serve as a useful adjunct tool to biopsy or as an isolated tool for neoplastic diagnosis when biopsy is not feasible. However, limitations of BAL for diagnostic purposes in malignancy should be recognized before interpretation of findings. Severe dysplastic changes may develop in airway epithelial cells in multiple clinical circumstances, and can be difficult to distinguish from malignant changes. Examples include but are not limited to: pneumonia, viral infections, adult respiratory distress syndrome (ARDS), IPF exacerbations, amiodarone lung injury, and following chemotherapy [157–159].

## Bronchoalveolar lavage in the diagnosis of infectious diseases

A primary concern in obtaining lower respiratory tract secretions for microbiologic analysis by BAL is contamination of the bronchoscope as it passes through the oropharynx and upper airway. Administration of lidocaine by inhalation and performance of BAL through a previously inserted endotracheal tube have been shown to reduce the incidence of contamination [8].

There has been extensive debate in the literature regarding indications for BAL in patients with suspected pneumonia. Ventilator-associated pneumonia (VAP), in particular, has undergone significant study. Mortality has been shown to correlate with early recognition and the initiation of appropriate therapy in this patient population [160,161]. This has supported the use of multiple diagnostic measures such as BAL to increase diagnostic yield [162].

BAL specimens have been extensively compared to samples obtained by blind endotracheal suction in ventilated patients. The results from these studies have been conflicting. Early studies supported a potential decrease in mortality with the use of BAL [163]. In subsequent studies, BAL was not shown to result in a convincing decrease in mortality, hospitalization length, or duration of intubation [164–166]. Preliminary studies also suggested that use of BAL may direct and subsequently decrease the quantity and duration of antimicrobial use [167]. This suggested that BAL could be a potential mechanism to decrease formation of multiresistant organisms. The Canadian Critical Care Trials Group later published a larger study which failed to show a decrease in antimicrobial use with BAL compared to blind endotracheal aspiration [168]. The comparative benefit of BAL remains an ongoing area of debate.

Use of BAL for the early diagnosis of suspected pulmonary infection in immunocompromised patients has been evaluated extensively [169,170]. Utility and safety of BAL in this patient population has been confirmed and is the preferred diagnostic modality [170–174]. Immunocompromised patients with clinical or radiographic evidence of pulmonary infection present a significant diagnostic challenge. Patient complexity typically results in a confusing clinical picture with multiple diagnostic possibilities. Despite these limitations, diagnostic yield has been shown to be as high at 77% for infectious causes [175,176].

Radiographic infiltrates in immunocompromised individuals may be secondary to infection from a wide range of viral, bacterial, or fungal sources. In addition, non-infectious causes such as diffuse pulmonary alveolar hemorrhage, radiation pneumonitis, and pulmonary drug toxicity must be considered [177]. BAL cellular findings are often limited by pancytopenia and subsequent friable airways with frequent bleeding. Additionally, culture results from BAL specimens are often limited by prior antimicrobial administration. Stolz and colleagues recently demonstrated neutrophil alveolitis on BAL in neutropenic, immunocompromised patients. Further, they showed neutrophil populations greater than 15% to indicate bacterial infection rather than non-bacterial sources [178]. Utility of BAL in this population continues to be an area of active clinical investigation.

## Summary

Since its introduction into clinical pulmonary medicine over 30 years ago, BAL continues to be a highly useful diagnostic technique throughout the spectrum of pulmonary disease.

## References

1 Hunninghake GW, Gadek JE, Kawanami O, *et al*. Inflammatory and immune processes in the human lung in health and disease: evaluation by bronchoalveolar lavage. *Am J Pathol* 1979; **97**: 149–206.

2 Reynolds HY, Newball HH. Analysis of proteins and respiratory cells obtained from human lungs by bronchial lavage. *J Lab Clin Med* 1974; **84**: 559–73.

3 Goldstein RA, Rohatgi PK, Bergofsky EH, *et al*. Clinical role of bronchoalveolar lavage in adults with pulmonary disease. *Am Rev Respir Dis* 1990; **142**: 481–6.

4 Helmers RA, Hunninghake GW. Bronchioalveolar lavage. In: Wang KP, ed. *Biopsy Techniques in Pulmonary Disorders*. New York: Raven Press; 1989: 15–28.

5 Technical recommendations and guidelines for bronchoalveolar lavage (BAL). Report of the European Society of Pneumology Task Group. *Eur Respir J* 1989; **2**: 561–85.

6 Haslam PL, Baughman RP. Report of ERS Task Force: guidelines for measurement of acellular components and standardization of BAL. *Eur Respir J* 1999; **14**: 245–8.

7 Haslam PL. Bronchoalveolar lavage. *Semin Respir Crit Care Med* 1984; **6**: 55–70.

8 Pang JA, Cheng AF, Chan HS, French GL. Special precautions reduce oropharyngeal contamination in bronchoalveolar lavage for bacteriologic studies. *Lung* 1989; **167**: 261–7.

9 Pingleton SK, Harrison GF, Stechschulte DJ, *et al*. Effect of location, pH, and temperature of instillate in bronchoalveolar lavage in normal volunteers. *Am Rev Respir Dis* 1983; **128**: 1035–7.

10 Helmers RA, Hunninghake GW. Bronchoalveolar lavage in the nonimmunocompromised patient. *Chest* 1989; **96**: 1184–90.

11 Davis GS, Giancola MS, Costanza MC, Low RB. Analyses of sequential bronchoalveolar lavage samples from healthy human volunteers. *Am Rev Respir Dis* 1982; **126**: 611–16.

12 Carre P, Laviolette M, Belanger J, Cormier Y. Technical variations of bronchoalveolar lavage (BAL): influence of atelectasis and the lung region lavaged. *Lung* 1985; **163**: 117–25.

13 Kelly CA, Kotre CJ, Ward C, *et al*. Anatomical distribution of bronchoalveolar lavage fluid as assessed by digital subtraction radiography. *Thorax* 1987; **42**: 624–8.

14 Baughman RP. Technical aspects of bronchoalveolar lavage: recommendations for a standard procedure. *Semin Respir Crit Care Med* 2007; **28**: 475–85.

15 King TE. The handling and analysis of bronchoalveolar lavage specimens. In: Baughman RP, ed. *Bronchoalveolar Lavage*. St. Louis: Mosby Year Book; 1992: 3–29.

16 Crystal RG, Reynolds HY, Kalica AR. Bronchoalveolar lavage. The report of an international conference. *Chest* 1986; **90**: 122–31.

17 Dohn MN, Baughman RP. Effect of changing instilled volume for bronchoalveolar lavage in patients with interstitial lung disease. *Am Rev Respir Dis* 1985; **132**: 390–2.

18 Lam S, Leriche JC, Kijek K, Phillips D. Effect of bronchial lavage volume on cellular and protein recovery. *Chest* 1985; **88**: 856–9.

19 Rennard SI, Ghafouri M, Thompson AB, *et al.* Fractional processing of sequential bronchoalveolar lavage to separate bronchial and alveolar samples. *Am Rev Respir Dis* 1990; **141**: 208–17.

20 Daniele RP, Elias JA, Epstein PE, Rossman MD. Bronchoalveolar lavage: role in the pathogenesis, diagnosis, and management of interstitial lung disease. *Ann Intern Med* 1985; **102**: 93–108.

21 BAL Cooperative Group Steering Committee. Bronchoalveolar lavage constituents in healthy individuals, idiopathic pulmonary fibrosis, and selected comparison groups. *Am Rev Respir Dis* 1990; **141**: S169–202.

22 Baughman RP, Lower EE. New treatment for sarcoidosis: where's the proof? *Eur Respir J* 1999; **14**: 1000–1.

23 Tilles DS, Goldenheim PD, Ginns LC, Hales CA. Pulmonary function in normal subjects and patients with sarcoidosis after bronchoalveolar lavage. *Chest* 1986; **89**: 244–8.

24 Von Essen SG, Robbins RA, Spurzem JR, *et al.* Bronchoscopy with bronchoalveolar lavage causes neutrophil recruitment to the lower respiratory tract. *Am Rev Respir Dis* 1991; **144**: 848–54.

25 Krause A, Hohberg B, Heine F, *et al.* Cytokines derived from alveolar macrophages induce fever after bronchoscopy and bronchoalveolar lavage. *Am J Respir Crit Care Med* 1997; **155**: 1793–7.

26 Hemmers T, Nusslein T, Teig N, *et al.* Prospective study of fever after bronchoalveolar lavage in children. *Klin Padiatr* 2006; **218**: 74–8.

27 Laviolette M, Carreau M, Coulombe R. Bronchoalveolar lavage cell differential on microscope glass cover. A simple and accurate technique. *Am Rev Respir Dis* 1988; **138**: 451–7.

28 Picard E, Goldberg S, Virgilis D, *et al.* A single dose of dexamethasone to prevent postbronchoscopy fever in children: a randomized placebo-controlled trial. *Chest* 2007; **131**: 201–5.

29 Cole P, Turton C, Lanyon H, Collins J. Bronchoalveolar lavage for the preparation of free lung cells: technique and complications. *Br J Dis Chest* 1980; **74**: 273–8.

30 Ognibene FP, Shelhamer J, Gill V, *et al.* The diagnosis of *Pneumocystis carinii* pneumonia in patients with the acquired immunodeficiency syndrome using subsegmental bronchoalveolar lavage. *Am Rev Respir Dis* 1984; **129**: 929–32.

31 Lin CC, Wu JL, Huang WC. Pulmonary function in normal subjects after bronchoalveolar lavage. *Chest* 1988; **93**: 1049–53.

32 Hattotuwa K, Gamble EA, O'Shaughnessy T, *et al.* Safety of bronchoscopy, biopsy, and BAL in research patients with COPD. *Chest* 2002; **122**: 1909–12.

33 Ouellette DR. The safety of bronchoscopy in a pulmonary fellowship program. *Chest* 2006; **130**: 1185–90.

34 Elston WJ, Whittaker AJ, Khan LN, *et al.* Safety of research bronchoscopy, biopsy and bronchoalveolar lavage in asthma. *Eur Respir J* 2004; **24**: 375–7.

35 Cordonnier C, Bernaudin JF, Fleury J, *et al.* Diagnostic yield of bronchoalveolar lavage in pneumonitis occurring after allogeneic bone marrow transplantation. *Am Rev Respir Dis* 1985; **132**: 1118–23.

36 Gurney JW, Harrison WC, Sears K, *et al.* Bronchoalveolar lavage: radiographic manifestations. *Radiology* 1987; **163**: 71–4.

37 Laviolette M. Lymphocyte fluctuation in bronchoalveolar lavage fluid in normal volunteers. *Thorax* 1985; **40**: 651–6.

38 Marcy TW, Merrill WW, Rankin JA, Reynolds HY. Limitations of using urea to quantify epithelial lining fluid recovered by bronchoalveolar lavage. *Am Rev Respir Dis* 1987; **135**: 1276–80.

39 Stover DE, White DA, Romano PA, Gellene RA. Diagnosis of pulmonary disease in acquired immune deficiency syndrome (AIDS). Role of bronchoscopy and bronchoalveolar lavage. *Am Rev Respir Dis* 1984; **130**: 659–62.

40 Crystal RG, Bitterman PB, Rennard SI, *et al.* Interstitial lung diseases of unknown cause. Disorders characterized by chronic inflammation of the lower respiratory tract (first of two parts). *N Engl J Med* 1984; **310**: 154–66.

41 Rankin JA, Naegel GP, Reynolds HY. Use of a central laboratory for analysis of bronchoalveolar lavage fluid. *Am Rev Respir Dis* 1986; **133**: 186–90.

42 Thompson AB, Robbins RA, Ghafouri MA, *et al.* Bronchoalveolar lavage fluid processing. Effect of membrane filtration preparation on neutrophil recovery. *Acta Cytol* 1989; **33**: 544–9.

43 Kelly C, Ward C, Bird G, *et al.* The effect of filtration on absolute and differential cell counts in fluid obtained at bronchoalveolar lavage. *Respir Med* 1989; **83**: 107–10.

44 Winquist AG, Orrico MA, Peterson LR. Evaluation of the cytocentrifuge Gram stain as a screening test for bacteriuria in specimens from specific patient populations. *Am J Clin Pathol* 1997; **108**: 515–24.

45 Armbruster C, Pokieser L, Hassl A. Diagnosis of *Pneumocystis carinii* pneumonia by bronchoalveolar lavage in AIDS patients. Comparison of Diff-Quik, fungifluor stain, direct immunofluorescence test and polymerase chain reaction. *Acta Cytol* 1995; **39**: 1089–93.

46 De Brauwer EI, Jacobs JA, Nieman F, *et al.* Bronchoalveolar lavage fluid differential cell count. How many cells should be counted? *Anal Quant Cytol Histol* 2002; **24**: 337–41.

47 Smith PA, Kohli LM, Wood KL, *et al.* Cytometric analysis of BAL T cells labeled with a standardized antibody cocktail correlates with immunohistochemical staining. *Cytometry B Clin Cytom* 2006; **70**: 170–8.

48 Welker L, Jorres RA, Costabel U, Magnussen H. Predictive value of BAL cell differentials in the diagnosis of interstitial lung diseases. *Eur Respir J* 2004; **24**: 1000–6.

49 Emad A, Emad Y. CD4/CD8 ratio and cytokine levels of the BAL fluid in patients with bronchiectasis caused by sulfur mustard gas inhalation. *J Inflamm (Lond)* 2007; **4**: 2.

50 Costabel U. *Atlas of Bronchoalveolar Lavage.* London: Chapman & Hall Medical; 1998.

51 Costabel U, Guzman J. Effect of smoking on bronchoalveolar lavage constituents. *Eur Respir J* 1992; **5**: 776–9.

52 Meyer KC, Soergel P. Variation of bronchoalveolar lymphocyte phenotypes with age in the physiologically normal human lung. *Thorax* 1999; **54**: 697–700.

53 Rose AS, Knox KS. Bronchoalveolar lavage as a research tool. *Semin Respir Crit Care Med* 2007; **28**: 561–73.

54 Hunninghake GW, Kawanami O, Ferrans VJ, *et al.* Characterization of the inflammatory and immune effector cells in the lung parenchyma of patients with interstitial lung disease. *Am Rev Respir Dis* 1981; **123**: 407–12.

55 Baughman RP, Drent M. Role of bronchoalveolar lavage in interstitial lung disease. *Clin Chest Med* 2001; **22**: 331–41.

56 Hunninghake GW, Crystal RG. Pulmonary sarcoidosis: a disorder mediated by excess helper T-lymphocyte activity at sites of disease activity. *N Engl J Med* 1981; **305**: 429–34.

57 Costabel U, King TE. International consensus statement on idiopathic pulmonary fibrosis. *Eur Respir J* 2001; **17**: 163–7.

58 Drent M, Grutters JC, Mulder PG, *et al.* Is the different T helper cell activity in sarcoidosis and extrinsic allergic alveolitis also reflected by the cellular bronchoalveolar lavage fluid profile? *Sarcoidosis Vasc Diffuse Lung Dis* 1997; **14**: 31–8.

59 Takahashi T, Azuma A, Abe S, *et al.* Significance of lymphocytosis in bronchoalveolar lavage in suspected ocular sarcoidosis. *Eur Respir J* 2001; **18**: 515–21.

60 Drent M, Jacobs JA, Cobben NA, *et al.* Computer program supporting the diagnostic accuracy of cellular BALF analysis: a new release. *Respir Med* 2001; **95**: 781–6.

61 Winterbauer RH, Lammert J, Selland M, *et al.* Bronchoalveolar lavage cell populations in the diagnosis of sarcoidosis. *Chest* 1993; **104**: 352–61.

62 Costabel U, Guzman J. Bronchoalveolar lavage in interstitial lung disease. *Curr Opin Pulm Med* 2001; **7**: 255–61.

63 Drent M, van Velzen-Blad H, Diamant M, *et al.* Relationship between presentation of sarcoidosis and T lymphocyte profile. A study in bronchoalveolar lavage fluid. *Chest* 1993; **104**: 795–800.

64 Kantrow SP, Meyer KC, Kidd P, Raghu G. The CD4/CD8 ratio in BAL fluid is highly variable in sarcoidosis. *Eur Respir J* 1997; **10**: 2716–21.

65 Drent M, Mansour K, Linssen C. Bronchoalveolar lavage in sarcoidosis. *Semin Respir Crit Care Med* 2007; **28**: 486–95.

66 Costabel U. CD4/CD8 ratios in bronchoalveolar lavage fluid: of value for diagnosing sarcoidosis? *Eur Respir J* 1997; **10**: 2699–700.

67 Grunewald J, Eklund A. Sex-specific manifestations of Lofgren's syndrome. *Am J Respir Crit Care Med* 2007; **175**: 40–4.

68 Drent M, Jacobs JA, de Vries J, *et al.* Does the cellular bronchoalveolar lavage fluid profile reflect the severity of sarcoidosis? *Eur Respir J* 1999; **13**: 1338–44.

69 Ziegenhagen MW, Rothe ME, Zissel G, Muller-Quernheim J. Exaggerated TNFalpha release of alveolar macrophages in corticosteroid resistant sarcoidosis. *Sarcoidosis Vasc Diffuse Lung Dis* 2002; **19**: 185–90.

70 Thomas PD, Hunninghake GW. Current concepts of the pathogenesis of sarcoidosis. *Am Rev Respir Dis* 1987; **135**: 747–60.

71 American Thoracic Society/European Respiratory Society International Multidisciplinary Consensus Classification of the Idiopathic Interstitial Pneumonias. This joint statement of the American Thoracic Society (ATS), and the European Respiratory Society (ERS) was adopted by the ATS board of directors, June 2001 and by the ERS Executive Committee, June 2001. *Am J Respir Crit Care Med* 2002; **165**: 277–304.

72 Nagao T, Nagai S, Kitaichi M, *et al.* Usual interstitial pneumonia: idiopathic pulmonary fibrosis versus collagen vascular diseases. *Respiration* 2001; **68**: 151–9.

73 Ryu YJ, Chung MP, Han J, *et al.* Bronchoalveolar lavage in fibrotic idiopathic interstitial pneumonias. *Respir Med* 2007; **101**: 655–60.

74 Papiris SA, Kollintza A, Kitsanta P, *et al.* Relationship of BAL and lung tissue CD4+ and CD8+ T lymphocytes, and their ratio in idiopathic pulmonary fibrosis. *Chest* 2005; **128**: 2971–7.

75 Flaherty KR, Travis WD, Colby TV, *et al.* Histopathologic variability in usual and nonspecific interstitial pneumonias. *Am J Respir Crit Care Med* 2001; **164**: 1722–7.

76 Nagai S, Kitaichi M, Itoh H, *et al.* Idiopathic nonspecific interstitial pneumonia/fibrosis: comparison with idiopathic pulmonary fibrosis and BOOP. *Eur Respir J* 1998; **12**: 1010–19.

77 Nagai S, Handa T, Ito Y, *et al.* Bronchoalveolar lavage in idiopathic interstitial lung diseases. *Semin Respir Crit Care Med* 2007; **28**: 496–503.

78 Veeraraghavan S, Latsi PI, Wells AU, *et al.* BAL findings in idiopathic nonspecific interstitial pneumonia and usual interstitial pneumonia. *Eur Respir J* 2003; **22**: 239–44.

79 Haslam PL, Dewar A, Butchers P, *et al.* Mast cells, atypical lymphocytes, and neutrophils in bronchoalveolar lavage in extrinsic allergic alveolitis. Comparison with other interstitial lung diseases. *Am Rev Respir Dis* 1987; **135**: 35–47.

80 Mohr LC. Hypersensitivity pneumonitis. *Curr Opin Pulm Med* 2004; **10**: 401–11.

81 Haslam PL. Bronchoalveolar lavage in extrinsic allergic alveolitis. *Eur J Respir Dis Suppl* 1987; **154**: 120–35.

82 Fournier E, Tonnel AB, Gosset P, *et al.* Early neutrophil alveolitis after antigen inhalation in hypersensitivity pneumonitis. *Chest* 1985; **88**: 563–6.

83 Pardo A, Barrios R, Gaxiola M, *et al.* Increase of lung neutrophils in hypersensitivity pneumonitis is associated with lung fibrosis. *Am J Respir Crit Care Med* 2000; **161**: 1698–704.

84 Bjermer L, Engstrom-Laurent A, Hallgren R, Rosenhall L. Bronchoalveolar lavage in persons acutely exposed to dust in the farm environment. *Am J Ind Med* 1990; **17**: 106.

85 Gariepy L, Cormier Y, Laviolette M, Tardif A. Predictive value of bronchoalveolar lavage cells and serum precipitins in asymptomatic dairy farmers. *Am Rev Respir Dis* 1989; **140**: 1386–9.

86 Ohtani Y, Kojima K, Sumi Y, *et al.* Inhalation provocation tests in chronic bird fancier's lung. *Chest* 2000; **118**: 1382–9.

87 Cormier Y, Belanger J, Laviolette M. Prognostic significance of bronchoalveolar lymphocytosis in farmer's lung. *Am Rev Respir Dis* 1987; **135**: 692–5.

88 Mossman BT, Bignon J, Corn M, *et al.* Asbestos: scientific developments and implications for public policy. *Science* 1990; **247**: 294–301.

89 Rebuck AS, Braude AC. Bronchoalveolar lavage in asbestosis. *Arch Intern Med* 1983; **143**: 950–2.

90 Dumortier P, de Vuyst P, Yernault JC. Mineralogical analysis of bronchoalveolar lavage fluids. *Z Erkr Atmungsorgane* 1988; **171**: 50–8.

91 De Vuyst P, Dumortier P, Moulin E, *et al.* Asbestos bodies in bronchoalveolar lavage reflect lung asbestos body concentration. *Eur Respir J* 1988; **1**: 362–7.

92 De Vuyst P, Jedwab J, Dumortier P, *et al.* Asbestos bodies in bronchoalveolar lavage. *Am Rev Respir Dis* 1982; **126**: 972–6.

93 Churg A. Fiber counting and analysis in the diagnosis of asbestos-related disease. *Hum Pathol* 1982; **13**: 381–92.

94 De Vuyst P, Dumortier P, Moulin E, *et al.* Diagnostic value of asbestos bodies in bronchoalveolar lavage fluid. *Am Rev Respir Dis* 1987; **136**: 1219–24.

95 Vathesatogkit P, Harkin TJ, Addrizzo-Harris DJ, *et al.* Clinical correlation of asbestos bodies in BAL fluid. *Chest* 2004; **126**: 966–71.

96 Fireman E, Lerman Y. Induced sputum in interstitial lung diseases. *Curr Opin Pulm Med* 2006; **12**: 318–22.

97 Teschler H, Thompson AB, Dollenkamp R, *et al.* Relevance of asbestos bodies in sputum. *Eur Respir J* 1996; **9**: 680–6.

98 Epstein PE, Dauber JH, Rossman MD, Daniele RP. Bronchoalveolar lavage in a patient with chronic berylliosis: evidence for hypersensitivity pneumonitis. *Ann Intern Med* 1982; **97**: 213–16.

99 Rossman MD, Kern JA, Elias JA, *et al.* Proliferative response of bronchoalveolar lymphocytes to beryllium. A test for chronic beryllium disease. *Ann Intern Med* 1988; **108**: 687–93.

100 Newman LS, Mroz MM, Balkissoon R, Maier LA. Beryllium sensitization progresses to chronic beryllium disease: a longitudinal study of disease risk. *Am J Respir Crit Care Med* 2005; **171**: 54–60.

101 Allen JN, Davis WB, Pacht ER. Diagnostic significance of increased bronchoalveolar lavage fluid eosinophils. *Am Rev Respir Dis* 1990; **142**: 642–7.

102 Bjermer L, Lundgren R, Hallgren R. Hyaluronan and type III procollagen peptide concentrations in bronchoalveolar lavage fluid in idiopathic pulmonary fibrosis. *Thorax* 1989; **44**: 126–31.

103 Blaschke E, Eklund A, Hernbrand R. Extracellular matrix components in bronchoalveolar lavage fluid in sarcoidosis and their relationship to signs of alveolitis. *Am Rev Respir Dis* 1990; **141**: 1020–5.

104 O'Connor C, Ward K, van Breda A, *et al.* Type 3 procollagen peptide in bronchoalveolar lavage fluid. Poor indicator of course and prognosis in sarcoidosis. *Chest* 1989; **96**: 339–44.

105 Ward K, O'Connor CM, Odlum C, *et al.* Pulmonary disease progress in sarcoid patients with and without bronchoalveolar lavage collagenase. *Am Rev Respir Dis* 1990; **142**: 636–41.

106 Costabel U, Guzman J, Bonella F, Oshimo S. Bronchoalveolar lavage in other interstitial lung diseases. *Semin Respir Crit Care Med* 2007; **28**: 514–24.

107 Lazor R, Cordier J. Idiopathic eosinophilic pneumonias. In: Costabel U, Du Bois RM, eds. *Diffuse Parenchymal Lung Disease. Prog Respir Res* Vol. 36. Basel: Karger; 2007: 238–49.

108 Philit F, Etienne-Mastroianni B, Parrot A, *et al.* Idiopathic acute eosinophilic pneumonia: a study of 22 patients. *Am J Respir Crit Care Med* 2002; **166**: 1235–9.

109 Pope-Harman AL, Davis WB, Allen ED, *et al.* Acute eosinophilic pneumonia. A summary of 15 cases and review of the literature. *Medicine (Baltimore)* 1996; **75**: 334–42.

110 Marchand E, Etienne-Mastroianni B, Chanez P, *et al.* Idiopathic chronic eosinophilic pneumonia and asthma: how do they influence each other? *Eur Respir J* 2003; **22**: 8–13.

111 Marchand E, Reynaud-Gaubert M, Lauque D, *et al.* Idiopathic chronic eosinophilic pneumonia. A clinical and follow-up study of 62 cases. The Groupe d'Etudes et de Recherche sur les Maladies "Orphelines" Pulmonaires (GERM"O"P). *Medicine (Baltimore)* 1998; **77**: 299–312.

112 Bouros D, Wells AU, Nicholson AG, *et al.* Histopathologic subsets of fibrosing alveolitis in patients with systemic sclerosis and their relationship to outcome. *Am J Respir Crit Care Med* 2002; **165**: 1581–6.

113 Silver RM, Miller KS, Kinsella MB, *et al.* Evaluation and management of scleroderma lung disease using bronchoalveolar lavage. *Am J Med* 1990; **88**: 470–6.

114 Goh NS, Veeraraghavan S, Desai SR, *et al.* Bronchoalveolar lavage cellular profiles in patients with systemic sclerosis-associated interstitial lung disease are not predictive of disease progression. *Arthritis Rheum* 2007; **56**: 2005–12.

115 Wells AU, Hansell DM, Haslam PL, *et al.* Bronchoalveolar lavage cellularity: lone cryptogenic fibrosing alveolitis compared with the fibrosing alveolitis of systemic sclerosis. *Am J Respir Crit Care Med* 1998; **157**: 1474–82.

116 Basset F, Soler P, Jaurand MC, Bignon J. Ultrastructural examination of broncho-alveolar lavage for diagnosis of pulmonary histiocytosis X: Preliminary report on 4 cases. *Thorax* 1977; **32**: 303–6.

117 Casolaro MA, Bernaudin JF, Saltini C, *et al.* Accumulation of Langerhans' cells on the epithelial surface of the lower respiratory tract in normal subjects in association with cigarette smoking. *Am Rev Respir Dis* 1988; **137**: 406–11.

118 Soler P, Moreau A, Basset F, Hance AJ. Cigarette smoking-induced changes in the number and differentiated state of pulmonary dendritic cells/Langerhans cells. *Am Rev Respir Dis* 1989; **139**: 1112–17.

119 Zamora MR, Warner ML, Tuder R, Schwarz MI. Diffuse alveolar hemorrhage and systemic lupus erythematosus. Clinical presentation, histology, survival, and outcome. *Medicine (Baltimore)* 1997; **76**: 192–202.

120 Collard HR, Schwarz MI. Diffuse alveolar hemorrhage. *Clin Chest Med* 2004; **25**: 583–92, vii.

121 Fontenot AP, Schwarz MI. Diffuse alveolar hemorrhage. In: King TE, Schwartz S, eds. *Interstitial Lung Disease*, 4th edn. Hamilton, ON, Canada: B.C. Decker; 2003: 632–56.

122 De Lassence A, Fleury-Feith J, Escudier E, *et al.* Alveolar hemorrhage. Diagnostic criteria and results in 194 immunocompromised hosts. *Am J Respir Crit Care Med* 1995; **151**: 157–63.

123 Springmeyer SC, Hoges J, Hammar SP. Significance of hemosiderin-laden macrophages in bronchoalveolar lavage fluid. *Am Rev Respir Dis* 1984; **131**: A76.

124 Stover DE, Zaman MB, Hajdu SI, *et al.* Bronchoalveolar lavage in the diagnosis of diffuse pulmonary infiltrates in the immunosuppressed host. *Ann Intern Med* 1984; **101**: 1–7.

125 Drew WL, Finley TN, Golde DW. Diagnostic lavage and occult pulmonary hemorrhage in thrombocytopenic immunocompromised patients. *Am Rev Respir Dis* 1977; **116**: 215–21.

126 Finley TN, Aronow A, Cosentino AM, Golde DW. Occult pulmonary hemorrhage in anticoagulated patients. *Am Rev Respir Dis* 1975; **112**: 23–9.

127 Huaringa AJ, Leyva FJ, Signes-Costa J, *et al.* Bronchoalveolar lavage in the diagnosis of pulmonary complications of bone marrow transplant patients. *Bone Marrow Transpl* 2000; **25**: 975–9.

128 Sherman JM, Winnie G, Thomassen MJ, *et al.* Time course of hemosiderin production and clearance by human pulmonary macrophages. *Chest* 1984; **86**: 409–11.

129 Bonfield TL, Russell D, Burgess S, *et al.* Autoantibodies against granulocyte macrophage colony-stimulating factor are diagnostic for pulmonary alveolar proteinosis. *Am J Respir Cell Mol Biol* 2002; **27**: 481–6.

130 Kitamura T, Tanaka N, Watanabe J, *et al.* Idiopathic pulmonary alveolar proteinosis as an autoimmune disease with neutralizing antibody against granulocyte/macrophage colony-stimulating factor. *J Exp Med* 1999; **190**: 875–80.

131 Uchida K, Nakata K, Trapnell BC, *et al.* High-affinity autoanti-bodies specifically eliminate granulocyte-macrophage colony-stimulating factor activity in the lungs of patients with idiopathic pulmonary alveolar proteinosis. *Blood* 2004; **103**: 1089–98.

132 Martin RJ, Coalson JJ, Rogers RM, *et al.* Pulmonary alveolar proteinosis: the diagnosis by segmental lavage. *Am Rev Respir Dis* 1980; **121**: 819–25.

133 Singh G, Katyal SL, Bedrossian CW, Rogers RM. Pulmonary alveolar proteinosis. Staining for surfactant apoprotein in alve-olar proteinosis and in conditions simulating it. *Chest* 1983; **83**: 82–6.

134 Costabel U, Guzman J. Pulmonary alveolar proteinosis: a new autoimmune disease. *Sarcoidosis Vasc Diffuse Lung Dis* 2005; **22** (Suppl 1): S67–73.

135 Danel C, Israel-Biet D, Costabel U, Klech H. Therapeutic appli-cations of bronchoalveolar lavage. *Eur Respir J* 1992; **5**: 1173–5.

136 Maygarden SJ, Iacocca MV, Funkhouser WK, Novotny DB. Pulmonary alveolar proteinosis: a spectrum of cytologic, histo-chemical, and ultrastructural findings in bronchoalveolar lavage fluid. *Diagn Cytopathol* 2001; **24**: 389–95.

137 Mikami T, Yamamoto Y, Yokoyama M, Okayasu I. Pulmonary alveolar proteinosis: diagnosis using routinely processed smears of bronchoalveolar lavage fluid. *J Clin Pathol* 1997; **50**: 981–4.

138 Brutinel WM, Martin WJ, 2nd. Chronic nitrofurantoin reaction associated with T-lymphocyte alveolitis. *Chest* 1986; **89**: 150–2.

139 Costabel U, Uzaslan E, Guzman J. Bronchoalveolar lavage in drug-induced lung disease. *Clin Chest Med* 2004; **25**: 25–35.

140 Fuhrman C, Parrot A, Wislez M, *et al.* Spectrum of CD4 to CD8 T-cell ratios in lymphocytic alveolitis associated with methotrexate-induced pneumonitis. *Am J Respir Crit Care Med* 2001; **164**: 1186–91.

141 Schnabel A, Richter C, Bauerfeind S, Gross WL. Bronchoalveolar lavage cell profile in methotrexate induced pneumonitis. *Thorax* 1997; **52**: 377–9.

142 Costabel U, Teschler H, Guzman J. Bronchiolitis obliterans organizing pneumonia (BOOP): the cytological and immuno-cytological profile of bronchoalveolar lavage. *Eur Respir J* 1992; **5**: 791–7.

143 Akoun GM, Cadranel JL, Blanchette G, *et al.* Bronchoalveolar lavage cell data in amiodarone-associated pneumonitis. Evalua-tion in 22 patients. *Chest* 1991; **99**: 1177–82.

144 Martin WJ, 2nd, Rosenow EC, 3rd. Amiodarone pulmonary toxicity. Recognition and pathogenesis (Part I). *Chest* 1988; **93**: 1067–75.

145 Coudert B, Bailly F, Lombard JN, *et al.* Amiodarone pneumo-nitis. Bronchoalveolar lavage findings in 15 patients and review of the literature. *Chest* 1992; **102**: 1005–12.

146 Popovich J, Jr., Kvale PA, Eichenhorn MS, *et al.* Diagnostic accuracy of multiple biopsies from flexible fiberoptic bronchos-copy. A comparison of central versus peripheral carcinoma. *Am Rev Respir Dis* 1982; **125**: 521–3.

147 Shure D, Fedullo PF. Transbronchial needle aspiration of peripheral masses. *Am Rev Respir Dis* 1983; **128**: 1090–2.

148 Bellocq A, Antoine M, Flahault A, *et al.* Neutrophil alveolitis in bronchioloalveolar carcinoma: induction by tumor-derived interleukin-8 and relation to clinical outcome. *Am J Pathol* 1998; **152**: 83–92.

149 Poletti V, Poletti G, Murer B, *et al.* Bronchoalveolar lavage in malignancy. *Semin Respir Crit Care Med* 2007; **28**: 534–45.

150 Poletti V, Romagna M, Allen KA, *et al.* Bronchoalveolar lavage in the diagnosis of disseminated lung tumors. *Acta Cytol* 1995; **39**: 472–7.

151 Wislez M, Massiani MA, Milleron B, *et al.* Clinical characteris-tics of pneumonic-type adenocarcinoma of the lung. *Chest* 2003; **123**: 1868–77.

152 Semenzato G, Poletti V. Bronchoalveolar lavage in lung cancer. *Respiration* 1992; **59** (Suppl 1): 44–6.

153 Morales FM, Matthews JI. Diagnosis of parenchymal Hodgkin's disease using bronchoalveolar lavage. *Chest* 1987; **91**: 785–7.

154 Wisecarver J, Ness MJ, Rennard SI, *et al.* Bronchoalveolar lavage in the assessment of pulmonary Hodgkin's disease. *Acta Cytol* 1989; **33**: 527–32.

155 Levy H, Horak DA, Lewis MI. The value of bronchial washings and bronchoalveolar lavage in the diagnosis of lymphangitic carcinomatosis. *Chest* 1988; **94**: 1028–30.

156 Radio SJ, Rennard SI, Kessinger A, *et al.* Breast carcinoma in bronchoalveolar lavage. A cytologic and immunocytochemical study. *Arch Pathol Lab Med* 1989; **113**: 333–6.

157 Beskow CO, Drachenberg CB, Bourquin PM, *et al.* Diffuse alveolar damage. Morphologic features in bronchoalveolar lavage fluid. *Acta Cytol* 2000; **44**: 640–6.

158 Rennard SI. Bronchoalveolar lavage in the diagnosis of cancer. *Lung* 1990; **168** (Suppl): 1035–40.

159 Stanley MW, Henry-Stanley MJ, Gajl-Peczalska KJ, Bitterman PB. Hyperplasia of type II pneumocytes in acute lung injury. Cytologic findings of sequential bronchoalveolar lavage. *Am J Clin Pathol* 1992; **97**: 669–77.

160 Iregui M, Ward S, Sherman G, *et al.* Clinical importance of delays in the initiation of appropriate antibiotic treatment for ventilator-associated pneumonia. *Chest* 2002; **122**: 262–8.

161 Luna CM, Aruj P, Niederman MS, *et al.* Appropriateness and delay to initiate therapy in ventilator-associated pneumonia. *Eur Respir J* 2006; **27**: 158–64.

162 Baughman RP. Nonbronchoscopic evaluation of ventilator-associated pneumonia. *Semin Respir Infect* 2003; **18**: 95–102.

163 Fagon JY, Chastre J, Wolff M, *et al.* Invasive and noninvasive strategies for management of suspected ventilator-associated pneumonia. A randomized trial. *Ann Intern Med* 2000; **132**: 621–30.

164 Elatrous S, Boukef R, Ouanes Besbes L, *et al.* Diagnosis of ventilator-associated pneumonia: agreement between quanti-tative cultures of endotracheal aspiration and plugged telescop-ing catheter. *Intensive Care Med* 2004; **30**: 853–8.

165 Ruiz M, Torres A, Ewig S, *et al.* Noninvasive versus invasive micr-obial investigation in ventilator-associated pneumonia: evalua-tion of outcome. *Am J Respir Crit Care Med* 2000; **162**: 119–25.

166 Sole Violan J, Fernandez JA, Benitez AB, *et al.* Impact of quan-titative invasive diagnostic techniques in the management and outcome of mechanically ventilated patients with suspected pneumonia. *Crit Care Med* 2000; **28**: 2737–41.

167 Heyland DK, Cook DJ, Marshall J, *et al.* The clinical utility of invasive diagnostic techniques in the setting of ventilator-associated pneumonia. Canadian Critical Care Trials Group. *Chest* 1999; **115**: 1076–84.

168 Canadian Critical Care Trials Group. A randomized trial of diagnostic techniques for ventilator-associated pneumonia. *N Engl J Med* 2006; **355**: 2619–30.

169 Hohenadel IA, Kiworr M, Genitsariotis R, *et al*. Role of bronchoalveolar lavage in immunocompromised patients with pneumonia treated with a broad spectrum antibiotic and antifungal regimen. *Thorax* 2001; **56**: 115–20.

170 Pisani RJ, Wright AJ. Clinical utility of bronchoalveolar lavage in immunocompromised hosts. *Mayo Clin Proc* 1992; **67**: 221–7.

171 Johnson PC, Hogg KM, Sarosi GA. The rapid diagnosis of pulmonary infections in solid organ transplant recipients. *Semin Respir Infect* 1990; **5**: 2–9.

172 Kahn FW, Jones JM. Analysis of bronchoalveolar lavage specimens from immunocompromised patients with a protocol applicable in the microbiology laboratory. *J Clin Microbiol* 1988; **26**: 1150–5.

173 Martin WJ, 2nd, Smith TF, Sanderson DR, *et al*. Role of bronchoalveolar lavage in the assessment of opportunistic pulmonary infections: utility and complications. *Mayo Clin Proc* 1987; **62**: 549–57.

174 Xaubet A, Torres A, Marco F, *et al*. Pulmonary infiltrates in immunocompromised patients. Diagnostic value of telescoping plugged catheter and bronchoalveolar lavage. *Chest* 1989; **95**: 130–5.

175 Peikert T, Rana S, Edell ES. Safety, diagnostic yield, and therapeutic implications of flexible bronchoscopy in patients with febrile neutropenia and pulmonary infiltrates. *Mayo Clin Proc* 2005; **80**: 1414–20.

176 Velez L, Correa LT, Maya MA, *et al*. Diagnostic accuracy of bronchoalveolar lavage samples in immunosuppressed patients with suspected pneumonia: analysis of a protocol. *Respir Med* 2007; **101**: 2160–7.

177 Cordonnier C, Escudier E, Verra F, *et al*. Bronchoalveolar lavage during neutropenic episodes: diagnostic yield and cellular pattern. *Eur Respir J* 1994; **7**: 114–20.

178 Stolz D, Stulz A, Muller B, *et al*. BAL neutrophils, serum procalcitonin, and C-reactive protein to predict bacterial infection in the immunocompromised host. *Chest* 2007; **132**: 504–14.

# 11

# Transbronchial Needle Aspiration for Cytology and Histology Specimens

## Ko-Pen Wang,[1] Atul C. Mehta,[2] and J. Francis Turner Jr[3]

[1] Chest Diagnostic Center and Lung Cancer Center at Harbor Hospital, Part-time Faculty of Interventional Pulmonology, Johns Hopkins Hospital, Baltimore, MD, USA
[2] Respiratory Institute, Cleveland Clinic, Cleveland, OH, USA
[3] Interventional Pulmonary and Critical Care Medicine, Nevada Cancer Institute and University of Nevada School of Medicine, Las Vegas, NV, USA

## Introduction

The use of transbronchial needle aspiration (TBNA) has been well documented in the literature [1–5]. Despite this, the American College of Chest Physicians survey of pulmonary specialists in North America, published in 1991, revealed that only 11.8% of the responding pulmonary specialists routinely used TBNA in malignant disease while 49.4% rarely used the procedure [6]. A subsequent study by the American Association for Bronchology in 1999 again demonstrated the infrequent use of TBNA with 54% (n = 270) performing TBNA in the preceding 12 months in less than 10 instances and 18% (n = 136) never utilizing TBNA in the prior year [7]. The *European Respiratory Journal* in 2002 published a study regarding the use of flexible bronchoscopy in the United Kingdom, which reviewed the responses of 328 consultants in adult respiratory medicine to a standardized questionnaire [8]. In this review, the overall use of flexible bronchoscopy was found to be variable, with TBNA in particular being utilized by only 27% of practitioners in the preceding 12 months, and the article noting that responders commented on their poor diagnostic yield. Since the second edition of this text, additional tools such as endobronchial ultrasound, CT fluoroscopy, and electromagnetic navigational bronchoscopy have become more widespread and reviewed, stimulating a renewed interest in transbronchial needle aspiration [9–11]. An editorial in *Chest* in 2002 supported the utilization of adjunctive instruments in synergy with the basic equipment and technique of transbronchial needle aspiration, thereby increasing the utilization of TBNA [12]. The use of these supportive instruments, such as endobronchial ultrasound and electromagnetic navigation bronchoscopy, are presented in detail in other chapters in this work.

We believe the use of TBNA to be a powerful tool in the diagnosis of both malignant and non-malignant diseases of the chest, but especially so in the diagnosis and staging of bronchogenic carcinoma [5,13]. This review is intended to outline the history of the technique with a subsequent discussion of the instrumentation, biopsy technique, relevant anatomy, indications, complications, as well as the limitations and potential for this tool in the era of flexible bronchoscopy.

## Historical overview

What was to become a landmark presentation in the history of transbronchial needle aspiration was presented by Dr Eduardo Schieppati in 1949 at the Argentine Congress of Bronchoesophagology. Schieppati went on to publish his data in the Review of the Argentine Medical Association in 1949 with subsequent publication of his findings in the English literature in the *Journal of Surgery, Gynecology, and Obstetrics* in 1958 [14,15]. His technique was to introduce a 1-mm steel needle through a rigid bronchoscope and perform transbronchial needle aspiration of the carina to aid in the diagnosis of patients thought to have either esophageal or bronchogenic carcinoma. Schieppati commented in his English language paper regarding the safety of this method and felt it to be "free of great risks" [15]. Despite the proximity of the great vessels and heart this proved to be a prophetic statement when Crymes et al. published their work outlining hemodynamic studies of the aorta, pulmonary artery, and left atrium by direct transbronchial needle puncture of these vascular structures [16]. Subsequently, transbronchial needle aspiration continued to be reported in the literature in limited numbers with the use of rigid bronchoscopy [17–22]. Another historic presentation in the

*Flexible Bronchoscopy*, Third Edition. Edited by Ko-Pen Wang, Atul C. Mehta, J. Francis Turner.
© 2012 Blackwell Publishing Ltd. Published 2012 by Blackwell Publishing Ltd.

history of bronchoesophagology was given at the American Bronchoesophagology Association in 1970 by Dr Shigeto Ikeda. Ikeda's presentation and subsequent publications regarding his groundbreaking work with flexible fiberoptics would serve not only to have an impact upon the ability to inspect the tracheobronchial tree, but also to allow greater utility in the application of transbronchial needle aspiration [23,24]. With the availability of the flexible bronchoscope, Dr Ko-Pen Wang of Johns Hopkins Hospital in Baltimore designed and utilized an innovative needle construction to perform transbronchial needle aspiration through this new flexible instrument [2].

Subsequent to this initial description, the usefulness of transbronchial needle aspiration was confirmed by bronchoscopists at other major institutions and continues to be used throughout the world [25–30].

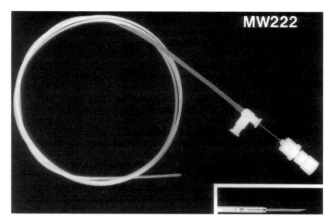

**Fig. 11.1** MW-222 transbronchial needle. The most proximal part "guide wire hub" does not need to be retracted for suction. However, it can be retracted partially to increase flexibility for peripheral lesions. This should be done before the instrument is introduced through the scope. In this instance, it is not necessary to re-advance the guide wire cap for suction.

## Instruments

The use of the rigid bronchoscope allows needle aspiration with long, thin, rigid needles, as described originally by Schieppati with the later use of modified Vim Biegeleisen and Vim-Silverman needles by Fox and Bridgeman [18,20]. Wang and associates in 1978 reported the first experience in the United States of a paratracheal lymph node aspiration utilizing a modified esophageal variceal needle introduced via a rigid bronchoscope [1]. This modification was very successful in obtaining diagnostic cytology specimens in patients with bronchogenic carcinoma [31]. Wang and associates then developed a prototype needle for use with the flexible equipment with subsequent modifications in design to allow greater use with the introduction of needles of different characteristics. The original Wang TBNA needles for use in the diagnosis of central and peripheral lesions were designated as three types: IA, IIA, IIIA. These incorporated a basic design of a 120-cm long semitranslucent catheter with an inner steel stylet ending in a 1.3-cm beveled or flat-tipped 22-gauge needle. These three needle types were subsequently modified, and designated as types IB, IIB, and IIIB, to ensure greater protection to the flexible bronchoscope and allow for greater utility in the diagnosis of central and peripheral lesions. All three types employ needles that are retractable, whether of the single lumen (type IB) or double lumen (types IIB and IIIB) design. Negative pressure for aspiration is transmitted from the luer lock side-hole at the proximal end of the catheter between the stylet and catheter in type IB and between the inner and outer catheter in type IIB and IIIB. In each of these three needle types protection of the working channel of the bronchoscope is ensured by the outer semitranslucent catheter having a metal hub at the distal tip. During insertion through the working channel the needle rests within the semitranslucent catheter with the beveled tip being surrounded by the outer metal hub at the distal end. All three of these MW needle types have an inner stylet, which enhances rigidity during puncture of the bronchial wall (Fig. 11.1). Type IB (MW-122) has a larger lumen to allow a greater suction capability but does not allow for partial withdrawal of the inner stylet for greater flexibility and is recommended for both central and peripheral lesions. Type IIB (MW-222) is of the double lumen retractable needle design, whereby the inner stylet may be partially withdrawn to allow more flexibility to reach apical or superior segmental lesions as needed. This needle does not have as much suction capability as the Type IB, but can be used in both peripheral and central lesions allowing the 22-gauge needle to obtain cytology specimens. The type IIIB needle (MW-322) consists of a double lumen minitrocar. As with the other types, this needle is retracted into the semitranslucent catheter during insertion through the working channel. When the distal end of the catheter protrudes beyond the end of the flexible bronchoscope and the needle is placed in the "out" position, the type IIIB is seen to contain a minitrocar inside the needle which protrudes distal to the beveled tip of the needle. This allows for insertion through the bronchial wall without plugging or contamination of the needle by the superficial bronchial mucosa. Upon penetration of the bronchial wall the inner minitrocar is withdrawn, allowing the beveled needle tip to act as a cutting edge and "core-out" a specimen for cytology. Subsequent to the development of the IB through IIIB types, a more flexible single lumen cytology catheter was developed to improve the ability to obtain cytology from peripheral masses, coin lesions, as well as aortopulmonary (AP) window adenopathy. This was designated as the MW-522 needle and, as with the other cytology needles of the MW series, contained a 22-gauge, 13-mm long beveled tip needle.

**Table 11.1** Wang transbronchial needles (Bard International Products)

| | Cytology specimen | | | Histology specimen | |
| Gauge | C | | P | C | P |
| --- | --- | --- | --- | --- | --- |
| | MW-122 | MW-222 | MW-522 | | |
| | MW-322 | | | | |
| | SW-121 | SW-221 | SW-521 | | |
| | W-120 | W-220 | W-520 | | |
| | | | | MW-319 | MWF-319 |

From: Wang KP, Gonullu U, Baker R. Transbronchial needle aspiration vs. transthoracic needle aspiration in the diagnosis of pulmonary lesions. *J Bronchol* 1994; **1**: 199–204.

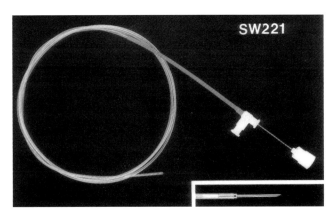

**Fig. 11.2** SW-221 needle. There are only two parts at the proximal end. When the needle is in retracted position, the distal end is flexible. When the needle is advanced and locked for puncture, the distal end is stiffer. All the rest of the cytology needles, central (MW-122 and SW-121) or peripheral (MW-522 and SW-521) are similar in appearance to this needle. In all spring needles, if the tip of the needle is still exposed when in retracted position, simply push it back against a hard sterile surface before use.

A more recent modification to the MW series has been to attach the needle to a spring allowing greater support and the development of momentum for increased puncture force. This series of needles, designated SW-121, 221, and 521, allows the marriage of the spring with a 21-gauge, 15-mm long needle (Table 11.1; Fig. 11.2). The SW-121, as its predecessor the MW-122, is of a single lumen design and has a fixed inner guide wire allowing more rigidity for sampling of central lesions in the mediastinum at the paratracheal, carinal, and hilar levels. The SW-221, also a single-lumen design, has a more flexible inner catheter to allow puncture of both central and peripheral areas. The SW-521 has the most flexible catheter, allowing cytology sampling to take place at peripheral masses, coin lesions, as well as the apical segments, and also has superior suction

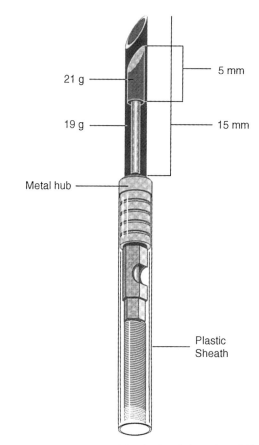

**Fig. 11.3** Schematic diagram of the distal end of transbronchial aspiration needle for histology specimen.

capability. A further development with SW series is that the inner guide wire protrudes halfway into the lumen of the needle. During aspiration this holding chamber formed in the distal half of needle allows the aspirated material to be "packed" thereby allowing improved "flushing" of the sample material onto a glass slide and utilization of the "smear technique". The SW series was noted to compare favorably with the results of the MW series in a recent study [32]. Three additional needles were developed in order to obtain histology core biopsies by this same transbronchial technique. The first needle released was the MW-418 [33]. This contained a 21-gauge inner needle and an 18-gauge outer needle. The 21-gauge inner needle protruded beyond the tip of the 18-gauge needle to prevent plugging of the 18-gauge needle during initial puncture. The 21-gauge trocar could then be withdrawn into the 18-gauge needle, again forming a chamber, whereby the histology biopsy was stored. This MW-418 was later modified to the MW-319 with a 21-gauge inner needle and 19-gauge outer needle, allowing easier use due to the smaller gauge of the outer needle (Fig. 11.3) [34]. A third needle design has been released in the form of the MWF-319, which is of the single-lumen design, but has a more flexible catheter allowing histology sampling of peripheral lesions. Additional needle designs have also been noted to be used with the standard TBNA technique discussed below and in the performance of endobronchial ultrasound in conjunction with TBNA [35,36].

## Biopsy technique

The technique of transbronchial needle aspiration for cytology or histology specimens is basically similar with minor modifications dependent on the needle used and location to be sampled. Prior to handing the catheter and needle to the bronchoscopist, the bronchoscopy technician should test the device to assure that insertion of the guide wire to the "locked position" results in deployment of the needle from the protective outer catheter and distal metal hub (Fig. 11.4). Once tested, the technician should again withdraw the needle into the protective outer catheter, assuring that the beveled tip is surrounded by the metal hub at the end of the semitranslucent outer catheter (Fig. 11.5). With this assured, the distal end of the catheter is handed to the bronchoscopist. The operator should again check that there is no protrusion of the bevel tip distal to the protective catheter and hub, and indeed the beveled tip remains covered by the metal hub at the distal end of the catheter. This double-checking will help ensure no damage to the working channel of the bronchoscope during subsequent insertion and also prevents laceration of the outer catheter by the beveled tip should the needle be proximal to the distal hub and thus be pushed through the wall of the plastic catheter. The needle

catheter device is then introduced into the working channel of the bronchoscope and smoothly threaded until metal hub at the distal end of the catheter is noted to protrude beyond the distal end of the flexible bronchoscope and is in the field of view. This should be performed when the distal end of the bronchoscope is straight and in approximately the midtracheal position, as this will help prevent inadvertent puncture of the catheter and working channel which may occur if the tip of the bronchoscope is in a flexed or extended position (Fig. 11.6). Also, initial deployment of the needle in the midtrachea will help prevent the distal end of the needle from encountering mucosa with subsequent bronchial mucosal contamination before the proper puncture site has been identified.

With the hub visualized, the needle is advanced and locked into place. The catheter is then gently withdrawn until only the very distal tip of the needle is seen in the visual field of the bronchoscope. For central lesions the MW and SW-121, 221, and 222 needles are utilized as their more rigid guide wires allow an improved puncture ability for central lesions such as the paratracheal, carinal, or hilar areas. With the puncture site identified, the bronchoscope, with needle tip protruding, is advanced to the target and the tip of the bronchoscope is flexed toward the puncture point. The bronchoscope is fixed at the patient's nose or mouth by the bronchoscopy assistant and the operator then advances the catheter with a quick thrusting motion allowing the needle to penetrate the intercartilaginous space. A summary of four insertions techniques has been well described by Mehta from the Cleveland Clinic (Fig. 11.7) [37].

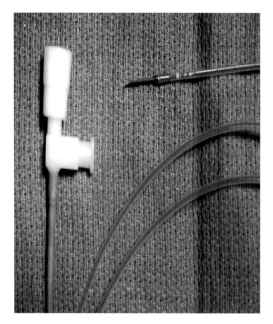

**Fig. 11.4** The Wang transbronchial needle seen with the guide advanced and the needle in the "out and locked" position.

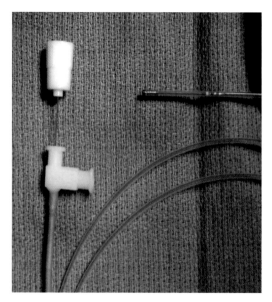

**Fig. 11.5** The Wang transbronchial needle with the guide withdrawn and needle in the semitranslucent outer catheter and needle tip surrounded by the metal hub.

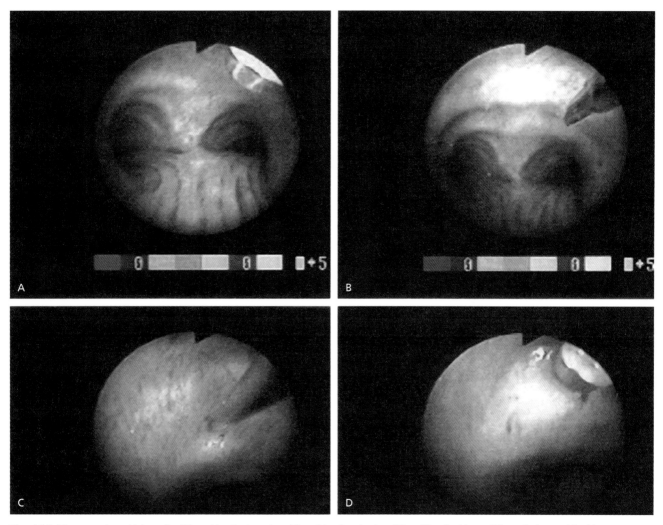

**Fig. 11.6** Wang transbronchial needle: (A) position for insertion; (B) position for piercing; (C) position for biopsy; (D) needle inserted for biopsy.

### The jabbing method

The needle is thrust through the intercartilaginous space with a quick, firm jab to the catheter, while the scope is fixed at the nose or mouth.

### The piggyback method

Once the needle is advanced and locked in position, the catheter is fixed against the proximal end of the insertion port using the index finger in a single-port scope or the digitus minimus in a dual-port scope to prevent recoil when resistance is met. The bronchoscope and catheter are then pushed forward as a single unit, until the entire needle penetrates the tracheobronchial wall [38].

### Hub-against-the-wall method

With the needle retracted, the distal end of the catheter (the metal hub) is placed in contact with the target and held firmly as the needle is pushed out of the catheter to penetrate the tracheobronchial wall.

### The cough method

While the bronchoscopist applies the jabbing or piggyback technique, the patient is asked to cough hard, which causes the needle to penetrate the wall [39].

Attempted penetration through a cartilaginous ring is met with increased resistance and the target site should be adjusted to avoid this. Often fibrous tissue may be encountered which makes penetration difficult as well. An additional technique may sometimes be employed, whereby after the needle tip is fixed in the mucosal tissue of the target site; the catheter is advanced until almost the entire length of the needle is distal to the end of the bronchoscope. With this technique, when the bronchoscope is pushed distally with the needle tip already imbedded in the mucosa, the needle will penetrate the bronchial wall in a more perpendicular orientation. This perpendicular angle will allow an increased depth of needle penetration at the target site and avoidance of the next lower cartilaginous ring. This is also of significant use in the biopsy of AP window adenopathy,

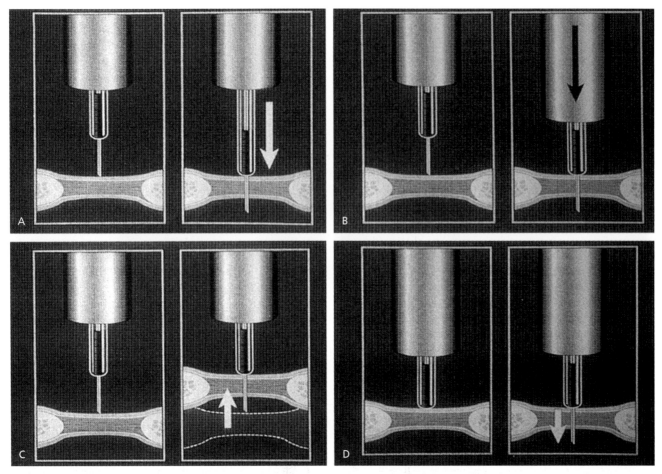

**Fig. 11.7** Different techniques used for tracheobronchial wall penetration by TBNA: (A) jabbing method; (B) piggy-back method; (C) cough method; (D) hub-against-the-wall method. From: Dasgupta A, Mehta AC. Transbronchial needle aspiration: an underused diagnostic technique. *Clin Chest Med* 1999; **20**: 41.

which requires perpendicular insertion of the needle to allow penetration between the aorta and pulmonary artery (Fig. 11.8). With the needle having punctured the bronchial wall and being completely embedded, the operator directs the bronchoscopy technician to apply suction at the proximal suction port. The negative pressure produced allows cells to be trapped in the inside needle chamber. Some operators, with suction maintained, will partially withdraw the needle reinserting it with this "jabbing" technique two or three times without ever allowing the needle to be fully withdrawn and thereby contaminated by bronchial epithelium. Suction is then eliminated by momentarily detaching the syringe from the proximal luer port of the catheter. With suction off the needle is withdrawn from the puncture site and with the bronchoscope again being straight, the catheter and needle are withdrawn from the working channel of the bronchoscope. The bronchoscopy assistant or operator will then take the still-protruding needle and place the tip immediately above and vertical to a glass slide. The specimen collected in the lumen of the needle is then "blown" onto

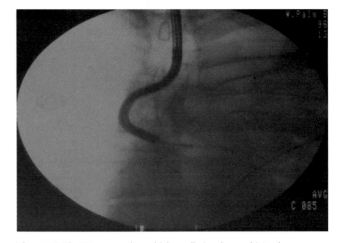

**Fig. 11.8** The Wang transbronchial needle is advanced into the aortopulmonary window.

the slide with positive pressure introduced through the proximal luer of the catheter by the syringe. Another glass slide is then used to press and smear the specimen with the slides immediately being placed in 95% alcohol. These smears are then sent to the cytology laboratory for staining without further preparation. A study comparing the smear technique with that of fluid specimens processed by the Millipore filtration technique indicated that the smear technique is superior in obtaining diagnoses to that of the Millipore technique [40]. The technique described is modified slightly in obtaining specimens from peripheral or coin lesions. In these instances, the catheter is introduced through the working channel in the same manner as described above until the hub of the catheter is noted to be in the field of view of the bronchoscope. With the hub of the catheter in the field of view and the biopsy needle still surrounded by the hub and catheter, the bronchoscope is advanced through the segmental and subsegmental openings, which lead to the peripheral target. Utilizing fluoroscopic guidance the catheter is then advanced with the needle still withdrawn to the peripheral target, remembering that when deployed the needle will protrude 15 mm beyond the tip of the catheter. The fluoroscope is then rotated to a selected

oblique view to better ensure that the catheter and, subsequently the needle, is indeed in contact with the target in two planes of view [41]. The needle tip will be noted to "dance" in the same orientation as the target with respiration and during agitation for sample collection. Without this assurance it is possible that the distal tip of the catheter and needle will be extended anteriorly or posteriorly to the lesion while appearing to have been in the correct biopsy position by only anterior–posterior fluoroscopy. When assured of the proper location the needle is then advanced and locked with aspiration for specimen retrieval. With suction off, the catheter is then withdrawn so the needle is just beyond the distal tip of the bronchoscope. The bronchoscope is then straightened to allow easy withdrawal without potential damage to the working channel of the bronchoscope. Slide preparation is then carried out in the standard smear fashion.

The technique for obtaining histology specimens from central and peripheral locations is similar to that described above (Fig. 11.9). For a central histology core biopsy the MW-319 needle is utilized [42]. As described above this needle has an inner 21-gauge trocar to allow easy penetration of the bronchial mucosa while protecting

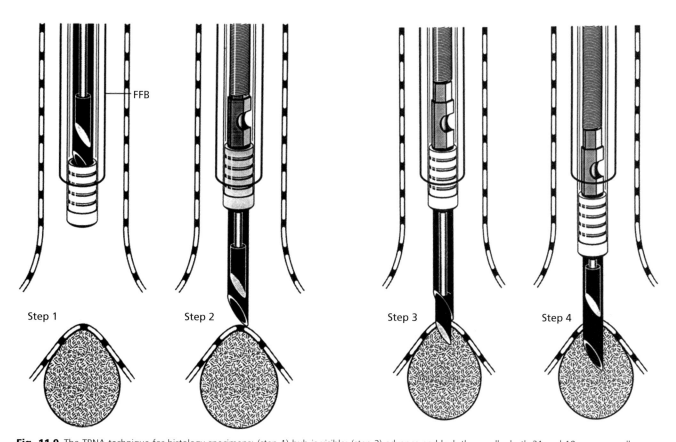

**Fig. 11.9** The TBNA technique for histology specimens: (step 1) hub is visible; (step 2) advance and lock the needle, both 21 and 19 gauge needles are advanced; (step 3) lodge needle tip into mucosa; (step 4) use pushing technique to penetrate bronchial wall. From: Dasgupta A, Mehta AC. Transbronchial needle aspiration: an underused diagnostic technique. *Clin Chest Med* 1999; **20**: 43.

contamination of the 19-gauge specimen chamber from bronchial epithelium. With the catheter having been advanced through the bronchoscope, the distal hub of the catheter is seen in the bronchial field of view. The needle-trocar combination is then advanced and locked with subsequent withdrawal of the catheter until only the distal tip of the needle with protruding trocar is seen. The target area is then approached and the tip of the trocar is imbedded in the bronchial mucosa. With the bronchoscope fixed at the nose or mouth by the assistant, the operator then imbeds the 19-gauge needle into the mucosa to penetrate the length of the needle. Once the entire length of the 19-gauge needle is imbedded, the bronchoscopy assistant withdraws the 21-gauge trocar by unlocking the hub of the trocar stylet and withdrawing it proximally. This is done without moving the hub that extended the combined histology-trocar needle allowing the 19-gauge needle to remain in the target while the trocar is withdrawn. Thus, with the trocar withdrawn, a chamber for the histology core biopsy is created inside the 19-gauge needle. Under the direct vision provided by the bronchoscope the length of the histology needle is then repeatedly drawn out to approximately one half to two-thirds of its length and forcefully reinserted. This action, although requiring some practice to perfect, enables the operator to "core-out" a 19-gauge histology specimen. By not withdrawing the tip of the histology needle the operator also avoids contamination of the specimen with the bronchial epithelium.

Suction is applied during specimen collection as with the cytology aspirations above. After several repeated advances the needle is completely withdrawn from the biopsy site with suction still applied. At this point the plunger withdrawing into the syringe is an indication that a good-sized core of tissue has been obtained (Fig. 11.10). With the suction removed and the needle withdrawn from the bron-

chial wall, the catheter is again withdrawn fully from the bronchoscope. The specimen is then flushed out with 3–5 mL of normal saline with positive pressure applied through the luer lock at the proximal end of the catheter. The normal saline is then decanted and sent for cytology with the core biopsy being placed in formalin. If multiple small fragments are obtained, after decanting the normal saline, they are bound together by placing a few drops of the patient's blood in the specimen cup allowing the fragments and tissue to clot forming a tissue fragment. The fragment formed by this "jello" technique can then be placed in formalin for histology [43]. The MWF-319 is more flexible than the MW-319 and is intended for histology core biopsy of more peripheral lesions. The technique for this peripheral histology needle (MWF-319) is as described for the central histology technique with the exception that the lesion is identified and approached using fluoroscopic guidance as discussed in obtaining cytology specimens of peripheral lesions.

## Relevant anatomy

The successful use of transbronchial needle aspiration involves not only a thorough understanding of instrumentation, technique, and preparation of slides for cytology, but also requires the bronchoscopist to have a detailed understanding of the relationship between the tracheobronchial tree and associated mediastinal and vascular structures. To aid the bronchoscopist in identifying endobronchial locations, four levels in the tracheobronchial tree were selected that are readily identified not only on CT scan of the chest, but also during endobronchial inspection. These four bronchoscopic levels are: (1) main carina, (2) right upper lobe bronchus, (3) bronchus intermedius, and (4) left upper lobe spur (Fig. 11.11; Table 11.2). These four levels correspond to 11 nodal stations that are readily and safely sampled by transbronchial needle aspiration. The 11 nodal stations correspond to those found to be most commonly and consistently involved with metastatic tumor [5]. It should be noted that the 11 nodal stations were developed to more easily identify where to place a TBNA needle for maximum diagnostic yield. These 11 stations do not include some commonly involved in adenopathy, as defined by the nodal staging system of the American Joint Commission on Cancer (AJCC). In the AJCC system those nodes not included in the 11 nodal stations described below include the subaortic lymph node, station 5; para-aortic lymph node, station 6; paraesophageal lymph node, station 8; and pulmonary ligament lymph node, station 9. In these instances, TBNA is not recommended for sampling of para-aortic, parapulmonary artery lymph nodes, or lymph nodes in the AP window, which are quite lateral to the trachea. These additional, often involved, lymph nodes are more readily sampled by transthoracic needle aspiration (TTNA) [41].

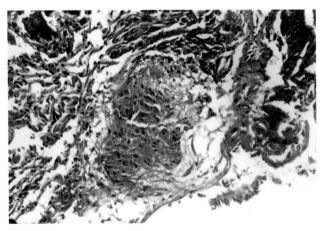

**Fig. 11.10** Histology specimen retrieved by 19-gauge transbronchial needle aspiration. From: Dasgupta A, Mehta AC. Transbronchial needle aspiration: an underused diagnostic technique. *Clin Chest Med* 1999; **20**:43.

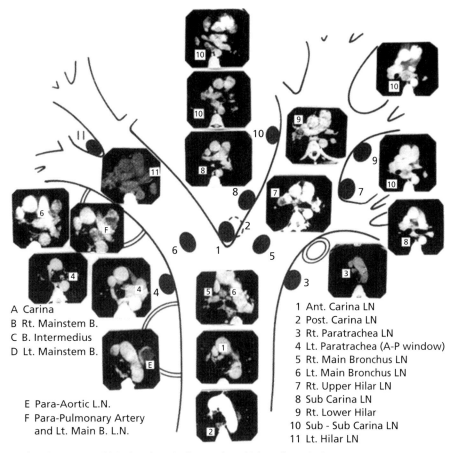

A Carina
B Rt. Mainstem B.
C B. Intermedius
D Lt. Mainstem B.

1 Ant. Carina LN
2 Post. Carina LN
3 Rt. Paratrachea LN
4 Lt. Paratrachea (A-P window)
5 Rt. Main Bronchus LN
6 Lt. Main Bronchus LN
7 Rt. Upper Hilar LN
8 Sub Carina LN
9 Rt. Lower Hilar
10 Sub - Sub Carina LN
11 Lt. Hilar LN

E Para-Aortic L.N.
F Para-Pulmonary Artery
  and Lt. Main B. L.N.

**Fig. 11.11** Nomenclature of mediastinum and hilar lymph nodes for transbronchial needle aspiration.

**Table 11.2** Wang TBNA staging system: TBNA site for mediastinum and hilar lymph nodes (defined by bronchoscopy)

|  | **Site** |
|---|---|
| 1 Anterior carina | First and second intercartilaginous interspaces from lower trachea at about 12–1 o'clock position |
| 2 Posterior carina | Posterior portion of carina at about 5–6 o'clock position |
| 3 Right paratracheal | Second to fourth intercartilaginous interspace of lower trachea at about 1–2 o'clock position |
| 4 Left paratracheal (aortic pulmonary window) | First or second intercartilaginous interspaces from lower trachea at about 9 o'clock position |
| 5 Right main bronchus | First or second intercartilaginous interspace from proximal right main bronchus at about 12 o'clock position |
| 6 Left main bronchus | First or second intercartilaginous interspace from proximal left main bronchus at about 12 o'clock position |
| 7 Right upper hilar | Anterior portion of right upper lobe spur |
| 8 Subcarina | Medial wall of right main bronchus at about 9 o'clock position, proximal to level of right upper lobe orifice |
| 9 Right lower hilar | Lateral or anterior wall of bronchus intermedius at about 3 o'clock position and 12 o'clock position, near or at level of right middle lobe orifice |
| 10 Sub-subcarina | Medial wall of bronchus intermedius at about 9 o'clock position, proximal to level of right middle lobe orifice |
| 11 Left hilar | Lateral wall of left lower lobe bronchus at about 9 o'clock, at level of superior segment orifice of left lower lobe |

From: Wang KP. Staging of bronchogenic carcinoma by bronchoscopy. *Chest* 1994; **106**: 588–93.

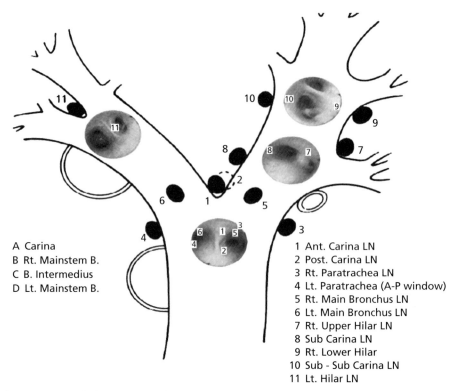

A Carina
B Rt. Mainstem B.
C B. Intermedius
D Lt. Mainstem B.

1 Ant. Carina LN
2 Post. Carina LN
3 Rt. Paratrachea LN
4 Lt. Paratrachea (A-P window)
5 Rt. Main Bronchus LN
6 Lt. Main Bronchus LN
7 Rt. Upper Hilar LN
8 Sub Carina LN
9 Rt. Lower Hilar
10 Sub - Sub Carina LN
11 Lt. Hilar LN

**Fig. 11.12** Location of mediastinum and hilar lymph nodes for transbronchial needle aspiration (defined by CT scan). From: Wang KP. Staging of bronchogenic carcinoma by bronchoscopy. *Chest* 1994; **106**: 590.

The 11 nodal stations are described in relation to their bronchoscopic levels, as identified by CT scan and during endoscopic visualization. On CT scan, the main carina is identified by the change of shape of the trachea to triangular or oval in appearance. At the carinal level there are six nodal stations: (1) anterior carina, (2) posterior carina, (3) right paratracheal, (4) left paratracheal or AP window, (5) right main bronchus, and (6) left main bronchus (Fig. 11.12; Table 11.3). Anterior carinal lymph nodes are those defined as lymph nodes in front of the main carina. This level often coexists with the visualization of the azygous arch. When this is seen the lymph node may be designated as an "azygous node" and is often slightly lateral to the midline towards the azygous vein. To puncture the anterior carinal node the needle is placed in the first or second intercartilagenous space from the lower part of the trachea at about the 12 to 1 o'clock position. Station 2 is the posterior carinal node, which is located posterior to the trachea at the level of the main carina. The CT scan will demonstrate this node often more posterior to the right main bronchus with the puncture site for TBNA being located at the medial posterior wall of the right main bronchus at about the 5 to 6 o'clock position. Although no major vessels exist in this area, care should be taken to insure the presence of adenopathy in this region as in the absence of an enlarged lymph node puncture of the azygoesophageal recess may occur, possibly producing a pneumothorax.

Station 3 defines the right paratracheal node. This is located anterior and lateral to the trachea and posterior-medial to the superior vena cava above the superior border of the azygos arch. To sample this station a puncture should be made at the second tracheal interspace above the carina at the anterior lateral or approximately 1 o'clock position. Station 4 is the left paratracheal node and is located lateral to the left lower border of the trachea. It lies below the aortic arch and immediately superior to the pulmonary artery, and therefore it is also termed the AP window lymph node. The AP window lymph node is sampled by placing the needle very close to the tracheal bronchial angulation, as horizontal as possible to the trachea, at approximately the 9 o'clock position. Stations 5 and 6 are the right main and left main bronchus nodes respectively. The main bronchus nodes are located inferior and lateral to the anterior carina. Station 5, the right main bronchus node, is sampled by placing the needle in the first or second intercartilaginous space from the proximal right main bronchus at about the 12 o'clock position, while the left main bronchus node is sampled in the first or second intercartilaginous space from the proximal left main bronchus at the 12 o'clock position.

The second level identified is where the right main bronchus nears the right upper lobe orifice as seen on CT scan or by endoscopic view. This allows visualization of nodal stations 7 (right upper hilar lymph node) and 8 (subcarinal lymph node) (Figs 11.13 and 11.14). On CT scans, the right

**Table 11.3** Wang TBNA staging system: location of mediastinum and hilar lymph nodes for TBNA (defined by CT scan)

| Location | |
|---|---|
| 1 Anterior carina | In front and between proximal portion of right and left main bronchi |
| 2 Posterior carina | Behind and between proximal portion of right and left main bronchi, or directly behind right main bronchus |
| 3 Right paratracheal | Behind superior vena cava and in front of anterolateral aspects of lower trachea near azygous arch |
| 4 Left paratracheal (aortic pulmonary window) | Lateral to trachea near tracheobronchial angulation, below aortic arch and above left main pulmonary artery |
| 5 Right main bronchus | In front of right main bronchus |
| 6 Left main bronchus | In front of left main bronchus |
| 7 Right upper hilar | In front and between right upper lobe bronchus and bronchus intermedius |
| 8 Subcarina | Between right and left main bronchi, at or near level of right upper lobe bronchus |
| 9 Right lower hilar | Lateral or in front of bronchus intermedius, at or near level of right middle lobe bronchus |
| 10 Subsubcarina | Between bronchus intermedius and left main bronchus, at or near level of right middle lobe bronchus |
| 11 Left hilar | Between left upper lobe and left lower lobe bronchus |

From: Wang KP. Staging of bronchogenic carcinoma by bronchoscopy. *Chest* 1994; **106**: 588–93.

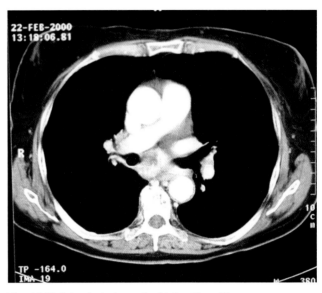

**Fig. 11.13** Subcarinal adenopathy (station 8) on CT scan.

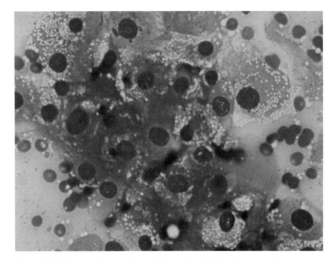

**Fig. 11.14** Smear from station 8 from Fig. 11.13, demonstrating metastatic renal cell carcinoma.

upper hilar node (station 7) is identified in front of and between the right upper lobe bronchus and the bronchus intermedius while the subcarinal lymph node (station 8) is identified between the right and left main bronchi at or near the level of the right upper lobe bronchus. During bronchoscopy when the right upper lobe bronchus is in view these two stations can be identified and targeted. To sample station 7, the needle is placed in the anterior portion of right upper lobe spur with sampling of station 8 accomplished by placing the needle at the medial wall of the right main bronchus at about the nine o'clock position just proximal to the level of the right upper lobe orifice.

The third level identified is at the level of the bronchus intermedius near the take-off of the right middle lobe orifice. At this level, station 9 (right lower hilar lymph node) and 10 (sub-subcarinal lymph node) are identified. The right

lower hilar lymph node (station 9) is located on the CT scan as lateral or in front of the bronchus intermedius at or near the level of the right middle lobe bronchus with the sub-subcarinal lymph node (station 10) located between the bronchus intermedius and left main bronchus at or near the level of the right middle lobe bronchus. During bronchoscopy, with the bronchus intermedius in view, stations 9 and 10 are identified and targeted. To sample station 9, a puncture should be made at the anterior or lateral wall of the bronchus intermedius at about the 3 o'clock position and the 12 o'clock position near or at the level of the right middle lobe orifice, with sampling of station 10 performed by inserting the needle at the medial wall of the bronchus intermedius at about the 9 o'clock position, just proximal to the level of the right middle lobe orifice. The fourth and final level is seen in the left main bronchus at the level of the spur between the left upper and lower lobes. On CT scan, the left hilar node is identified between the left upper lobe and left lower lobe bronchus and labeled station 11. To sample station 11 a puncture should be made along the lateral wall of the left lower lobe bronchus at approximately the 9 o'clock position at the level of the superior segment orifice of the orifice of the left lower lobe.

While blind sampling of the eleven nodal stations may be performed without serious complication (with the exception of station 2 as noted above), particularly in the presence of endobronchial abnormalities such as mucosal irregularities or widening of the main or secondary carina, it is helpful to correlate the proposed puncture site with a CT of the chest. Upon review it will be noted that there will exist minor variations in locations regarding the described anatomy. The CT of the chest will then provide a road map to identifying involvement of the various stations. It will also be noted that stations 1, 3 and 5, defined as the right mediastinal lymph node chain, are often all involved in metastatic disease and are difficult to separate from one another. It will further be noted that when sampling the AP window, if the needle is placed too high the aorta may be punctured and if placed too low the pulmonary artery may be punctured, making it important to puncture station 4 as horizontal to the trachea as possible. Puncture of the right upper and lower hilar nodes can be seen to sometimes result in bloody aspiration because of the proximity of the superior pulmonary vein in the case of the right upper hilar node and right main pulmonary artery to the right lower hilar node.

As noted above, the range of each station can be variable. The important criteria for stations 1 and 2 are that they are anterior or posterior to the carina, although they can extend from the tip of the carina to the proximal portion of the right and left main bronchus, and occasionally to the level of the right upper lobe bronchus. The right paratracheal lymph node (station 3) can extend superiorly proximal to the brachiocephalic artery. The left paratracheal station (AP, station 4) can be at the level of the lower trachea at the tracheobronchial angulation or along the left main bronchus. When the right upper lobe bronchus is visible on the CT scan, any lymph node anterior to the right upper lobar spur is defined as the right upper hilar node. Also, nodal stations 9 and 10 can often be seen on CT scan to extend below the right middle lobe bronchus. The left hilar lymph node (station 11) can be located near the tip of the left upper spur or may be as low as the superior segment of the left lower lobe [5,44].

This 11 nodal station system, as defined by Wang, is not meant to be a major modification of the existing AJCC and ATS systems [5]. Rather, it is to be utilized as a framework whereby endoscopic visualization may be correlated with defined lymph node stations in existing traditional systems and correlated with CT findings. AJCC stations 1, 2, 3, and 4 are combined as station 3 in this system, owing to the fact that stations 1, 2, and 3 in the AJCC system are rarely involved without involvement of station 4. AJCC stations 5 and 6 are able to be sampled only by TTNA or mediastinotomy and are thus eliminated in this 11-station system. Station 7 is expanded to include the anterior and posterior carina as well as sub- and sub-subcarinal lymph nodes as these are considered central mediastinal N2 stations. Stations 8 and 10 may represent some paraesophageal or pulmonary ligament lymph nodes. Only stations 7, 9, and 11 are considered as N1 hilar lymph nodes, which is equivalent to station 11 interlobar lymph node by the AJCC and ATS systems. Station 5 and 6, the right and left main bronchus nodes, are considered as N2 mediastinal in our system which are N2 in the ATS system and the most recent AJCC system.

## Indications

The original intent of transbronchial needle aspiration was described by Schieppati in the English language version of his work in 1958. In this article he stated "this method permits the exploration of important lymphatic areas which are difficult to approach by any other means" [15]. With the improvement in the design of available needles and their modification to be used through the flexible bronchoscope, the utility of transbronchial needle aspiration has greatly expanded. With this expansion, the potential for the diagnostic and therapeutic use of the transbronchial needle technique has also become more powerful. The technique section of this paper has briefly outlined the multiple staging areas available to be sampled, as well as commenting on obtaining specimens from those peripheral lesions. This section will summarize the indications and potential for the technique for those endoscopic and pathologic abnormalities that are most often encountered by the bronchoscopist [30].

### Endobronchial lesions
TBNA is useful in the diagnosis of intraluminal masses, necrotic, or submucosal lesions [31,45]. This is best exemplified by those tumors that are more vascular in nature or tend to bleed easily, such as carcinoids. In this instance the needle puncture will cause less bleeding than brushing or biopsy techniques (Figs 11.15 and 11.16). TBNA may also be used to sample necrotic or submucosal lesions without repeatedly sampling the superficial necrotic area or normal mucosa. Shure and Fedullo studied 31 patients with endobronchial lesions using a combination of wash, brush, forceps, and TBNA techniques. They found that a successful diagnosis was obtained in 71% with TBNA alone [46]. A subsequent study under the direction of Mehta's bronchoscopy suite by Dasgupta *et al.* revealed that TBNA was able to provide a diagnosis in 95.6% of patients with endobronchial lesions, surpassing the combined yield of all other

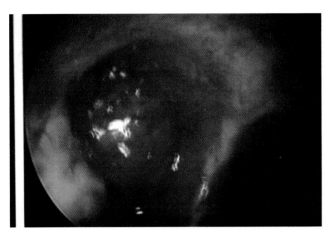

**Fig. 11.15** Endobronchial polypoid lesion obstructing the left main bronchus.

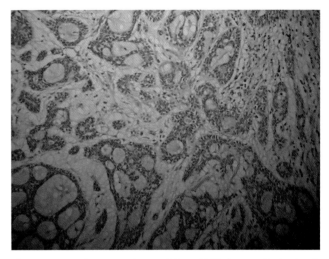

**Fig. 11.16** Cytology smear from endobronchial lesion seen in Fig. 11.15 demonstrating adenocystic carcinoma.

**Table 11.4** Diagnostic yield from individual procedures and their combinations

| Procedures | EML (n = 32) Number (%) | SPD (n = 23) Number (%) | Total (n = 55) Number (%) | Exclusively diagnostic Number (%) |
|---|---|---|---|---|
| BW | 10 (31) | 5 (22) | 15 (27) | 0 (0) |
| BB | 19 (59) | 11 (48) | 30 (55) | 2 (6) |
| EBB | 23 (72) | 10 (43) | 33 (60) | 1 (3) |
| TBNA | 25 (78) | 22 (96) | 47 (85) | 11 (20) |
| EBB + BB | 26 (81) | 14 (61) | 40 (73) | |
| | 27 (84) | 22 (96) | 49 (89) | |
| TBNA + BB | 30 (94) | 22 (96) | 52 (95) | |
| EBB + BB + TBNA | 31 (97) | 22 (96) | 53 (96) | |

SPD, submucosal and peribronchial disease; EML, exophytic mass lesion.

From: Dasgupta A, Jain P, Minai OA. Utility of transbronchial needle aspiration in the diagnosis of endobronchial lesions. *Chest* 1999; **115**: 1237–41.

procedures (Table 11.4) [47]. The comparison of CDT (conventional diagnostic procedures) which included forceps biopsy, wash, and brush plus the utilization of TBNA in patients with exophytic mass lesions, submucosal disease, and peribronchial disease was again reviewed in 2005 [48]. This review of 115 lung cancer cases from 2001 to 2003 demonstrated an overall significant improvement in the diagnostic yield when TBNA was performed in addition to CDT ($P < 0.001$). Also, the increased sensitivity in peribronchial disease with TBNA, from 52 to 87% ($P < 0.001$), was statistically significant, with a notable improvement in the sensitivity in exophytic mass lesions and submucosal disease from 85 to 100% and 84 to 97%, respectively.

### Cystic lesions of the lung

Up to 20% of all mediastinal masses in adults are due to cystic lesions whose origins are predominately pericardial,

bronchogenic, and enteric [49,50]. Bronchogenic and esophageal cysts, as well as possible mediastinal abscesses, are able to be sampled easily for diagnosis, and using needles with excellent suction ability (e.g. MW-122) therapeutic aspiration may also be accomplished [51–55].

Mediastinal cysts result from anomalous budding of the primitive foregut and early tracheobronchial tree and makeup to 9% of all primary mediastinal tumors in surgical series [56–58]. Each type of foregut cyst has typical histologic features and characteristic anatomic locations within the chest and may present as an incidental finding on chest films or routine esophagrams [59]. Distinction between types of congenital cysts is sometimes difficult, however, as they share overlapping anatomic locations and histologic features [50]. Also, when inflammation and hemorrhage occur in the foregut cyst, the type-specific lining may be replaced by non-specific granulation tissue with non-specific cysts accounting for 17 to 20% of all foregut cysts [57,60].

Bronchogenic cysts are the most common intrathoracic foregut cysts, accounting for 54 to 63% of cases in surgical series [57,59,60]. Early in embryogenesis the lung begins as a ventral diverticulum that arises from the primitive foregut. This diverticulum then undergoes a series of buddings that result in the tracheobronchial tree and alveoli. Aberrant buds give rise to cystic structures that may or may not communicate with the bronchial tree and rarely occur in an endobronchial location [50,60]. These bronchogenic cysts are typically lined by ciliated columnar epithelium and pseudostratified squamous epithelium and may also contain bronchial glands or bronchial cartilage [50,59,60]. Bronchogenic cysts may be either parenchymal or mediastinal in location and most commonly occur in paratracheal, carinal, hilar, and paraesophageal sites.

Esophageal duplication cysts are uncommon and constitute 0.5 to 2.5% of all esophageal masses and make up 10 to 15% of all alimentary tract duplications [61,62]. Most esophageal duplication cysts are discovered in children, but up to 25 to 30% are not found until adulthood [61].

The primitive foregut begins to elongate at about the fourth week of embryologic development with the proliferation of lining cells producing a nearly solid tube. By the sixth week, however, small holes or vacuoles begin to arise in the tube and coalesce to form the lumen of the esophagus. Duplication cysts arise when isolated vacuoles fail to coalesce with the rest of the lumen [56,59,61,62].

Histologically, esophageal duplication cysts contain a double layer of smooth muscle without cartilage [50]. They may also contain gastric mucosa leading to peptic ulceration or hemorrhage [50,59]. Technetium 99 m sodium pertechnetate scans show uptake of tracer in some duplications,

indicating the presence of ectopic gastric mucosa [63]. Esophageal duplication cysts may be found adjacent to the esophagus throughout its course, with 60% located around the lower third of the esophagus. The remainder are found near the upper or middle third of the esophagus in equal numbers [61]. Although a paraesophageal location is common for duplication cysts, they may also be intramural in location.

Neurenteric cysts are part of the split notochord syndrome, which occurs when a portion of the yolk sac and primitive foregut herniates through a gap and attaches itself to the dorsal ectoderm or primitive skin tissue [59]. Neurenteric cysts have a smooth muscle wall, similar to the gastrointestinal tract, but a variable epithelial lining. Associated spinal defects such as hemivertebrae, butterfly vertebrae, and scoliosis are common, usually with the position of the cyst below the vertebral abnormality [59,64]. A connection may or may not exist between the neurenteric cyst and the thoracic spine meninges, but communication with the actual subarachnoid space is unusual.

Although usually asymptomatic, mediastinal cysts may produce symptoms by compressing adjacent structures, such as the esophagus with resultant dysphagia, or the tracheobronchial tree leading to dyspnea or persistent cough. Bleeding or infection may cause the cyst to enlarge, exacerbating symptoms [61].

The majority of benign mediastinal cysts have a characteristic CT appearance as a well-defined, cystic mass, with homogenous low CT attenuation in the range of water density (0 to 20 Hounsfield units, HU) (Figs 11.17–11.19). The cystic mass shows a thin or imperceptible wall and demonstrates no enhancement with intravenous contrast injection. A number of other disease processes may produce mediastinal masses with low CT attenuation. They include

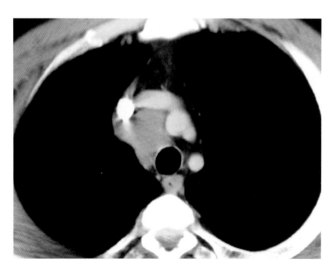

**Fig. 11.17** A right paratracheal mass with CT features of benign mediastinal cyst with homogenous attenuation measuring 10 to 20 HU is identified. Courtesy of CDR, Robert Browning, MD.

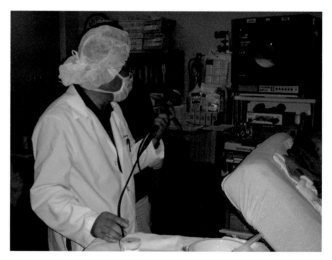

**Fig. 11.18** Dr Ko-Pen Wang preparing bronchoscope for diagnostic-therapeutic TBNA of right paratracheal mass seen in Fig. 11.17. Courtesy of CDR, Robert Browning, MD.

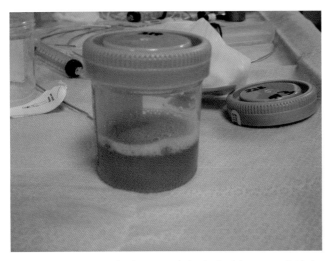

**Fig. 11.19** The paratracheal cyst was drained, obtaining serous fluid via TBNA aspiration. Courtesy of CDR, Robert Browning, MD.

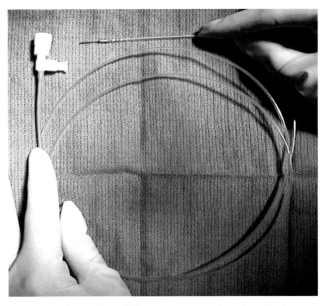

**Fig. 11.20** The transbronchial or transesophageal needle aspiration system. A beveled needle is attached to a semitransparent sheath. An inner steel stylet traverses the sheath providing rigidity during aspiration procedure. Proximal side port used for syringe.

metastases from testicular tumors, cystic metastases from ovarian or gastric cancer, abscesses, resolving hematomas, treated or untreated lymphoma, hydatid cysts, lymphoceles, seromas, and some neurogenic tumors [65,66]. The CT attenuation of these masses is rarely as low as water density, and seldom do these mediastinal masses fulfill the other CT criteria for diagnosing a benign mediastinal cyst [55,67,68]. Although most benign mediastinal cysts demonstrate CT attenuation values in the range of 0 to 20 HU, occasionally a mediastinal cyst will be found with a higher CT density than water. This is most often due to the presence of milk of calcium, proteinaceous fluid, mucus, or blood debris within the cyst [69–71]. One can often suspect the correct diagnosis of benign mediastinal cyst, however, even in these cases because of the characteristic shape and location of the lesion, its homogenous appearance, and the complete absence of contrast enhancement [72].

MRI appearances of the mediastinal cysts include the presence of a well-defined, rounded mass in the middle and posterior mediastinum [73,74]. MRI may also demonstrate the presence of hemorrhage in some mediastinal cysts.

When the presumptive diagnosis of a benign mediastinal cyst is made with imaging procedures, the asymptomatic individual or elderly patient may be followed conservatively with serial CT examinations to ensure stability of the size and character of the lesion over time. A more definitive answer, however, is required when the patient is symptomatic, if signs and symptoms suggest possible malignancy, or the lesion changes in size or shape over time. Abnormalities in the paratracheal and carinal areas have traditionally been diagnosed and treated with mediastinoscopy or thoracotomy, however, by utilizing transbronchial or transesophageal needle aspiration both a diagnosis and therapy may be accomplished [51,52,54,55,67,75,76]. This application of

TBNA was well described by McDougal and Fromme, who reported a patient with severe airway obstruction from a subcarinal cyst complicating ventilation during general anesthesia. They elected to decompress the cyst via flexible bronchoscopy allowing for more effective ventilation during general anesthesia [53]. This technique was also utilized in a patient with central airway stenosis secondary to a mediastinal cyst using a 22-gauge TBNA needle and without recurrence at 1-year follow-up [77].

The procedure is performed in the operating room or endoscopy suite with conscious sedation utilizing an opiod and bensodiazepine, such as fentanyl and midazolam, along with sequential topical anesthesia of the nasal cavity, nasopharynx, and oropharynx with 2% Xylocaine [75].

Based on the CT findings, the flexible bronchoscope is introduced to the appropriate level. The biopsy sheath system consisting of a semitransparent polyethylene sheath 120 cm long with an attached 18-, 21-, or 22-gauge needle, 12 mm in length (C.R. Bard, Inc., Billerica, MA) (Fig. 11.20) is passed through the scope until the needle projects just beyond the end of the scope. The stylet is retracted slightly and the needle aimed at the target site. The stylet is then further retracted and the cyst is aspirated using a 30- or 50-mL syringe containing 3 mL normal saline or Hank's balanced solution attached to the proximal luer-lock port. Cytopathology and cultures of the aspirated material are obtained [75]. A follow-up CT examination of the mediastinal lesion is used to determine the success of the aspiration procedure and to exclude complications such as bleeding, abscess formation, or pneumomediastinum.

## Granulomatous disease

Granulomatous conditions, such as sarcoidosis, are effectively diagnosed by TBNA [78–81]. Utilizing a cytology TBNA needle (22 gauge), Garwood and colleagues enrolled 50 consecutive patients being evaluated for sarcoidosis [79]. In this study, 82 lymph nodes with a median size of 16 mm were punctured, demonstrating non-caseating granulomas in 85% with a final diagnosis of sarcoidosis. Granulomatous disease, sometimes, requires a larger biopsy specimen in order to be able to view the proper architecture for diagnosis, as suggested by Mehta and Meeker commenting on the Cleveland Clinic experience, to obtain histology specimens with TBNA [80]. TBNA for histology core biopsy was performed using the 18-gauge or newer 19-gauge histology needle (MW-319). Histology samples were judged to be adequate in 25 of these patients, with 16 being diagnostic. In these 25 patients, nine procedures were performed to diagnose benign disease; four of nine biopsies were diagnostic with two being "exclusively diagnostic" of sarcoidosis. The remaining positive sample was diagnostic of histoplasmosis. Of the four "non-diagnostic" specimens, one patient was diagnosed with sarcoidosis and three were found to have benign conditions (mesothelioma, silicosis, empyema). There were no false positives with the overall positive predictive value of the test (including both benign and malignant conditions) being 100% with a specificity of 100% and sensitivity of 61%. Morales *et al.* employed TBNA in 51 consecutive patients suspected of having sarcoidosis. In patients with stage I and II disease, TBNA was able to establish a diagnosis in 53 and 48%, respectively, with Leonard *et al.* combining the techniques of transbronchial biopsy, BAL, and TBNA for a diagnostic sensitivity of 100% in sarcoidosis [82,83]. Thus with the introduction the 19-gauge histology biopsy needle, TBNA has proven to be useful in the diagnosis of benign granulomatous conditions with one author commenting that it may become a preferred procedure in conditions such as sarcoidosis, lymphoma, and other conditions presenting with mediastinal mass [54,55,84].

## Infectious disease

TBNA in the diagnosis of infectious disease has also proved valuable [85–92]. Harkin *et al.* performed 44 procedures in 41 HIV-infected patients with mediastinal or hilar adenopathy, reported in 1998. Mycobacterial disease was present in 52% of these patients with TBNA providing the diagnosis in 87%, with a follow-up study in 2006 reviewing a 15-year experience demonstrating TBNA having a yield of 82% in mycobacterial disease, 75% in fungal disease, and providing the only diagnostic specimen in 35% of cases [90,93]. TBNA has also been shown useful in the diagnosis of additional infections, including *Pneumocystis carinii*, histoplasmosis, and cryptococcus [94,95] (Figs 11.21 and 11.22).

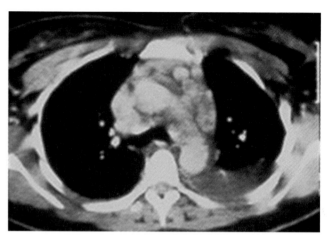

**Fig. 11.21** CT scan demonstrating mediastinal adenopathy and left parenchymal consolidation with subsequent TBNA of a station 4 lymph node.

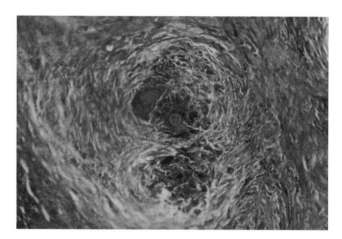

**Fig. 11.22** TBNA smear from station 4 of the CT scan seen in Fig. 11.21, demonstrating coccidiomycosis.

## Peripheral pulmonary lesions

Since the publication of the second edition of Flexible Bronchoscopy, the utilization of TBNA in the diagnosis of peripheral pulmonary lesions has been more widely utilized, with the supplementary use of image guidance techniques, such as radial ultrasound and electromagnetic navigational bronchoscopy. Peripheral pulmonary lesions, particularly solitary pulmonary nodules without evidence of mediastinal adenopathy, are most often approached for diagnosis by TTNA or excisional biopsy by VATS procedure or traditional thoracotomy. In 1994, Wang *et al.* published a prospective study of 329 patients undergoing transbronchial needle aspiration for cytology or histology where TBNA was found to establish the diagnosis of malignant or benign disease in 68% [96] (Table 11.5). Of those lesions limited to the periphery, without mediastinal involvement, the diagnostic yield

**Table 11.5** TBNA and TTNA results for 329 patients

| | Total TBNA cases (329; 100%) | | | Total TTNA cases (105; 31.9%) | | |
| --- | --- | --- | --- | --- | --- | --- |
| | C | Both C and P | P | C | Both C and P | P |
| No. of cases | 169 | 329 | 160 | 18 | 105 | 87 |
| Diagnosed | 151 (89.3%) | 224 (68.1%) | 73 (45.6%) | 15 (83.3%) | 73 (69.5%) | 58 (66.7%) |
| Undiagnosed | 18 (10.7%) | 105 (31.9%) | 87 (54.4%) | 3 (16.7%) | 32 (31.5%) | 29 (33.3%) |

C, central lesion—mediastinal and hilar lymph node; P, peripheral lesion—lung parenchymal nodule or mass.

From: Wang KP, Gonullu U, Baker R. Transbronchial needle aspiration vs. transthoracic needle aspiration in the diagnosis of pulmonary lesions. *J Bronchol* 1994; **1**: 199–204.

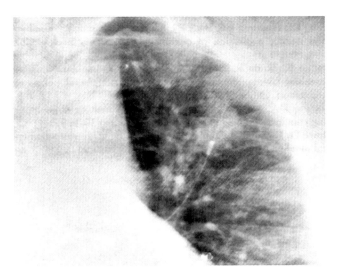

**Fig. 11.23** Chest X ray demonstrating left upper lobe nodule with TBNA placed for diagnosis.

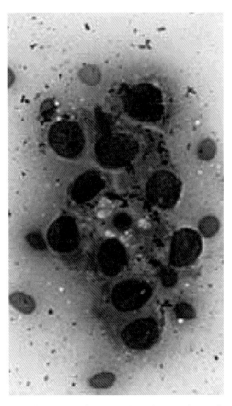

**Fig. 11.24** Cytology smear demonstrating adenocarcinoma from the TBNA performed in Fig. 11.23.

of TBNA was 45.6%. While the diagnostic yield of TTNA, compared with TBNA, in those pulmonary lesions without mediastinal or hilar involvement was greater at 66.7%, the rate of pneumothorax complication was much higher and the authors concluded in those patients having pulmonary lesions without mediastinal or hilar involvement, TBNA should be considered first (Figs 11.23 and 11.24). It should also be noted in this study that 8.8% of diagnosis by TBNA was of benign lesions. Of these 20 benign diagnoses, 16 were sarcoidosis (80%), two were bronchogenic cysts (10%), one was mycetoma (5%), and one was due to tuberculosis (5%). In evaluating a peripheral lesion for the utility of TBNA, the sensitivity of the technique will often be related to the tumor–bronchus relationship, the size of the target, and the location in the pulmonary field. Four types of tumor–bronchus relationship have been described (Fig. 11.25) [37]. Type I has a patent bronchial lumen to the mass. Type II has tumor mass surrounding and invading the bronchus. Type III has extrinsic compression of the bronchus by the tumor.

Type IV has extrinsic compression of the bronchus by tumor spread to the peribronchial lymph nodes or the submucosa. The role of TBNA in each of these classifications is beneficial and additive to traditional cytology and transbronchial forceps, which cannot penetrate the bronchial wall. In 1999, a review of TBNA use at the University Hospital in Basal, Switzerland, Reichenberger *et al.* utilized TBNA in the diagnosis of peripheral pulmonary lesions in 172 patients [97]. In 87 patients (51%), a final diagnosis was established by bronchoscopy, with TBNA used in 152 of the 172 patients (89%). TBNA demonstrated a positive result in 35% of

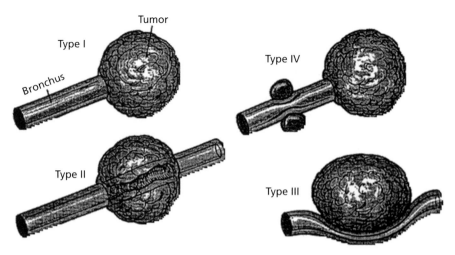

**Fig. 11.25** Tumor–bronchial relationship. From: Dasgupta A, Mehta AC. Transbronchial needle aspiration: an underused diagnostic technique. *Clin Chest Med* 1999; **20**: 45.

cases, in comparison to 17% for transbronchial biopsy, 22% for bronchial washing, and 30% for bronchial brushing. TBNA was diagnostic in 27.5% of malignant lesions less than 3 cm in diameter and in 65% for lesions greater than 3 cm. The use of TBNA increased the diagnostic yield of bronchoscopy from 35 to 51% without additional risk of complications. Baaklini *et al.* studied the effectiveness of TBNA taking into account the location of the lesion (outer one-third versus inner two-thirds) in the pulmonary parenchyma and the size of the lesion [98]. They found that overall the diagnostic accuracy of bronchoscopy in malignant and benign lesions was 64% (97 of 151) and 35% (9 of 26), respectively. The ability to obtain a diagnosis was related to the size of the lesion size ($P < 0.001$) and distance from the hilum. Lesions less than 2 cm had a diagnostic yield of 14% (2 of 14) when located in the peripheral one-third versus 31% (5 of 16) when located in the inner two-thirds of the lung. Transbronchial biopsy, washing, and brushing were complementary in obtaining a diagnosis with flexible bronchoscopy. The studies by Wang, Reichenberger, and Baalini were performed with standard imaging techniques such as fluoroscopy. The development of additional imaging modalities has led to renewed interest in TBNA for peripheral lesions. In a prospective study, 362 patients were identified as having a peripheral pulmonary lesion [99]. The addition of TBNA to EBUS plus biopsy and wash compared to EBUS plus biopsy and wash alone resulted is a significant improvement in diagnostic yield ($P = 0.015$). Electromagnetic navigation-guided (ENB) bronchoscopy has also been developed, with encouraging studies [100,101]. A recent study using ENB without fluoroscopy showed an improved diagnostic ability with an overall yield of 77.2% when the divergence from the target was less than 4 mm, and an overall yield of 56–73% in T1 and T2 lesions, respectively [102].

## Staging of bronchogenic carcinoma

We feel that the potential for the most powerful application of this technique lies in the staging bronchogenic carcinoma. A complete review of the lymphatic anatomy of the lung and mediastinum is given in the chapter on relevant anatomy. It is well recognized that the spread of bronchogenic carcinoma to the mediastinal lymph nodes has a major effect on the prognosis for patients. Carcinomas of the lung most commonly first metastasize to the immediate surrounding segmental and bronchial lymph nodes with eventual extension to hilar, central mediastinal, and, finally, contralateral nodes. As the prognostic value of this spread is important, not only to the individual patient, but also to the study of lung cancer, a detailed staging system has been developed over the years [103–107]. In 1973, the American Joint Committee on Cancer utilized the TNM classification system for the staging of bronchogenic carcinoma. This was later revised to eliminate problems with the combination of various stages. The seventh edition of the TNM system has been published after review of detailed proposals by the International Staging Project of the International Association for the Study of Lung Cancer (IASLC) [108]. This revised staging system has been adopted by the AJCC and the International Union Against Cancer. The AJCC has recommended that each patient with bronchogenic carcinoma receive a clinical diagnostic staging to aid in their treatment and prognosis. As reviewed in the relevant anatomy section, the 11 nodal staging system is not in conflict with the AJCC system of staging, but is a modification to allow bronchoscopists to easily correlate endoscopic landmarks with CT imaging to improve the diagnostic yield of TBNA and thereby staging without more invasive operative procedures, such as mediastinotomy or thoracotomy. Although it has been suggested that CT or MRI may be a way of non-invasively staging the extent of disease, an extensive review of the literature in 1994 by Grover concluded that the use of CT in the staging of N2 disease had a sensitivity of 70–90%, specificity of 60–90%, and an accuracy of only 66–90%, depending on the definitions used for determining negative or positive adenopathy and on subsequent follow-up with surgical staging [109]. Building on advances in both nuclear medicine and CT imaging, integrated positron emission tomography with CT (PET/CT) has shown improvement in non-invasive staging in regards to T, N, and M staging. A review of pooled data for N-staging demonstrated an accuracy of 87% versus 82% for PET and 73% for CT [110].

As noted in the Lung Cancer Guideline published by the American College of Chest Physicians in 2007, the non-invasive staging of bronchogenic carcinoma provides important information utilizing both CT and PET imaging [111]. CT scanning is noted to provide anatomic detail with PET scanning having an improved sensitivity and specificity compared to CT scanning. However, as noted in the guidelines, abnormal imaging must be confirmed by tissue to assure accurate staging.

As "tissue is the issue," TBNA by flexible bronchoscopy is both sensitive and specific in the sampling for mediastinal involvement [112,113]. The sensitivity and specificity of transbronchial needle aspiration has been well documented in the literature [26–29,96,114]. In a seminal prospective study by Wang *et al.*, the diagnostic yield was 89.3% for mediastinal lesions and 45.6% for those lung lesions without abnormal mediastinal or hilar areas [96]. The overall diagnostic rate was 68.1%. Although lower yields have been reported, a series of complimentary educational interventions to promote consistency in TBNA performance over a 3-year period at Indiana University and the Bowman-Gray School of Medicine, demonstrated a significant increase in TBNA yield from 21.4 to 47.6% [115]. Subsequent investigations have confirmed that increased experience with TBNA results in increased yield [116,117].

Thus, by combining the information gleaned from evaluation by synergistic imaging techniques and during endoscopic evaluation, the most contralateral nodal station to the supposed primary is first sampled, prior to any bordering adenopathy or complete tracheobronchial inspection. This will allow for the least chance of possible contamination of the working channel and needle before attempting to sample more adjacent adenopathy or the lesion itself. A positive diagnosis from the most contralateral adenopathy will effectively stage the patient according to the TNM classification. Although a negative aspirate at a particular station does not completely rule out that nodal station's involvement as expressed in the sensitivity of the procedure, false positives have been rarely reported [118]. We believe the proper application of this technique to be a reliable and effective, minimally invasive tool in the staging of bronchogenic carcinoma.

## Complications and limitations

The major complication of TBNA is perforation of the working channel of the bronchoscope. This can be successfully avoided by close attention to technique and the needle's position. The use of TBNA overall is very safe with no reported major complications. Although minor fever has been reported after TBNA to approximately 38°C (100.4°F) blood cultures drawn at 5 and 30 minutes following needle aspiration were not associated with any clinically detectable bacteremia and no antimicrobial prophylaxis was felt to be required [119]. A prospective study of 67 patients who underwent a total of 351 fine needle passes with subsequent blood cultures demonstrated no significant bacteremia and fever in only 3% [120]. One case of purulent pericarditis from polymicrobial mouth flora in a patient with multiple myeloma after TBNA of a subcarinal mass has been reported, with the patient surviving the infection [121]. A second case of mediastinitis and purulent pericarditis, presumed secondary to EBUS-TBNA, was presented in abstract form in 2008 [122]. Although the rare occurrence of a pneumothorax associated with puncture of the posterior carinal node or with TBNA of a peripheral lesion has been noted, as well as a case of hemomediastinum after transbronchial needle aspiration, no major sequelae have resulted [123]. The major limitations of this procedure are of two types and are related to equipment and operator experience. Damage to the working channel of the bronchoscope was reported when non-retractable needles were first utilized and although scope damage has been reported with a 19-gauge needle, careful use of the instruments makes this problem unusual [124,125].

The diagnostic sensitivity of TBNA has also been commented upon as limiting the usefulness of this technique. A detailed understanding by the operator of the target to be approached and application of the existing technology, however, will serve to increase yield. CT guidance for TBNA of mediastinal adenopathy was also evaluated by Rong and Cui, who proposed multiple static CT images while the patient was undergoing bronchoscopy to localize the needle tip location [126]. They reported a significant increase in sensitivity, from 20 to 60%, and noted that this technique may also increase the specificity of the procedure as three patients were found to have mediastinal abscesses. Also, as noted above by Haponik, educational initiatives to train bronchoscopists in this technique are successful in increasing success [115]. Therefore, it is incumbent upon the bronchoscopist to have an understanding of the technical and prognostic implications of TBNA for benign and malignant disease and in the staging of bronchogenic carcinoma and to work closely with the pathologist in the interpretation of these results. It is standard practice in our bronchoscopy suites for the bronchoscopy technicians to be specially trained in the smear technique and for the bronchoscopist to consult with the attending pathologist regarding the facts of the case and subsequently review our own cytologic and histologic material. This is to assure that the bronchoscopist and cytopathologist are clear as to the specimen's station of origin, as well as the adequacy of the specimen obtained. Diette and Davenport have concluded that the availability of rapid, on-site evaluation of samples (ROSE) by a cytopathologist improved the diagnostic yield when sampling lung nodules or hilar and mediastinal adenopathy [127,128]. A subsequent study by Baram et al. of 44 bronchoscopies with TBNA showed that the diagnostic sensitivity (79–98%), accuracy (85–99%), and procedural time were similar between those procedures performed with and without ROSE; however, fewer additional biopsies allowed for a decrease in use of radiology and pathology resources [129].

The number of punctures performed with the TBNA technique to obtain the maximum yield has been reviewed as well. Shure recommended at least three TBNA aspirates be performed for each target site, consistent with original reports by Wang [29,130]. In a prospective study of 79 patients, Chin et al. performed 451 aspirates with a mean of 5.7 aspirates per patient and a positive diagnosis of malignancy in 57% [131]. It was notable that in patients where ROSE was used (55 patients) a positive diagnosis was obtained in 71%, versus 25% (six patients) where ROSE was not employed. Importantly, 77% of diagnostic aspirates for malignancy were obtained in the first four attempts, and 93% of diagnostic aspirates were obtained in the first four attempts at a single nodal location. This study demonstrated improved yield from subcarinal (64%) and right paratracheal (38%) lymph nodes, with fewer samples needed for a diagnosis of small cell carcinoma compared to non-small cell carcinoma. Herth and Becker comparing conventional TBNA to EBUS-TBNA noted the average number of aspirates needed were four with EBUS-TBNA, statistically improving the yield [132].

With the use of EBUS-TBNA, Lee et al. prospectively enrolled 106 patients with lymph nodes between 5 and 20 mm on axial CT scan, judged to be accessible for biopsy [133]. The stations approached were noted to be the right and left paratracheal nodes and subcarinal nodes (AJCC 2 R,L; 4 R,L, 7) with the medial short axis size on CT scan to be 8.6 mm. The sampling adequacy was 90.1% for one aspiration and reached 100% for three aspirations. In this study the positive predictive value was 100%, with a sensitivity and specificity of predicating mediastinal metastasis being 93.8 and 100%, respectively, with the conclusion that optimal results can be obtained in three aspirations with EBUS-TBNA for mediastinal staging of non-small cell carcinoma. In addition, Kanoh et al. have found that with the utilization of endobronchial ultrasound and a double-channel bronchoscope the mean number of penetrations needed for diagnosis was only 1.24 [134].

TBNA must also be utilized with a clear understanding of the sensitivity and specificity of the technique itself. As discussed above, although false positives are not of serious concern with proper technique and specimen handling, false negative results are possible as defined by the overall sensitivity of the procedure. In this regard, should a negative result be obtained by TBNA, and there remains a clinical suspicion of malignancy, the patient should be referred for more invasive diagnostic or therapeutic procedures such as mediastinotomy or thoracotomy.

Transbronchial needle aspiration is, therefore, an essential instrument in the accurate diagnosis of both benign and malignant disease. Moreover, accuracy in the staging of bronchogenic carcinoma and the possible therapeutic applications, as discussed, make the application of TBNA an essential component of the bronchoscopic procedure.

## References

1 Wang KP, Terry P, Marsh B. Bronchoscopic needle aspiration biopsy of paratracheal tumors. *Am Rev Respir Dis* 1978; **118**: 17–21.

2 Wang KP, Haponik EF, Gupta PK, Erozan YS. Flexible transbronchial needle aspiration: Technical Considerations. *Ann Otol Rhinol Laryngol* 1984; **93**: 233–6.

3 Wang KP. Transbronchial needle aspiration. "How I Do It." *J Bronchol* 1994; **1**: 63–8.

4 Wang KP. Transbronchial needle aspiration to obtain histology specimen. *J Bronchol* 1994; **1**: 116–22.

5 Wang KP. Staging of bronchogenic carcinoma by bronchoscopy. *Chest* 1994; **106**: 588–93.

6 Prakash UBS, Offord KP, Stubbs SE. Bronchoscopy in North America: The ACCP survey. *Chest* 1991; **100**: 1668–75.

7 Colt HG, Prakash UBS, Offord KP. Bronchoscopy in North America. Survey by the American Association for Bronchology, 1999. *J Bronchol* 2000; **7**: 8–25.

8 Smyth CM, Stead RJ. Survey of fiberoptic bronchoscopy in the United Kingdom. *Eur Respir J* 2002; **19**: 458–63.

9 Herth FJ, Becker HD, Ernst A. Ultrasound-guided transbronchial needle aspiration. *Chest* 2003; **123**: 604–7.

10 Ost D, Shah R, Anasco E, et al. A randomized trial of CT fluoroscopic-guided bronchoscopy vs. conventional bronchoscopy in patients with suspected lung cancer. *Chest* 2008; **134**: 507–13.

11 Gildea TR, Mazzone PJ, Karnak D, et al. Electromagnetic navigation diagnostic bronchoscopy. *Am J Respir Crit Care Med* 2006; **174**: 982–9.

12 Turner JF. Endobronchial ultrasound and peripheral pulmonary lesions. localization and histopathological correlates using a miniature probe and the flexible bronchoscope. *Chest* 2002; **122**: 1874–5.

13 Alberts WM. Diagnosis and management of lung cancer executive summary. ACCP evidence-based clinical practice guidelines (2nd edition). *Chest* 2007; **132**: 1S–19S.

14 Schiepatti E. La puncion mediastinal atraves del espolon traquea review. *Rev Asoc Med Argent* 1949; **663**: 497–9.

15 Schiepatti E. Mediastinal lymph node puncture through the tracheal carina. *Surg Gynecol Obstet* 1958; **110**: 243–6.

16 Crymes TP, Fish RG, Smith DE, *et al.* Complications of transbronchial left atrial puncture. *Am Heart J* 1959; **58**: 46.

17 Versteegh RM, Swierenga J. Bronchoscopic evaluation of the operability of pulmonary carcinoma. *Acta Otolaryngol* (Stockh) 1963; **56**: 603–11.

18 Fox RT, Lees WM, Shields TW. Transcarinal bronchoscopic needle biopsy. *Ann Thorac Surg* 1965; **1**: 92–6.

19 Simecek C. Cytological investigation of intrathoracic lymph nodes in carcinoma of the lung. *Thorax* 1966; **21**: 369–71.

20 Bridgeman AH, Duffield GD, Takaro T. An appraisal of newer diagnostic methods for intrathoracic lesions. *Dis Chest* 1968; **53**: 321–7.

21 Atay Z, Brandt HJ. Die Bedeutung Der Zytodiagnostik Der Perbronchialen Feinnadelpunktion von mediastinalen oder ilaren Tumoren. *Dtsch Med Wochenschr* 1977; **102**: 345–8.

22 Lemer J, Malberger E, Konig-Nativ R. Transbronchial fine needle aspiration. *Thorax* 1982; **37**: 270–4.

23 Ikeda S. Flexible Bronchofiberscope. *Ann Otol* 1970; **79**: 916.

24 Ikeda S. The development and progress of endoscopes in the field of bronchoesophagology. *J Jap Bronchoesophagol Soc* 1988; **39**: 85–96.

25 Wang KP. "How I Do It: "Transbronchial Needle Aspiration. *J Bronchol* 1994; **1**: 63–8.

26 Shure D, Fedullo PF. The role of transcarinal needle aspiration in the staging of bronchogenic carcinoma. *Chest* 1984; **96**: 693–6.

27 Shure D, Fedullo PF. Transbronchial needle aspiration and diagnosis of submucosal and peribronchial bronchogenic carcinoma. *Chest* 1985; **88**: 49–51.

28 Schenk DA, Bryan CL, Bower JH, Myers DL. Transbronchial needle aspiration and the diagnosis of bronchogenic carcinoma. *Chest* 1987; **92**: 83–5.

29 Schure D. Transbronchial biopsy and needle aspiration. *Chest* 1989; **95**: 1130–8.

30 Wang KP. Flexible bronchoscopy with transbronchial needle aspiration: biopsy for cytology specimens. In: Wang KP, ed. *Biopsy Techniques on Pulmonary Disorders*. New York: Raven Press; 1989: 63–71.

31 Wang KP, Terry PB. Transbronchial needle aspiration in the diagnosis and staging of bronchogenic carcinoma. *Am Rev Respir Dis* 1983; **127**: 344–7.

32 Wang KP, Ndukwu AI, Davis D, *et al.* Direct smear for cytological examination of transbronchial needle aspiration specimens. *Harbor Med Rev* 1991; **2**: 10–11.

33 Wang KP. Flexible transbronchial needle aspiration biopsy for histologic specimens. *Chest* 1985; **88**: 860–3.

34 Gittlen SD, Wang KP. TBNA for histology: Can it be improved? *Chest* 1989; **96**: 1765.

35 Yung RC. Efficacy and safety of the new Excelon transbronchial needle experience with the first 50 cases. *Chest* 2004; **126**: 820S.

36 Yasufuku K, Chiyo M, Sekine Y, *et al.* Real-time endobronchial ultrasound-guided transbronchial needle aspiration of mediastinal and hilar lymph nodes. *Chest* 2004; **126**: 122–8.

37 Dasgupta A, Mehta AC. Transbronchial needle aspiration. an underused diagnostic technique. *Clin Chest Med* 1999; **20**: 39–51.

38 Wang KP. Flexible bronchoscopy with transbronchial needle aspiration: biopsy for cytology specimens. In: Wang KP, ed. *Biopsy Techniques in Pulmonary Disorders*. New York: Raven Press; 1989: 69.

39 Olsen JD, Thomas DA, Young MB, *et al.* Cough and transbronchial needle aspiration. (Letter to the Editor). *Chest* 1986; **89**: 315.

40 Wang KP, Ztselcuk ZT, Erozan Y. Transbronchial needle aspiration for cytology specimens. *Monaldi Arch Chest Dis* 1994; **49**: 265–7.

41 Wang KP, Turner JF, Girgiana F. "How I Do It." Transthoracic needle aspiration biopsy. *J Bronchol* 1995; **2**: 243–7.

42 Wang KP. Flexible bronchoscopy with transbronchial needle aspiration: biopsy for cytology specimens. In: Wang KP, ed. *Biopsy Techniques in Pulmonary Disorders*. New York: Raven Press; 1989: 75.

43 Wang KP. Transbronchial needle aspiration to obtain histology specimen. *J Bronchol* 1994; **1**: 116–22.

44 Wang KP. Transbronchial needle aspiration and percutaneous needle aspiration for staging and diagnosis of lung cancer. *Clin Chest Med* 1995; **16**; 535–52.

45 Buriski G, Calverley P, Douglas NJ, *et al.* Bronchial needle aspiration in the diagnosis of bronchial carcinoma. *Thorax* 1981; **36**: 508–11.

46 Shure D, Fedullo PF. Transbronchial needle aspiration in the diagnosis of submucosal and peribronchial bronchogenic carcinoma. *Chest* 1985; **88**: 49–51.

47 Dasgupta A, Jain P, Minai OA. Utility of transbronchial needle aspiration in the diagnosis of endobronchial lesions. *Chest* 1999; **115**: 1237–41.

48 Caglayan B, Akturk UA, Fidan A. Diagnosis of endobronchial malignant lesion. *Chest* 2005; **128**: 704–8.

49 Silverman NA, Sabiston DC. Mediastinal masses. *Surg Clin North Am* 1980; **60**: 757–77.

50 Salyer DC, Salyer WR, Eggleston JC. Benign developmental cysts of the mediastinum. *Arch Pathol Lab Med* 1977; **101**: 136–9.

51 Wang KP, Nelson S, Scatarige J, *et al.* Transbronchial needle aspiration of a mediastinal mass: therapeutic implication. *Thorax* 1983; **38**: 557–7.

52 Schwartz DB, Beals TF, Wimbish KJ, *et al.* Transbronchial fine needle aspiration of bronchogenic cysts. *Chest* 1985; **88**: 573–5.

53 McDougall JC, Fromme GA. Transcarinal aspiration of a mediastinal cyst to facilitate anesthetic management. *Chest* 1990; **97**: 490 2.

54 Wang KP, Terry P, Marsh B. Bronchoscopic needle aspiration biopsy of paratracheal tumors. *Am Rev Respir Dis* 1978; **118**: 17–21.

55 Kuhlman JE, Fishman EK, Wang KP. *et al.* Esophageal duplication cyst: CT and transesophageal needle aspiration. *Am J Respir* 1985; **145**: 531–2.

56 Morrison IM. Tumors and cysts of the mediastinum. *Thorax* 1958; **13**: 294–307.

57 Wychulis AR, Payne WS, Clagett OT, Woolner LB. Surgical treatment of mediastinal tumors: a 40-year experience. *J Thoracic Cardiovasc Surg* 1971; **62**: 379–92.

58 Heithoff KB, Sane SM, Williams HJ, *et al.* Bronchopulmonary foregut malformations: a unifying etiological concept. *AJR Am J Roentgenol* 1976; **126**: 46–55.

59 Kirwan WO, Walbaum PR, McCormick RJM. Cystic intrathoracic derivatives of the foregut and their complications. *Thorax* 1973; **28**: 424–8.

60 Sirivella S, Ford WB, Zikria EA, *et al*. Foregut cysts of the mediastinum: results in 20 consecutive surgically treated cases. *J Thorac Cardiovasc Surg* 1985; **90**: 776–82.

61 Whitaker JA, Deffenbaugh LD, Cooke AR. Esophageal duplication cyst. *Am J Gastroenterol* 1980; **73**: 329–32.

62 Hocking M, Young DG. Duplications of the alimentary tract. *Br J Surg* 1981; **68**: 92–6.

63 Ferguson CC, Young LN, Sutherland JB, Macpherson RI. Intrathoracic gastric cyst: preoperative diagnosis by technetium pertechnetate scan. *J Pediatr Surg* 1973; **8**: 827–8.

64 Reed JC, Sobonya RE. Morphologic analysis of foregut cysts in the thorax. *AJR Am J Roentgenol* 1974; **120**: 851–60.

65 Yousem DM, Scatarige JC, Fishman EK, Siegelman SS. Low-attenuation thoracic metastases in testicular malignancy. *AJR Am J Roentgenol* 1986; **146**: 291–3.

66 Glazer HS, Siegel MJ, Sagel SS. Low-attenuation mediastinal masses on CT. *AJR Am J Roentgenol* 1989; **152**: 1173–7.

67 Kuhlman JK, Fishman EK, Wang KP, *et al*. Mediastinal cysts: diagnosis by CT and needle aspiration. *AJR Am J Roentgenol* 1988; **150**: 75–8.

68 Weiss LM, Fagelman D, Warhit JM. CT demonstration of an esophageal duplication cyst. *J Comput Assist Tomogr* 1983; **7**: 716–18.

69 Nakata H, Nakayama C, Kimoto T, *et al*. Computed tomography of mediastinal bronchogenic cysts. *J Comput Assist Tomogr* 1982; **6**: 733–8.

70 Medelson DS, Rose JS, Efremidis SC, *et al*. Bronchogenic cysts with high CT numbers. *AJR Am J Roentgenol* 1983; **140**: 463–5.

71 Nakata H, Sato Y, Nakayama T, *et al*. Bronchogenic cyst with high CT number: analysis of contents. *J Comput Assist Tomogr* 1986; **10**: 360–2.

72 Salonen O. CT characteristics of expansions in the middle and posterior mediastinum. *Comput Radiol* 1987; **11**: 95–100.

73 Lupetin AR, Dash N. MRI appearance of esophageal duplication cyst. *Gastrointest Radiol* 1987; **12**: 7–9.

74 Rhee RS, Ray CG, Kravetz MH, *et al*. Cervical esophageal duplication cyst: MR imaging. *J Comput Assist Tomogr* 1988; **12**: 693–5.

75 Scatarige JC, Wang KP, Siegelman SS. Transbronchial needle aspiration biopsy of the mediastinum. In: Siegelman SS, ed. *Contemporary Issues in Computed Tomography*, vol. 4. Computed tomography of the chest. New York: Churchill Livingstone; 1984: 59–79.

76 Schwartz AR, Fishman EK, Wang KP. Diagnosis and treatment of a bronchogenic cyst using transbronchial needle apsiration. *Thorax* 1986; **41**: 326–7.

77 Nakajima T, Yasufuku K, Shibuya K, *et al*. Endobronchial ultrasound-guided transbronchial needle aspiration for the treatment of central airway stenosis caused by a mediastinal cyst. *Eur J Cadiothorac Surg* 2007; **32**: 538–40.

78 Pauli G, Pelletier A, Bohner C, *et al*. Transbronchial needle aspiration in the diagnosis of sarcoidosis. *Chest* 1984; **85**: 482–4.

79 Garwood S, Judson M, Silvestri G. Endobronchial ultrasound for the diagnosis of pulmonary sarcoidosis. *Chest* 2007; **132**: 1298–304.

80 Mehta AC, Meeker DP. Transbronchial needle aspiration for histology specimens. In: Wang KP, Mehta AC, eds. *Flexible Bronchoscopy*. Massachusetts: Blackwell Science. 1995: 199–205.

81 Parrish S, Turner JF. Diagnosis of sarcoidosis. *Dis Mon* 2009; **55**: 693–703.

82 Morales CF, Patefield AJ, Strollo PJ, *et al*. Flexible transbronchial needle aspiration in the diagnosis of sarcoidosis. *Chest* 1994; **106**: 709–11.

83 Leonard C, Tormey VJ, O'Keane C, *et al*. Bronchoscopic diagnosis of sarcoidosis. *Eur Repsir J* 1997; **10**: 2722–4.

84 Trisolini R, Lazzari L, Cancelleri A, *et al*. The value of flexible transbronchial needle aspiration in the diagnosis of stage i sarcoidosis. *Chest* 2003; **124**: 2126–30.

85 Simecek C. Diagnosis of mycobacterial mediastinal lymphadenopathy by transbronchial needle aspiration (Letter). *Chest* 1992; **102**: 1919.

86 Baron KM, Arauda CP. Diagnosis of mediastinal mycobacterial lymphadenopathy by transbronchial needle aspiration. *Chest* 1991; **100**: 1723–4.

87 Serda JG, de Castro RF, Sanchez-Alarcos FJM, *et al*. Transcarinal needle aspiration in the diagnosis of mediastinal adenitis in a patient infected with the human immunodeficiency virus. *Thorax* 1990; **45**: 414–15.

88 Malabonga VM, Basti J, Kamholz SL. Utility of bronchoscopic sampling techniques for cryptococcal disease in AIDS. *Chest* 1991; **99**: 370–2.

89 Harkin TJ, Karp J, Ciotoli C, *et al*. Transbronchial needle aspiration in the diagnosis mediastinal mycobacterial infection (abstract). *Am Rev Respir Dis* 1993; **147** (Suppl): 801a.

90 Harkin TJ, Ciotolo C, Addrizzo-Harris DJ, *et al*. Transbronchial needle aspiration (TBNA) in patients infected with HIV. *Am J Respir Crit Care Med* 1998; **157**: 1913–18.

91 Baron KM, Aranda CP. Diagnosis of mediastinal mycobacterial lymphadenopathy by transbronchial needle aspiration. *Chest* 1991; **100**: 1723–4.

92 Bilaceroglu S, Gunel O, Eris N, *et al*. Transbronchial needle aspiration in diagnosing intrathoracic tuberculous lymphadenitis. *Chest* 2004; **126**: 259–67.

93 Herscovici P, Harkin TJ, Nadich DP. Transbronchial needle aspiration in HIV infected patients with intrathoracic adenopaty: A 15-year experience at a major teaching hospital. *Chest* 2006; **130**: 275S.

94 Wang KP. Transbronchial needle aspiration to obtain histology specimen. *J Bronchol* 1994; **1**: 116–22.

95 Malabonga VM, Basti J, Kamholz SL. Utility of bronchoscopic sampling technique for cryptococcal disease in AIDS. *Chest* 1991; **99**: 370–2.

96 Wang KP, Gonullu U, Baker R. Transbronchial needle aspiration vs. transthoracic needle aspiration in the diagnosis of pulmonary lesions. *J Bronchol* 1994; **1**: 199–204.

97 Reichenberger F, Weber J, Tamm M, *et al*. The value of transbronchial needle aspiration in the diagnosis of peripheral pulmonary lesions. *Chest* 1999; **116**: 704–8.

98 Baaklini WA, Reinoso MA, Gorin AB. Diagnostic yield of fiberoptic bronchoscopy in evaluating solitary pulmonary nodules. *Chest* 2000; **117**: 1049–54.

99 Chao T, Chien M, Lie C, *et al*. Endobronchial ultrasonography-guided transbronchial needle aspiration increases the diagnos-

tic yield of peripheral pulmonary lesions; a randomized trial. *Chest* 2009; **136**: 229–36.

100 Schwarz Y, Greif J, Becker HD, *et al.* Real-time electromagnetic navigation bronchoscopy to peripheral pulmonary lesions using overlaid CT images: the first human studies. *Chest* 2006; **129**: 988–94.

101 Gildea TR, Mazzone PJ, Karnak D, *et al.* Electromagnetic navigation bronchoscopy: a prospective study. *Am J Respir Crit Care Med* 2006; **174**: 982–9.

102 Makris D, Scherpereel A, Bouchindhomme B, *et al.* Electromagnetic navigation diagnostic bronchoscopy for small peripheral lung lesions. *Eur Resp J* 2007; **29**: 1187–92.

103 Mountain CF. A new international staging system for lung cancer. *Chest* 1986; **89**: 225S–233S.

104 Mountain CF. Revisions in the international system for staging lung cancer. *Chest* 1997; **111**: 1710–17.

105 Mountain CF. Prognostic implications of the International Staging System for lung cancer. *Semin Oncol* 1988; **15**: 236.

106 Mountain CF. Value of the new TNM staging system for lung cancer. *Chest* 1989; **96** (Suppl 1): 47S.

107 Naruke T, Goya T, Tsuchiya R, *et al.* Prognosis and survival in resected lung carcinoma based on the new international staging system. *J Thorac Cardiovasc Surg* 1988; **96**: 440.

108 Goldstraw P. The 7th edition of TNM in lung cancer: what now. *J Thorac Oncol* 2009; **4**: 671–3.

109 Grover FL. The role of CT and MRI in staging of the mediastinum. *Chest* 1994; **106**: 391S–6S.

110 De Wever W. Stroobants S, Coolen J, *et al.* Integrated PET/CT in the staging of nonsmall cell lung cancer: technical aspects and clinical integration. *Eur Respir J* 2009; **33**: 201–12.

111 Silvestri GA, Gould MK, Margolis ML. Noninvasive staging of non-small cell lung cancer. ACCP evidenced-based clinical practice guidelines (2nd edition). *Chest* 2007; **132**: 178S–201S.

112 Turner JF, Wang KP. Staging of mediastinal involvement in lung cancer by bronchoscopic needle aspiration. Pro: needle aspiration. *J Bronchol* 1996; **3**: 74–6.

113 Turner, JF, Del Rosario A. Staging of bronchogenic carcinoma. An interventional pulmonary perspective. In: Simoff M, Sterman D, Ernst A, eds. *Thoracic Endoscopy; Advances in Interventional Pulmonology.* Blackwell Science; 2006.

114 Utz JP, Patel AM, Edell ES. The role of transcarinal needle aspiration in the staging of bronchogenic carcinoma. *Chest* 1993; **104**: 1012–16.

115 Haponik EF, Cappellari JO, Chin R, *et al.* Education and experience improve transbronchial needle aspiration performance. *Am J Respir Crit Care Med* 1995; **141**: 1998–2002.

116 De Castro FR, Cappellari JO, Loez F, *et al.* Relevance of training in transbronchial fine-needle aspiration technique. *Chest* 1997; **111**: 103–5.

117 Hsu LH, Liu CC, Ko JS. Education and experience improve the performance of transbronchial needle aspiration. A learning curve at a cancer center. *Chest* 2004; **125**: 532–40.

118 Schenk DA, Bower JH, Bryan CL, *et al.* Transbronchial needle aspiration staging of bronchogenic carcinoma. *Am Rev Respir Dis* 1986; **134**: 146–8.

119 Witte EMC, Opal SM, Gilbert JG, *et al.* Incidence of fever and bacteremia following transbronchial needle aspiration. *Chest* 1986; **89**: 85–7.

120 Compere C, Duysinx B, Dediste A, *et al.* Prospective risk assessment of bacteremia associated with real-time ultrasound-guided transbronchial needle aspiration (EBUS-TBNA). *Chest* 2007; **132**: 439.

121 Epstein SK, Winslow CJ, Brecher SM, *et al.* Polymicrobial bacterial pericarditis after transbronchial needle aspiration. Case report with an investigation on the risk of bacterial contamination during fiberoptic bronchoscopy. *Am Rev Respir Dis* 1992; **146**: 523–5.

122 Ostman H, Shepherd RW. Mediastinitis and purulent pericarditis following endobronchial ultrasound transbronchial needle aspiration of lymph node. *Chest* 2008; **134**: c26001.

123 Kucera F, Wolfe GK, Perry ME. Hemomediastinum after transbronchial needle aspiration (Letter). *Chest* 1990; **98**: 466.

124 Sherling BE. Complications with a transbronchial histology needle. *Chest* 1990; **98**: 783–4.

125 Mehta AC, Curtis PS, Scalzitti ML, *et al.* The high price of bronchoscopy. *Chest* 1990; **98**: 448–54.

126 Rong F, Bing C. CT scan directed transbronchial needle aspiration biopsy for mediastinal nodes. *Chest* 1998: **114**; **1**: 36–9.

127 Davenport RD. Rapid on-site evaluation of transbronchial aspirates. *Chest* 1990; **98**: 59–61.

128 Diette B, White P, Terry P. Utility of on-site cytopatholgy assessment for bronchoscopic evaluation of lung masses and adenopathy. *Chest* 2000; **117**: 1186–90.

129 Baram D, Garcia RB, Richman PS. Impact of rapid on-site cytologic evaluation during transbronchial needle aspiration. *Chest* 2005; **128**: 869–73.

130 Wang K, Brower R, Haponik EF, *et al.* Flexible transbronchial needle aspiration for staging of bronchogenic carcinoma. *Chest* 1983; **84**: 571–6.

131 Chin R, McCain TW, Lucia MA, *et al.* Transbronchial needle aspiration in diagnosing and staging lung cancer. How many aspirates are needed? *Am J Respir Crit Care Med* 2002; **166**: 377–81.

132 Herth F, Becker HD, Ernst A. Conventional vs endobronchial ultrasound-guided transbronchial needle aspiration. *Chest* 2004; **125**: 322–5.

133 Lee HS, Lee GK, Lee HS, *et al.* Real-time endobronchial ultrasound-guided transbronchial needle aspiration in mediastinal staging of non-small cell lung cancer: how many aspirations per target lymph node station? *Chest* 2008; **134**: 368–74.

134 Kanoh K, Miyazawa T, Kurimoto N, *et al.* Endobronchial ultrasonography guidance for transbronchial needle aspiration using a double-channel bronchoscope. *Chest* 2005; **128**: 388–93.

## 12

# The Utilization of Autofluorescence in Flexible Bronchoscopy

## Taichiro Ishizumi[1] and Stephen C. T. Lam[2]

[1] Department of Thoracic Surgery, Tokyo Medical University, Tokyo, Japan
[2] University of British Columbia and Provincial Lung Tumor Group, British Columbia Cancer Agency, Vancouver, BC, Canada

## Introduction

Lung cancer is the most common cause of cancer deaths worldwide [1]. It is projected that by 2020, lung cancer will be the fifth biggest killer among all diseases [2]. Improvement in survival has been very modest. Less than 16% of lung cancer patients survive 5 years or more [3], owing to late diagnosis and a paucity of effective therapies. In contrast to the poor survival of patients with advanced disease, the survival of those with carcinoma *in situ* (Stage 0) or microinvasive disease is up to 90% [4–6]. Most central type early stage lung cancers can be successfully treated by minimally invasive endoscopic methods, such as photodynamic therapy, electrocautery treatment, or cryotherapy [7–9]. It is therefore important to be able to detect preinvasive and microinvasive bronchial cancers.

Early central type lung cancers remain difficult to detect with white light bronchoscopy even with the improved image capability of videobronchoscopy because these lesions are small and relatively flat [10]. Advances in photonic imaging offers unique capabilities to use visible and near-infrared light to determine the morphological, functional, biochemical, or even molecular changes in the airways for detection of early bronchial cancers. In this chapter, the principles of photonic imaging, how these principles have been applied to detect early bronchial cancers, the clinical trial results, and future directions will be discussed.

## Principles of photonic imaging

When the bronchial surface is illuminated by light, the light can be reflected from the surface (specular reflection), absorbed, induce autofluorescence, travel in the bronchial tissue and back-scattered at the same wavelength as the incident light (elastic scattering), or scatter at a different wavelength (inelastic or Raman scattering) due to light energy modification by the vibrational state of molecules [11]. White-light bronchoscopy (WLB)—the simplest and most commonly used bronchoscopic imaging method—makes use of the specular reflection, back scattering, and absorption properties of broadband visible light from approximately 400 to 700 nm to define the structural features of the bronchial surface and discriminate between normal and abnormal tissues. To highlight the vasculature, narrow-band blue light, centered at 415 nm, and green light, centered at 540 nm, corresponding to the maximal hemoglobin absorption peaks, are used instead. The blue light highlights the superficial capillaries while the green light can penetrate deeper to highlight the larger blood vessels in the submucosa. This is called narrow-band imaging (NBI) and is often used in conjunction with high magnification videobronchoscopy [12–14]. NBI provides more detailed images of the microvasculature in preneoplastic and neoplastic lesions, reflective of the altered angiogenesis process.

Autofluorescence bronchoscopy (AFB) makes use of fluorescence and absorption properties to provide information about the biochemical composition and metabolic state of bronchial tissues [15]. Most endogenous fluorophores are associated with the tissue matrix or are involved in cellular metabolic processes. The most important fluorophores are structural proteins, such as collagen and elastin, and those involved in cellular metabolism, such as nicotinamide adenine dinucleotide (NADH) and flavins. Other fluorophores include the aromatic amino acids, various porphyrins, and lipopigments. The fluorescence properties of bronchial tissue is determined by the distribution of fluorophores, their distinct excitation and emission spectra, their metabolic state, the tissue architecture, and the wavelength-dependent light attenuation due to the concentration as well as distribution of non-fluorescent chromophores such as

*Flexible Bronchoscopy*, Third Edition. Edited by Ko-Pen Wang, Atul C. Mehta, J. Francis Turner.
© 2012 Blackwell Publishing Ltd. Published 2012 by Blackwell Publishing Ltd.

hemoglobin [11]. Upon illumination by violet or blue light (380 to 460 nm), normal bronchial tissues fluoresce strongly in the green (480 to 520 nm). As the bronchial epithelium changes from normal to dysplasia, and then to carcinoma *in situ* and invasive cancer, there is a progressive decrease in green autofluorescence but proportionately less decrease in the red fluorescence intensity. These differences between normal, preneoplastic, and neoplastic tissues are due to breakdown of stromal collagen cross-links, increase in cellular metabolic activity leading to changes in NADH, FAD coenzymes, increased absorption of the excitation violet/blue light by hemoglobin due to angiogenesis, as well as changes in the light scattering process from an increase in nuclear size, cellular density, and distribution of the cells associated with lung cancer development. The excitation wavelength that produces the highest tumor to normal tissue intensity and chromatic contrast is 405 nm [16,17]. The fluorescence differences between 480 nm and 700 nm in normal, preneoplastic, and preneoplastic tissues serve as the basis for the design of several autofluorescence endoscopic imaging devices for localization of early lung cancer in the bronchial tree [15]. Commercially available AFB devices make use of a combination of autofluorescence and reflectance imaging to optimize the image quality.

## Autofluorescence bronchoscopy devices

Endoscopic fluorescence diagnosis using exogenous fluorescence drug such as hematoporphyrin derivatives was developed by Profio in 1982 [18]. These drugs are expensive and require intravenous injection several hours to 2 days before bronchoscopic examination. Fluorescence diagnosis using tissue autofluorescence alone was reported by Palcic and Lam in 1991 [19,20]. The first real-time device, the LIFE-Lung System (Xillix Technologies, Vancouver, Canada) became commercially available in 1998 [21]. The device used a helium–cadmium laser for illumination (442 nm) and detected the emitted red and green autofluorescence light with two image-intensified charge-coupled device (CCD) cameras. Normal areas appear green and abnormal areas appear reddish brown due to reduced green autofluorescence in preneoplastic and neoplastic lesions [21,22]. With advances in technology, most devices now use a filtered lamp for illumination and non-image intensified sensors for imaging [23–27]. Switching between white-light and fluorescence examination no longer requires removing the light guide from different light sources but rather by pressing a switch button. Instead of mounting the camera onto the eyepiece of a fiberoptic bronchoscope, the CCD sensor at the tip of a videoendoscope is used for imaging [24,28]. Small amounts of reflected light (blue, green, or near infrared) is employed to form a reflectance image which is then used to

enhance the chromatic contrast and to normalize the green autofluorescence image to correct for non-uniformity caused by optical and geometrical factors, such as variable distances and angles between the endoscope tip to the bronchial surface. Depending on the type of reflected light used to combine with the fluorescence image for display, abnormal areas appear brownish red, red, purple, or magenta while normal areas appear green or light blue [21–28] (Table 12.1). Some devices allow simultaneous display of the white-light and fluorescence images [28,29]. An example of this technique is shown in Fig. 12.1. Thus, white-light and fluorescence examination has become an integrated procedure, providing information using all the optical properties of bronchial tissues with the exception of Raman scattering. A summary of the devices is shown in Table 12.1. There is only one study comparing different devices such as D-Light with LIFE-Lung [30]. The study showed comparable results with a slightly longer examination time for the LIFE-Lung device due to the use of two separate light sources. The LIFE-Lung system was the very first device that received regulatory approval for marketing; it has been replaced by a second generation device [23].

## Results of clinical trials

In addition to several single-center studies [31], there have been two randomized trials [32,33], and three large, multicenter trials [21,23,34] comparing WLB and AFB. The results are summarized in Table 12.2. The studies show an improvement in the detection rate of high-grade dysplasia, carcinoma *in situ* (CIS), and microinvasive cancer with AFB compared to WLB. The sensitivity of WLB is dependent on the study population and the experience of the endoscopist accounting for the variation in the reported relative sensitivity of AFB versus WLB. In general, there is a twofold improvement in the relative sensitivity with AFB. The specificity of AFB is lower due to false-positive fluorescence with inflammation, mucous gland hyperplasia, and interobserver error.

The specificity of AFB can be improved by quantifying the red to green fluorescence ratio (R/G) of the target lesion during the bronchoscopic procedure [35]. Analysis of the R/G ratios of 3362 bronchial biopsies from 738 subjects with various pathology grades showed that when a R/G ratio of 0.56 or higher was used as the threshold, the sensitivity of detecting moderate/ severe dysplasia and CIS was 85% at a specificity of 80% [35]. Combining the R/G ratios with the visual score improved the specificity further to 88%. Similar results were found in a multicenter trial where the R/G ratios were hidden from the bronchoscopists when making the visual classification of the bronchial mucosal changes [23]. Quantitative imaging helps to decrease intra- and interobserver variation.

**Table 12.1** Autofluorescence bronchoscopy devices

| Device | Bronchoscope | Excitation light | Fluorescence | Reflectance | Image composition | Abnormal lesion |
|---|---|---|---|---|---|---|
| Onco-LIFE | Fiberscope | 395–445 nm | 500–720 nm | 675–720 nm | Green fluorescence<br>Red reflectance | Reddish brown/red on green background |
| SAFE-3000 | Videoendoscope | 408 nm | 430–700 nm | 408 nm | Green/ red fluorescence<br>Blue reflectance | Purple on bluish green background |
| AFI | Videoendoscope | 395–445 nm | 460–490 nm | 550 nm, 610 nm | Green fluorescence<br>Green and red reflectance | Magenta/ purple on green background |
| DAFE | Fiberscope | 390–470 nm | 500–590 nm | 650–680 nm | Green fluorescence<br>Red reflectance | Red on green background |
| D-light | Fiberscope | 380–460 nm | ≥480 nm | 380–460 nm | Green/ red fluorescence<br>Blue reflectance | Purple on bluish green background |
| ClearVu Elite | Fiberscope | 400–450 nm | 470–700 nm | 720–800 nm | Green fluorescence<br>Red reflectance | Reddish brown/ red on green background |

Onco-LIFE /Pin-point (Novadq, Richmond, BC Canada); SAFE 3000 (Pentax-Hoya Corp., Tokyo, Japan); AFI (Olympus Corp; Tokio, Japan); DAFE (Wolf, Knittlingen, Germany); D-Light (Storz, Tuttingen, Germany); ClearVu Elite (Perceptronix Medical Inc., Vancouver, Canada).

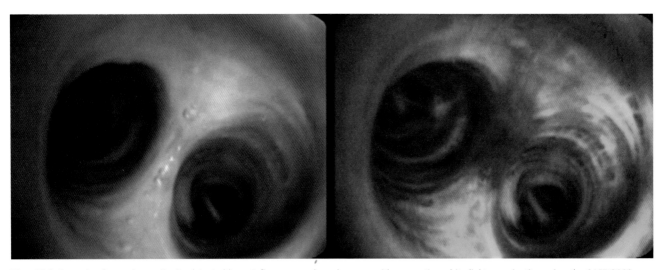

**Fig. 12.1** Example of a carcinoma *in situ* detected by autofluorescence bronchoscopy with a negative white light examination using the SAFE 3000 system (Pentax-Hoya Corp. Tokyo, Japan). The white light and autofluorescence images are displayed simultaneously in real time. Normal area appears green while the tumor area shows decrease in green autofluorescence. Courtesy of Professor Norihiko Ikeda, Tokyo Medical University.

Technology is available to improve the specificity of AFB further by combining optical coherence tomography (OCT) with AFB. OCT works like ultrasound except that near-infrared light is used instead of sound to probe structures below the bronchial surface. It is a non-contact method which delivers near-infrared light to the tissue and allows imaging of cellular and extracellular structures from analysis of the backscattered light with a spatial resolution of approx-imately 3 to 15 μm and a depth penetration of approximately 2 mm to provide near-histological images in the bronchial wall [36,37]. Quantitative measurement of the epithelial thickness showed that invasive carcinoma was significantly different from CIS and dysplasia was significantly different from metaplasia or hyperplasia [37]. In addition, nuclei of the cells became more discernible in lesions that were moderate dysplasia or worse, compared to lower-grade

**Table 12.2** Results of multicenter clinical trials and randomized studies of autofluorescence bronchoscopy

| Study | Device | No. of Subjects | Sensitivity (%) | | Specificity (%) | |
|---|---|---|---|---|---|---|
| | | | WLB | AFB | WLB | AFB |
| Lam S 1998 [21]* | LIFE-Lung | 173 | 9 | 66 | 90 | 66 |
| Ernst 2005 [34]* | D-Light | 293 | 11 | 66 | 95 | 73 |
| Hirsch 2001 [32]† | LIFE-Lung | 55 | 18 | 73 | 78 | 46 |
| Häussinger 2005 [33]† | D-Light | 1173 | 58 | 82 | 62 | 58 |
| Edell 2009 [23]* | Onco-LIFE | 170 | 10 | 44 | 94 | 75 |

WLB, white-light bronchoscopy; AFB, autofluorescence bronchoscopy.
*Multicenter clinical trial.
†Randomized trial.

**Table 12.3** Combined autofluorescence bronchoscopy and spiral CT for early detection of lung cancer

| Study | Study population | Percent detected by autofluorescence alone |
|---|---|---|
| McWilliams et al. [40] | 1594 volunteer smokers ≥50 years of age and ≥30 pack-years | 20 |
| Loewen et al. [41] | 402 subjects with two or more features: ≥20 pack-years; COPD, asbestos exposure or previous curatively treated upper aerodigestive cancer | 23 |
| Lam B et al. [42] | 85 smokers attending smoking cessation clinic with sputum atypia | 28 |

lesions. Systems under development with ultrahigh resolution, Doppler capability, and polarization sensitivity, which can measure tissue microstructures in greater detail and quantify microvascular blood flow, will likely be able to eliminate false-positive biopsies [38,39]. AFB serves as a rapid scanning tool to detect abnormal mucosal changes in large surface areas while OCT provides the means to characterize the abnormality in question prior to taking a biopsy.

## Role of autofluorescence bronchoscopy in the early detection of lung cancer

Low-dose thoracic CT scanning is a sensitive tool to detect peripheral lung cancers that are surrounded by low-density air-containing lung. However, it is not as sensitive for detecting early central lung cancers that are surrounded by soft tissue. Three studies examined the role of combined AFB and spiral CT to detect early lung cancers [40–42]. The results are summarized in Table 12.3. All three studies showed that approximately 20% of lung cancers are detected by AFB alone with a negative spiral CT [40–42]. The majority of these CT-occult cancers are early squamous cell carci-

nomas. However, two of these studies were in subjects with sputum atypia, either by image cytometry or by conventional cytology [40,42], and the third study was in patients with previous curatively treated upper aerodigestive cancer or chronic obstructive pulmonary disease [41]. The role of AFB as part of a multimodal early lung cancer detection program in high-risk smokers is currently under investigation by the Pan-Canadian Early Lung Cancer Detection Study.

## Clinical applications

Improved localization rates of lesions by AFB were reported for patients with abnormal sputum cytology findings [42,43]. In addition, AFB contributes to objective diagnosis of tumor extent. Pathological examination of the bronchus of resected lungs due to lung cancer revealed AFB diagnosed the extent of tumor invasion more accurately than white light examination alone [44]. It is helpful for defining the bronchial resection margin preoperatively and to detect synchronous lung cancer [45,46].

Current evidence supports the use of AFB in the following clinical situations:

**1** patients with severe atypia or malignant cells in their sputum cytology and a negative chest X ray or CT scan;
**2** as part of a diagnostic bronchoscopy in patients suspected to have lung cancer where a bronchoscopy is indicated; and
**3** patients with carcinoma *in situ*/ microinvasive cancer being considered for curative endobronchial therapy.

## Summary

Autofluorescence bronchoscopy plays an important role in the localization of preinvasive and early invasive bronchial lesions, delineation of the extent of tumor spread, and for guiding bronchoscopic biopsy. Localization of early central lesions enables minimally invasive endobronchial treatment without removing adjacent normal lung tissue. False-positive fluorescence can occur in areas with inflammation or severe mucus gland hyperplasia. Quantifying the red to green fluorescence ratio of target sites can improve the specificity. The role of autofluorescence bronchoscopy as part of a multimodal early lung cancer detection program needs to be investigated further.

## References

1 Parkin DM, Bray F, Ferlay J, *et al*. Global cancer statistics, 2002. *CA Cancer J Clin* 2005; **55**: 74–108.

2 Murray CJ, Lopez AD Alternative projections of mortality and disability by cause 1990–2020: Global burden of disease study. *Lancet* 1997; **349**: 1498–504.

3 Jemal A, Siegel R, Ward E, *et al*. Cancer statistics, 2009. *CA Cancer J Clin* 2009; **59**: 225–49.

4 Saito Y, Nagamoto N, Ota S, *et al*. Results of surgical treatment for roentgenographically occult bronchogenic squamous cell carcinoma. *J Thorac Cardiovasc Surg* 1992; **104**: 401–7.

5 Cortese DA, Pairolero PC, Bergstralh EJ, *et al*. Roentgenographically occult lung cancer: a 10-year experience. *J Thorac Cardiovasc Surg* 1983; **86**: 373–80.

6 Bechtel JJ, Petty TL, Saccomanno G. Five year survival and later outcome of patients with X-ray occult lung cancer detected by sputum cytology. *Lung Cancer* 2000; **30**: 1–7.

7 Kato H, Okunaka T, Shimatani S. Photodynamic therapy for early stage bronchogenic carcinoma. *J Clin Laser Med Surg* 1996; **14**: 235–8.

8 Sutedja G, Postmus PE. Bronchoscopic treatment of lung tumors. *Lung Cancer* 1994; **119**: 1–7.

9 Deygas N, Froudarakis M, Ozenne G, *et al*. Cryotherapy in early superficial bronchogenic carcinoma. *Chest* 2001; **120**: 26–31.

10 Chhajed PN, Shibuya K, Hoshino H, *et al*. A comparison of video and autofluorescence bronchoscopy in patients at high risk of lung cancer. *Eur Respir J* 2005; **25**: 951–5.

11 Wagnieres G, McWilliams A, Lam S. Lung cancer imaging with fluorescence endoscopy. In: Mycek M, Pogue B, eds. *Handbook of Biomedical Fluorescence*, Marcel Dekker: New York; 2003: 361–96.

12 Shibuya K, Hoshino H, Chiyo M, *et al*. High magnification bronchovideoscopy combined with narrow band imaging could detect capillary loos of angiogenic squamous dysplasia in heavy smokers at high risk for lung cancer. *Thorax* 2003; **58**: 989–95.

13 Vincent B, Fraig M, Silvestri G. A Pilot study of narrow-band imaging compared to white light bronchoscopy for evaluation of normal airways and premalignant and malignant airways disease. *Chest* 2007; **131**: 1788–94.

14 Gono K, Obi T, Yamaguchi M, *et al*. Appearance of enhanced tissue features in narrow-band endoscopicimaging. *J Biomed Opt* 2004; **9**: 568–78.

15 Lam S. The role of autofluorescence bronchoscopy in diagnosis of early lung cancer. In: Hirsch FR, Bunn Jr. PA, Kato H, Mulshine JL, eds. *IASLC Textbook of Prevention and Early Detection of Lung Cancer*. Taylor & Francis; 2005.

16 Hung J, Lam S, LeRiche JC, Palcic B . Autofluorescence of normal and malignant bronchial tissue. *Lasers Surg Med* 1991; **11**: 99–105.

17 Zellweger M, Grosjean P, Goujon D, *et al*. In vivo autofluorescence spectroscopy of human bronchial tissue to optimize the detection and imaging of early cancers. *J Biomed Opt* 2001; **6**: 41–51.

18 Balchum OJ, Doiron DR, Profio AE. Fluorescence bronchoscopy for localizing bronchial cancer and carcinoma in situ. *Recent Results Cancer Res* 1982; **82**: 97–120.

19 Palcic B, Lam S, Hung J, MacAulay C. Detection and localization of early lung cancer by imaging techniques. *Chest* 1991; **99**: 742–3.

20 Lam S, MacAulay C, Hung J, LeRiche J, *et al*. Detection of dysplasia and carcinoma in situ with a lung imaging fluorescence endoscope device. *J Thorac Cardiovasc Surg* 1993; **105**: 1035–40.

21 Lam S, Kennedy T, Unger M, *et al*. Localization of bronchial intraepithelial neoplastic lesions by fluorescence bronchoscopy. *Chest* 1998; **113**: 696–702.

22 Lam S, MacAulay C, LeRiche JC, Palcic B. Detection and localization of early lung cancer by fluorescence bronchoscopy. *Cancer* 2000; **89** (11 Suppl): 2468–73.

23 Edell E, Lam S, Pass H, *et al*. Detection and localization of intraepithelial neoplasia and invasive carcinoma using fluorescence-reflectance bronchoscopy: an international, multicenter clinical trial. *J Thorac Oncol* 2009; **4**: 49–54.

24 Chiyo M, Shibuya K, Hoshino H, *et al*. Effective detection of bronchial preinvasive lesions by a new autofluorescence imaging bronchovideoscope system. *Lung Cancer* 2005; **48**: 307–13.

25 Häussinger K, Stanzel F, Huber RM, *et al*. Autofluorescence detection of bronchial tumors with the D-light/AF. *Diagn Ther Endosc* 1999; **5**: 105–12.

26 Goujon D, Zellweger M, Radu A, *et al*. In vivo autofluorescence imaging of early cancers in the human tracheobronchial tree with a spectrally optimized system. *J Biomed Opt* 2003; **8**: 17–25.

27 Tercelj M, Zeng H, Petek M, *et al*. Acquisition of fluorescence and reflectance spectra during routine bronchoscopy examinations using the ClearVu Elite device: pilot study. *Lung Cancer* 2005; **50**: 35–42.

28 Ikeda N, Honda H, Hayashi A, *et al*. Early detection of bronchial lesions using newly developed videoendoscopy-based autofluorescence bronchoscopy. *Lung Cancer* 2006; **52**: 21–7.

29 Lee P, Brokx HAP, Postmus PE, Sutedja TG. Dual digital video-autofluorescence imaging for detection of preneoplastic lesions. *Lung Cancer* 2007; **58**: 44–9.

30 Herth FJ, Ernst A, Becker HD. Autofluorescence bronchoscopy—a comparison of two systems (LIFE and D-Light). *Respiration* 2003; **70**: 395–8.

31 Kennedy TC, McWilliams AM, Edell E, *et al*. Bronchial intraepithelial neoplasia/ early central airways lung cancer: ACCP evidence-based clinical practice guidelines (2nd Edition). *Chest* 2007; **132**: 221S–233S.

32 Hirsch FR, Prindiville SA, Miller YE, *et al* Fluorescence versus white-light bronchoscopy for detection of preneoplastic lesions: a randomized study. *J Natl Cancer Inst* 2001; **93**: 1385–91.

33 Häussinger K, Becker H, Stanzel F, *et al*. Autofluorescence bronchoscopy with white light bronchoscopy compared with white light bronchoscopy alone for the detection of precancerous lesions: a European randomised controlled multicentre trial. *Thorax* 2005; **60**: 496–503.

34 Ernst A, Simoff P, Mathur P, *et al*. D-light autofluorescence in the detection of premalignant airway changes; a multicenter trial. *J Bronchol* 2005; **12**: 133–8.

35 Lee P, van den Berg RM, Lam S, *et al*. Color fluorescence ratio for detection of bronchial dysplasia and carcinoma in situ. *Clin Cancer Res* 2009; **15**: 4700–05

36 Tsuboi M, Hayashi A, Ikeda N, *et al*. Optical coherence tomography in the diagnosis of bronchial lesions. *Lung Cancer* 2005; **49**: 387–94.

37 Lam S, Standish B, Baldwin C, *et al*. In-vivo optical coherence tomography imaging of pre-invasive bronchial lesions. *Clin Cancer Res* 2008; **14**: 2006–11.

38 Yang VX, Vitkin IA. Principles of Doppler optical coherence tomography. In: Regar E, van Leeuwen T, Serruys P, eds. *Handbook of Optical Coherence Tomography in Cardiology*. Oxford, UK: Taylor and Francis Medical; 2006.

39 Yang VXD, Tang S, Gordon ML, *et al*. Endoscopic Doppler optical coherence tomography in the human GI tract: initial experience. *Gastrointest Endosc* 2005; **61**: 879–90.

40 McWilliams AM, Mayo JR, Ahn MI, *et al*. Lung cancer screening using multi-slice thin-section computed tomography and autofluorescence bronchoscopy. *J Thorac Oncol* 2006; **1**: 61–8.

41 Loewen G, Natarajan N, Tan D, *et al*. Autofluorescence bronchoscopy for lung cancer surveillance based on risk assessment. *Thorax* 2007; **62**: 335–40.

42 Lam B, Lam SY, Wong M, *et al*. Sputum cytology examination followed by autofluorescence bronchoscopy: A practical way of identifying early stage lung cancer in central airway. *Lung Cancer* 2009; **64**: 289–94.

43 Sato M, Sakurada A, Sagawa M, *et al*. Diagnostic results before and after introduction of autofluorescence bronchoscopy in patients suspected of having lung cancer detected by sputum cytology in lung cancer mass screening. *Lung Cancer* 2001; **32**: 247–53.

44 Ikeda N, Hiyoshi T, Kakihana M, *et al*. Histopathological evaluation of fluorescence bronchoscopy using resected lungs in cases of lung cancer. *Lung Cancer* 2003; **41**: 303–9.

45 Piérard P, Faber J, Hutsebaut J, *et al*. Synchronous lesions detected by autofluorescence bronchoscopy in patients with high-grade preinvasive lesions and occult invasive squamous cell carcinoma of the proximal airways. *Lung Cancer* 2004; **46**: 341–7.

46 Sutedja TG, Codrington H, Risse EK, *et al*. Autofluorescence bronchoscopy improves staging of radiographically occult lung cancer and has an impact on therapeutic strategy. *Chest* 2001; **120**: 1327–32.

# 13    Endobronchial Ultrasound

## Heinrich D. Becker

Thoraxclinic-Heidelberg, Academic Teaching Hospital, University of Heidelberg, Heidelberg, Germany

## Introduction

Within the central airways, the endoscopist's view is restricted to the lumen and to the internal surface. Intramural processes and those adjacent to the airways, as well as mediastinal structures, can only be assessed from indirect signs, including discoloration, displacement, and destruction of anatomical structures. In the 1980s, despite early enthusiasm with the broader application of computed tomography (CT), clinical staging of lung cancer corresponded to pTNM stage (pathological tumor size and invasion, regional lymph node involvement, and distant metastasis) in only 60% of cases. We therefore began to consider endoscopic ultrasound as a potentially useful technology for the airways [1]. As external mediastinal ultrasound and transesophageal endosonography proved insufficient for exploration of the mediastinal structures, in 1989 we approached the Olympus Co. for the development of endobronchial ultrasound (EBUS), first using miniaturized radial scanning probes which were applied in the gastrointestinal tract (EUS) [2,3], and cardiovascular endosonography, preliminary experience of which had been reported in endovascular sonography of the pulmonary artery to exclude tumor invasion [4]. After extensive experience with dedicated radial ultrasound probes, in addition bronchoscopes with integrated linear electronic transducers were developed with Doppler function for visualization of vessels and real-time observation of transbronchial needle aspiration.

## Endobronchial ultrasound systems

There are two basic devices of EBUS systems: miniaturized probes with radial mechanical transducers and linear electronic tranducers, which are integrated into the tip of bronchoscopes. In the radial probes the transducer is attached to a wire that is rotated by a motor to send out waves perpendicular to the axis of the bronchi and provides a 360° surround view of the airways and adjacent mediastinal structures. The linear electronic transducers provide a sectorial view along the axis of the bronchi and by Doppler function can give information on intravascular blood flow. Currently, mechanical transducers have higher frequencies of 20 and 30 MHz, which give higher resolution of structures, but less penetration into distant structures. Electronic transducers have frequencies of 5–10 MHz, with less resolution but higher penetration (Figs 13.1 and 13.2).

## Miniaturized probes with mechanical transducers

Systems have been available commercially since 1999 (Olympus UM-2R/3R with MH-240 driving unit and EU-M20 and 30 processors). The system is complete with balloon catheters (MAJ-643R) which are attached to the probe and to the driving unit (Olympus UM-BS20-26R). The balloon is fixed at the tip of the probe by an O-ring that slips into a notch at the tip of the probe. In the case of over-inflation or excessive pressure, the balloon slips from the tip and a small amount of water is released into the airways, preventing the balloon from rupturing and latex particles dislodging into the lung. The development of the balloon provided three essential features for imaging within the airways: first, it provided circular contact, giving a 360° view for exact anatomical orientation; second, the 20-MHz frequency allows detailed analysis of the tracheobronchial wall in high resolution; and third, the water shifts the focus towards the periphery, thus the parabronchial mediastinal structures can also be analyzed, which frequently are the grey zone in CT [5]. The biopsy channel of the bronchoscope should be at least 2.8 mm. For the periphery of the lung, a smaller probe with a guide sheath is available (UM-S20-20R) of 1.4 mm diameter, which combined with a guide

*Flexible Bronchoscopy*, Third Edition. Edited by Ko-Pen Wang, Atul C. Mehta, J. Francis Turner.
© 2012 Blackwell Publishing Ltd. Published 2012 by Blackwell Publishing Ltd.

EBUS-Bronchoscope          Miniaturprobe

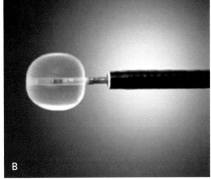

**Fig. 13.1** (A) Tip of an ultrasonic bronchoscope with transducer and dedicated needle introduced via the biopsy channel and (B) miniaturprobe with balloon sheath and inflated balloon introduced via the biopsy channel of a videobronchoscope.

sheath passes via 2.0-mm biopsy channels. A 30-MHz probe provides images with higher resolution (30 MHz UM-S30-25R), and by another device three-dimensional images can be generated as the probe is moving along its length axis during image acquisition (20MHZ 3D EU-IP2). Later, the Hitachi Co. also developed a 20-MHz radial probe with a balloon sheath (PL2220-20).

## Ultrasonic bronchoscopes

The current ultrasonic bronchoscope from Olympus is a hybrid endoscope with fiberoptic imaging, which is picked up by an electronic camera in the handle. It has an electronic transducer of 7.5 MHz at its tip with a maximum diameter of 6.9 mm and a 2.0-mm biopsy channel, which allows passage of a dedicated biopsy needle of 22 gauge (7.5 MHz CP-EBUS XBF-UC260F-OL). If necessary, a balloon can be attached to the tip for better contact. The bronchoscope requires an electronic processor (EU-C2000). As the mechanical and the electronic systems are complementary, there is now a processor available that integrates both (XEU-M60A). Another EBUS videoscope by Hitachi/Pentax (EB1970UK) has a color chip at the tip, variable ultrasound frequencies (from 5 to 10 MHz), and an 2.0-mm biopsy channel, allowing the passage of a dedicated 22-gauge biopsy needle. The diameter at the tip of the endoscope is slightly larger (7.3 mm).

## Special considerations for handling

Miniprobes are delicate and fragile devices, which have to be handled skillfully and with care. The transducer and the connecting driving wire are protected from friction inside the plastic sheath by a gel solution. The devices should be stored in a hanging position with the connector upwards and the tip of the probe downward. The probe should never be advanced inside the biopsy channel with the tip of the bronchoscope in a sharply bent position. It should also not

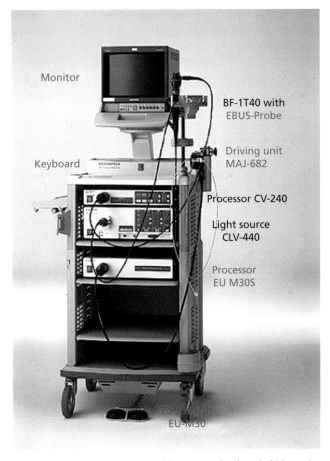

**Fig. 13.2** Ultrasound equipment with processor, key board, driving unit, and monitor, with the miniatureprobe already introduced via the biopsy channel of the bronchoscope, which is connected to the light source and processor.

be activated then as the transducer might be fixed while the wire is still rotating and could then shear off. Force should be never used while advancing the probe, neither advancing the tip nor pressing the probe sideways against the wall.

The optic of the EBUS bronchoscope provides an approximately 30° forward view, which means that the tip of the bronchoscope can not be seen during maneuvering of the instrument. Thus the direction of advancement has to be anticipated, which can give problems in passage of the larynx and into the periphery. In addition, the longer stiff part of the tip and its larger diameter can give problems in narrow airways or at curves. When performing transbronchial needle aspiration it is essential that the tip of the catheter that is protecting the needle is visible before the needle is advanced; otherwise the biopsy channel can be damaged and then the endoscope might be destroyed by moisture [5].

### Imaging artefacts

In the miniature probes the image construction begins in a radial way at the nine o'clock position and the rotation is slow enough to create a motion artefact, as due to pulsation or respiration the wall can change its position during one revolution. This creates an artificial interruption in the continuity of the bronchial wall and motion of the wall can be suggested. As the artefacts are not synchronous with respiration and pulsation they can easily be recognized as such. The strong echo of the balloon occasionally causes multiple ring reflections. Strong reflections of surrounding structures can create multiple reflex echoes, mirror or comet artefacts. This applies especially to the adjacent surface of the lung, the vertebral column, calcified cartilages, or lymph nodes. Triangular distortions of lymph nodes and attenuation of the outer contours of echogenic structures is also very common with the 20-MHz probes. Air bubbles in the balloon can cause shadows or image distortion, resembling a "rabbit's ear".

### Sonographic anatomy

The complex structure of the airway wall, as described in anatomy textbooks, can be clearly seen with the 20-MHz probe. There is continuing debate on the number of layers that are visible with the 20-MHz EBUS. The descriptions range from three to five and seven layers [6–8]. By *in vitro* experiments on resected human specimens we found a complex seven-layer structure, for which a high-resolution setting is necessary: the first, innermost hyperechoic layer is composed of a combination of the reflections from the balloon and the mucosa. The next hypoechoic layer is the submucosa. Under normal conditions it can be easily differentiated from the mucosa and from the third layer, the hyperechoic internal surface of the cartilage, which anatomically can be described as tabula interna or endochon-

drium, as I term this layer. This borderline structure is important as tumors that do not transgress it, by histopathological definition, are early cancers and can be efficiently treated by bronchoscopic means such as photodynamic therapy (PDT) or endobronchial high-dose radiation (HDR or brachytherapy), as has been demonstrated by Miyazu *et al.* According to their investigation, the mucosa epithelium is 0.05 mm thick and the first marginal echo is 0.68 mm thick [9]. The internal spongiform structure of the cartilage appears as hypoechoic in EBUS, whereas the outer surface (tabula externa or perichondrium) is hyperechoic again. It is a little-known fact that the central airways are surrounded by a double layer of loose and dense connective tissue [10], representing the sixth (hypoechoic) and seventh (hyperechoic) layer. This seven-layer structure has been confirmed in a further prospective, experimental study [11].

*In vivo* this complex structure can only be seen under high magnification, whereas at medium and low magnification, in particular, the delicate hypoechoic layers condense with the strong echoes of the supporting cartilages. With the Linear 7.5-MHZ and 12-MHz transducers of the ultrasonic bronchoscope these layers are invisible. The multilayer structure progressively comes down to five and three layers with passage towards the peripheral bronchi as the cartilages become scarce and finally disappear altogether. Shaw *et al.* compared the thickness of the bronchial wall in segmental bronchi as described by EBUS (1.3 mm) to high resolution CT scan and found no significant difference [12].

Spatial orientation within the mediastinum is not easy. This is due to the complex anatomy as well as to motion artefacts, pulsation, and, in addition, to the uncommon planes of the images. The plane of the circumferential image of the miniprobe is perpendicular to the axis of the probe. Whereas the horizontal planes inside the trachea are comparable to those in CT, following the oblique course of the airways down from the bifurcation, the images are tilting more and more with passage through the left main bronchus, until an almost coronary plane is reached at the distal left main bronchus. Entering the apical segments of the upper lobes the horizontal images become almost inverse.

In order to enhance orientation, it is useful to recognize key anatomical landmarks, and their relationship to the airways and to each other, rather than to observe the position of the probe (Fig. 13.3). Familiarity with the mediastinal anatomy is essential for orientation [13]. The image has to be set accordingly, so that landmark structures that are found only ventrally or dorsally to the bronchi, such as the esophagus or the pulmonary artery, are in the correct position. It is helpful to place the tip of the bronchoscope in direct contact with the balloon to look inside and follow the direction of the transducer when the tip of the bronchoscope is flexed sideways or up and down and adjust the ultrasonic image accordingly with the scroll ball or the reverse button on the keyboard. Vessels can be easily recognized due to

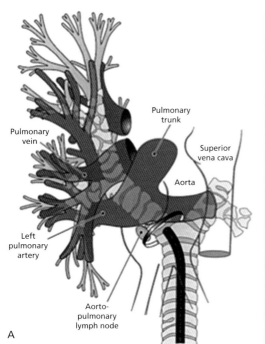

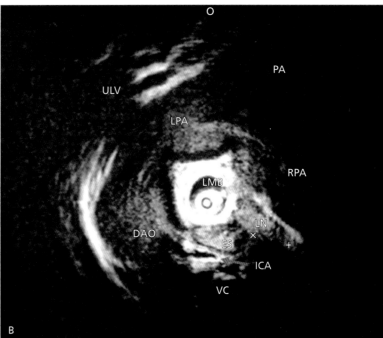

**Fig. 13.3** Ultrasonic mediastinal anatomy at the level of the proximal left main bronchus. (A) A situational sketch with approximately the plain of the radial ultrasonic image (courtesy Atul Mehta). (B) The corresponding ultrasonic image with the probe inside the left main bronchus (LMB). Anterior the left (LPA) and right main pulmonary (RPA) artery are seen. Dorsally, more to the left the descending aorta (DAO) is passing behind the left main bronchus and medially the multilayer structure of the esophagus is seen (ES) with some air and fluid inside. Anterolaterally to it a paraesophageal/ subcarinal lymph node is located in position 7 (LN ). Behind the esophagus and in front of the vertebral column (VC) an intercostal artery (ICA) crosses from the descending aorta to the right (arrow). In front of the left pulmonary artery the upper lobe vein (ULV) is crossing to the left atrium.

their low echogenicity and pulsations; arteries show a pulsation that is congruent with the pulse oximetry signals, whereas veins show the typical double motion as can be observed on the large peripheral veins. A Doppler function currently is not available for the miniprobes; however, lymph nodes can be easily differentiated from vessels due to their higher echogenicity.

As the water in the balloon shifts the focus more distally, with the 20-MHz probe the depth of penetration into the mediastinum can be well up to 5 cm. Thus, from the distal left main bronchus the left atrium and the mitral valve can frequently be seen. Near the bifurcation, from the left main bronchus the main pulmonary artery and its left and right branches are visualized ventrally. Dorsally, the descending aorta, the multilayer structure of the esophagus, and the vertebral column appear from left to right, behind the proximal left main bronchus, as clear landmarks for orientation. Ventrally to the right main bronchus appears the right pulmonary artery, which is accompanied by the ascending aorta to the left and by the cava vein to the right. Somewhat more proximally in the distal trachea, at the level of the right tracheobronchial angle, the azygos vein is located dorsally to the right besides the esophagus, where it circumflexes the trachea to the anterior and joins the cava vein. Further distally, at the level of the intermediate bronchus, the pulmonary artery and vein cross ventrally. Close to the middle lobe, the artery for the apical segment of the lower lobe crosses laterally backwards. This is important to know as it is easily punctured during transbronchial needle aspiration (TBNA) of lymph node 10 on the right side. Dorsally, the bright reflection corresponds to the adjacent pleura of the apical segment of the lower lobe and medially the pulmonary vein enters the atrium. The branching of the vessels at the segmental levels of the bronchi is less consistent and shows a lot of variation. Localization of the vessels, however, can be important to avoid contamination of TBNA specimens by blood and perforation during laser treatment of tumors, especially in both upper lobes. The lung tissue itself is highly reflective and shows a "snow storm-like" feature with the alveoli and capillary vessels. Some authors described alterations in the pattern by interstitial lung diseases [14], and benign infiltrates can be easily differentiated from malignant nodular lesions and cystic structures. Using computer-assisted analysis of the structures in the form of a histogram, in a prospective study we were able to accurately diagnose malignancies in over 90% of cases.

## Clinical application

EBUS with the radial scanning miniaturprobe is easily applied, has a negligible complication rate, and usually adds 6.3 minutes to a regular bronchoscopy, as we showed in a prospective study, with a total of 19.9 minutes for the whole procedure [15]. Complications were rare and of only minor nature: 5% of patients required additional oxygen. Transient minor arrhythmias were observed in 18 out of 103 patients (17%), who underwent complete blockage of the left main bronchus by the balloon. Rarely, minor self-limiting bleeding occurred during placement of the probe in the periphery of the lung. We improved the cost-effectiveness of the procedure, by re-sterilization and re-using the probes as long as they resisted the stress and strain, which was several hundred procedures in our hands, but at least up to 100 in general. EBUS has begun to be reimbursed in the USA. However, the system is also cost-effective without reimbursement as it can help to avoid more invasive and expensive procedures. We performed several prospective studies to validate EBUS for various indications [16–20]. Meantime the results have been confirmed by other authors and it has been shown that EBUS is comparable, and in many instances even superior, to other procedures. Recently, the dedicated ultrasonic bronchoscope with electronic linear transducer has drawn the main attention of physicians and helped to spread EBUS worldwide, especially with regard to staging of the mediastinum. These instruments are complementary, not in competition.

## Indications for clinical application of the radial ultrasound probe

Due to its specific properties, namely the high resolution of the image with the 20-MHz probe and the small diameter, there are several indications for application of the radial scanning ultrasound probe that are not met by other devices.

### Benign diseases

Several reports on the use of EBUS in the diagnosis of benign diseases have been published. Soja *et al.* found a greater total wall thickness in asthma as compared to normal, owing to an increase in the mucosal and submucosal layers as well as the smooth muscles, which corresponded to the impairment of FEV1 [21]. Also in COPD Deveci *et al.* found a thickening of the bronchial wall in advanced stages and in smokers more so than in non-smokers [22] According to Murgu *et al.* different forms of collapse of the airways could be differentiated by EBUS. In dynamic collapse the cartilage layer is normal and in contrast the membranaceous layer is thinner than in normal subjects. In postintubation and post-tracheotomy collapse, both the cartilaginous and the membranaceous layers are thickened and in chronic relapsing polychondritis the cartilages are thickened and irregular,

whereas the membranaceous layers are normal [23]. In addition, Miyazu *et al.* found significant fragmentation and edema of cartilages in chronic relapsing polychondritis [24]. Irani *et al.* studied the layer structure in lung transplant recipients for diagnosis of rejection and found the submucosal layer significantly thinner in the transplanted bronchus, which they attributed to a decrease in blood flow. In contrast, during inflammation the wall was thickened, may be due to inflammatory infiltrates or due to increased vascularization [25]. In a study by Herth *et al.* of the early detection of lung cancer comparing autofluorescence and narrow-band imaging (NBI), in more than 90% the histology was negative when the layer structure was intact in EBUS [26].

### Staging of lung cancer

The purpose of staging is to provide a precise classification in accordance with the current TNM system as a rational basis for treatment. Bronchoscopic criteria are documented in the UICC classification [27]. Radiologically invisible endobronchial tumors have to be located in persons who are at high risk or who have positive sputum cytology. Once they are detected, decision on the appropriate therapy is made on the basis of histological differentiation and local tumor spread and depth of penetration into the wall. Lymph node involvement is diagnosed by CT, EBUS, and TBNA. In addition to their extent and size, the relationship of tumors to parabronchial mediastinal structures, central airways, lung, and pleura is important. Here, EBUS can provide additional information, especially in regions that are not easily accessible by the bronchoscope or other diagnostic procedures.

*Primary lung cancer: endobronchial extent, early cancer.* By pathological definition, *in situ* lung cancer is limited to the mucosa, not transgressing the lamina propria, and early lung cancer is limited within the confinements of the inner layers of the bronchial wall and does not infiltrate or transgress the cartilage. Until recently, it was assumed that this equals radiological invisibility by high-resolution CT. However, it has been known for a long time, from earlier radiographic studies, that only 75% of bronchoscopically visible tumors are detected by radiology [28]. Radiographically invisible tumors included lesions that have penetrated into the wall and, from the beginning of the application of EBUS at our institution, we frequently find radiologically invisible lesions that have even penetrated transmurally and also those showing local lymph node metastasis, which had escaped all previous diagnostic procedures.

In all malignant lesions that were detected using video bronchoscopy, autofluorescence, and NBI, by application of the 20-MHz radial probe we found sonographic alterations in the texture of the bronchial wall, either thickening of specific layers or destruction of the architecture. As autofluorescence is unspecific and also positive in benign lesions, such as scars, granulomas, and inflammation, EBUS can significantly improve specificity and reliably clarify the nature of the lesion [29]. In our experience, correlation with the histology was improved from 58 to 92%. Even in macroscopically intact mucosa, submucosal and intramural tumor spread can be detected by EBUS. Tumors that do not show any signs of infiltration of the deeper layers or involvement of lymph nodes can be classified as early cancers and can be treated successfully with curative intent using endoscopic methods, such as PDT, endoluminal HDR (brachytherapy), or even laser and argon plasma coagulation [30]. This is in contrast to former studies on treatment by electrocautery and PDT, which reported recurrence rates of up to 50% [31]. It has been shown in a prospective study by Miyazu *et al.* [9] that this is not due to inefficient treatment, but due to insufficient local staging with conventional imaging technologies. All tumors that they staged by EBUS as limited within the internal layers of the bronchial wall, were associated with complete remission in long-term follow-up. This demonstrates that, currently, EBUS is the only reliable technique for staging of early lung cancer. Thus, we expect that, in the future, cancer detection by molecular biological markers in sputum, blood, or mouth swab, localization by autofluorescence and NBI, and local staging by EBUS with a miniature radial scanning probe will be the three pillars of early detection and local, minimally invasive treatment for central early lung cancer [32] (Figs 13.4 and 13.5).

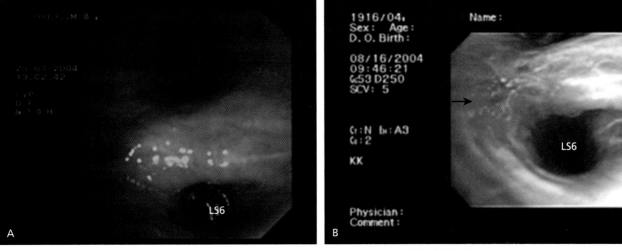

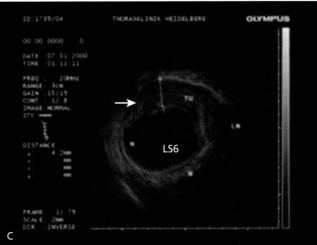

**Fig. 13.4** Early lung cancer. (A) On the left side, the carina at entrance to B6 (LS 6) is somewhat widened and shows an irregular surface with scattering of the light reflection. (B) In autofluorescence (AFI system, Olympus Co.) the area becomes clearly visible by its magenta color as compared to the normal green fluorescence. (C) Endobronchial ultrasound shows a thickening of the mucosa/ submucosa of 4mm as compared to the normal walls (N). If the radiologically invisible lymph node (LN) adjacent to B6 has been proved to be negative by transbronchial needle aspiration (TBNA), in the case of inoperability local destruction by endoscopic means (Nd-YAG laser, APC) could be considered. Otherwise high-dose radiation by Ir192 brachytherapy would be preferable as it can also cover the lymph node.

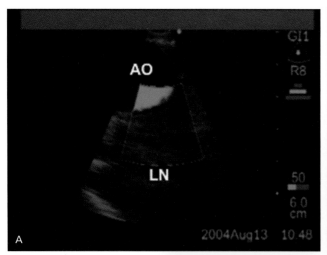

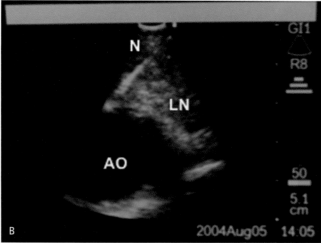

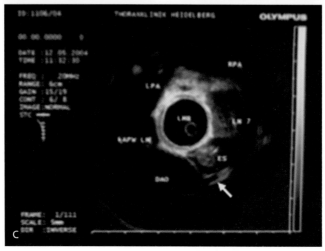

**Fig. 13.5** Transbronchial needle aspiration (TBNA). To avoid biopsy of lymph nodes (LN) behind a vessel such as the aorta (AO) in (A), or biopsy of lymph nodes adjacent to a vessel (AO) as in (B), visualization of the needle's (N) pathway is essential. (C) If there are clear landmarks, as for the lymph node (LN) in position 7L, localization by CT scan or by the radial probe is sufficient for successful biopsy. APW LN, lymph node in aortopulmonary window; DAO, descending aorta with offset of intercostal artery (yellow arrow); ES, esophagus; LPA, left pulmonary artery; RPA right pulmonary artery.

*Local staging of more advanced cancer.* CT is still the gold standard for diagnosis of local tumor spread. However, clinical staging corresponds with postoperative staging in only 60–70% [33]. In locally advanced bronchial carcinoma EBUS also provides useful information. In patients with complete obstruction of the airway we can localize the base and the surface of the occluding tumor, diagnose the extent to which the tumor has penetrated into the wall and into the mediastinum, and by passing the stenosis with the probe we can assess whether the airways distally to the stenosis are patent. Not infrequently, the airways are plugged with sticky proteinaceous secretions that cannot be differentiated from tumor on CT. Particularly with regard to surgical strategy, it is important to know the exact extent with regard to prospective resection lines. Involvement of the main bronchi, the carina, and the trachea requires elaborate techniques for resection and not infrequently precludes operability. The combination of autofluorescence and EBUS has proved useful for the detection of submucosal tumor spread. In particular, diagnosing involvement of the pulmonary vessels has great influence on decisions for interventions [20]. Perfusion of the lung can be shut down completely by the Euler–Liljestrand reflex, even if the pulmonary artery is patent, and in former times one had to resort to angio-CT to exclude obstruction. With the radial probe one is able to see minor infiltrations of the wall and pulsations of the wall as well as fluid inside the vessel. However, in this respect the Doppler function of the linear scanning probe is an additional advantage, provided the stenosis can be passed with the endoscope.

*Mediastinal infiltration: trachea, pulmonary vessels, esophagus, and large vessels.* Diagnosis of infiltration of the large mediastinal vessels—the aorta, vena cava, main pulmonary artery, and vein—is crucial and can be difficult by radiographic methods. Tumors located in trachea, main bronchus, and left hilum are in close vicinity to the esophagus and we have been able to detect direct infiltration by EBUS in several cases.

In addition, tumor invasion of the aortic arch, the descending aorta, and the main pulmonary artery can be seen from both main bronchi and the trachea. Infiltration of these structures usually excludes surgical procedures. However, if one can see a distinct sonographic interface between the tumor and these structures, operability is possible, as has been shown in many of our patients. Only with the high resolution of the radial probes, infiltration of the external layers of the trachea and main bronchi can be reliably diagnosed and distinguished from impression without infiltration. In our prospective study, CT had a sensitivity of only 25% and specificity of 80% (accuracy 51%) as compared to EBUS, which had an accuracy of 94%, sensitivity of 89%, and specificity of 100% [17]. For this purpose the resolution of the EBUS linear scope is insufficient.

*Lymph nodes: location, size, structure, infiltration, and biopsy.* Detection, localization, structure analysis, and especially real time *ultrasound-controlled* transbronchial needle biopsy or aspiration (TBNA) is the one indication for which the radial scanning probe has been replaced by the linear electronic scanning ultrasonic bronchoscope (EBUS-scope or so-called "puncture scope"). However, in contrast to the esophagus, which is mobile within the mediastinal structures and can change its position in relation to the lymph nodes, the airways always remain in stable contact with their vicinity and have distinct landmarks. This is why by CT guidance, and especially with the radial scanning probe, lymph nodes can be localized, and after withdrawal of the probe from the biopsy channel the biopsy needle is inserted according to the anatomical landmarks. Even with this *ultrasound-guided* technique we were successful in more than 80% of procedures [18].

Currently, staging of lymph nodes and diagnosing mediastinal masses is the domain of the ultrasonic bronchoscope [34]. Usually, the procedure is performed under local anesthesia, sometimes via an orotracheal tube or laryngeal mask. For the transnasal route the diameter is too large. Once the lymph node is identified, the dedicated needle is fixed to the working channel of the bronchoscope and the sheath is adjusted so that the tip of the catheter with the hub is visualized through the endoscope. Only then can the needle be advanced without risk of damaging the biopsy channel. The needle can then be advanced into the lesion under direct observation up to 4 cm. It takes a curved path to stay within the range of the ultrasound

sectorial view. Apart from the para-aortic/ subaortic, and paraesophageal region, all lymph nodes are within reach. In some case series by dedicated interventional teams, positive results have been achieved in 89–98%, thus reaching diagnostic accuracy as by mediastinoscopy. Especially in combination with transesophageal ultrasound-controlled needle biopsy (EUS-TBNA) the accuracy can even be higher, thus giving the potential for replacing mediastinoscopy in a considerable number of patients [35]. In some cases, we successfully applied the CP bronchoscope for this purpose. Lymph node stations 5 and 6 still need video-assisted thoracoscopy or anterior mediastinostomy for evaluation. Visual control of the needle enables puncture of lymph nodes less than 10 mm in size [36]. Especially after previous mediastinoscopy, restaging by EBUS-TBNA after induction chemotherapy seems to be easier than re-mediastinoscopy. By rapid onsite evaluation of the samples, results of EBUS-TBNA can be further improved as in a negative sample the procedure can be repeated on the spot. Recently, a prospective multicenter study has been published, which might represent a more realistic picture within a general population including non-dedicated interventional centers [37]. This reported an overall diagnostic yield of 75%, which represents what might be expected when starting an EBUS-TBNA program. Recently, two studies by Kurimoto's and Yasufuku's groups examined whether accuracy could be improved by analysis of the internal structure of lymph nodes [38,39] (Fig. 13.5).

*Mediastinal lesions.* If lesions within the mediastinum are in contact with the central airways they can also be explored with the radial probe and approached by TBNA. If the wall is infiltrated, deep transmural biopsies (so-called button-hole biopsies) can be performed without risk (Fig. 13.6). However, as the depth of penetration with 20 MHz is limited, exploration with the linear probe is superior in many instances. We have been able to diagnose infiltration of the lateral wall of the trachea and the anterior wall of the esophagus. If in doubt as to whether an esophageal lesion is a primary cancer, lymph node invasion, or leiomyoma, the radial probe can be inserted into the esophagus and after reaching the cardia the balloon is inflated and the esophagus is explored during retraction. Whereas malignant lesions show a destruction of the wall, leiomyomas expand within the layer structures of the wall in a spiral arrangement without destroying the architecture and can be very reliably differentiated. Bronchogenic or other mediastinal cysts are easily seen by their low echogenic structure. Sometimes the are septated and in case of bleeding, infection, or more solid content they show irregular echoes inside. In contrast to reports after transesophageal puncture, so far we have not observed severe complications after transbronchial needle aspiration due to infection. This might be due to the less contaminated environment within the airways.

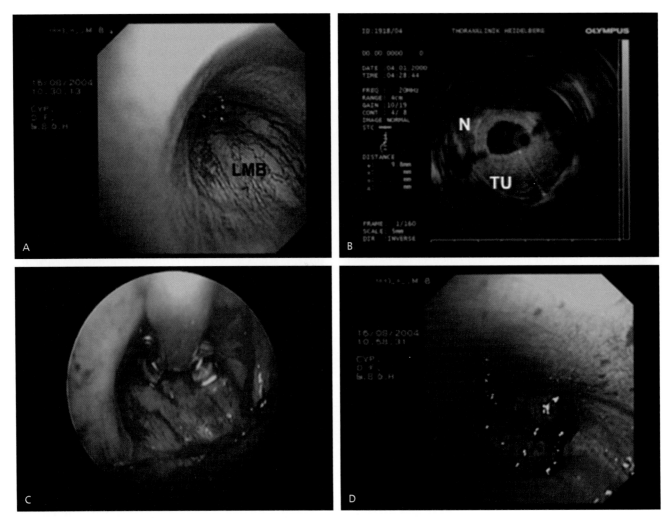

**Fig. 13.6** External infiltration of the bronchial wall. (A) The left main bronchus (LMB) is occluded subtotally by lymph node compression from dorsal. The mucosa is intact and only shows some vascular engorgement. (B) By ultrasonography the intact mucosa can be seen as an uninterrupted white line, whereas the deeper layers are completely invaded by tumor (TU) as compared to the normal wall (N) and to the pulmonary artery. Due to the oval deformation, the balloon is lacking contact at the dorsolateral wall. In these cases the tumor can be biopsied by the rigid forceps (C) right through the intact muscosa without any risk, a so called "button hole biopsy". (D) After biopsy the tumor is protruding through the defect, which is lined by the thinned mucosa.

*Intrapulmonary lesions.* Ultrasound is strongly reflected by air. Therefore, in the beginning we were skeptical about its application within the lung. However, Hürther and Hanrath in their early publications reported that EBUS is useful for the detection of peripheral lesions [6,7], and it even appeared to be possible to analyze the lung tissue [14]. Later, we were also able to localize solid and cystic lesions within the periphery of the lung with the radial probe. Localization for biopsy was successful in up to 80% and particularly superior to fluoroscopy in lesions of less than 3 cm and those that were hidden behind the heart or other anatomical structures and pleural effusion [19] (Fig. 13.7).

If the probe is introduced via a catheter as an extended working channel and can be placed exactly inside the lesion, biopsies are positive in up to 100%. Particularly in combina-tion with electromagnetic navigation, placement has become so reliable that currently we use EBUS for placement of Ir192 probes to treat inoperable peripheral lesions by brachy-therapy. The high resolution provided by 20 MHz allows detailed imaging of the anatomic infrastructure of these lesions, which correlates significantly to the histological diagnosis [40]. Applying computer-assisted analysis of the EBUS images, we were able to predict the nature of such lesions in 92% of cases [41] (Fig. 13.8).

In patients with infiltrations or atelectasis, EBUS is useful in exploring the cause such as bronchial compression by lymph nodes, benign strictures, tumor infiltration, or com-pression of the lung by pleural effusion or solid formations. The diagnosis and localization of cavitating lesions due to tuberculosis, necrotizing tumors, and mycetomas is helpful in guiding placement of pigtail catheters for drainage and instillation of drugs.

*Pleura and neighboring organs.* If there is an acoustic window due to atelectasis, pleural fluid, or a solid lesion, the pleura and neighboring structures, such as solid structures on the visceral and parietal pleura or on the pericardium, can be visualized. In cases where pleural effusion reaches the central airways, we successfully performed transbronchial thoracocentesis for diagnostic purposes by needle aspiration (Fig. 13.9).

## EBUS in therapeutic bronchoscopy

In our institution, approximately 20% of all procedures are performed for therapeutic interventions. In 48% of these ultrasound provides useful additional information, which has strategic importance for planning of the procedure in

43% of cases [20]. Exploration of central airway stenoses with EBUS in order to assess the cause and extent of a lesion and its relation to surrounding structures is helpful in making a decision on the appropriate technique—for example mechanical dilation, laser or argon plasma coagulation, and stenting—and for controlling the effect during follow-up [42]. Before resecting granulomas and scars, evaluation of the wall and vascularization is important to avoid perforation and bleeding (Fig. 13.10).

As described above, local staging of small cancers in preparation for bronchoscopic therapy has become essential. Complications in healing of anastomoses after bronchoplastic procedures can be difficult to diagnose by bronchoscopy alone. Edema, superficial necrosis, and the beginning of dehiscence can be differentiated by EBUS and it is especially useful to detect involvement of the adjacent pulmonary artery by localized abscess formation in order to indicate

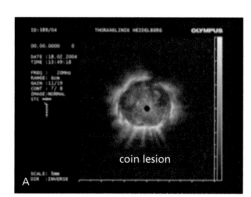

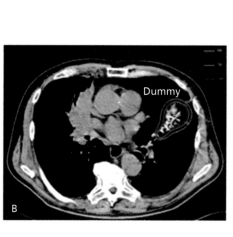

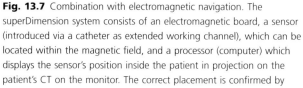

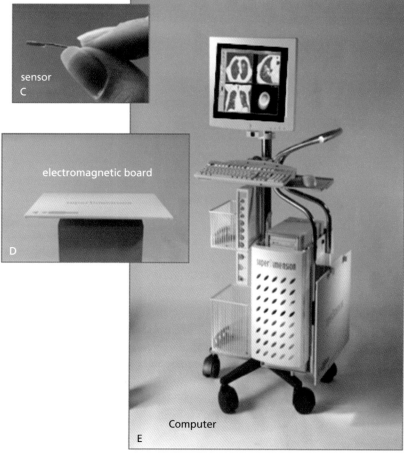

**Fig. 13.7** Combination with electromagnetic navigation. The superDimension system consists of an electromagnetic board, a sensor (introduced via a catheter as extended working channel), which can be located within the magnetic field, and a processor (computer) which displays the sensor's position inside the patient in projection on the patient's CT on the monitor. The correct placement is confirmed by

insertion of the miniprobe via the EWC (coin lesion). Afterwards, a brachytherapy catheter can be inserted and left in place for potentially curative treatment if the lesion's diameter is well within range of a curative dosage as calculated from the isodose lines by insertion of a dummy probe.

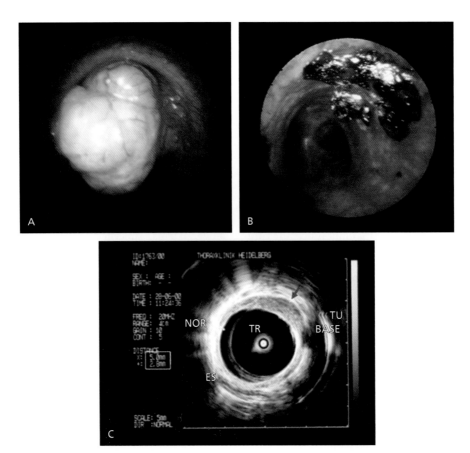

**Fig. 13.8** Adenoid cystic carcinoma of the trachea. (A) The pedunculated tumor is attached to the right lateral wall of the trachea. (B) After combined mechanical and laser resection only flat carbonized residuals remain. (C) However, ultrasound shows extensive tumor residuals within the wall (arrow). The thickness is 5mm as compared to the normal contralateral side with 2.8mm. Thus additional treatment is necessary. TR trachea; ES esophagus; NOR normal wall; TU BASE tumor residuals at base.

prophylactic surgical repair, before hemoptysis signals a fatal hemorrhage.

### EBUS in pediatric bronchoscopy

EBUS has also proved useful in pediatric bronchoscopy as conventional radiological imaging in these patients can be even less reliable due to the smaller organs, motion artefacts, and restrictions with regard to radiation exposure. In 412 children (3% of our population) with a median age of 4.2 years that we examined in an observation period between January 1998 and December 2001, EBUS was applied in 140 cases (34%), an almost equivalent frequency to that in adults. The indications were analysis of structures in stridor and intermittent dyspnea, which especially in this age group can be caused by vascular malformations, especially pulmonary sling syndrome. We diagnosed 11 of these cases by EBUS, some even after radiological diagnosis had failed. Solid lesions, perforating lymph nodes, atelectasis, and pneumonia were other indications. Children tolerated the procedure as well as adults and it did not take any longer [43].

### Training and the learning curve for EBUS

Compared to other bronchoscopic techniques, EBUS takes a considerably longer time to learn and to apply. This is primarily due to the fact that pulmonologists have only very recently been exposed to ultrasound technology and the interpretation of images. Secondly, handling of the equipment, especially the fragile radial scanning miniprobe, needs considerable skill. This is all the more demanding as for imaging the time that the airways can be occluded by the balloon probe is usually restricted, and especially when performed under local anesthesia the procedure might have to be repeatedly interrupted for re-oxygenation. And, lastly, as was described in the section above on anatomy, orientation within the complex mediastinal structures is difficult. For these reasons it took a long time for EBUS to be accepted and become distributed more widely. It was only with the introduction of the linear ultrasonic bronchoscope, a more familiar instrument than the radial probe, that currently EBUS is spreading with increasing speed world-wide and has become ". . . the highest impact technology in 2007" [44].

In our experience, after instruction by reading, lectures, and digital media, training by hands on is essential. This initial exposure can be achieved in training courses, which usually last 1 or 2 days. However, after this, more extensive experience is necessary to get more detailed insight. Depending on the primary experience, usually at least 1 week of additional experience in a dedicated training center is useful to obtain anatomical orientation and make the initial steps for image interpretation. Posters illustrating the mediastinal anatomy and the corresponding ultrasound images, including the location of lymph nodes, are available for this purpose and digital media (CDs and DVDs) are available for interactive learning. This has to be reinforced by personal practical experience with patients, for which approximately 50 procedures are necessary. According to Falcone *et al.* [45], 20 procedures are necessary for image interpretation, and sufficient experience can be gained after 6–24 months, depending on the frequency of examinations, illustrating the difficulty of this method as compared to other techniques. The development of interactive virtual training models could be very efficient in shortening the learning curve, since currently neither training on phantom models nor in animal models is capable of replacing experience in real patients.

## Cost-effectiveness

As with all new procedures, cost-effectiveness is an important issue. For Europe, we performed a cost assessment using the example of lymph node staging by the radial scanning probe. The costs for acquisition and write-off for the equipment, costs for physician and other staff, and the costs of the disposable materials amount to approximately €138 per procedure (excluding costs for bronchoscopy, which are the same for all calculation models). If 100 patients with enlarged lymph nodes undergo mediastinoscopy for preoperative staging the total costs amount to €162,000, calculated on the basis of €1620 per procedure. If staging is performed by conventional CT-guided TBNA, the costs comprising disposables, needles, and staff amount to €57 per procedure. Calculating an optimistic accuracy rate of 60%, 40 patients will need an additional mediastinoscopy, increasing the total costs to €70,000. By improving the results of TBNA to 80% by EBUS guidance, only 20 additional mediastinoscopies are needed, which adds up to a total of €51,000. This demonstrates that EBUS-guided TBNA is the most cost-

effective strategy for lymph node staging [46]. With the introduction of the ultrasonic bronchoscope and in combination with EUS, mediastinoscopy might be almost completely replaced in the future. However, recently, reimbursement of EBUS has been cancelled in the US. In addition, a study in Canada showed that repair costs for damage to the ultrasonic bronchoscopes vastly exceed that for regular bronchoscopes (approximately US$7500 versus US$40 per repair, or US$100 versus US$20 per procedure), which must be taken into account when planning to set up a program [47].

## Future prospects

As EBUS currently is spreading world wide, it is beginning to replace other methods. These include staging of early lung cancer and TBNA. The ultrasonic endoscope is attracting wide attention as the technique is more similar to that with which bronchoscopists are already familiar. However, it should be borne in mind that both methods are complementary rather than competitive. Exploration by 30-MHz probes might become useful in exploration of the small mucosal vessels in bronchoplastic procedures, inflammation, and neoplasia. Special processing algorithms and elastography could be useful for tissue characterization [48,49]. Combination with electromagnetic navigation is improving our methods for diagnosis and treatment of peripheral lesions, including radio frequency ablation and injection of chemotherapeutic agents in addition to brachytherapy, and tumor response can be assessed by computer analysis of images [50]. The role of EBUS in local staging of early cancers detected by screening programs has been described. Also, in screening programs for peripheral lesions by low-dose spiral CT, EBUS will play an important role, as a large number of these lesions are benign and do not need interventions. Ultrasound might also be applied for tissue destruction as its inherent energy can be focused in high-intensity focused ultrasound (HIFU) and transformed into heat. As the EBUS image changes with water content of the tissue, computed analysis of changes in impedance could serve as control for the effectiveness of treatment. The same technique could be applied to transmural treatment of mediastinal lesions after localization by the radial probe or under direct vision via the channel of the ultrasonic bronchoscope (Figs 13.9 and 13.10).

In conclusion, EBUS is currently complementing and in some respects beginning to replace other technologies. By application of EBUS, diagnostic and therapeutic decisions can be made immediately during bronchoscopy without the need for further time-consuming and costly procedures. As has been shown by the introduction of the ultrasonic bronchoscope, interest in this new technique has increased significantly, and we are currently observing the beginning

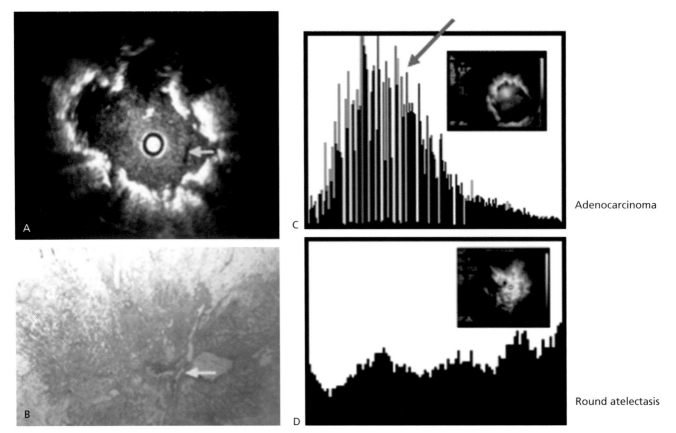

**Fig. 13.9** Histogramm of two peripheral lung lesions. (A) The high resolution of the 20-MHz radial probe provides detailed analysis of the structures with bright dots from airspaces and black lines from vessels (arrows) and the irregular margins to the surrounding lung tissue, as also seen in the histology specimen (B). The comparatively homogenous lesion (C) shows a peak on the dark side of the histogramm, when all pixels are counted, which is highly suggestive for malignancy, in this case an adenocarcinoma. In contrast the benign lesion, a round atelectasis, shows an even distribution of the echo signals (D). Probably, the dark peak corresponds to the neovascularisation of malignant lesions. Images for A and B courtesy of N. Kurimoto.

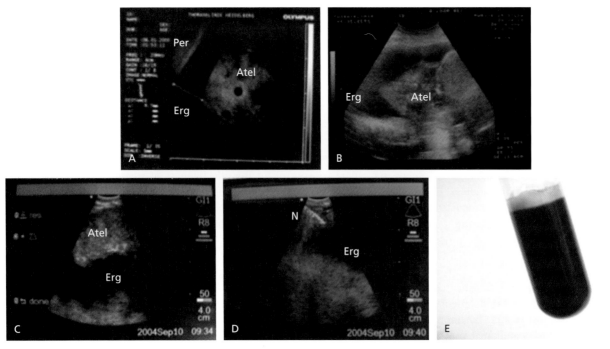

**Fig. 13.10** Ultrasonic view to lung tissue and pleura. In (A) the miniatureprobe is inserted into an atelectasis (Atel). The lung is surrounded by pleural effusion (Erg), which separates the lung from the pericardium (Per). (B) The deep penetration of the lower frequency by the ultrasonic bronchoscope provides a deeper view, showing a lower lobe atelectasis (Atel) above the liver and extensive pleural effusion (Erg). In (C) vegetations can be seen on the parietal pleura, protruding into the effusion (Erg) that is surrounding the atelectasis (atel). (D) If the effusion (Erg) is adjacent to the bronchus, the needle (N) can be used under ultrasonic control for thoracocentesis. (E) In this case the hemorrhagic effusion contained cells of an adenocarcinoma.

rather than the end of a development that will provide an ever-increasing range of instruments and applications.

## References

1 Becker HD. Short history of the development of endobronchial ultrasound—a story of success. In: Bolliger CT, Herth FJF, Miyazawa T, Beamis JF, eds. *Clinical Chest Ultrasound: From the ICU to the Bronchoscopy Suite*. Prog Respir Res. Basel: Karger; 2009; 99, 128–39.

2 Becker HD. EBUS—A new dimension in bronchoscopy. Editorial. *Respiration* 2006; **73**: 583–6.

3 Koga T, Ogata K, Hayashida R, Hattori R. Usefulness of transluminal ultrasonography in the evaluation of bronchial stenosis secondary to tuberculosis. *J Jpn Soc* 1994; **16**: 477–82.

4 Frank N, Holzapfel P, Wenk A. Neue Endoschall Minisonde in der täglichen Praxis. *Endosk Heute* 1994; **3**: 238–44.

5 Becker HD (2006) Endobronchial ultrasound with miniprobe radial scanning. In: CF Dietrich, ed. *Endoscopic ultrasound—an introductory manual and atlas*. Stuttgart-New York: Thieme; 2006: 334–51.

6 Hürther T, Hanrath P. Endobronchial sonography in the diagnosis of pulmonary and mediastinal tumors. *Dtsch Med Wochenschr* 1990; **115**: 1899–905.

7 Hürther T, Hanrath P. Endobronchial sonography: feasibility and preliminary results. *Thorax* 1992; **47**: 565–7.

8 Kurimoto N, Murayama M, Yoshioka S, *et al.* Assessment of usefulness of endobronchial ultrasonography in determination of depth of tracheobronchial tumor invasion. *Chest* 1999; **115**: 1500–6.

9 Miyazu Y, Miyazawa T, Kurimoto N, *et al.* Endobronchial ultrasonography in the assessment of centrally located early-stage lung cancer before photodynamic therapy. *Am J Respir Crit Care Med* 2002; **165**: 832–7.

10 Netter FH. *The Ciba collection of medical illustrations. Respiratory system.* Ardsley, NY: CIBA-GEIGY Corporation; 1979: 23.

11 Shirakawa T, Miyazawa T, Becker HD. The layer structure of central airways as described by endobronchial ultrasonography (EBUS). *J Bronchol* 2008; **15**: 129–33.

12 Shaw TJ, Wakely SL, Peebles CR, *et al.* Endobronchial ultrasound to assess airway wall thickening: validation in vitro and in vivo. *Eur Respir J* 2004; **23**: 813–17.

13 Becker HD. Bronchoscopy for airway lesions. In: Wang KP, Mehta AC, eds. *Flexible Bronchoscopy*. Blackwell Scientific Publications, 1995: 136–59.

14 Omori S, Takiguchi Y, Hiroshima K, *et al.* Peripheral pulmonary diseases: evaluation with endobronchial US; initial experience. *Radiology* 2002; **24**: 603–8.

15 Herth F, Becker HD, Manegold C, Drings P. Endobronchial ultrasound (EBUS): assessment of a new diagnostic tool in bronchoscopy for staging of lung cancer. *Onkologie* 2001; **24**: 151–4.

16 Becker HD. Options and results in endobronchial treatment of lung cancer. *Minim Invasive Ther Allied Technol* 1996; **5**: 165–78.

17 Herth F, Ernst A, Schulz M, Becker HD. Endobronchial ultrasound reliably differentiates between airway infiltration and compression by tumor. *Chest* 2003; **123**: 458–62.

18 Herth FJ, Becker HD, Ernst A. Ultrasound-guided transbronchial needle aspiration: an experience in 242 patients. *Chest* 2003; **123**: 604–7.

19 Herth FJ, Ernst A, Becker HD. Endobronchial ultrasound-guided transbronchial lung biopsy in solitary pulmonary nodules and peripheral lesions. *Eur Respir J* 2002; **20**: 118–21.

20 Herth FJ, Becker HD, LoCocero J III, Ernst A. Endobronchial ultrasound in therapeutic bronchoscopy. *Eur Respir J* 2002; **20**: 118–21.

21 Soja J, Grzanka P, Sladek K, *et al.* The use of endobronchial ultrasonography in assessment of the bronchial wall remodeling in asthma patients. *Chest* 2009; **136**: 797–804.

22 Deveci F, Murat A, Turgut T, *et al.* Airway wall thickness in patients with COPD and healthy current smokers and healthy non-smokers: assessment with high resolution computed tomographic scanning. *Respiration* 2004; **71**: 602–10.

23 Murgu S, Kurimoto N, Colt H, *et al.* Endobronchial ultrasound morphology of expiratory central airway collapse. *Respirology* 2008; **13**: 315–9.

24 Miyazu Y, Miyazawa T, Kurimoto N, *et al.* Endobronchial ultrasonography in the diagnosis and treatment of relapsing polychondritis with tracheobronchial malacia. *Chest* 2003; **124**: 2393–5.

25 Irani S, Hess T, Hofer M, *et al.* Endobronchial ultrasonography for the quantitative assessment of bronchial mural structures in lung transplant recipients. *Chest* 2006; **129**: 349–55.

26 Herth FJF, Becker HD, LoCicero J, Ernst A. Endobronchial ultrasound improves classification of suspicious lesions detected by autofluorescence bronchoscopy. *J Bronchol* 2003; **4**: 249–52.

27 Mountain CF. Revisions in the international system for staging lung cancer. *Chest* 1997; **111**: 1710–7.

28 Naidich DP. Staging of lung cancer. Controversy: computed tomography versus bronchoscopic needle aspiration: pro computed tomography. *J Bronchol* 1996; **3**: 73.

29 Herth F, Becker HD, LoCicero J, Ernst A. Endobronchioal ultrasound improves classification of suspicious lesions detected by autofluorescence bronchoscopy. *J Bronchol* 2003; **10**: 249–52.

30 Becker HD. Endobronchial ultrasound: a new perspective in bronchology. *J Ultraschall Med* 1996; **17**: 106–12.

31 Becker HD. The role of endobronchial ultrasound (EBUS) in diagnosis and treatment of centrally located early lung cancer. In: Hirsch FR, Bunn Jr PA, Kato H, Mulshine L, eds. *Textboook of Prevention and detection of Early Lung Cancer*. London and New York: Taylor and Francis; 2006: 161–75.

32 Lam S, Becker IID. Future diagnostic procedures. *Chest Surg Clin N Am* 1996; **6**: 363–80.

33 Becker HD, Kayser K, Schulz V, *et al. Atlas of Bronchoscopy. Technique, Diagnosis, Differential Diagnosis, Therapy.* Philadelphia – Hamilton: B.C. Decker, Inc.; 1991.

34 Yasufuku K, Nakajima T. Convex probe endobronchial ultrasound. In: Bolloger CT, Herth JFJ, Mayo PH, Miyzawa T, Beamis JF, eds. *Clinical Chest Ultrasound: From the ICU to the Bronchoscopy Suite*. Prog Respir Res, Vol. 37. Basel: Karger; 2009: 147–52.

35 Annema JT, Rabe KF. Esophageal ultrasound. In: Bolloger CT, Herth JFJ, Mayo PH, Miyazawa T, Beamis JF, eds. *Clinical Chest Ultrasound: From the ICU to the Bronchoscopy Suite*. Prog Respir Res, Vol. 37. Basel: Karger; 2009: 166–70.

36 Herth JFJ, Eberhardt R. Flexible Bronchoscopy and its Role in the Staging of Non-Small Cell Lung Cancer. *Clin Chest Med* 2010; **31**: 87–100.

37 Ernst A, Simoff M, Ost D, *et al.* A multicenter, prospective, advanced diagnostic bronchoscopy outcomes registry. *Chest* 2010; **138**: 165–70.

38 Kurimoto N, Osada H, Miyazwa T, *et al.* Targeting the area in metastatic lymph nodes in lung cancer for endobronchial ultrasonography-guided transbronchial needle aspiration. *J Bronchol* 2008; **15**: 134–8.

39 Fujiwara T, Yasufuku K, Nakajima T, *et al.* The utility of sonographic fetures during endobronchial ultrsound-guided transbronchial needle aspiration for lymph node staging in patients with lung cancer. *Chest* 2010; **138**: 641–7.

40 Kurimoto N, Murayama M, Yoshioka S, Nishisaka T. Analysis of the internal structure of peripheral pulmonary lesions using endobronchial ultrasonography. *Chest* 2002; **122**: 1887–94.

41 Becker HD, Herth F, Shirakawa T. Computer assisted analysis of endosonographic images of solitary pulmonary nodules (SPN). *Eur Respir J* 2001; **20**: 462.

42 Shirakawa T, Ishida A, Miyazu Y, *et al.* Endobronchial ultrasound for difficult airway problems. In: Bolloger CT, Herth JFJ, Mayo PH, Miyzawa T, Beamis JF, eds. *Clinical Chest Ultrasound: From the ICU to the Bronchoscopy Suite*. Prog Respir Res, Vol. 37. Basel: Karger; 2009: 189–201.

43 Link B, Liman YST, Becker HD, Dienemann H. Endobronchial juvenile hemangioma in infancy: removal by main bronchus cuff resection. *Chirurg* 2001; **72**: 584–7.

44 Kovitz K. Literature review. Lecture at the meeting of the American Association for Bronchology, Chicago, Oct. 2007.

45 Falcone F, Fois F, Grosso D. Endobronchial ultrasound. *Respiration* 2003; **70**: 179–94.

46 Herth F, Ernst A, Becker HD. Initial EBUS-guided TBNA is the most cost-effective means of lymph node staging—a German experience trial. *Chest* 2002; **122**: 104.

47 Herrgott CA, MacEachern P, Stather DR, Tremblay A. repair costs for endobronchial ultrasound bronchoscopes. *J Bronchol Intervent Pulmonol* 2010; **17**: 223–7.

48 Basset O, Sun Z, Mestas JL, Gimenez G. Texture analysis of ultrasonic images of the prostate by means of co-coccurence matrices. *Ultrasound Imaging* 1993; **15**: 218–37.

49 Wagner RF, Insana MF, Brown DG. Unified approach to the detection an classification of speckle texture in diagnostic ultrasound. *Opt Eng* 1986; **25**: 738–4.

50 Becker HD, Herth F, Schwarz Y, Ernst A. Bronchoscopic biopsy of peripheral lung lesions under electromagnetic guidance. A pilot study. *J Bronchol* 2005; **12**: 1, 9–13.

# 14 Application and Limitations of Virtual Bronchoscopic Navigation

**Fumihiro Asano**

Department of Pulmonary Medicine and Bronchoscopy, Gifu Prefectural General Medical Center, Gifu, Japan

## Bronchoscopic diagnosis of peripheral pulmonary lesions

The diagnostic yield of peripheral lesions by bronchoscopy has been an unsatisfactory 78%, according to the guidelines of the American College of Chest Physicians (ACCP) published in 2007, and has been reported to be 34% for lesions less than 2 cm [1]. Factors affecting the transbronchial diagnosis of isolated peripheral pulmonary lesions include the size [2,3], site [2], presence or absence of an involved bronchus [4], and whether the disease is malignant or benign [3], as well as the instrument used and skill [5] and experience of the bronchoscopist.

## Computed tomography two-dimensional mapping

Volumetric data with three-dimensional continuity can be obtained by helical computed tomography (CT), but images are usually presented as two-dimensional planar axial slices. Planar two-dimensional axial CT is the basis for not only routine airway imaging, but also lung parenchymal and mediastinal diagnostic imaging. Presently, CT scan-based (axial slice) two-dimensional road mapping is used for bronchoscopic path selection, but it is difficult to identify the bronchial path to the lesion, and path selection is inaccurate even at the third to fourth-generation bronchus levels [6].

## Virtual bronchoscopy

Virtual bronchoscopy (VB) is a method to present computer-generated three-dimensional images of the tracheal and bronchial lumens reconstructed from continuous volumetric data obtained by helical CT [7]. An advantage of VB is that it can be performed as many times as necessary, non-invasively, without additional exposure, through the use of CT volume data sets.

VB is performed by either the surface or volume rendering method, but an important point in the preparation of virtual images is the determination of the threshold. The interface generated by the determination of a threshold is the tracheal or bronchial wall observed by VB. Therefore, virtual images change, based on how the threshold is determined, and divisions may be omitted, or holes may be observed in the bronchial wall, suggesting divisions, particularly in the peripheral airway [8]. It is important to verify the presence or absence of divisions in the axial, sagittal, and coronary images and to compare the results with the virtual images.

## Virtual bronchoscopy mapping

Virtual mapping is a method that uses positional information on lesions generated by VB. There have been clinical reports of its application for visible lesions at the proximal bronchial level and lymph node biopsy from the proximal bronchial level (TBNA) [9]. It is more useful than two-dimensional CT mapping for bronchial path selection, but there have been few reports of its use for the examination of peripheral lesions, with the exception of case reports of bronchoscopy for virtual mapping of the subsegmental level [10]. In the 1990s, multidetector CT was not widely available, it was difficult to prepare accurate virtual images to peripheral regions, and there was no thin bronchoscope that would have allowed the effective use of such images.

Virtual mapping is problematic as a potential method of supporting bronchoscopists. In actual bronchoscopy, unlike in VB, the bronchoscope tip can be moved only up or down, and the bronchoscope should therefore be appropriately

*Flexible Bronchoscopy*, Third Edition. Edited by Ko-Pen Wang, Atul C. Mehta, J. Francis Turner.
© 2012 Blackwell Publishing Ltd. Published 2012 by Blackwell Publishing Ltd.

rotated at the time of its advancement. Therefore, the virtual images differ from the real images based on the angle of this rotation. Unless the bronchoscope is advanced while both images are matched with each other at each branching, the risk of disorientation is high.

## Virtual bronchoscopic navigation

This author and colleagues previously reported a method of presenting virtual images, including mapping information along with real images, to guide an ultrathin bronchoscope to the target as virtual bronchoscopic navigation (VBN) [11]. In the cases reported, the ultrathin bronchoscope could be guided to the target using virtual images prepared to the tenth-generation bronchus. The categorization of bronchi in the Japanese reports cited in this chapter, including those related to VBN, is based on the Japanese method, in which subsegmental branches are regarded as third-generation bronchi. In the early stages, printouts of a series of virtual images were held in the hand and rotated to fit the real images, but we have begun to use the VBN system, which is described below. Dolina and Merrit have reported that using virtual images interactively with real images is more useful than conventional mapping [6,12].

Previous studies on VBN for the diagnosis of peripheral pulmonary lesions are shown in Table 14.1. We performed CT-guided ultrathin bronchoscopy using VBN in 36 peripheral pulmonary lesions [13]. After the ultrathin bronchoscope (2.8 mm external diameter, 1.2 mm diameter of the forceps channel) was guided using virtual images, we examined whether the bronchoscope was actually on the intended route to the lesion by thin-section CT. Virtual images could be prepared to a mean of the 6.1st-generation bronchi. Ultrathin bronchoscopes allowed examination to a mean of the 6.9th-generation bronchi. Since virtual images satisfactorily reflected the real morphology of the bronchial divisions, ultrathin bronchoscopes could be guided to 30 (83.3%)

of the 36 lesions along the intended routes without fluoroscopy, demonstrating the usefulness of VBN. Guidance was impossible in six lesions because of rotation of the bronchoscope and inappropriate determination of the threshold, and these failures led to the development of a VBN system.

Shinagawa and colleagues performed a similar procedure in 26 peripheral pulmonary lesions less than 2 cm in diameter and reported that 17 lesions (65.4%) could be diagnosed [14].

Using a similar method, we transbronchially marked, with barium, 31 lesions 1 cm or less in diameter showing a pure ground-glass opacity pattern, which we planned to remove by thoracoscopic surgery. Using virtual images prepared to a median of the sixth-generation bronchi, ultrathin bronchoscopes could also be guided to a median of the sixth-generation bronchi to the intended marking sites. Since ultrathin bronchoscopes were inserted into areas near the lesions, catheters could be guided accurately and readily to the intended sites, and marking was possible with a median of 4 mm from the lesions and within 1 cm from 27 lesions. The barium-marked lesions could be removed in all patients by thoracoscopic partial resection. Since this method is free of complications such as pneumothorax and hemorrhage, unlike percutaneous procedures, and is technically simple and multiple lesions can be treated [15].

Moreover, a method concomitantly using VBN and endobronchial ultrasonography with a guide-sheath (EBUS-GS) has also been reported as a procedure using a modality other than CT to determine the route to transport the biopsy device to the lesion. EBUS-GS was reported by Kurimoto and colleagues [16]. By this method, the arrival of the biopsy device at the lesion is confirmed using an ultrasound probe with a guide sheath, and samples are collected from the same site through the guide sheath. Asahina and colleagues performed this technique in 30 peripheral pulmonary lesions 3 cm or less in diameter, and reported that 24 lesions (80%) could be delineated by EBUS and 19 lesions (63.3%) could be diagnosed [17].

**Table 14.1** Virtual bronchoscopic navigation for the diagnosis of peripheral pulmonary lesions

| Author | Confirmation of arrival | No. examined lesions | Diagnostic yield (%) | No. of lesions <2 cm | Diagnostic yield for lesions <2 cm (%) | Examination time (min) |
|---|---|---|---|---|---|---|
| Asano et al. [13] | CT and X-ray fluoroscopy | 36 | 86.1 | 26 | 80.8 | n/a |
| Shinagawa et al. [14] | CT fluoroscopy | 26 | 65.4 | 26 | 65.4 | 29.3 |
| Asahina et al. [17] | EBUS | 30 | 63.3 | 18 | 44.4 | 25.7 |
| Asano et al. [19] | CT and X-ray fluoroscopy | 38 | 81.6 | 26 | 80.8 | 24.9 |
| Shinagawa et al. [20] | CT fluoroscopy | 71 | 70.4 | 71 | 70.4 | 24.5 |
| Tachihara et al. [21] | X-ray fluoroscopy | 96 | 62.5 | 77 | 54.5 | 24.1 |
| Asano et al. [18] | EBUS | 32 | 84.4 | 15 | 73.3 | 22.3 |
| Ishida et al. [22] | EBUS | 99 | 80.8 | 58 | 75.9 | 24.0 |
| Summary | | 428 | 73.6 | 317 | 67.5 | |

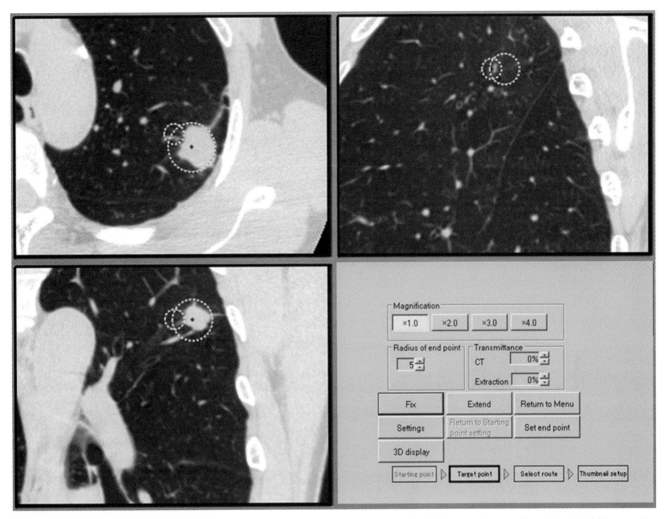

**Fig. 14.1** VBN system (Bf-NAVI) setting of the target and terminal point. A small lesion in the distal left S1+2. The target (large dotted circle) is set on the lesion by viewing the axial, sagittal, and coronal images. The terminal point (small dotted circle) is set at the distal end of the extracted involved bronchus.

## Virtual bronchoscopic navigation system

As mentioned above, using VBN poses several challenges: (1) some skill and effort are needed for preparation of the virtual images, and (2) the technique cannot sufficiently cope with the problem caused by rotation of the broncho-scope. We have therefore developed a system that allows the automatic preparation of virtual images of the bronchial path and presents them with real images for comparison. This system (Bf-NAVI; Cybernet Systems, Olympus Medical Systems) has both virtual image preparation [18] and navigation functions [19].

Images are prepared through the following processes:

**1** Inputting of CT data; DICOM data of CT are input into the system.

**2** Setting of the starting point; once the starting point is set at the trachea, the threshold is automatically adjusted, and the bronchi are extracted.

**3** Setting of the target and terminal point; the lesion and extracted bronchi nearest the lesion are determined as the target and terminal point, respectively (Fig. 14.1). When they are determined, the route to the terminal point is automatically sought and displayed.

**4** Checking of the route; the route is also presented as a bronchial tree. As the point on the route is moved from the starting point to the terminal point, the corresponding cross-sectional images are presented (Fig. 14.2). When the route is determined, the virtual images on the route are automatically prepared.

**5** Thumbnail registration; while serially displaying virtual images from the starting point to the terminal point, the bronchus into which the bronchoscope should be inserted is marked at each bronchial division, and the images are registered as thumbnails (Fig. 14.3). This system can confirm areas for which VB images could not be produced because of the absence of the automatic extraction of bronchi. VB images of these areas can be added by manual extraction.

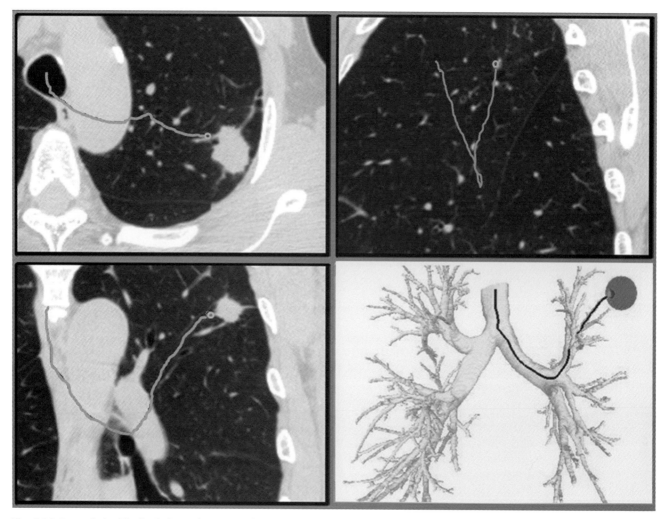

**Fig. 14.2** Route display. The line indicates the route to the terminal point. The panel in the lower left shows a bronchial tree. The circle indicates the target. Each cross-sectional image corresponding to the points on the line is presented.

After using this function, the bronchi are further extracted peripherally.

Navigation is performed by matching the virtual image showing the target bronchus with the real image using the four functions of: (1) presenting the target bronchus, (2) rotating images, (3) advancing or retreating images, and (4) displaying thumbnails. The direction of the lesion is also indicated in the image for additional reference (Fig. 14.4). Since the bronchoscope is advanced according to virtual images indicating the target, any bronchoscopist can lead the bronchoscope to the target in a short time. The system can also be used educationally for simulation before the examination.

The following results have been reported concerning the VBN system. We performed CT-guided ultrathin bronchoscopy using the VBN system in 38 small pulmonary lesions 3 cm or less in diameter. We successfully led the bronchoscope along the intended route without fluoroscopy in 36 (94.7%) lesions, and diagnosed 31 (81.6%) lesions [19].

In addition, Shinagawa and colleagues reported a significant shortening of the time until the beginning of biopsy and examination time through the use of the VBN system compared with standard VBN, although this was based on a retrospective evaluation [20].

Tachihara and colleagues performed biopsy under fluoroscopy using the VBN system in 96 peripheral pulmonary lesions 3 cm or less in diameter, and reported a diagnostic yield of 62.5% and an examination time of 24.1 minutes [21].

We performed biopsies by combining this system with a thin bronchoscope (4.0 mm external diameter, 2.0 mm diameter of the forceps channel) and EBUS-GS in 32 peripheral pulmonary lesions (including 11 fluoroscopically invisible lesions) [18]. Virtual images could be prepared to a median of the fifth-generation bronchi, and divisions showed agreement between the virtual and real images in all patients. Thirty lesions (93.8%) could be delineated by EBUS, and 27 lesions (84.4%) could be diagnosed.

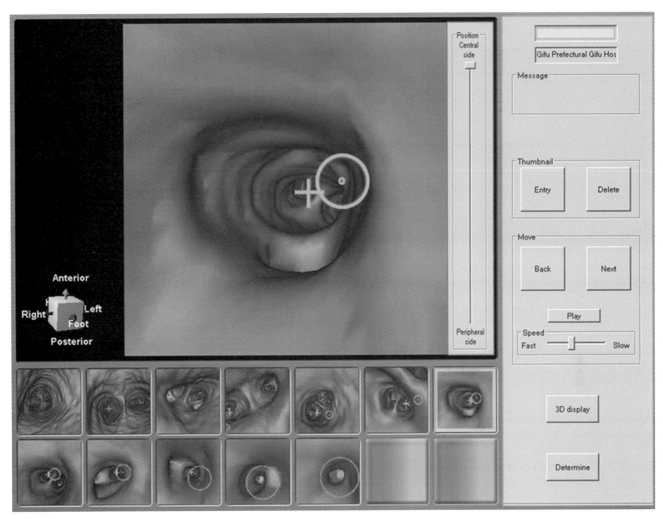

**Fig. 14.3** Virtual images on the route. VB images of the route are automatically produced. The bronchus in which the bronchoscope should be inserted at each division is marked with a cross by advancing the virtual images from the starting point to the terminal point, and registered as thumbnails (below). The circle indicates the direction of the target.

## Virtual Navigation in Japan (NINJA) study

To objectively demonstrate the effectiveness of the VBN system, we performed a multicenter, collaborative, randomized study (NINJA Study) [22]. Two hundred patients with peripheral pulmonary lesions 3 cm or less in diameter were randomized to VBN and no-VBN groups, and biopsy was performed by EBUS-GS. The thin bronchoscope was guided using the VBN system in the VBN group, and according to axial CT images in the non-VBN group. In the VBN group, virtual images could be prepared to a median of the sixth-generation bronchi, and the rate of agreement with the real images was 98%. The diagnostic yield in the VBN group (80.8%) was significantly higher than in the non-VBN group (67.4%) at $P < 0.05$. The time until the initiation of the biopsy and the examination time (median, 8.1 and 24 minutes, respectively) were significantly shortened in the

VBN compared with the non-VBN group ($P < 0.05$). The VBN system was confirmed to improve the diagnostic yield and shorten the examination time.

## Summary of VBN studies

Reports of VBN studies are summarized in Table 14.1. The diagnostic yield was 65.4–86.1% by CT-guided ultrathin bronchoscopy, 63.3–84.4% by EBUS-GS, 62.5% by fluoroscopy, and 73.6% by all techniques combined. Comparison of the diagnostic yield is difficult, as it is affected not only by lesion size but also the disease in question, site, percentage of benign diseases, and presence or absence of bronchial involvement. However, when limiting the lesion size to 2 cm or less, the diagnostic yield was 65.4–80.8% by CT-guided ultrathin bronchoscopy, 44.4–75.9% by EBUS-GS, 54.5% by fluoroscopy, and 67.5% for all techniques. These diagnostic

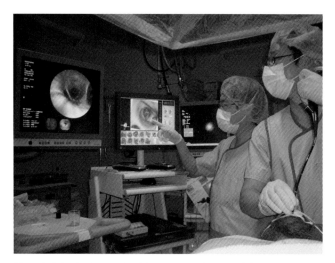

**Fig. 14.4** Navigation. Using this system, VB images of the target bronchus are displayed in comparison with the real images. Since the bronchoscope is advanced according to VB images indicating the target, anyone can guide the bronchoscope to the target in a short time.

yields were higher than the 34% mentioned in the ACCP guidelines. The diagnostic yield appears to be the highest for CT-guided ultrathin bronchoscopy among the three techniques, but a controlled study is needed for more exact comparisons. Fluoroscopy is the most widely used technique today, but there has been only one report of the use of fluoroscopy with VBN. Further evaluation of its effectiveness is necessary because it is simpler than the other methods. EBUS-GS requires a special instrument, but as the technique is simple and can identify lesions undetectable by fluoroscopy, it is considered to be the most promising and may make fluoroscopy unnecessary for some patients. No complications associated with VBN have been reported.

## Advantages and limitations

The advantages of VBN are: (1) it facilitates the guidance of the bronchoscope by indicating the bronchial route to the lesion, (2) the time needed for the guidance can be markedly shortened, because the position of the bronchoscope and direction of its advancement need not be checked by fluoroscopy or other imaging modalities, (3) it is expected to have educational benefits because the preparation of virtual images itself serves to stimulate the field of bronchoscopy, and (4) it contributes to the reduction in invasiveness of the examination and improvement in the diagnostic yield as it can be easily performed, even by an inexperienced bronchoscopist. The low cost is another major advantage of the technique.

However, while this method is simple and practical, the necessity of manually fitting the virtual images to the real

ones remains a problem. Research and development efforts to automatically match virtual and real images have been made to date [23,24]. As an example of clinical application, McLennan and colleagues performed a randomized, controlled prospective trial using a system that superimposes virtual bronchoscopic images showing the location of the lesion and route to it over actual images in real time [25]. In 87 patients who underwent mediastinal lymph node biopsy, they reported that the successful sampling rate from the paratracheal or perihilar lymph nodes improved significantly from 68.6 to 100% through the use of the system. Merritt and colleagues also applied the same system to peripheral lesions and reported that the accuracy of biopsy from peripheral lesions in distal bronchi could be significantly improved [12]. Despite problems such as respiratory movements and the difficulty of securing a good visual field in the examination of peripheral lesions, the clinical application of the system was awaited. In 2009, LungPoint was clinically introduced in the US as another VBN system. LungPoint does not have the manual bronchi extraction function, but it is straightforward to use. Although further improvement in performance is necessary, VB images automatically synchronize with real images. Eberhardt and colleagues performed biopsy using this VBN system in 25 peripheral pulmonary lesions (<42 mm), and reported a diagnostic yield of 80% [26].

The second problem with the VBN system is that there is no method to confirm the arrival of the bronchoscope at the target, as in electromagnetic navigation (EMN) [27]. VB images are also employed in EMN, but virtual images of central bronchi are used only for the matching of CT data indicating the position of the lesion with that in the actual patient, and the subsequent guidance of the biopsy device, and confirmation of its arrival are performed using an EMN sensor. Since VBN has no such sensor, it must be combined with fluoroscopy, CT, or EBUS to confirm the arrival. However, the guidance of an ultrathin bronchoscope to a bronchus immediately proximal to the lesion has been confirmed in a report using CT, and as the lesion can be reached simply by inserting forceps, the examination is sufficiently possible even under fluoroscopy. In addition, bronchoscopes 4 mm in diameter at the minimum are presently necessary for use in EBUS-GS, but according to our experience, most lesions can be reached simply by the insertion of an echo probe or forceps into the bronchoscope.

By VBN, the bronchoscope can be advanced according to the corresponding virtual images. Therefore, the bronchoscopic process is markedly facilitated regardless of the skill of the bronchoscopist, leading to an improvement in the diagnostic yield and shortening of the examination time. Since VBN is inexpensive and facilitates the guidance of the bronchoscope, which is a basic aspect of bronchoscopy of peripheral lesions, its wider use is anticipated.

## Acknowledgments

I would like to express my deep gratitude to the late Dr Koichi Yamazaki and to Dr Naofumi Shinagawa (First Department of Internal Medicine, Hokkaido University Hospital), Dr Takashi Ishida (Department of Pulmonary Medicine, Fukushima Medical University Hospital), and Dr Hiroshi Moriya (Department of Radiology, Sendai Kousei Hospital) for their collaboration.

## References

1 Rivera MP, Mehta AC. Initial diagnosis of lung cancer: ACCP evidence-based clinical practice guidelines (2nd edition). *Chest* 2007; **132**: 131S–148S.

2 Chechani V. Bronchoscopic diagnosis of solitary pulmonary nodules and lung masses in the absence of endobronchial abnormality. *Chest* 1996; **109**: 620–5.

3 Baaklini WA, Reinoso MA, Gorin AB, *et al.* Diagnostic yield of fiberoptic bronchoscopy in evaluating solitary pulmonary nodules. *Chest* 2000; **117**: 1049–54.

4 Naidich DP, Sussman R, Kutcher WL, *et al.* Solitary pulmonary nodules. CT-bronchoscopic correlation. *Chest* 1988; **93**: 595–8.

5 Minami H, Ando Y, Nomura F, *et al.* Interbronchoscopist variability in the diagnosis of lung cancer by flexible bronchoscopy. *Chest* 1994; **105**: 1658–62.

6 Dolina MY, Cornish DC, Merritt SA, *et al.* Interbronchoscopist variability in endobronchial path selection: a simulation study. *Chest* 2008; **133**: 897–905.

7 Vining DJ, Liu K, Choplin RH, Haponik EF. Virtual bronchoscopy. Relationships of virtual reality endobronchial simulations to actual bronchoscopic findings. *Chest* 1996; **109**: 549–53.

8 De Wever W, Vandecaveye V, Lanciotti S, Verschakelen JA. Multidetector CT-generated virtual bronchoscopy: an illustrated review of the potential clinical indications. *Eur Respir J* 2004; **23**: 776–82.

9 McAdams HP, Goodman PC, Kussin P. Virtual bronchoscopy for directing transbronchial needle aspiration of hilar and mediastinal lymph nodes: a pilot study. *AJR Am J Roentgenol* 1998; **170**: 1361–4.

10 Moriya H, Koyama M, Honjo H, Hashimoto N. Interactive virtual bronchoscopy as a guide for transbronchial biopsy in two cases. *J Jpn Soc Bronchol* 1998; **20**: 610–13.

11 Asano F, Matsuno Y, Matsushita T, *et al.* Transbronchial diagnosis of a pulmonary peripheral small lesion using an ultrathin bronchoscope with virtual bronchoscopic navigation. *J Bronchol* 2002; **9**: 108–111.

12 Merritt SA, Gibbs JD, Yu KC, *et al.* Image-guided bronchoscopy for peripheral lung lesions: a phantom study. *Chest* 2008; **134**: 1017–26.

13 Asano F, Matsuno Y, Takeichi N, *et al.* Virtual bronchoscopy in navigation of an ultrathin bronchoscope. *J Jpn Soc Bronchol* 2002; **24**: 433–8.

14 Shinagawa N, Yamazaki K, Onodera Y, *et al.* CT-guided transbronchial biopsy using an ultrathin bronchoscope with virtual bronchoscopic navigation. *Chest* 2004; **125**: 1138–43.

15 Asano F, Shindoh J, Shigemitsu K, *et al.* Ultrathin bronchoscopic barium marking with virtual bronchoscopic navigation for fluoroscopy-assisted thoracoscopic surgery. *Chest* 2004; **126**: 1687–93.

16 Kurimoto N, Miyazawa T, Okimasa S, *et al.* Endobronchial ultrasonography using a guide sheath increases the ability to diagnose peripheral pulmonary lesions endoscopically. *Chest* 2004; **126**: 959–65.

17 Asahina H, Yamazaki K, Onodera Y, *et al.* Transbronchial biopsy using endobronchial ultrasonography with a guide sheath and virtual bronchoscopic navigation. *Chest* 2005; **128**: 1761–5.

18 Asano F, Matsuno Y, Tsuzuku A, *et al.* Diagnosis of peripheral pulmonary lesions using a bronchoscope insertion guidance system combined with endobronchial ultrasonography with a guide sheath. *Lung Cancer* 2008; **60**: 366–73.

19 Asano F, Matsuno Y, Shinagawa N, *et al.* A virtual bronchoscopic navigation system for pulmonary peripheral lesions. *Chest* 2006; **130**: 559–66.

20 Shinagawa N, Yamazaki K, Onodera Y, *et al.* Virtual bronchoscopic navigation system shortens the examination time—feasibility study of virtual bronchoscopic navigation system. *Lung Cancer* 2007; **56**: 201–6.

21 Tachihara M, Ishida T, Kanazawa K, *et al.* A virtual bronchoscopic navigation system under X-ray fluoroscopy for transbronchial diagnosis of small peripheral pulmonary lesions. *Lung Cancer* 2007; **57**: 322–7.

22 Ishida T, Asano F, Yamazaki K, *et al.* Virtual bronchoscopic navigation combined with endobronchial ultrasound to diagnose small peripheral pulmonary lesions: A randomized trial. *Thorax* (in press).

23 Mori K, Deguchi D, Sugiyama J, *et al.* Tracking of a bronchoscope using epipolar geometry analysis and intensity-based image registration of real and virtual endoscopic images. *Med Image Anal* 2002; **6**: 321–36.

24 Higgins WE, Helferty JP, Lu K, *et al.* 3D CT-video fusion for image-guided bronchoscopy. *Comput Med Imaging Graph* 2008; **32**: 159–73.

25 McLennan G, Ferguson JS, Thomas K, *et al.* The use of MDCT-based computer-aided pathway finding for mediastinal and perihilar lymph node biopsy: a randomized controlled prospective trial. *Respiration* 2007; **74**: 423–31.

26 Eberhardt R, Kahn N, Gompelmann D, *et al.* LungPoint—a new approach to peripheral lesions. *J Thorac Oncol* 2010; **5**: 1559–63.

27 Schwarz Y, Greif J, Becker HD, *et al.* Real-time electromagnetic navigation bronchoscopy to peripheral lung lesions using overlaid CT images: the first human study. *Chest* 2006; **129**: 988–94.

# 3 Therapeutic Bronchoscopy

# 15 Application of Laser, Electrocautery, Argon Plasma Coagulation, and Cryotherapy in Flexible Bronchoscopy

## Praveen N. Mathur

Department of Medicine, Indiana University Medical Center, Indianapolis, IN, USA

## Introduction

Benign or malignant tracheobronchial obstruction can lead to acute respiratory distress or even asphyxia and death. Endobronchial obstruction may present as an endobronchial lesion, or an extraluminal obstruction, or sometimes a combined endobronchial and extraluminal form.

If curative resection is not possible, various endoscopic methods for palliation are available, such as Nd:YAG laser therapy, cryotherapy, electrocautery, and argon plasma coagulation. In cases of extraluminal lesions, palliation is performed by balloon dilatation, stent placement, and/or external beam radiation, which are discussed in other chapters.

Patients presents with dyspnea, cough, chest discomfort, hemoptysis, stridor, or a localized wheeze. The history may include known cancer, aspiration of a foreign body, prior airway surgery or intubation, recurrent pneumonia, or other underlying illnesses involving the airways, such as sarcoidosis or tuberculosis.

These lesions may be detected on chest radiography or CT scan, but direct airway visualization with bronchoscopy is often needed to define the lesion. Bronchoscopy will determine the appropriateness of treatment, for example by removing a foreign body or using a laser to debulk a tracheal tumor. When treatment is not emergent, therapy may be determined by the histology of an obstructing lesion, potential curative therapy, properties of the lesion such as location, endobronchial mass with complete or partial obstruction, extrinsic compression, malacia, etc., and patient tolerance and acceptance. It is extremely important as to whether appropriate equipment and experienced operators are available.

## Nd: YAG laser

### Background

Using theories proposed on radiant energy in 1917 [1], Schawlow and Townes [2] formulated the hypothesis of laser light, with the subsequent development of a ruby laser reported by Maimon in 1960 [3].

Laser technology makes use of the power of radiant energy and properties of light amplification; laser being an acronym for "light amplified by the stimulated emission of radiation." For the stimulated emission of light to occur, there must be developed an adequate population of excited electrons with subsequent release of photons to produce the lasers light. This phenomenon is termed population inversion and requires an outside energy source to excite a designated medium. Almost any solid, liquid, or gas may act as a medium, and placing the substance to be excited in a chamber with mirrors at either end further facilitates population inversion. The effectiveness of laser light as opposed to naturally occurring light is associated with three important properties: wavelength, spatial coherence, and temporal coherence [4].

Whereas naturally occurring light comprises light of varying wavelengths, laser light contains only one color or a narrow band of wavelengths. Spatial coherence is achieved in laser because laser light diverges only minimally from its source, thereby maintaining its intensity. For temporal coherence, the packets of energy produced travel in uniform time with equal alignment. These three characteristics apply whether the medium is a solid, gas, or liquid.

The amount of energy that is delivered to a lesion depends on the power setting of the laser expressed in Watts, the distance from the laser tip to the target, and the duration of

*Flexible Bronchoscopy*, Third Edition. Edited by Ko-Pen Wang, Atul C. Mehta, J. Francis Turner.
© 2012 Blackwell Publishing Ltd. Published 2012 by Blackwell Publishing Ltd.

impact [5]. Light directed at a surface may also be reflected, scattered, transmitted, or absorbed [4]. The depth of penetration, therefore, depends not only on the properties of the light but also the inherent properties of the tissue, the characteristics of the light produced, and also on the medium used. The two most commonly used media in interventional bronchology are the carbon dioxide ($CO_2$) and neodymiun:yttrium–aluminum–garnet (Nd:YAG) lasers.

In the $CO_2$, laser light is produced in the infrared spectrum at a wavelength of 10,600nm. The $CO_2$ laser has an exact interaction with soft tissue, owing to its almost complete absorption by most tissues. When the $CO_2$ laser contacts tissue, the water content of the tissue is raised to temperatures of 100°C with subsequent vaporization. The $CO_2$ laser can be used as a precise cutting tool, with only minimal blood loss, owing to a relatively shallow depth of penetration. The most widely used laser light for tracheobronchial lesions is the Nd:YAG laser, which is produced by the stimulation of an yttrium–aluminum–garnet glass, coated with neodymium. The Nd:YAG laser has a wavelength of 1064nm and is easily transmitted through pale tissues, with sizeable scatter and a potential penetration of up to 5 to 10mm from the focal point.

The $CO_2$ laser, owing to its long wavelength, requires an articulating arm and a series of mirrors; however, it is now available on a probe. $CO_2$ laser therapy is most commonly used in the management of laryngeal lesions involving the area around the glottic opening. The $CO_2$ laser can serve as an excellent scalpel as scattering is minimal, tissue vaporization is rapid, and there is minimal damage to tissue. When used appropriately, laser energy can be directed precisely onto a target tissue, avoiding damage to healthy tissue. However, it does not have good coagulation properties. The Nd:YAG lasers, unlike the $CO_2$ laser, can cause deep tissue vasoconstriction, with a penetration depth of up to 10mm, but it has very good coagulation properties.

## Contraindications

Laser therapy of the tracheobronchial tree may be contraindicated because of the location of the lesion in relation to contiguous anatomy and the associated clinical condition of the patient (Table 15.1). Anatomic contraindications are relevant when the depth of injury causes destruction of tissue demarcating the boundaries between the target and such associated structures as the esophageal lumen, mediastinum, and vascular structures. Clinical contraindications are relevant in patients who may not tolerate the conscious or general anesthesia because of severe cardiac or pulmonary disease, or who have an uncorrectable coagulopathy. In addition, patients in whom atelectasis distal to the obstruction has been present for more than 4 to 6 weeks will probably not benefit from endoscopic laser resection because re-expansion of the involved lung is unlikely.

**Table 15.1** Contraindications for laser/cryotherapy/electrocautery

**Anatomic contraindications**

Extrinsic obstruction without endobronchial lesion

Lesion incursion into bordering major vascular structure (e.g. pulmonary artery) with potential for fistula formation

Lesion incursion into bordering esophagus with potential for fistula formation

Lesion incursion into bordering mediastinum with potential for fistula formation

**Clinical contraindications**

Candidate for surgical resection

Unfavorable short-term prognosis without hope for palliation of symptoms

Inability to undergo conscious sedation or general anesthesia

Coagulation disorder

Total obstruction more than 4 to 6 weeks

## Complications

Complications of laser therapy are related to the laser equipment or instruments, the anesthesia used, and perioperative causes. However, despite the possibility of severe, often fatal, complication, the overall risk is low in trained hands, with one series reporting only 60 complication and 12 deaths associated with Nd:YAG laser therapy in 2610 resections.

Pulmonary complications of the anesthesia during laser therapy may be related to anoxia, hypercarbia, or fire. A potential catastrophic intraoperative complication of laser therapy is endotracheal fire. The use of combustible anesthetic gases must be avoided, and the use of supplemental oxygen should be less than 40%. Although the metal rigid bronchoscope cannot catch fire, the use of the Nd:YAG laser through an endotracheal tube deserves special consideration. With the oxygen mixture, the possible additional fuel source provided by an endotracheal tube, and the potential for producing sparks when the laser light hits carbonized tissue, endotracheal fire is a serious concern. An immediate danger to the patient and operating room personnel is that of intratracheal explosion, with the anesthetic gases or oxygen producing a "torch effect". Following ignition of the endotracheal tube, longer-term complication may result from the subsequent lower airway inhalation injury, with mucosal sloughing and airway obstruction caused by granulation tissue. Similarly, a silicone stent should be removed prior to use of laser.

Fatal hemorrhage is associated with perforation into an involved or contiguous vascular structure. Apart from creating a fistula into the artery resulting in massive hemorrhage, perforation may also occur into adjacent structures with development of pneumothorax, pneumomediastinum, and tracheoesophageal fistula. Systemic air embolism has been reported and is associated with the development of vascular communication with the tracheobronchial tree.

## Technique

Physicians prefer to use rigid bronchoscopy with general anesthesia, although procedures can be performed through the flexible fiberoptic bronchoscope using topical anesthesia alone [6]. Oxygenation and ventilation are provided, using either spontaneous-assisted ventilation, jet ventilation, or laryngeal mask assisted ventilation

Laser resection is performed first with photocoagulation of the tumor. Coagulated tissue is then removed by the use of the beveled edge of the rigid bronchoscope, forceps, and suction. Complete laser vaporization of tissue may also be performed, but has a high risk of endobronchial fire. The laser beam should always be aligned parallel to the bronchial wall and never be discharged perpendicular to the airway wall. Laser pulses of 1 second or less are usually employed. When using a flexible bronchoscope the removal of devitalized tissue can be slow and difficult due a small forceps. In addition, the flexible bronchoscope can itself be combustible.

## Precautions

The patient's eyes should be protected with saline-soaked pads and aluminum foil to avoid injury from accidental laser scatter, and all personnel should wear protective goggles. A few precautions are necessary to minimize the risk of combustion: the fraction of inspired oxygen should be kept below 40%. Flammable materials should be kept far away from the operating field, such as endotracheal tubes. Silicone stents should be removed prior to the use of laser. The laser should always be placed on standby mode when tissue is removed from the bronchoscope. If a flexible bronchoscope is employed, the laser must be kept a sufficient distance beyond the tip of the bronchoscope to avoid combustion. Power settings greater than 40 watts are never necessary.

## Indications and outcome

The indications depend on the anatomic characteristics of the obstructing lesion and the clinical conditions, as outlined in Table 15.2 [7].

Benign and malignant airway endobronchial lesions causing symptomatic or obstructive complications do benefit from endoscopic laser photoresection [8–13] (Fig. 15.1). Laser therapy has also been performed for stenosis related to prolonged intubation [14], stricture produced by inflammatory granulation tissue caused by mycobacterial infection, anastomosis granulation tissue following lung transplantation [15], suture granulomas [16], and in systemic inflammatory conditions caused by collagen vascular diseases such

**Table 15.2** Indications for laser/cryotherapy/electrocautery

Benign or malignant airway lesion associated with:

Dyspnea

Uncontrolled cough

Impending asphyxiation

Stridor

Inability to wean from ventilator owing to obstruction

Postobstructive pneumonia

Symptomatic or unresolving atelectasis

Nearly complete (>50%) obstruction of one major bronchus

Recurrent hemoptysis

Closure of bronchopleural fistula not responsive to conventional therapy

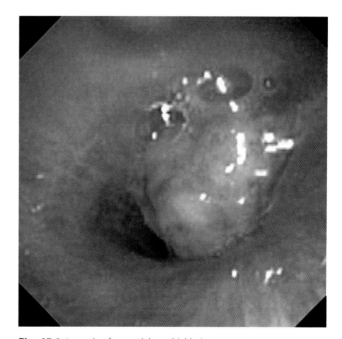

**Fig. 15.1** Example of an endobronchial lesion.

as Wegner's granulomatosis, Beçhet's syndrome, and relapsing polychondritis [17,18]. Endobronchial laser therapy has also been performed in patients with symptomatic obstruction secondary to broncholithiasis [19].

Benign or low-grade tumors, such as hamartomas, spindle cell carcinomas, endobronchial Kaposi's sarcomas, and even diffuse papillomatosis, have also benefited from Nd:YAG laser photoablation. Shah [20] reported a large series of benign tumor resections of the tracheobronchial tree in 185 patients with benign tumors; 317 procedures were performed with the results of laser resection thought to be very good in 62% and good in 38%, with minimal complications.

Toty *et al.*, in an early experience, were able to restore adequate respiratory function in 16 of 24 patients presenting in acute respiratory distress with recently detected tracheal carcinoma [14]. Seventeen of 48 patient with recurrent carcinoma received palliation from endobronchial therapy, nine of these patients, first seen in acute respiratory distress, were alive a year later after two to five sessions and eight were alive or were kept alive for 6 months at the end of this trial. Hetzel reported their experience with 100 patients referred for palliative treatment of tracheobronchial malignancy [21]. They showed objective improvement in the peak flow and alleviation of hemoptysis in 63% of patients with airway obstruction and 29% of those patients with collapsed lung.

Kvale *et al.*, in their early experience, reported 55 patients who received 82 treatments with laser therapy for obstructing lesions of the central airways, with 10 of having benign lesions and 45 having carcinoma of the lobar or main stem bronchus or trachea [11]. Eichenhorn performed Nd:YAG laser therapy in 19 patients with inoperable non-small cell carcinoma and symptomatic bronchial obstruction, with the goal of debulking the airways before conventional external-beam radiation therapy [8]. Patients with satisfactory debulking and subsequent radiation therapy had a significantly better outcome compared to those with unsatisfactory laser therapy (mean survival 340 days compared with less than 100 days; P < 0.006).

Desai *et al.* showed a significant increase in survival among the subset of 15 patients who underwent emergency palliative photoresection as the initial therapeutic intervention compared to the subset of 11 patients who received palliative radiation alone [22].

In a review paper of laser bronchoscopy by Ramser and Beamis, 85% of 100 patients had relief of symptoms and achieved preoperative goals [7]; 87% of these procedures were performed for lesions in main stem bronchi, with no fatalities reported and an overall complication rate of 6.5%. Rare tumors of the tracheobronchial system have also been noted to benefit from laser resection. Although comparisons using survival as an endpoint have dealt largely with historical control groups, the palliation of symptoms and the ability to remove some patients from mechanical ventilation provides evidence to document the efficacy of laser therapy. Mehta outlined the use of lasers with the flexible bronchoscope [23], in group of patients who underwent a combination of Nd:YAG photoresection with subsequent external-beam radiation therapy or external-beam radiation therapy plus brachytherapy. Although the number of such patient was small (17 of 300 patients), their survival rate was significantly greater than that of historical controls treated with radiation therapy only (P = 0.022).

Cavaliere supplemented their earlier extensive case series with the report of their 13-year experience outlining the treatment of 2008 patients with malignant airway obstructions using combined therapy with Nd:YAG laser, stents, and brachytherapy [24]. In patients treated with laser resection, 93% achieved immediate airway patency and consequent improvement in their quality of life.

## Summary

A primary goal of laser therapy is the safe, effective, and rapid palliation of symptoms owing to tracheal or bronchial obstruction. Laser therapy has proved to be beneficial in the therapy of benign and malignant obstructive lesions of the airway.

## Electrocautery

### Background

Electrocautery uses an electric current to produce heat and to destroy tissue. Strauss and colleagues used electrocautery for treating gastrointestinal tumors in 1913, and in 1935 reported their experience on over 40 cases [25].

Electrocautery uses alternating current at a high frequency (105 to 107 Hz) to generate heat that coagulates, vaporizes, or cuts tissue depending on the power. The power applied to the electrocautery device (measured in watts) corresponds to the heat generated in the tissue, as related by the equation:

$$power = (current)^2 \times resistance$$

Coagulation involves high amperage and low voltage, whereas vaporization uses high voltage and low amperage. Cutting tissue with the ability to coagulate blends these two settings. At a temperature of approximately 70°C tissue coagulates and over 200°C tissue carbonizes. The degree of destruction depends on the applied power, the electrical properties of the tissue, the device–tissue contact time, and the device–tissue contact surface area.

When a tissue is heated sufficiently, cellular water evaporates, thereby destroying the cell and then the tissue. Heating to higher temperatures leads to chemical breakdown of the cell and tissue constituents and eventual vaporization/carbonization. Electrocautery devices are monopolar; that is, they require the bronchoscope, the generator, and the patient to be grounded to complete the circuit, or otherwise shocks and burns may occur. The bronchoscope should be insulated. The generator should at least have an isolated power output to minimize current leakage and possible injury, if it is not grounded.

## Indications

The indications and contraindication for electrocautery are similar to those for Nd:YAG laser [26,27] (Tables 15.1 and 15.2). Similar to laser therapy, electrocautery produces rapid debulking of tumor and can be a modality to relieve impending respiratory failure at a lower cost.

## Equipment and technique

Insulated flexible bronchoscopes with working channels of 2.0 or 2.6 mm are used. Electrocautery blunt-tip probes and snares are compatible with the flexible bronchoscopes most commonly used. The generator should regulate the high-frequency current, so that the operator can adjust the setting depending on whether the procedure is intended to coagulate, cut, cut and coagulate, or vaporize. The monopolar unit must be grounded with an electrode pad.

The operator can use either closed forceps or the blunt electrocautery probe to manipulate the lesion and thus to assess its size, mobility, friability/bleeding potential, and to locate any attachment to the airway. Elongated or flat lesions may be suited for the blunt probe, whereas polypoid lesions may be amenable to the snare. The snare is used to cut and remove tissue and a blended current is used to cut and coagulate but not vaporize. With the loop open, the snare is placed over the tissue as close to the base as possible. As the loop is tightened a snug feeling is felt in the handgrip that controls the snare. At this point the unit is activated and the loop is slowly tightened. In this fashion the heat cuts and coagulates the tissue, not the mechanical effect of the wire. When the procedure is complete the snugness is gone and the loop is retracted into the catheter. The severed tissue can be removed with the snare or forceps.

## Outcomes

In a study of 56 patients, Homasson stated that hemoptysis was controlled in 75% of the cases, dyspnea was alleviated in 67%, and cough or stridor was relieved in 55% [28]. Petrou *et al.* reported that 28 of 29 patients had symptomatic improvement after removal of a lesion with a snare [29]. Sutedja *et al.* showed that 15 of 17 treated patients had immediate restoration of a patent airway; eight had relief of dyspnea, and four had control of hemoptysis [30]. Most series [31–33] involve predominantly malignancies, and success was defined as removing greater than 50% of the tumor; success rates of 70 to 95% have been reported.

## Complications

Two endobronchial fires have been reported during electrocautery procedures [34]; both were associated with high inspired oxygen concentrations, and in one a silicon stent ignited. Several investigators have reported hemorrhage, in most cases minor. One death secondary to hemorrhage occurred. Operator and patient burns and electrical

shocks are mentioned frequently as possible complications; however, published data are scant. Another concern is using electrocautery in a patient with a pacemaker or an automatic implantable defibrillator because the devices may malfunction and cause a dysrythmia. Electrocautery, when used in animal models, has been shown to result in airway stenosis, and cartilage damage can occur [28]. This cartilage damage can lead to bronchomalacia.

## Summary

Like laser therapy, electrocautery seems to be an effective palliation treatment for an endobronchial lesion. It is a cheaper alternative to laser therapy. Complications seem to be limited in number and severity.

## Argon plasma coagulation

Argon plasma coagulation (APC) is an electrosurgical technique similar to laser or electrocautery, used to remove an obstructing lesion and/or to achieve homeostasis.

APC was developed more than 20 years ago to improve surgical hemostasis. In the early 1990s, a flexible probe was introduced that facilitated its use during endoscopic procedures. APC was initially used during gastrointestinal endoscopy to achieve hemostasis during polypectomy [35], APC has been used during bronchoscopic procedures to debulk malignant airway tumors, control hemoptysis, remove granulation tissue from stents or anastomoses, and treat a variety of other benign disorders [36–40]. Although this is also a form of electrocautery, it is a non-contact form. The indication and contraindication are similar to those of laser and electrocautery.

## Procedure

Similar to electrocautery, a grounding pad should be placed on the patient back. The settings should be power of 30 watts and an argon flow rate of 0.8 to 1 L/min. The argon flow rate will determine the length of the flame. As the argon will seek biological tissue or any combustible object, the flame length is important in its airway application. This equipment is often used by multiple operators therefore, prior to each use, the setting should be set for your own needs. The probe tip should be several centimeters beyond the bronchoscope's tip. This insures that the bronchoscope will not be burned. The probe tip should be within 1 cm of the target lesion. The electric current will not be conducted if the probe is further from the target lesion. The probe tip should not contact the target lesion.

Argon gas is expelled from the probe and then a high-voltage electric current is passed along the probe. When the electric current contacts the argon gas, the argon gas becomes ionized and conducts a monopolar current to the target lesion [38]. This argon plasma is applied to the surface in 1

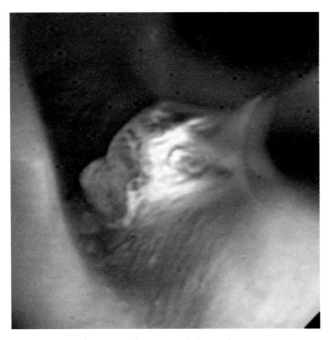

**Fig. 15.2** Use of an argon plasma coagulation probe.

to 3-second bursts (Fig. 15.2). The net tissue effect is similar to electrocautery.

In the process of debulking a endobronchial lesion, the eschar is first formed with the application of APC and then removed with forceps or a cryotherapy probe. APC is then applied to the underlying fresh tissue. This process is repeated until the tumor is removed. If brisk bleeding is encountered, the argon gas can used without the ignition of the gas to blow blood away, thus improving visualization.

### Outcome

A prospective cohort study of 364 patients who underwent APC (482 procedures) reported a success rate of 67%, defined as hemostasis and/or full or partial airway re-canalization [40]. The most common indications were airway obstruction (51%) and hemostasis (33%), of which malignancy was the underlying cause in nearly 90%. Of note, rigid bronchoscopy was used in 90% of the interventions. In a retrospective cohort study of 60 patients who underwent APC (70 procedures), treatment was immediately successful in 59 patients [37]. All of the patients had either hemoptysis or airway obstruction, with treatment success defined as resolution of hemoptysis and/or decreased airway obstruction. Hemoptysis did not recur over a mean follow-up of 97 days and improved dyspnea persisted over a mean follow-up of 53 days. Malignant disease existed in 95% of patients, and all of the procedures were performed with flexible bronchoscopy. A similar study of 47 patients reported a success rate of 92%, which was maintained over a mean follow-up of 6.7 months [36]. However, an average

of more than three sessions per patient was required to achieve this result.

APC has successfully treated benign disorders such as granulation tissue due to stents or airway anastomosis [40,41].

### Complications

Complications of APC are infrequent (less than 1% of procedures). They include airway burn and airway perforation, which can cause pneumomediastinum, subcutaneous emphysema, and pneumothorax [40]. Gas embolism has also been described in a case series, leading to three cases of cardiovascular collapse and one case of death [42]. Such a complication is a reflection of the lack of experience by the operator. A burned bronchoscope has also been reported.

Similar to laser and elctrocautery, limiting the inspired oxygen concentration, the applied power (less than 80 watts), and the application time (less than 5 seconds), probably minimizes the risk of airway perforation or fire. Keeping the probe tip several centimeters away from any combustible material likely prevents airway fire. Similarly, keeping the probe tip several centimeters away from the bronchoscope tip probably prevents the bronchoscope from being burned.

### Summary

Of all the modalities, only APC, electrocautery, and laser therapy can remove tissue rapidly and, therefore, have an immediate effect. APC is superior to electrocautery and laser photoresection in achieving homeostasis APC can be used during flexible or rigid bronchoscopy. Complications of APC are infrequent, occurring in less than 1% of procedures.

---

## Cryotherapy

Documents from 3500 BC described the use of cold as treatment for swelling and war wounds [43]. Hippocrates described the use of cold to treat orthopedic injuries [43]. Arnott described the use of salt solutions containing crushed ice at a temperature of about −8 to −12°C to freeze advanced cancers in accessible sites, producing a reduction in tumor size and improvement of pain [44,45]. The Joule–Thomson effect, which is the sudden expansion of a gas from a high to a low-pressure region, is the basis for the function of cryoprobes, especially in pulmonary medicine.

Neel showed the destructive effect of cold had been confirmed. The destruction of mucosa, submucosal glands, and serosa is complete, but the framework of connective tissue and cartilage remains for structural support, with healing of the tracheobronchial tree and regrowth of cuboidal epithelium beginning within 14 days of freezing [46–53]. The first study from the Mayo Clinic, consisting of 28 patients with endobronchial tumors, concluded that cryotherapy did serve as a good alternative for palliation [54–57].

Cryotherapy deals with the destruction of biological materials through the cytotoxic effects of freezing. The damage induced by freezing occurs at several levels, including the molecular, cellular, and structural levels and the whole tissue. The effect of freeze injury is influenced by many factors and the survival of cells is dependent on the cooling rate [58–60], the thawing rate [61], the lowest temperature achieved [62], and repeated freezing thawing cycles [63,64]. Certain tissues are cryosensitive (skin, mucous membrane, granulation tissue), and others are cryoresistant (fat, cartilage, fibrous or connective tissue). The cryosensitivity depends on the water content of the cells. Tumor cells may be more sensitive than normal cell [64].

## Cooling agents

Several cooling agents can be used as cryogen. These are generally used in the liquid phase so that on vaporization they remove heat at a constant temperature (heat of vaporization). Several studies have shown that the core temperature needed for a lesion to be destroyed is between −20 and −40°C. Freezing to −40°C or below at the rapid rate of −100°C per minute will cause more than 90% cell death.

Two cryogens available to the pulmonologists are liquid nitrogen and nitrous oxide. Nitrous oxides ($N_2O$) are the commonest cooling agents used in tracheobronchial cryotherapy. The vapor haze of $N_2O$ occurs at the metal tip of the cryoprobes where it expands from a high pressure to atmospheric pressure (Joule–Thomson effect). This expansion lowers the temperature of the fluid and produces droplets of liquid, reaching an equilibrium of −89°C at atmospheric pressure.

## Cryotherapy equipment

There are three parts to the cryomachine: the console, the cryoprobe, and the transfer line that connect the console and gas cylinder to the probe. Cryoprobes are rigid, semirigid, or flexible; rigid and semirigid cryoprobes can only be used through a rigid bronchoscope, but flexible cryoprobes can be used through the channel of the fiberoptic bronchoscope and the rigid bronchoscope. The efficacy of a cryoprobe depends in part on its diameter, thus if a fiberoptic bronchoscope is used, the operative lumen must be as large as possible (2.6 to 3.2 mm). There is no distortion of the optical equipment by cold, but during freezing the entire bronchoscope is cooled and this effect may be increased with retrofreezing if the cryoprobe is defective.

Monitoring of the freezing remains a problem [65] and there is no ideal solution. The empirical method relies on the experience of the operator, and the operator relies on the change in color/consistency of the frozen tissue, and the length of freezing. In clinical studies [66], using rigid, semirigid, or flexible cryoprobes, each freeze–thaw cycle is about 30 seconds. The thaw phase is almost immediate with rigid probes that have a system of reheating, but with the flexible

probes thawing is by body temperature, thus increasing the freeze–thaw cycle times.

## Indication

Cryotherapy is indicated for tracheobronchial obstruction. The selection criteria are similar to laser, APC, or electrocautery (Tables 15.1 and 15.2), except when there is an urgency to treat. In addition, cryotherapy can be used for extraction of foreign bodies, blood clots, or mucous plugs.

## Bronchoscopy

Endoscopic therapy is performed using a flexible cryoprobe [57], which is passed through the working channel. The cryoprobe tip is visualized and directly applied to the tumor area. The cryoprobe is started with a foot pedal once in the lumen of the airway, about 4 mm away from the tip of the bronchoscope. An ice ball appears within 30 seconds on the tip of the probe; one to three freeze–thaw cycles, each lasting for 1 minute, are applied to the same or immediate area. The tip of the probe can be applied perpendicularly, tangentially, or driven into the tumor mass. The tissues are frozen at −30 −40°C. The destruction due to cryotherapy is readily visible. The cryoprobe is deactivated by removal of the foot from the foot pedal. At the end of each freeze cycle, the ice ball is observed until thawing is completed before removal of the tip from the airway lesion (Fig. 15.3). With infiltrating lesions, cryotherapy can be used with lateral tangential contact.

The most suitable types of lesions are polypoid, benign or malignant. The metallic tip of the cryoprobe is placed on the

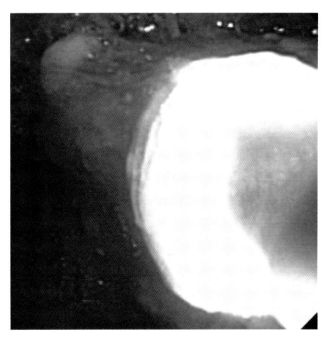

**Fig. 15.3** Use of a cryoprobe.

tumor or pushed into it, which produces circumferential freezing of maximal volume. Three freeze thaw cycles are carried out at each site. The probe is then moved 5–6 mm and another three cycles carried out in the adjoining area. Administration of corticosteroid is not routine. The hemostatic effect of freezing is often sufficient to stop hemoptysis.

## Outcomes

Walsh *et al.* reported the effects of cryotherapy on dyspnea, hemoptysis, cough, and stridor [67]. In his study, symptoms, lung function, chest radiography, and bronchoscopic findings were recorded serially before and after 81 cryotherapy sessions in 33 consecutive patients. Most patients improved in overall symptoms, stridor, and hemoptysis, and there was an overall improvement in dyspnea. Similarly, Maiwand *et al.* reported 600 patients with cryotherapy [68]. Following cryotherapy, 78% of the patients noticed a subjective improvement in their condition. These patients had less coughs (64%), dyspnea (66%), hemoptysis (65%), and stridor (70%) [69]. Homasson *et al.* reported that hemoptysis stopped in 80% of cases and dyspnea was less in 50% of case [54]. Mathur *et al.* reported similar finding in a smaller number of patients when cryotherapy was used with a fiberoptic bronchoscope [57,70]. Objective improvement of pulmonary function was seen in 58% of patients, and these changes in lung function correlated with symptoms shown by Walsh [67].

In order to make cryotherapy immediately effective and avoid a second clean-up procedure to effect recanalization, Hetzel *et al.* demonstrated cryorecanalization in 60 patients with exophytic tumors [71]. Tumor tissue was frozen on the tip of the probe and subsequently removed from the surrounding respiratory tract tissue through retraction of the probe; 83% of patients were successfully or partially successfully treated. Bleeding occurred in six patients and required argon plasma coagulator treatment. The same group extended their experience in a larger group of patients 225 patients with symptomatic airway stenosis [72]. Successful cryorecanalization was achieved in 91.1%. Argon plasma coagulation was used 16.4% for bleeding. A bronchus blocker was required in 8.0% of patients. The flexible cryoprobe for treatment of symptomatic endobronchial tumor stenosis is successful for immediate treatment but the safety has to questioned. This, potentially, can be dangerous in inexperienced hands. This method has been helpful in obtaining larger biopsy samples [73].

Cryotherapy has been used to obtain transbronchial lung biopsies, as currently biopsy lack sufficient quality due to crush artifact and are generally too small for the diagnosis of diffuse lung diseases. Forty-one patients with diffuse lung disease were selected for transbronchial biopsy. During flexible bronchoscopy, conventional transbronchial biopsies using forceps were carried out first. Then, a flexible cryo-

probe was introduced into the selected bronchus under fluoroscopic guidance. Once brought into position, the probe was cooled and then retracted with the frozen lung tissue attached on the probe's tip. The mean specimen area was 5.82 mm$^2$ (0.58–20.88 mm$^2$) taken by forceps compared to 15.11 mm$^2$ obtained using the cryoprobe (2.15–54.15 mm$^2$, $P < 0.01$). Two patients had a pneumothorax, which resolved with tube thoracostomy. Transbronchial cryobiopsy enabled large biopsy samples of lung parenchyma to be obtained. Further trials are needed to compare this technique with VATS, as well as investigation of the number of complications

There has been a renewed interest in the treatment of early stages of lung cancers. The French experience [74], reported by the GECC (study group on cryosurgery), was based on 36 patients with 44 lesions (*in situ* or microinvasive tumors); 42% of these patients had been treated for an invasive ear, nose, throat or bronchial cancer. At 1 year, complete clinical and histological control of the tumor was achieved in 88.8%, with a mean follow-up of 32 months. The mean survival of this population was 30 months.

## Cryotherapy–radiotherapy

Like laser therapy, cryotherapy will relieve bronchial obstruction and prevent local complications, which is the cause of most of deaths. Certain studies have suggested a possible synergy between the effect of cryotherapy and that of external irradiation due to blood flow [68]. In two similar prospective studies, Vergnon *et al.* [75] and Homasson [54] treated patients with cryotherapy associated with radiotherapy. A satisfactory outcome was defined as greater than 50% tumor destruction. Vergnon's group consisted of 29 patients, each of whom presented with a symptomatic, unresectable obstruction, either for local or functional reasons. One or two sessions of cryotherapy were carried out; cryotherapy was considered satisfactory in 16 cases and unsatisfactory in 13 cases, with persistent tumor lesions. Twenty-one patients received 65 Gy and eight patients in poor general condition received 45 Gy. In the unsatisfactory cryotherapy group, patients died quickly of local complications, with a median survival of 5 months. In the satisfactory cryotherapy group, the median survival was 11 months and a significant improvement in survival was obtained.

## Benign tracheobronchial lesions

Benign lesions have been treated with cryotherapy with very good results, particularly for granulomatous tissues; 100% had favorable results with no recurrence months or even years after treatment. Granulation tissue is very sensitive to the effects of cold. When surgery is not possible, treatment with cryotherapy can yield good results, and several cases of carcinoid, cylindromas, and laryngotracheal papillomas have been successfully treated.

## Removal of foreign bodies

Foreign bodies have been extracted with success using cryotherapy. It is most useful to remove friable or biological matter, such as pills, peanuts, tooth, chicken bones, etc. It is also extremely helpful in the removal blood clots, mucus plugs, and slough.

## Future work

In the treatment of lung cancers, local cryotherapy has been used for palliative care. However, cryotherapy can also be used as an adjuvant treatment, for instance in association with chemotherapy. Forest has demonstrated differential biological effects of these therapies and the benefit of combining them [76–80]. As vascular changes occur after cryotherapy, intratumoral angiogenesis was also studied. Tumors were treated with cryotherapy or chemotherapy, by injection of vinorelbine, or both. Tumor growth was studied in each group and the treated : control ratios were compared. Tumors treated by cryochemotherapy presented a significantly reduced volume and lower treated : control ratio, confirming the benefit of a combined treatment. Such studies improve the understanding of the full role of cryotherapy.

## Conclusion

Cryotherapy for endobronchial lesions has been shown to be an effective and safe therapy in a number of pathologies. In particular, the technique is extremely useful in patients with carcinoma of the lung and airway obstruction. More than a third of the patients had an improvement in symptoms and respiratory function. These benefits are achieved by using a technique that is safe, easy to perform, inexpensive, and has few complications.

## References

1 Einstein A. Zur quantientheoric der strahlung. *Physikalishe Zeitschrift* 1917; **18**: 121–8.

2 Schawlow AL, Townes CH. Infrared and optical masers. *Phy Rev* 1958; **112**: 1940–9.

3 Maimon TI-I. Stimulated optical radiation in ruby. *Nature* 1960; **187**: 493–4.

4 Herd RM, Dover JS, Amdt KA. Lasers in dermatology. *Dermatol Clin* 1997; **15**: 355–73.

5 Dumon MC, Dumon JF. Laser bronchoscopy. In: Feinsilver SH, Fein AM, eds. *Textbook of Bronchoscopy.* Baltimore, Williams & Wilkins; 1995: 393–9.

6 Prakash UBS, Offord KP, Stubbs SE. Bronchoscopy in North America: The ACCP survey. *Chest* 1991; **100**: 1668–75.

7 Ramser ER, Beamis JF. Laser bronchoscopy. *Clin Chest Med* 1995; **16**: 415–26.

8 Eichenhorn MS, Kvale PA, Miks VM, *et al.* Initial combination therapy with YAG laser photoresection and irradiation for inoperable non-small cell carcinoma of the lung. *Chest* 1986; **89**: 782–5.

9 Gelb AF, Epstein JD. Neodymium-yttrium-aluminum-garnet laser in lung cancer. *Ann Thorac Surg* 1987; **43**: 164–7.

10 Macha HN, Becker KO, Kemmer HP. Pattern of failure and survival in endobronchial laser resection. *Chest* 1994; **105**: 1668–72.

11 Kvale PA, Eichenhom MS, Radke JR, *et al.* YAG laser photoresection of lesions obstructing the central airways. *Chest* 1985; **87**: 283–8.

12 Ross DJ, Mohsenifar Z, Koemer SK. Survival characteristics after neodymium: YAG laser photoresection in advanced stage lung cancer. *Chest* 1990; **98**: 581–5.

13 Stanopoulos IT, Beamis JF, Martinez FJ, *et al.* Laser bronchoscopy in respiratory failure from malignant airway obstruction. *Crit Care Med* 1993; **21**: 386–91.

14 Toty L, Personne C, Colchen A, *et al.* Bronchoscopic management of tracheal lesions using the neodymium yttrium aluminum garnet laser. *Thorax* 1981; **36**: 175–8.

15 Madden BP, Kumar P, Sayer R, *et al.* Successful resection of obstructing airway granulation tissue following lung transplantation using endobronchial (Nd : YAG) therapy. *Eur J Cardiothorac Surg* 1997; **12**: 480–5.

16 Brutinel WM, Cortese DA, Edell ES, *et al.* Complications of Nd: YAG laser therapy. *Chest* 1988; **94**: 903–4.

17 Sacco O, Fregonese B, Oddone M, *et al.* Severe endobronchial obstruction in a girl with relapsing polychondritis: Treatment with Nd YAG laser and endobronchial silicon stent. *Eur Respir J* 1997; **10**: 494–6.

18 Witt C, John M, Martin H, *et al.* Bechet's syndrome with pulmonary involvement-combined therapy for endobronchial stenosis using neodymium-YAG laser, balloon dilation and immunosuppression. *Respiration* 1996; **63**: 195–8.

19 Cahill BC, Harmon KR, Sumway SJ, *et al.* Tracheobronchial obstruction due to silicosis. *Am Rev Respir Dis* 1992; **145**: 719–21.

20 Shah H, Garbe L, Nussbaum E, *et al.* Benign tumors of the tracheobronchial tree. Endoscopic characteristics and role of laser resection. *Chest* 1995; **107**: 1744–51.

21 Hetzel MR, Nixon C, Edmondstone WM, *et al.* Laser therapy in 100 tracheobronchial tumors. *Thorax* 1985; **40**: 341–5.

22 Desai SJ, Mehta AC, VanderBrug Medendorp S, *et al.* Survival experience following Nd: YAG laser photoresection for primary bronchogenic carcinoma. *Chest* 1988; **94**: 939–44.

23 Mehta AC, Lee FYW, DeBoer GE. Flexible bronchoscopy and the use of lasers. In: Wang KP, Mehta AC, eds. *Flexible Bronchoscopy.* Cambridge: Blackwell Science; 1995: 274.

24 Cavaliere S, Venuta F, Foccoli P, *et al.* Endoscopic treatment of malignant airway obstructions in 2,008 patients. *Chest* 1996; **110**: 1536–42.

25 Strauss AA, Strauss SF, Crawford RA. Surgical diathermy of carcinoma of the rectum, Its clinical end results. *JAMA* 1935; **104**: 1480–4.

26 Hooper RG, Jackson FN. Endobronchial electrocautery. *Chest* 1985; **87**: 712–14.

27 Hooper RG, Jackson FN. Endobronchial electrocautery. *Chest* 1988; **94**: 595–8.

28 Homasson JP: Endobronchial electrocautery. *Semin Respir Crit Care Med* 1997; **18**: 535–43.

29 Petrou M, Kaptan D, Goldstraw P. Bronchoscopic diathermy resection and stent insertion: A cost effective treatment for tracheobronchial obstruction. *Thorax* 1993; **48**: 1156–9.

30 Sutedja C, Van Kralingen K, Schramet FMNH, *et al.* Fiberoptic bronchoscopic electrosurgery under local anesthesia for rapid palliation in patients with central airway malignancies: A preliminary report. *Thorax* 1994; **49**: 1243–6.

31 Carpenter RJ, Neel T, Sanderson DR. Comparison of endoscopic cryosurgery and electrocoagulation of bronchi. *Trans Am Acad Ophthalmol Otolaryngol* 1977; **84**: 313–23.

32 Sutedja C, Schramel PMNH, Smit HJF, *et al.* Bronchoscopic electrocautery as an alernative for Nd: YAG laser in patients with intraluminal tumor. *Eur Resp* 1996; **9** (Suppl 23): 258–9s.

33 Lavandier M, Carre T, Rivoire B, *et al.* High frequency electrocautery in the management of tracheobronchial disorders. *Respir Crit Care Med* 1996; **75**: A477.

34 Yankauer S. Two cases of lung tumor treated bronchoscopically. *N Y Med J* 1922; **21**: 741–2.

35 Grund KE, Storek D, Farin G. Endoscopic argon plasma coagulation (APC) first clinical experiences in flexible endoscopy. *Endosc Surg Allied Technol* 1994; **2**: 42–46.

36 Crosta C, Spaggiari L, De Stefano A, *et al.* Endoscopic argon plasma coagulation for palliative treatment of malignant airway obstructions: early results in 47 cases. *Lung Cancer* 2001; **33**: 75–80.

37 Morice RC, Ece T, Ece F, Keus L. Endobronchial argon plasma coagulation for treatment of hemoptysis and neoplastic airway obstruction. *Chest* 2001; **119**: 781–7.

38 Vonk-Noordegraaf A, Postmus PE, Sutedja TG. Bronchoscopic treatment of patients with intraluminal microinvasive radiographically occult lung cancer not eligible for surgical resection: a follow-up study. *Lung Cancer* 2003; **39**: 49–53.

39 Reichle G, Freitag L, Kullmann HJ, *et al.* [Argon plasma coagulation in bronchology: a new method—alternative or complementary?] *Pneumologie* 2000; **54**: 508–16.

40 Platt RC. Argon plasma electrosurgical coagulation. *Biomed Sci Instrum* 1997; **34**: 332–7.

41 Colt HG. Bronchoscopic resection of Wallstent-associated granulation tissue using argon plasma coagulation. *J Bronchol* 1998; **5**: 209.

42 Reddy C, Majid A, Michaud G, *et al.* Gas embolism following bronchoscopic argon plasma coagulation: a case series. *Chest* 2008; **134**: 1066–9.

43 Breasted JH. *The Edwin Smith Surgical Papyrus.* Chicago: University of Chicago Oriental Institute; 1930: 3, 217.

44 Arnott J. *On the Treatment of Cancer by Regulated Application of an Anaesthetic Temperature.* London: J. Churchill; 1851.

45 Arnott J. *On the Treatment of Cancer by Congelation and an Improved Mode of Pressure.* London: J. Churchill; 1855.

46 Grana L, Kidd J, Swenson O. Cryogenic techniques within tracheobronchial tree. *J Cryosurg* 1969; **2**: 62.

47 Thomford NR, Wilson WH, Blackburn ED, Pace WG. Morphological changes in canine trachea after freezing. *Cryobiology* 1970; **7**: 19–26.

48 Skivolocki WP, Pace WG, Thomford NR. Effect of cryotherapy on tracheal tumors in rats. *Arch Surg* 1971; **103**: 341–3.

49 Neel HB, Farrell KH, DeSanto LW, *et al.* Cryosurgery of respiratory structures 1. Cryonecrosis of trachea and bronchus. *Laryngoscope* 1973; **83**: 1062–71.

50 Gorenstein A, Neel HB, Sanderson DR. Transbronchoscopic cryosurgery of respiratory strictures. Experimental and clinical studies. *Ann Otol Rhinol Laryngol* 1976; **85**: 670–8.

51 Carpenter RJ, Neel HB, Sanderson DR. Cryosurgery of bronchopulmonary structures. An approach to lesions inaccessible to the rigid bronchoscope. *Chest* 1977; **72**: 279–84.

52 Gage AA. Cryotherapy for cancer. In: Rand R, Rinfret R, Rinfret A, Von Leden H, eds. *Cryosurgery.* Springfield, Ill: Thomas Charles C. Publisher; 1968: 376–87.

53 Sanderson DR, Neel HB, Payne WS, Woolner LB. Cryotherapy of bronchogenic carcinoma. Report of a case. *Mayo Clin Proc* 1975; **50**: 435–7.

54 Homasson JP, Renault P, Angebault M, *et al.* Bronchoscopic cryotherapy for airway strictures caused by tumors. *Chest* 1986; **90**: 159–64.

55 Maiwand MO. Cryotherapy for advanced carcinoma of the trachea and bronchi. *Br Med J* 1986; **293**: 181–2.

56 Astesiano A, Aversa S, Ciotta D, *et al.* Distruzione crioterapica dei tumori invasivi tracheobronchiali. Casistica personale. *Min Med* 1986; **77**: 2159.

57 Mathur PN, Wolf KM, Busk MF, *et al.* Fiberoptic bronchoscopic cryotherapy in the management of tracheobronchial obstruction. *Chest* 1996; **110**: 718–23.

58 Fahy GM, Saur J, Williams RJ. Physical problems with the vitrification of large biological systems. *Cryobiology* 1990; **27**: 492–510.

59 Gage AA, Guest K, Montes M, *et al.* Effect of varying freezing and thawing rates in experimental cryosurgery. *Cryobiology* 1985; **22**: 175–82.

60 Smith JJ, Fraser J. An estimation of tissue damage and thermal history in cryolesion. *Cryobiology* 1974; **11**: 139–47.

61 Miller RH, Mazur P. Survival of frozen-thawed human red cells as a function of cooling and warming velocities. *Cryobiology* 1976; **13**: 404–14.

62 Gage AA. Critical temperature for skin necrosis in experimental cryosurgery. *Cryobiology* 1982; **19**: 273–82.

63 Rand RW, Rand RP, Eggerding FA, *et al.* Cryolumpestomy for breast cancer: an experimental study. *Cryobiology* 1985; **22**: 307–18.

64 Rubinsky B, Ikeda M. A cryomicroscope using directional solidification for the controlled freezing of biological tissue. *Cryobiology* 1985; **22**: 55.

65 Homasson JP, Thiery JP, Angebault M, *et al.* The operation and efficacy of cryosurgical, nitrous oxide-driven cryoprobe. Cryoprobe physical characteristics : their effects on cell cryodestruction. *Cryobiology* 1994; **31**: 290–304.

66 Le Pivert PJ, Binder P, Ougier T. Measurement of intratissue bioelectrical low frequency impedance : a new method to predict per-operatively the destructive effect of cryosurgery. *Cryobiology* 1977; **14**: 245–50.

67 Walsh DA, Maiwand MO, Nath AR, *et al.* Bronchoscopic cryotherapy for advanced bronchial carcinoma. *Thorax* 1990; **45**: 509–13.

68 Maiwand MO, Homasson JP. Cryotherapy for tracheobronchial disorders. *Clin Chest Med* 1995; **16**: 427–43.

69 Homasson JP. Cryotherapy in pulmonology today and tomorrow. *Eur Resp J* 1989; **2**: 799–801.

70 Sheski FD, Mathur PN. Endobronchial cryotherapy for benign tracheobronchial lesions. *Chest* 1998; **114**: 261–2s.

71 Hetzel M, Hetzel J, Schumann C, *et al*. Cryorecanalization: a new approach for the immediate management of acute airway obstruction. *J Thorac Cardiovasc Surg* 2004; **127**: 1427–31.

72 Schumann C, Hetzel M, Babiak AJ, *et al*. Endobronchial tumor debulking with a flexible cryoprobe for immediate treatment of malignant stenosis. *J Thorac Cardiovasc Surg* 2010; **139**: 997–1000.

73 Franke KJ, Szyrach M, Nilius G, *et al*. Experimental study on biopsy sampling using new flexible cryoprobes: influence of activation time, probe size, tissue consistency, and contact pressure of the probe on the size of the biopsy specimen. *Lung* 2009; **187**: 253–9.

74 Deygas N, Froudarakis ME, Ozenne G, *et al*. Cryotherapy in early superficial bronchogenic carcinoma. *Eur Respir J* 1998; **12** (Suppl 28): 266S.

75 Vergnon JM, Schmitt T, Alamartine E, *et al*. Initial combined cryotherapy and irradiation for unresectable non-small cell lung cancer. *Chest* 1992; **102**: 1436–40.

76 Forest V, Peoc'h M, Campos L, *et al*. Effects of cryotherapy or chemotherapy on apoptosis in a non-small-cell lung cancer xenografted into SCID mice. *Cryobiology* 2005; **50**: 29–37.

77 Forest V, Campos L, Péoc'h M, *et al*. [Development of an experimental model for the study of the effects of cryotherapy on lung tumours]. *Pathol Biol* (Paris) 2005; **53**: 199–203.

78 Forest V, Peoc'h M, Ardiet C, *et al*. In vivo cryochemotherapy of a human lung cancer model. *Cryobiology* 2005; **51**: 92–101.

79 Forest V, Peoc'h M, Campos L, *et al*. Benefit of a combined treatment of cryotherapy and chemotherapy on tumour growth and late cryo-induced angiogenesis in a non-small-cell lung cancer model. *Lung Cancer* 2006; **54**: 79–86.

80 Forest V, Hadjeres R, Bertrand R, Jean-François R. Optimisation and molecular signalling of apoptosis in sequential cryotherapy and chemotherapy combination in human A549 lung cancer xenografts in SCID mice. *Br J Cancer* 2009; **100**: 1896–902.

# 16

# Flexible Bronchoscopy and the Application of Endobronchial Brachytherapy, Fiducial Placement, and Radiofrequency Ablation

**Michael A. Jantz**

Division of Pulmonary, Critical Care, and Sleep Medicine, University of Florida, Gainesville, FL, USA

It is estimated that 222,520 people will be diagnosed with, and 157,300 people will die of, cancer of the lung and bronchus in 2010 in the United States [1]. Many patients will require radiation therapy as part of their treatment, given that most patients will have stage III or stage IV disease at the time of diagnosis. Brachytherapy, with or without external beam radiotherapy, has been utilized in the treatment of lung cancer when endobronchial disease is present and has also been used in the treatment of patients with endobronchial metastases from extrapulmonary malignancies. Some patients may have early stage lung cancer or oligometastatic disease from other primaries and are not able to undergo surgical resection due to inadequate pulmonary reserve or other comorbidities. Image-guided radiation therapy is playing an important part in the treatment of these patients. Some of these image-guided radiation therapy systems require fiducial markers for tumor tracking. The use of bronchoscopic placement of fiducial markers is continuing to expand. Radiofrequency ablation is also being utilized to treat patients with early stage lung cancer who cannot undergo surgical resection, as well as patients with lung metastases. Although very limited experience with radiofrequency ablation delivered via bronchoscopy exists, the possibility to doing so in conjunction with navigation bronchoscopy is intriguing. A review of these topics will be covered in this chapter.

## Brachytherapy

The majority of patients with lung cancer present with locally advanced or metastatic disease and thus are not candidates for curative surgical resection. Many patients have tumor located in the proximal airways, causing dyspnea, cough, hemoptysis, atelectasis, and/or postobstructive pneu-

monia. External beam radiotherapy is effective in reversing atelectasis in 21–74% of patients [2,3]. Recurrence of tumor may occur in up to 50% of patients following external beam radiotherapy [4]. The majority of these patients will not be eligible for additional external beam radiotherapy. Endobronchial brachytherapy may be utilized to alleviate symptoms from endobronchial obstruction and improve local control as well as provide curative therapy in patients with carcinoma *in situ*. Brachytherapy, given very localized effects, may be provided to patients who have already received the maximum dose of external beam radiation. Brachytherapy may be used in conjunction with external beam radiotherapy or other bronchoscopic techniques such as laser therapy, electrocautery, cryotherapy, and stent placement to alleviate symptoms of malignant airway obstruction.

Brachytherapy, derived from the Greek term brachys meaning "short", refers to the placement of a highly radioactive source inside or near a tumor mass. This chapter will focus on endobronchial brachytherapy, as opposed to placement of the radioactive source into the tumor bed during surgical resection or percutaneous placement inside the tumor mass (interstitial brachytherapy). In 1922, Yankauer described two cases of lung cancer treated by radon capsule implantation via rigid bronchoscopy [5]. In the 1960s, cobalt-60 seeds were frequently used as the radiation source. In addition to radon-222 and cobalt-60, other radionuclides used for endobronchial brachytherapy have included cesium-137, gold-198, iodine-125, and palladium-103. Risk of radiation exposure to medical personnel and the need for rigid bronchoscopy for implantation hampered the widespread adoption of endobronchial brachytherapy. In the 1980s, two major developments led to renewed interest in endobronchial brachytherapy. First, was the development of flexible bronchoscopes, which allowed for the insertion

*Flexible Bronchoscopy*, Third Edition. Edited by Ko-Pen Wang, Atul C. Mehta, J. Francis Turner.
© 2012 Blackwell Publishing Ltd. Published 2012 by Blackwell Publishing Ltd.

of small-diameter after-loading catheters into every bronchial segment. Second, was the availability of high-activity iridum-192 and development of the remote after-loader for placing the iridium-192 seeds in the catheters.

As compared to conventional external beam radiotherapy, brachytherapy offers the potential advantage of providing a higher dose of radiation to the tumor while sparing normal tissues. Radioactive isotopes are characterized by the inverse square law, which means that the radiation dose rate decreases as a function of the inverse square of the distance from the source center. The standard unit for radiation absorbed dose is the gray (Gy). Endobronchial brachytherapy can be divided into three dose rate regimens. Low dose rate (LDR) is defined as less than 2 Gy/h, intermediate dose rate (IDR) 2–12 Gy/h, and high dose rate (HDR) greater than 12 Gy/h. LDR brachytherapy usually requires 8–48 h of treatment time while HDR can be achieved in a few minutes of treatment time.

The following patient characteristics should, in general, be present to consider brachytherapy:

**1** Histologic diagnosis of malignancy.

**2** Significant endobronchial tumor component causing symptoms such as dyspnea, hemoptysis, cough, and/or postobstructive pneumonitis.

**3** Involvement of proximal airways such as trachea, mainstem bronchi, or lobar bronchi.

**4** Able to pass catheter into, and preferably beyond, the obstructing endobronchial lesion.

**5** Unable to undergo resection due to cancer stage or inadequate pulmonary function.

**6** Sufficient life expectancy to benefit from palliation, typically greater than 3 months.

Potential candidates for endobronchial brachytherapy include patients with unresectable lung cancer, recurrent lung cancer, and cancers metastatic to the airway. Lesions to be treated should be located in the proximal airways and visible by bronchoscopy. The bronchoscopist should be able to pass the catheter into the obstructing lesion and ideally beyond the lesion. While brachytherapy may be used to treat extrinsic airway compression, intrinsic airway tumor obstruction is the more common indication. Patients with extrinsic airway compression may be better treated with stent placement. In the setting of subtotal bronchial stenosis, recannalization techniques such as laser or electrocautery resection or balloon dilatation may need to be performed to allow for catheter passage beyond the obstruction. Concern has been raised of a higher risk of fistula formation with the combination of laser resection and endobronchial brachytherapy. As such, some authors recommend a 1 to 2-week interval between laser recannalization and performing brachytherapy, while others combine the procedures in the same sitting [6–8].

Palliation of symptoms caused by tumor airway obstruction is the primary indication for brachytherapy. Brachytherapy has been also used as an adjunct to external beam radiotherapy as curative intent treatment for non-small cell carcinoma of the lung. Brachytherapy has been utilized as a boost before, during, and after external beam radiation. In the setting of atelectasis due to obstruction of a major bronchus, brachytherapy can help reduce the amount of radiation to normal lung parenchyma as a result of large external beam fields. In one study, endobronchial brachytherapy reduced normal tissue irradiation by an average of 32% [9]. In addition, endobronchial brachytherapy may provide curative treatment for patients with carcinoma *in situ* of the bronchus.

Contraindications to endobronchial brachytherapy include airway–esophageal, airway–mediastinal, and bronchopleural fistulas. Brachytherapy is probably not indicated in patients who are asymptomatic unless the treatment is with curative intent. Patients with major airway obstruction and impending respiratory failure should be treated with other bronchoscopic techniques prior to embarking on a treatment course with brachytherapy. These techniques may include mechanical tumor debulking, laser therapy, electrocautery, cryotherapy, and/or stent placement. High-grade obstructing lesions of the trachea should be treated with alternative methods prior to brachytherapy due to concerns of postradiation edema causing complete airway obstruction.

LDR brachytherapy uses low-activity iridium-192 seeds encased in a nylon ribbon. The delivery catheter is loaded by the radiation oncologist manually after positioning in the target bronchus. The catheter and seeds are left in place for 24–72 h. Although LDR brachytherapy requires no expensive equipment, major disadvantages include the need for inpatient treatment and intolerance to the in-dwelling catheter. HDR brachytherapy utilizes a highly active iridium-192 source. A HDR remote after-loading brachytherapy system consists of a housing unit for the radioactivity source, a source drive mechanism, and treatment planning computer system. The source is driven along the length of the delivery catheter by a computer-controlled cable. The source will stop at dwell points for a designated time to deliver the prescribed dose. The number of dwell points and interval between dwell points is determined by the computer to provide the optimal radiation dose to the tumor volume. Treatment is delivered to the patient in a heavily shielded room. Treatment times with HDR brachytherapy are very short, lasting 5–20 min. HDR brachytherapy has the advantages of greater patient comfort, being able to provide treatment as an outpatient procedure, and no radiation exposure to medical personnel, although initial equipment costs are higher. Given these advantages, HDR brachytherapy has replaced LDR brachytherapy at most institutions.

## Technique and treatment planning

A brachytherapy prescription will include the radiation dose per fraction, the number of fractions, and the prescribed depth, that is the radial distance from the source at which the dose is prescribed. The biologic effect of a given radiation course is determined not only by the total radiation dose, but also by the dose per fraction, the dose rate, and total time over which the entire course of radiation is given [10]. Using a larger fraction size, for a given total dose of radiation, will result in a higher effective dose to the tumor as compared to a smaller fraction size. The biologic effect on late-responding tissues will increase more rapidly than the biologic effect on the tumor cells, however, for a given increase in fraction size. Potential gains in treatment efficacy with a larger fraction dose need to be balanced with a potential increase in the risk of complications [10]. Dose and fractionation schemes for HDR brachytherapy can vary among institutions. Treatment regimens have ranged from 15 Gy in a single fraction to four to five fractions of 4 Gy each. A total dose higher than 30–40 Gy does not seem to be necessary for sufficient tumor control and may be associated with a higher risk of fatal hemorrhages [11]. The interval between fractions ranges from 1 to 3 weeks with a 1-week interval being most commonly used. The American Brachytherapy Society has recommended either three weekly fractions of 7.5 Gy each, two weekly fractions of 10 Gy each, or four weekly fractions of 6 Gy, each prescribed at a distance of 1 cm from the source for HDR brachytherapy when used as a sole modality for palliation [12]. When used as a boost to external beam radiation for palliation, two fractions of 7.5 Gy each, three fractions of 5 Gy each, or four fractions of 4 Gy, each at 1 cm every 1 to 2 weeks, is recommended for HDR brachytherapy. For curative therapy, HDR brachytherapy of three fractions of 5 Gy each or two fractions of 7.5 Gy each at 1 cm as a boost to external beam radiation, given as 60 Gy in 30 fractions or 45 Gy in 15 fractions, is recommended. If HDR brachytherapy is used alone in previously unirradiated patients, the recommendation is five fractions of 5 Gy each or three fractions of 7.5 Gy each, at 1 cm. With regards to LDR brachytherapy, the American Brachytherapy Society recommends a total dose of 30 Gy at 1 cm when used as the primary modality and 20 Gy at 1 cm when used as an adjunct to external beam radiotherapy [12]. The prescribed depth or number of fractions may be reduced depending on prior radiation or location, such as the left upper lobe bronchus. Consideration for decreasing the brachytherapy dose should be given if the patient has received radiosensitizing chemotherapy. Endobronchial brachytherapy should be delivered with at least a 1 cm margin on each end of the tumor target.

The first step in endobronchial brachytherapy is to review pertinent imaging. Bronchoscopy is performed in a standard fashion with topical anesthesia and sedation medications per the bronchoscopist's standard practice. Bronchoscopy is typically performed by the transnasal route to facilitate catheter stability during patient transport and treatment. Attention should be paid to adequate topical anesthesia of the larynx

and catheter insertion site to minimize coughing and potential catheter dislodgement. The proximal, and if possible, distal ends of the tumor target are visualized with the bronchoscope. Treatment of complex tumors at a carina may be facilitated by placement of multiple catheters. After inspection of the tumor and determination of the number of required catheters, a 5–6 Fr catheter(s) is/are inserted through the working channel of the bronchoscope and passed beyond the area of endobronchial tumor under direct bronchoscopic visualization (Fig. 16.1). A radiopaque internal guidewire can assist in placing the catheter and confirming catheter position with fluoroscopy. The bronchoscope is slowly withdrawn as the catheter/guidewire is advanced by an equal amount by the bronchoscopist or assistant and the catheter/guidewire stabilized at the nose. The bronchoscope is then reinserted and visual confirmation of appropriate catheter positioning is performed. With the guidewire in place, fluoroscopy can also be used to confirm correct positioning (Fig. 16.1). After appropriate positioning is established, the catheter is taped to the nose. This process is repeated if an additional catheter is needed with the additional catheter usually placed into another bronchial segment. The catheter may be placed with the tip 2 cm beyond the distal end of the tumor or can be placed as far distally as possible to wedge it into a smaller peripheral bronchus. The distal end of the irradiation target length may need to be estimated from previous chest radiographs or CT scans when the distal end of the tumor cannot be visualized with the bronchoscope. More distal catheter placement may be advantageous when the catheter placement is done in the bronchoscopy suite, as opposed to the radiation suite, to lessen the chance of catheter dislodgement during patient transport. Wedging the catheter may also be useful if LDR brachytherapy is performed given the prolonged treatment time. With distal placement care should be taken not to use excessive force while inserting the catheter/guidewire and cause a pneumothorax. As noted, a recannalization technique may need to be employed to facilitate catheter placement in a subtotally occluded airway (Fig. 16.1). Although a variety of outer sheaths, balloons, and cages have been designed to hold the application catheter in the center of the airway and avoid "hot spots" on the bronchial mucosa, these are not typically used by most practitioners.

After bronchoscopic placement of the catheter(s) and patient transport to the radiation oncology treatment area, dummy seeds consisting of radiopaque markers are inserted into the catheter. Orthogonal radiographs are taken to confirm correct placement and facilitate treatment planning. A treatment plan is designed with planning software (Fig. 16.2). The dummy seeds are removed and the catheters are then loaded with the radioactive source for the predetermined amount of time. After each treatment session, the catheters are removed and the patient is discharged home. Potential acute side-effects of

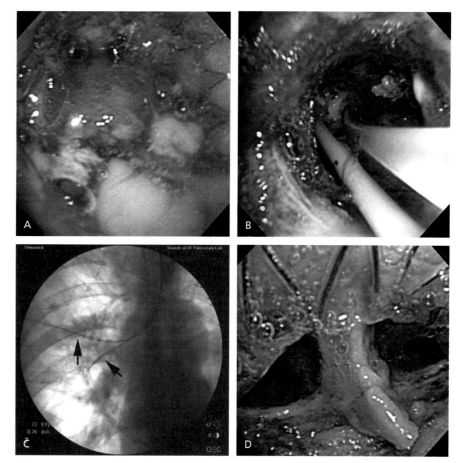

**Fig. 16.1** Brachytherapy catheter placement. (A) Tumor recurrence at end of a bronchial stent. (B) Insertion of two brachytherapy catheters following argon plasma coagulation deobstruction. (C) Fluoroscopic image following placement of catheters with guidewires (arrows). (D) Appearance of airway with stent placement at bronchoscopic follow-up.

the procedure include coughing, bronchospasm, increased bronchial secretions, hemoptysis from abrasion of the tumor, and pneumothorax from catheter/guidewire puncture of the lung.

## Results for malignant disease

A number of randomized trials involving the use of HDR have been published. In a study by Huber and coworkers evaluating two different treatment regimens of HDR brachytherapy, patients with lung cancer were randomized to treatment with HDR brachytherapy at a dose of 3.8 Gy at 1 cm weekly for four treatments (group 1, N = 44) or 7.2 Gy at 1 cm every 3 weeks for two treatments (group 2, N = 49) [13]; 88.9% of patients in group 1 and 92.7% of patients in group 2 had undergone previous treatment, including external beam radiotherapy in 47.2% and 39.0%, respectively. Twelve patients in group 1 and seven patients in group 2 did not receive full treatment due to death or deterioration. There was minimal change of the mean Karnofsky performance scores; 60.7 to 63.8 and 60.0 to 65.7 for group 1 and group 2, respectively. Median survival times were essentially equal in both groups, 19 weeks versus

18 weeks respectively, while 1-year survival rates were 11.4% in group 1 and 20.4% in group 2 (P = ns). Fatal hemoptysis occurred in 22 and 21% of patients, respectively; 18.2% of group 1 required further therapy as did 22.4% of group 2.

Huber and colleagues also conducted a randomized trial comparing external beam radiotherapy alone to external beam radiotherapy plus HDR brachytherapy in patients with inoperable non-small cell lung cancer [14]. Patients receiving external irradiation only (N = 42) were treated with 50 Gy with four to five fractions per week plus a 10-Gy boost. Patients receiving external irradiation plus brachytherapy (N = 56) received the same dose of external beam radiation and 4.8 Gy at 1 cm dose of brachytherapy 1 week prior to external beam, and a second dose 3 weeks after completing external beam treatment. Twenty-five patients (44.6%) patients did not receive the second brachytherapy treatment. According to the authors, the main reason for this deviation from protocol was that the treatment was on an outpatient basis where patients, some from very far away, were irradiated and did not come back 3 weeks after termination of the external irradiation due to complete relief of

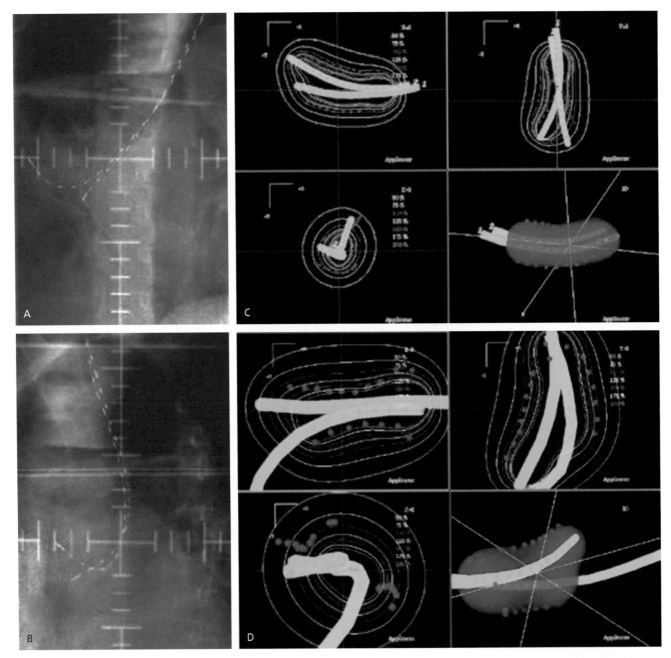

**Fig. 16.2** Treatment planning. (A and B) Planning chest X ray with two catheters and dummy strands in place. (C and D) Treatment planning with isodose distribution and isodose cloud. Figures courtesy of Robert Zlotecki, MD, Professor of Radiation Oncology, University of Florida, Gainesville FL.

symptoms. No changes in Karnofsky performance scores were noted in either group. Overall median survival was 28 weeks in the external beam radiotherapy only group and 27 weeks in the external beam–brachytherapy group ($P = 0.42$). In patients treated per protocol, the median survival was 33 weeks for external beam irradiation only and 43 weeks for external beam irradiation plus brachytherapy ($P = 0.08$). In the subgroup of patients with squamous cell carcinoma (n = 68), there was a non-significant trend

for improved median survival in the external beam–brachytherapy group, 40 weeks versus 33 weeks. Fatal hemoptysis occurred in six patients receiving external beam alone and 11 patients receiving external beam plus brachytherapy.

A second randomized study comparing the addition of HDR brachytherapy to external beam radiotherapy versus external beam radiotherapy alone in patients with inoperable non-small cell lung cancer was reported by Langendijk and colleagues [15]. For radical external beam radiation therapy patients with performance status at or less than 2 and no supraclavicular node involvement (79%) were treated with 60 Gy, whereas palliative radiation therapy in patients with performance status of 3 or supraclavicular node involvement (21%) consisted of a dose of 30 Gy. In the group receiving brachytherapy as well, the dose was 7.5 Gy on day 1 and day 8. Forty-eight patients were randomized to external beam radiotherapy alone and 47 were randomized to external beam–brachytherapy. In the group of patients with an atelectasis before radiotherapy, nine out of 26 (35%) improved with external beam alone, while 17 out of 30 (57%) improved with external beam–brachytherapy. Response rates were 37% versus 46% ($P = 0.29$) for dyspnea, 38% versus 24% for cough, and 82% versus 86% for hemoptysis in the external beam only group and external beam plus brachytherapy group, respectively. The median survival after external beam irradiation only was 8.5 months and external beam irradiation plus brachytherapy 7.0 months ($P = 0.21$). Six patients treated with external beam only died of massive hemoptysis (13%) compared to seven patients treated with external beam–brachytherapy (15%).

A third randomized study, comparing external beam radiotherapy plus brachytherapy versus external beam radiotherapy alone, in patients with locally advanced non-small cell lung cancer with endobronchial involvement, was conducted by Sur and coworkers with an update published in abstract form [16,17]. After receiving 30–40 Gy of external beam radiation in 10–20 fractions, 65 patients were randomized to further external beam radiation of 20 Gy in 10 fractions or to receive two weekly fractions of 6 Gy at 1 cm HDR brachytherapy. Symptom-free survival was 129 days in the external beam alone group versus 77 days in the external beam plus brachytherapy group ($P = 0.009$). Overall survival at 1 year was similar at 29.4 and 29.7%, respectively.

A randomized trial by Stout and colleagues compared HDR endobronchial brachytherapy to external beam radiotherapy for palliation in 99 patients with inoperable non-small cell lung cancer [18]. Forty-nine patients received a single treatment of brachytherapy at a dose of 15 Gy at 1 cm and 50 patients received 30 Gy of external beam radiation over 10–12 fractions. Positive responses to symptom end points, as assessed by clinicians at 8 weeks for the brachytherapy group versus the external beam radiation group, respectively, were 59 and 78% for dyspnea, 50 and 67% for cough, 78 and 89% for hemoptysis, 61 and 80% for chest pain, 57 and 74% for tiredness, and 63 and 78% for anorexia. Although the improvements in symptoms as assessed by clinicians favored the external beam radiotherapy group, the results were not statistically significant. Assessments of positive response by patients at 8 weeks for the brachytherapy group and the external beam radiation group were 38 and 49% for dyspnea, 45 and 65% for cough, 71 and 90% for hemoptysis, 43 and 77% for chest pain ($P < 0.05$),

30 and 65% for tiredness ($P < 0.05$), and 43 and 77% for anorexia ($P < 0.05$), respectively. A higher percentage of patients in the external beam radiotherapy only group achieved good global palliation in assessments by clinicians (91 versus 76%, $P = 0.09$) and by patients (83 versus 59%, $P = 0.029$). Fifty-one percent of the brachytherapy group required subsequent external beam radiation at a median time of 125 days (range 15–511) while 28% of the external beam radiotherapy group required subsequent brachytherapy at a median time of 304 days (range 98–1037). Median survival was 287 days in the external beam radiation group compared to 250 days in the brachytherapy group while 1-year survival rates were 38 versus 22%, respectively ($P = 0.04$).

Mallick and coworkers compared three different doses of HDR brachytherapy with or without external beam radiation in a randomized study of patients with advanced non-small cell lung cancer [19]. Fifteen patients were treated with two sessions of brachytherapy with a dose of 8 Gy at 1 cm plus 30 Gy of external beam radiation, 15 patients were treated with a single fraction of brachytherapy with a dose of 10 Gy at 1 cm plus 30 Gy of external beam radiation, and 15 patients received a single fraction of brachytherapy with a dose of 15 Gy at 1 cm without external beam radiation. Reductions in obstruction scores were 57.7, 55.8, and 44.4%, respectively ($P = 0.54$). Overall symptomatic response rates were 91% for dyspnea, 84% for cough, 94% for hemoptysis, and 83% for obstructive pneumonia. Improvements in dyspnea, cough, hemoptysis, and obstructive pneumonia were similar among the three groups, although the duration of relief from hemoptysis was significantly shorter in the group receiving brachytherapy alone. Improvements in the EORTC QLQ-C30 (European Organization for Research and Treatment of Cancer quality of life questionnaire) global health status scores were similar between the three groups, as were the QLQ-lung cancer-13 (QLQ-LC13) scores. The QLQ-C30 improved from 35 to 67 and the QLQ-LC13 improved from 30 to 10, overall.

A number of non-randomized studies have evaluated different dosing schemes of HDR brachytherapy, and HDR brachytherapy with or without external beam radiotherapy. In a study by Muto and colleagues, 320 patients with stage IIIA or IIIB non-small cell lung cancer were treated with 10 Gy in one fraction (n = 84), two fractions of 7 Gy (n = 47), or three fractions of 5 Gy (n = 189) [20]. Patients were also treated with 60 Gy of external beam radiation. Improvements in dyspnea were noted in 80, 85, and 94% of patients, respectively; cough in 58, 72, and 89%, respectively; and hemoptysis in 100, 99, and 99%, respectively. Mean survival was 9.7 months, with no difference in survival between the groups. Radiation bronchitis, with or without concomitant bronchial stenosis, was found at 6 months in 80% of the 10 Gy single fraction group, 48% of the 7 Gy two fraction group, and 17% of the 5 Gy three fraction group. Fatal hemoptysis occurred in 2.5, 6.5, and 3.2% of patients, respectively. Bronchoesophageal fistulas were noted in 1–2% of patients. Mallick and coworkers treated 95 patients with stage IIIA or IIIB non-small cell lung cancer with HDR brachytherapy plus external beam radiotherapy or HDR brachytherapy alone [21]. Sixty-five patients received two fractions of 8 Gy at 1 cm plus 30 Gy of external beam radiation in 10 fractions, 15 patients received one fraction of 10 Gy at 1 cm plus 30 Gy of external beam radiation in 10 fractions, and 15 patients received a single fraction of 15 Gy at 1 cm alone. Changes in obstruction scores were 57, 54, and 44%, respectively ($P = 0.066$). Overall response rates were 93% for dyspnea, 81% for cough, 97% for hemoptysis, and 91% for obstructive pneumonia. The symptom responses for dyspnea, cough, and obstructive pneumonia were similar between the groups although the group receiving brachytherapy alone had less improvement in hemoptysis (83.3 versus 100%, $P = 0.041$). The overall EORTC QLQ-30 scores improved from 35 to 67 while the overall QLQ-LC13 scores improved from 30 to 10. The median time to symptom progression ranged from 6 to 11 months. A total of 648 patients with locally advanced non-small cell lung cancer were treated with two different dose schedules of HDR brachytherapy by Skowronek and colleagues, depending on clinical stage and ECOG (Eastern Cooperative Oncology Group) performance status [22]; 303 patients received three fractions of 7.5 Gy at 1 cm weekly and 345 patients, most of whom had a performance status greater than 2, received a single fraction of 10 Gy at 1 cm. There was a trend for improved survival times in patients treated with three fractions of 7.5 Gy but this was not significant in multivariate analysis. Mantz and coworkers compared HDR brachytherapy plus external beam radiotherapy to external beam radiotherapy only in a matched pair analysis of patients with medically inoperable non-small cell lung cancer [23]. Thirty-nine patients were treated with brachytherapy at total doses ranging from 10 to 30 Gy in two to four fractions and external beam radiation at total dose ranging from 54.0 to 75.6 Gy. Each patient was matched with two patients with similar stage and external beam radiation dose. At 5 years, patients treated with brachytherapy plus external beam radiotherapy achieved a local control rate of 58% compared with 32% local control for patients treated with external beam alone. Three-year overall survival rates were 15 and 9%, respectively. No differences in acute and late toxicity were noted.

A number of descriptive case series studies of brachytherapy have been published. These are listed in Table 16.1. Improvements in dyspnea ranged from 24 to 100% of patients. Cough improved in 24 to 88% of patients. Hemoptysis was controlled in a higher percentage of patients than dyspnea or cough, with response rates of 69 to 100%. Improvement in atelectasis or obstructive pneumonitis was more variable, with radiographic responses ranging from 20 to 85%. Median survival times ranged from 5 to 21 months, depending on whether therapy was palliative or curative intent. Different survival times, as noted in Table 16.1, were observed in different patients groups within some studies and were related to previous treatment versus no previous treatment, the use of concurrent external beam radiotherapy, and dose/fractions of brachytherapy. Some studies evaluated change in performance status, in addition to symptoms, following brachytherapy. Nori and associates treated 32 patients with malignant airway obstruction with brachytherapy [49]. Seventeen patients were treated with brachytherapy as a boost to external beam radiotherapy (group 1) and 15 patients were treated for endobronchial recurrence after prior external beam irradiation (group 2). Most patients received three to four fractions of HDR brachytherapy at a dose of 4 to 5 Gy at 1 cm per fraction. Evaluated 1 month after treatment, the mean ECOG (Eastern Cooperative Oncology Group) performance status improved from 2.2 to 1.2. Prior to intervention, 14 patients had grade 3 or 4 status whereas five patients had this level of severely decreased performance status afterwards. Median survival was 17.7 months for group 1 and 7.5 months for group 2. Twenty-nine patients with symptomatic endobronchial recurrence following maximal external irradiation for bronchogenic carcinoma were treated with HDR brachytherapy by Hernandez and colleagues [41]. Patients received three fractions every 2 weeks at a single fraction dose of 7.5 to 10 Gy at 1 cm. Twenty-six patients completed the protocol. ECOG performance status (mean grade 1.9 at study entry) improved in 24%, remained unchanged in 42%, and worsened in 34%. Mehta and colleagues treated 31 patients with primary lung cancer and metastatic malignancies with HDR brachytherapy, delivering four fractions of 4 Gy at 1 cm over 2 days [52]. The ECOG performance status improved from 2.1 to 1.6. Cotter and coworkers evaluated changes in performance status in 65 patients with airway obstructions from primary lung cancer [56]. Patients were treated with external beam radiotherapy at doses of 55 to 66 Gy and either intermediate dose rate brachytherapy (135 to 300 cGy/h) in 17 patients or HDR brachytherapy (15 to 74 cGy/s) in 48 patients. Total implant doses ranged from 2.7 to 10 Gy. An improvement in ECOG performance status was noted in 66% of patients overall. Improvement was noted in 39% (5/13) of patients receiving total doses less than 70 Gy, 72% (13/18) of patients receiving total doses between 70 and 84 Gy, and 74% (20/27) of patients receiving total doses of greater than 85 Gy. Mean survival of all patients was 12.4 months and did not significantly differ when stratified for total dose of administered radiotherapy.

Some studies have also evaluated changes in pulmonary function after brachytherapy. Changes in pulmonary function and ventilation and perfusion following HDR brachytherapy in 19 patients were evaluated by Goldman and coworkers [45]. Patients were treated with a single fraction

**Table 16.1** Descriptive case series studies of high dose rate brachytherapy

| Author, year [reference] | N | Treatment* | Symptom improvement (number of patients) | | | | | Performance status | Median survival[†] |
|---|---|---|---|---|---|---|---|---|---|
| | | | Overall | Cough | Dyspnea | Hemoptysis | Atelectasis/ pneumonitis | | |
| Manali et al. 2010 [24] | 34 | 7.1 Gy × 1–3 ± EBRT | 56% | | | | | | 7.8 months |
| Hauswald et al. 2010 [25] | 41 | 5 Gy × 1–5 | 58% | | | | | | 6.7 months |
| Ozkok et al. 2008 [26] | 158 | 5–7.5 Gy q1w × 2–3 + EBRT | | 57% | 85% | 88% | | | 6–11 months |
| Hennequin et al. 2007 [27] | 106 | 5–7 Gy qw × 6 | | | | | | | 21.4 months |
| Escobar-Sacristán et al.., 2004 [28] | 81 | 5 Gy q1w × 4 | 85% | 88% (30/34) | 75% (18/24) | 96% (23/24) | | | |
| Gejerman et al. 2002 [29] | 41 | 5–7.5 Gy q1–2w × 1–5 ± EBRT | 72% | | | | | | 5.2 months |
| Anacak et al. 2001 [30] | 30 | 5 Gy q2w × 3 + EBRT | | 43% (12/28) | 80% (12/15) | 95 (20/21) | | | 11 months |
| Petera et al. 2001 [31] | 67 | 5–7.5 Gy q1–2w × 1–5 ± EBRT | | 52% (23/44) | 59% (29/51) | 76% (13/17) | 50% (27/54) | | 5.0–8.2 months |
| Harms et al. 2000 [32] | 55 | 5 Gy × 2–5 ± EBRT | 75% | | | | | | 5, 20 months |
| Kelly et al. 2000 [33] | 175 | 15 Gy q2w × 1–3 | 66% | | | | | | 6 months |
| Marsiglia et al. 2000 [34] | 34 | 5 Gy q1w × 6 | | | | | | | (78% at 2 years) |
| Taulelle et al. 1998 [35] | 189 | 8–10 Gy q1w × 3–4 | | 54% | 54% | 74% | | | 7 months |
| Ofiara et al. 1997 [36] | 30 | 8 Gy q2w × 3 | | 46% (11/24) | 33% (8/24) | 79% (11/14) | 43% (9/21) | | |
| Ornadel et al. 1997 [37] | 117 | 15 Gy × 1 ± LR | | 59% | 73% | 73% | | 75% improved | |
| Nomoto et al. 1997 [38] | 39 | 6 Gy q1w × 3 + EBRT or 10 Gy × 1 | | | | | | | 8 months |
| Pérol et al. 1997 [39] | 19 | 7 Gy q1w × 3–5 | | | | | | | 28 months |
| Delclos et al. 1996 [40] | 81 | 15 Gy @ 6–7.5 mm q2w × 1–3 | 84% (68/81) | | | | | | 5 months |
| Hernandez et al. 1996 [41] | 29 | 7.5–10 Gy q2w × 1–3 | | 24% (7/29) | 24% (7/29) | 69% (11/16) | 28% (5/18) | 24% improved | |
| Macha et al. 1995 [42] | 365 | 5 Gy q2w × 1–6 | | | | | | | 5–9 months |

*Continued*

**Table 16.1** *Continued*

| Author, year [reference] | N | Treatment* | Symptom improvement (number of patients) | | | | | Performance status | Median survival[†] |
|---|---|---|---|---|---|---|---|---|---|
| | | | Overall | Cough | Dyspnea | Hemoptysis | Atelectasis/pneumonitis | | |
| Trédaniel *et al.* 1994 [43] | 51 | 7 Gy in 2 fx over 2 days q2w × 3 | 70% (21/30) | 85% | 55% | 85% | | | 5 months, not reached |
| Chang *et al.* 1994 [44] | 76 | 7 Gy q2w × 3 ± EBRT | | 79% (37/47) | 87% (47/54) | 95% (20/21) | 88% (15/17) | | 5 months |
| Goldman *et al.* 1993 [45] | 19 | 15 Gy × 1 | 89% (17/19) | 37% (7/19) | 89% (17/19) | 100% (6/6) | 69% (9/13) | | |
| Gollins *et al.* 1994 [46] | 406 | 10–20 Gy × 1 ± EBRT | | 45% (172/380) | 45% (172/380) | 84% (128/152) | 43% (89/207) | | 4.3–6.6 months |
| Speiser and Spratling, 1993 [47] | 342 | 7.5–10 Gy @ 0.5–1 cm q1w × 3 ± EBRT | | 85% | 86% | 99% | | | 5.6–9.5 months |
| Pisch *et al.* 1993 [48] | 39 | 10 Gy q 2w × 1–2 | | 80% (16/20) | | 93% (13/14) | 20% (3/15) | | |
| Nori *et al.* 1993 [49] | 32 | 5 Gy q1w × 3 ± EBRT | | 86% (6/7) | 100% (10/10) | 100% (15/15) | 44% | Improved in 11/14 pt's ECOG ≥ 2 | 7.5, 17.5 months |
| Bedwinek *et al.* 1992 [50] | 38 | 6 Gy q1w × 3 | 76% (29/38) | | | | 64% (9/14) | | 6.5 months |
| Gauwitz *et al.* 1992 [51] | 24 | 15 Gy @ 6 mm q2w × 3 | 88% (21/24) | | | | 83% (15/18) | | 7.4 months |
| Mehta *et al.* 1992 [52] | 31 | 4 Gy @ 2 cm × 4 over 2d | 79%[¹] | 73% (19/26) | 75% (18/24) | 100% (10/10) | 85% (12/14) | ECOG 2.1→1.6 | |
| Sutedja *et al.* 1992 [53] | 31 | 10 Gy q2w × 1–3 ± LR | | | 82% (18/22) | | | | 3, 7 months |
| Aygun *et al.* 1992 [54] | 62 | 5 Gy q1w × 3–5 + EBRT | | | | | | | 10, 20 months |
| Burt *et al.* 1990 [55] | 50 | 15–20 Gy × 1 | | 50% (9/18) | 64% (21/33) | 86% (24/28) | 33% (11/24) | | |

Gy, gray; EBRT, external beam radiotherapy; LR, laser resection; ECOG, Eastern Cooperative Oncology Group; q, every; w, week.

*Treatment at 1 cm unless specified.

†Median survival may be reported for different groups within case series depending on dose fraction and curative versus palliative intent.

of 15 Gy at 1 cm. Pulmonary function testing performed 6 weeks later demonstrated mean increases in $FEV_1$ (forced expiratory volume in 1 s) from 1.45 to 1.61 L (55.5 to 62.3% of predicted) and $FVC$ (forced vital capacity) from 2.17 to 2.48 L (63.9 to 74.0% of predicted) ($P < 0.05$ for both). There was no significant change in total lung capacity, residual volume, or diffusion capacity. Radionuclide lung scans 6 weeks after treatment showed improvement in ventilation of the abnormal lung from 17.0 to 27.7% and in perfusion from 15.1 to 21.9% ($P < 0.005$). The mean 5 minute walking distance increased from 305 meters to 329 meters ($P < 0.01$). Patients with occlusion of a mainstem bronchus had greater improvement than patients with lobar bronchus occlusion. Macha and colleagues evaluated pulmonary function in a subset of 40 patients with obstruction of a mainstem bronchus treated with HDR brachytherapy at a dose of 5 Gy at 1 cm every 2 weeks for one to six fractions [42]. $FEV_1$ increased from 1.50 L to 2.15 L while $FVC$ increased from 2.61 L to 3.41 L. Pulmonary function was assessed after LDR brachytherapy in 38 patients by Mehta and coworkers [57]. The average $FEV_1$ improved from 1.47 to 1.88 L and $FVC$ improved from 2.21 to 3.09 L.

Brachytherapy has been utilized for curative intent therapy in patients who are not candidates for surgical resection. Fourteen patients with limited endobronchial disease, including 11 patients with residual positive bronchial margins following surgery, were treated with four fractions of 5 Gy at 1 cm by Macha and coworkers [42]. Mean survival time was 23 months. Tredaniel and colleagues treated 29 patients with lung cancer limited to the bronchial wall and lumen [43]. Patients were treated with 7 Gy at 1 cm fractions on two consecutive days with repeat treatment every 15 days to a maximum of six fractions. Histologic complete responses were noted in 18/25 patients who underwent bronchoscopic assessment. The mean overall actuarial survival was not achieved after 23 months of follow-up. Nineteen patients with limited endobronchial non-small cell carcinomas, lesions at or less than 1 cm, were treated with HDR brachytherapy by Pérol and coworkers [39]. Patients received weekly fractions of 7 Gy at 1 cm for a total of three to five fractions. Twelve of 16 patients (75%) evaluated bronchoscopically at 1 year had histologic evidence of tumor control. Overall survival rates were 78% at 1 year and 58% at 2 years with a median value of 28 months. Partial fibrous stenosis of the treated bronchus occurred in 10 of 18 patients, including 8 of 12 patients receiving five fractions. Two patients treated with five fractions developed bronchial wall necrosis. Hennequin and colleagues treated 106 patients with lung cancer limited to the bronchus who developed disease relapse after surgery (n = 43) or external beam radiotherapy (n = 27) or who had respiratory insufficiency precluding other therapy (n = 36) with six weekly fractions of 7 Gy (initial regimen) or 5 Gy (subsequent regimen) [27]. At 5 years, the local control, overall survival, and cause-specific survival rates were 51.6, 24, and 48.5%, respectively. Two patients died of hemoptysis and three from bronchial necrosis. Marsiglia and coworkers observed a local control rate of 85% and a survival rate of 78% at 2 years in 34 patients with early stage endobronchial non-small cell lung cancer treated with six weekly fractions of 5 Gy [34]. A median survival time of 20 months was observed in the subset of 19 patients with stage I non-small cell lung cancer treated with three to five weekly fractions of 5 Gy at 1 cm HDR brachytherapy and 50–60 Gy of external beam radiation therapy by Aygun and colleagues [54]. Results similar to those presented have been noted in patients with roentgenographically occult lung cancer treated with external beam radiotherapy and LDR brachytherapy [58,59].

Brachytherapy has also been utilized as palliative treatment for endobronchial metastases from non-bronchogenic malignancies. Eleven patients with endobronchial metastases were treated with three to four weekly fractions of 5–6 Gy at 1 cm in one study [60]. Improvement in signs and symptoms of obstruction occurred in eight patients. Bronchoscopic evaluation revealed complete response in three patients and partial response (≥60% decrease in obstruction) in five patients. In another study, 37 patients with endobronchial metastases were treated with a single fraction of 10–15 Gy at 1 cm [61]. Dyspnea improved in 42% of patients, cough in 50%, and hemoptysis in 67%. Survival ranged from 9 to 1145 days with a mean of 280 days. Survival was longer in patients without overt extrabronchial metastases. Although not specifically evaluated in the studies, various case series of brachytherapy have also included patients with endobronchial metastases.

Additional bronchoscopic modalities have been combined with brachytherapy. Chella and colleagues randomized 15 patients with central non-small cell lung cancer (NSCLC) to treatment with neodymium–yytrium–aluminum–garnet (Nd:YAG) laser therapy alone and 14 patients to Nd:YAG laser resection followed by HDR brachytherapy [62]. The brachytherapy treatment dose was 5 Gy at 0.5 cm weekly to a total dose of 15 Gy and treatment began 15–18 days after laser treatment. Median survival was 7.4 months in the laser resection alone group and 10.3 months in the laser plus HDR brachytherapy group (P = ns). The Speiser obstruction index improved to a similar degree in both groups. The period free from symptoms in the responsive patients was 2.8 months for Nd:YAG treatment alone and 8.5 months for combined Nd:YAG and HDR treatment (P < 0.05). Improvements in spirometry were similar for the two groups: $FEV_1$ 1.35 to 2.16 L and 1.43 to 2.32 L, respectively; $FVC$ 2.08 to 3.34 L and 2.11 to 3.47 L, respectively. Further bronchoscopic interventions were required in 15 of the Nd:YAG laser alone treated patients versus three of the Nd:YAG plus brachytherapy group. Jang and colleagues conducted a retrospective review of patients with primary lung cancer (n = 67) or metastatic cancer (n = 13) treated with laser resection (n = 22), HDR brachytherapy (n = 37), or a combination (n = 21) [63]. The vast majority were treated with a single fraction of brachytherapy with a mean dose of 12.5 Gy. Overall median survival rates were 111 days in the laser therapy group, 115 days in the brachytherapy group, and 264 days in the combined group, which was statistically significant for the brachytherapy versus combined treatment groups but not for the laser therapy versus combined treatment groups. A retrospective review of 33 patients with squamous cell carcinoma treated with Nd:YAG laser therapy alone and 13 patients treated with Nd:YAG plus LDR brachytherapy was reported by Shea and coworkers [64]. Mean survival times were 16.4 weeks and 40.8 weeks, respectively (P = 0.001). Other authors have suggested that progression-free survival times may be increased with the combination of laser therapy and brachytherapy, albeit in uncontrolled case series [7,37]. Seventy-nine patients with primary lung cancer were treated by HDR brachytherapy by Kohek and coworkers [65]. Patients received 5 Gy per session with total doses ranging from 5 to 25 Gy (mean 11.6). In 26 patients with complete or nearly complete obstruction, Nd:YAG laser resection was performed to allow for catheter placement. External beam radiotherapy was administered to 48 patients following brachytherapy at a total dose of 50 to 70 Gy. The mean Karnofsky performance score improved from 68.2 to 77.2 in 58 of the 79 patients. Dyspnea was relieved in 67% of patients (41 of 61), hemoptysis in 86% (6 of 7), and cough in 70% (50 of 71). In the 41 patients with atelectasis, radiologic evidence of reaeration was noted in 29 patients (70%). The median survival of the 48 patients who received additional external beam radiotherapy was 13 months while the median survival of the 31 patients who did not was 6 months ($P < 0.01$). Ornadel and associates evaluated 117 patients treated with HDR brachytherapy for recurrent malignant airway obstruction after prior therapy [37]. Patients underwent a single fraction of 15 Gy at 1 cm, except for four patients who received additional fractions. Nd:YAG laser resection was performed in 51 patients prior to brachytherapy. Fifty-four percent of patients had an improvement in ECOG performance status of at least 1 grade ($P = 0.0417$). Dyspnea improved in 50% ($P = 0.0063$). The mean $FEV_1$ improved from 1.30 to 1.38 L ($P = 0.0504$) and the mean FVC improved from 1.92 to 2.06 L ($P = 0.041$). Median survival was 12 months. Macha and colleagues evaluated 56 patients with malignant obstruction of the trachea or mainstem bronchus following treatment with three fractions of HDR brachytherapy at a dose of 7.5 Gy at 1 cm [66]. Twenty-nine patients with mainstem bronchial occlusion underwent Nd:YAG laser resection prior to catheter placement. Pulmonary function tests, available for 20 patients although it was not specified how many of these received laser resection, demonstrated increases in mean values of $FEV_1$ from 1.62 to 2.13 L, and $FVC$ from 2.61 to 3.31 L ($P < 0.001$ for both). The severity of dyspnea was reduced in 44 patients (79%). In the 25 patients with atelectasis, radiographic evidence of reaeration was noted in 22 (88%).

Brachytherapy has also been combined with photodynamic therapy (PDT). Freitag and colleagues treated 32 patients with inoperable or recurrent endobronchial non-small cell lung cancer with PDT followed by HDR brachytherapy 5–6 weeks after completing PDT [67]. The brachytherapy regimen consisted of five weekly fractions of 4 Gy at 1 cm beginning 6 weeks after PDT. Complete response was achieved in 24 patients (75%) after initial PDT and in all but one patient after brachytherapy (97%). Cancer recurred in six patients at time intervals ranging from 6 to 26 months. Moderate scarring of the bronchus 2–3 months after treatment was usually observed although no interventions were required. No other complications were noted. Nine patients were non-small cell lung cancer underwent PDT and HDR brachytherapy treatment by Weinberg and coworkers [68]. Seven patients received three weekly fractions of 5 Gy at 0.5 cm followed by PDT, while two patients received PDT first. Intervals between the two treatments ranged from 9 to 63 days. Local control was achieved in seven patients. Bronchial scarring and/or benign local tissue reactions were noted in eight patients.

Simultaneous stent placement with HDR brachytherapy has also be described by Allison and colleagues [69]. Ten patients with symptomatic endobronchial recurrence following chemotherapy and external beam radiotherapy for stage III non-small cell lung cancer underwent placement of a self-expanding metallic stent and HDR brachytherapy during the same bronchoscopy. Patients were treated with three weekly fractions of 6 Gy at 0.5 cm. The Karnofsky performance status improved in all patients. Local control was observed in all patients with survival times ranging from 4 to 18 months. No complications were noted.

Brachytherapy via bronchoscopy has recently been used to treat small peripheral lung cancers. Kobayashi and colleagues treated two patients with peripheral lung cancers using CT guidance for HDR brachytherapy [70]. The first patient, with a left upper lobe 2.3 × 2.2 cm adenocarcinoma, initially had the lesion marked using CT-guided bronchoscopic barium instillation in the peripheral bronchus directly under the visceral pleura. Nine days later the patient underwent repeat bronchoscopy with placement of a 5 Fr applicator at the site of the barium marker under fluoroscopy. An 8 Gy at 1 cm dose of brachytherapy was then administered. This was repeated twice more, at weekly intervals. The second patient, with a right upper lobe 2.6 × 1.8 cm adenocarcinoma, was treated with a single fraction of 15 Gy at 1 cm. In this case the brachytherapy catheter was placed under CT-guided bronchoscopy without barium marking. Follow-up at 18 and 10 months, respectively, demonstrated excellent treatment effects. Seven patients with peripheral T1–T2 lung cancer underwent transbronchial brachytherapy using fluoroscopy and CT-guidance by Imamura and coworkers [71]. Transbronchial brachytherapy was attempted in an eighth patient but was unsuccessful due to inability to access the tumor. The brachytherapy regimens included five fractions of 5 Gy, three fractions of 7 Gy, and two fractions of 12.5 Gy. Also included in this study were five patients who under percutaneously delivered brachytherapy. Complete response was noted in three patients, partial response in four, and stable disease in five patients. Disease recurrence occurred in three patients 12–32 months after treatment, including the single patient with a T2 tumor and one patient being treated with salvage brachytherapy after conformal external beam radiotherapy. The results for patients treated with transbronchial brachytherapy were not separately reported from those receiving percutaneous brachytherapy. Harms and colleagues described the use of navigation bronchoscopy in combination with brachytherapy in a patient with a right upper lobe lung cancer [72]. Navigation bronchoscopy was used with the superDimension system (superDimension Ltd, Herzliya, Israel) to position the extended working channel at the tumor. Confirmation of positioning of the extended working channel catheter was confirmed using endobronchial ultrasound (EBUS) with a radial probe (Olympus Co., Tokyo, Japan). A 6 Fr brachytherapy catheter was then placed through the extended working channel and the extended working channel was removed. Three fractions of brachytherapy at a dose of 5 Gy were given over a 1-week period, leaving the brachytherapy catheter in place during the treatment time. The catheter was well tolerated by the patient and repeat imaging prior to treatment showed no catheter migration. Repeated bronchoscopic biopsies were negative for recurrence. In a similar approach, using electromagnetic navigation bronchoscopy and catheter position confirmation with peripheral radial EBUS, by the same investigators at Heidelberg University and collaborators at the University of Texas, Tyler, reported the treatment of 32 patients with peripheral lung cancer in abstract form [73]. Patients were treated with a total of 15–30 Gy of HDR brachytherapy. Patients treated at Heidelberg University had the brachytherapy catheter left in place for up to 8 days while patients at the University of Texas, Tyler, underwent two separate brachytherapy catheter insertions within 2 weeks. The catheter could not be placed in one patient and one patient had a pneumothorax that did not require treatment. Twenty-seven of the 32 patients had histologically confirmed complete remission with at least 2 years of follow-up.

## Results for benign disease

HDR brachytherapy has also been utilized in the management of obstructive endobronchial granulation tissue following lung transplantation and stent placement for benign disease. Kennedy and colleagues treated two patients with 3 Gy at 1 cm of brachytherapy for recurrent granulation tissue in the left mainstem bronchi despite prior treatment with stent placement (Wallstent; Boston Scientific Corp, Natick MA), Nd:YAG laser resection, and balloon dilatation [74]. The patients underwent stent placement 3 and 4 months after lung transplant, respectively, and were treated with brachytherapy 4 and 7 months after stent insertion, respectively. One patient required bronchoscopy every 10–14 days while the other required bronchoscopy every 28–35 days to manage the stenoses prior to brachytherapy. One patient required a second course of brachytherapy (3 Gy) 3 weeks after the first treatment due to recurrent granulation tissue. Both patients were free of granulation tissue at 6 and 7 months of follow-up. Four patients with airway stenosis were treated with two to four fractions of 3 Gy at 1 cm over a time span of 1–30 months by Halkos and coworkers [75].

The patients had been treated for anastomotic stenosis with stent placement 4–12 months after transplant; silicone in two, metallic in one (Wallstent), and silicone followed by metallic (Wallstent) in one patient, as well as Nd:YAG laser therapy, electrocautery therapy, and balloon dilatation. Brachytherapy was performed 9 months to 5 years after transplant. Successful treatment was noted in three patients while one patient had no benefit despite four fractions of brachytherapy and subsequently died of pneumonia and respiratory failure. Madu and colleagues treated five patients with recurrent obstructive granulation tissue, four with lung transplant anastomotic-related stenosis, and one patient with recurrent tracheal granulation tissue secondary to prior tracheostomy tube placement [76]. The time to first stenosis ranged from 1 to 10 months and treatment with prior interventions included stent placement, balloon dilatation, endobronchial steroid injection, Nd:YAG laser, electrocautery, and topical mitomycin-C application. Brachytherapy was administered with two to three weekly fractions of 7 Gy for the lung transplant patients and two weekly fractions of 5 Gy for the patient with post-tracheostomy tube granulation tissue. At a median follow-up of 12 months, the average number of interventional procedures decreased from 11 (range 6–17) to 3 (range 0–7) after brachytherapy. The $FEV_1$ increased in all four lung transplant patients after brachytherapy treatment. One patient died during a subsequent bronchoscopy for stent placement, likely secondary to a cerebral air embolism. Six patients with granulation tissue following Wallstent metallic stent placement for benign subglottic/tracheal stenosis (n = 5) and right mainstem bronchial stenosis (n = 2) were treated with HDR brachytherapy by Kramer and colleagues [77]. Five patients were treated secondary to recurrent granulation tissue requiring multiple procedures and two patients, interestingly, were treated prophylactically. The brachytherapy consisted of a single fraction of 10 Gy at 1 cm and was performed after Nd:YAG laser resection of granulation tissue. At follow-up ranging from 4 to 30 months, two patients had no granulation tissue while four had minimal and one had recurrent moderate granulation tissue noted 5–30 months after brachytherapy. Radiation necrosis was noted in one patient. Of the two patients treated prophylactically, one had no granulation tissue and one had minimal granulation tissue. The same investigators, in a study of 115 patients undergoing treatment for benign tracheal stenosis, reported the use of a single HDR brachytherapy fraction of 10 Gy at 1 cm to treat recurrent granulation tissue in 28 of 33 patients who underwent metallic stent placement (Wallstent and SMART nitinol stent; Cordis Corp, Bridgewater NJ). All patients were reported as requiring less therapeutic bronchoscopies after brachytherapy but no further details were provided. No complications were noted. Tendulkar and coworkers treated eight patients with refractory endobronchial granulation tissue following stent placement for lung transplant anastomotic problems (n = 6),tracheobronchomalacia(n = 1), and Wegener's granulomatosis (n = 1) [78]. Patients received one or two fractions of 7.1 Gy at 1 cm HDR brachytherapy. The interval between lung transplant and brachytherapy ranged from 7 to 50 months. The interval between the last therapeutic bronchoscopy and performing brachytherapy ranged from 1 to 215 days. Within the first 6 months after brachytherapy, six patients were judged to have a good-to-excellent response whereas two patients had a fair-to-poor response. The mean number of procedures in the 6 months pre- and post-treatment decreased from 3.1 to 1.8. $FEV_1$ increased from 36% of predicted to 46% of predicted. Of the four patients alive at 1 year, only one maintained an excellent response. Of note, this patient had electrocautery resection of granulation tissue the day before receiving brachytherapy. The investigators speculated that brachytherapy may be effective for this application if performed 24–48 hours after an intervention to remove the granulation tissue. In terms of complications, one patient had an anastomotic dehiscence 5 months after brachytherapy and one patient had fatal hemoptysis from a bronchoarterial fistula 4 months after brachytherapy.

## Complications

Endobronchial brachytherapy is a generally well-tolerated procedure with few acute side effects. Most of the acute toxicity is related to the bronchoscopy for catheter placement and cough during the time the brachytherapy catheter is in place. Massive hemoptysis is the most common life-threatening complication. The incidence of massive hemoptysis has ranged from 0 to 32%, with most series reporting values between 3 and 10%. Tumor progression likely plays a role in many patients and sorting out the contribution of this versus massive hemoptysis as a direct complication of brachytherapy is difficult. Different risk factors for the development of massive hemoptysis have been reported, including upper lobe tumor location, endobronchial tumor length, prior radiation therapy, prior laser therapy, large fraction size, and presence of hemoptysis prior to treatment. Bedwinek and colleagues, in their analysis of 38 patients previously treated with external beam radiation, observed fatal pulmonary hemorrhage in 12 patients (32%) 2–56 weeks after receiving three fractions of 6 Gy HDR brachytherapy [50]. This complication observed in patients who were treated in the upper lobes and right mainstem bronchus. Other investigators have also noted increase risk for massive hemoptysis with treatment of the upper lobes. This observation is likely due in part to the right pulmonary artery lying directly over the anterior surface of the right mainstem bronchus and right upper lobe, while the left pulmonary artery lies directly over the anterior left mainstem bronchus and left upper lobe. The angulation of the brachytherapy catheter at the take-off of the upper lobe bronchi may produce a "hot spot" along the bronchial wall

and adjacent pulmonary artery. Ornadel and colleagues treated 117 patients with HDR brachytherapy, 51 of whom also underwent prior Nd:YAG laser resection [37]. Eleven patients suffered fatal hemoptysis. Patients who had received Nd:YAG laser treatment were more likely to have fatal hemoptysis although laser therapy was performed if there was significant endobronchial disease likely to cause lung collapse or if patients were in severe respiratory distress and, thus, differences in tumor-related factors may have existed. In an analysis of 406 patients treated with a single dose of 15 Gy or 20 Gy HDR brachytherapy, Gollins and coworkers identified 32 patients (8%) who died of massive hemoptysis 7 days to 26 months after therapy [11]. A Cox multivariate regression analysis showed that increased brachytherapy dose (20 Gy vs. 15 Gy), prior laser treatment at the site of brachytherapy, and second brachytherapy treatment at the same site increased the risk of fatal massive hemoptysis. The concurrent use of brachytherapy and external beam radiation did not quite reach statistical significance in the regression analysis with a $P$ value of 0.08. Twenty out of 25 evaluable patients (80%) who died of massive hemoptysis had evidence of residual or recurrent tumor. Hennequin and colleagues reviewed 149 patients who received two to six fractions of 4–7 Gy HDR brachytherapy for complications [79]. Hemoptysis was observed in 11 cases (7.4%), 10 of which were lethal, 1 to 48 weeks after brachytherapy. All but one patient were considered to have progressive disease. In univariate analysis, treatment for palliation (as opposed to curative intent) and endobronchial tumor length were significantly associated with hemoptysis. Tumor location, treatment volume parameters, and associated bronchoscopic treatments were not correlated with hemoptysis in this study. In multivariate analysis, only the therapeutic group retained statistical significance. In a study by Hara and coworkers, 7 of 36 patients treated with HDR brachytherapy developed fatal hemoptysis [80]. Local failure or persistent malignancy and laser resection were found to be statistically significantly associated with massive hemoptysis as was direct contact between the catheter and tracheobronchial walls at the vicinity of the great vessels. Brachytherapy fraction and total doses, length of treated bronchial segment, and concurrent or previous external beam radiation were not correlated. Eight of 84 patients (9.5%) developed fatal hemoptysis 0.5–8 months following HDR brachytherapy in a series by Carvalho and colleagues [81]. The only factor with significantly correlated with fatal hemoptysis was larger irradiated volumes. Langendijk and coworkers reviewed 938 patients who were treated with external beam radiotherapy and/or HDR brachytherapy [82]. The incidence of fatal massive hemoptysis was 4.3% in patients treated with external beam (18/421), 13.1% in patients treated with external beam but would have been eligible for brachytherapy (55/419), 25.8% in patients receiving external beam plus brachytherapy (16/62), 15.4% in patients receiving brachytherapy alone (2/13), and 43.4% in patients treated with brachytherapy following recurrence after external beam (10/23). In multivariate analysis, fraction size (15 Gy vs. 10 Gy or 7.5 Gy) (relative risk, RR 5.3), upper lobe location (RR 2.7), intrabronchial tumor extension into main bronchus (RR 2.7), and hemoptysis prior to radiotherapy (RR 2.1) were associated with fatal hemoptysis in patients receiving brachytherapy. A summary of studies reporting on complications, including massive hemoptysis, is presented in Table 16.2.

Radiation bronchitis and stenosis have been well described as a complication of brachytherapy (see Table 16.2). This was initially described by Speiser and Spratling in 1993 [85]. In their series of patients treated with HDR brachytherapy, the incidence was 9% in patients receiving 10 Gy at 5 mm for three fractions, 12% in those receiving 10 Gy at 1 cm for

**Table 16.2** Complications following high dose rate brachytherapy

| Author, year [reference] | N | Treatment* | Prior/ concurrent EBRT | Prior laser | Massive hemoptysis | Radiation bronchitis (any grade) | Radiation bronchitis grade III/IV | Fistula | Airway stenosis |
|---|---|---|---|---|---|---|---|---|---|
| Manali et al. 2010 [24] | 34 | | 68% | 26% | 3% | 21% | | | |
| Hauswald et al. 2010 [25] | 41 | 5 Gy × 1–5 | 100% | | 15% | 5% | | 5% | |
| Weinberg et al. 2010 [68] | 9 | 5 Gy @ 5 mm q1w × 3 + PDT | 36% | 11% | 0% | 78% | | 0% | 22% |
| Ozkok et al. 2008 [26] | 158 | 5–7.5 Gy q1w × 2–3 | 100% | | 11% | 5% | | | |
| Carvalho et al. 2007 [81] | 84 | 5–7.5 Gy × 1–5 | 55% | 24% | 10% | | | | |
| Hennequin et al. 2007 [27] | 106 | 5–7 Gy q1w × 6 | 47% | | | 8% | 4% | | |
| Escobar-Sacristan et al. 2004 [28] | 81 | 5 Gy q1w × 4 | 63% | 2% | 0% | | 1% | 1% | 1% |
| Mantz et al. 2004 [23] | 39 | 4–9 Gy q1w × 2–4 | 100% | 0% | 0% | | | | 2.6% |
| Langendijk et al. 2001 [15] | 47 | 7.5 Gy q1w × 2 | 100% | 0% | 15% | | | | 4% |
| Hara et al. 2001 [80] | 36 | 4–45 Gy total dose | 81% | 22% | 19% | | | | |
| Anacak et al. 2001 [30] | 30 | 5 Gy q2w × 3 | 100% | | 11% | 70% | 7% | | 13% |
| Petera et al. 2001 [31] | 67 | 5–7.5 Gy q1–2w × 1–5 | 84% | | 3% | 7% | 1.5% | 1.5% | 4% |
| Muto et al. 2000 [20] | 84 | 10 Gy × 1 | 100% | 5% | 2.5% | 80% | 37% | 1% | |
| | 47 | 7 Gy × 2 | | | 6.5% | 48% | 13% | 2% | |
| | 50 | 5 Gy × 3 | | | 5.5% | 22% | 17% | 3% | |
| | 139 | 5 Gy @ 5 mm × 3 | | | 2.5% | 16% | 8% | 0% | |
| Stout et al 2000 [18] | 49 | 15 Gy × 1 | 0% | 0% | 8% | | | | |
| Marsiglia et al. 2000 [34] | 34 | 5 Gy q1w × 6 | 0% | | | 3% | | | |
| Kelly et al. 2000 [33] | 175 | 15 Gy q2w × 1–3 | NS | 11% | 5% | | | 0.5% | 0.5% |
| Taulelle et al. 1998 [35] | 189 | 8–10 Gy q 1w × 3–4 | 62% | 14% | 7% | 22% | 6% | 1.6% | 6% |
| Hennequin et al. 1998 [79] | 149 | 4–7 Gy × 2–6 | 75% | 6% | 7% | 9% | | | 1% |

*Continued*

**Table 16.2** *Continued*

| Author, year [reference] | N | Treatment* | Prior/ concurrent EBRT | Prior laser | Massive hemoptysis | Radiation bronchitis (any grade) | Radiation bronchitis grade III/IV | Fistula | Airway stenosis |
|---|---|---|---|---|---|---|---|---|---|
| Langendijk *et al.* 1998 [82] | 98 | 7.5 Gy × 2 or 10–15 Gy ×1 | 87% | NS | 29% | | | | |
| Ornadel *et al.* 1997 [37] | 117 | 15 Gy × 1 | 79% | 44% | 9% | | | | |
| Huber *et al.* 1997 [14] | 56 | 4.8 Gy × 2 | 100% | 16% | 19% | | | | |
| Pérol *et al.* 1997 [39] | 19 | 7 Gy q1w × 3–5 | | 0 | 11% | 56% | 11% | | |
| Nomoto *et al.* 1997 [38] | 39 | 6 Gy q1w × 3 + EBRT or 10 Gy × 1 | NS | | 8% | | | | |
| Delclos *et al.* 1996 [83] | 81 | 15 Gy @ 6–7.5 mm q2w × 1–3 | 100% | NS | 1% | | 2% | 1% | 2% |
| Gollins *et al.* 1996 [11] | 406 | 15 Gy × 1 20 Gy × 1 | 20% | 2% | 6% 16% | 44% 60% | 13% 20% | 0% | 2% |
| Hernandez *et al.* 1996 [41] | 29 | 7.5-10 Gy q2w × 1–3 | 100% | 10% | 4% | 0% | | | 0% |
| Gustafson *et al.* 1995 [84] | 46 | 7 Gy q1w × 3 | 30% | 0 | 7% | | | | |
| Huber *et al.* 1995 [13] | 44 49 | 3.8 Gy q1w × 4 7.2 Gy q 3w × 2 | 47% 39% | 33% 46% | 22% 21% | | | | |
| Macha *et al.* 1995 [42] | 365 | 5 Gy q2w × 1–6 | Most | Most | 21% | | | 2% | |
| Trédaniel *et al.* 1994 [43] | 51 | 7 Gy in 2 fx over 2 days q2w × 3 | 63% | 8% | 10% | 14% | | | |
| Chang et al 1994 [44] | 76 | 7 Gy q2w × 3 | 80% | 3% | 4% | | | | |
| Speiser and Spratling 1993 [85] | 47 144 151 | 10 Gy @ 5 mm × 3 10 Gy × 3 7.5 Gy × 3 | 41% | 24% | 4% 7% 9% | 9% 12% 13% | 9% 9% 2% | | |
| Cotter *et al.* 1993 [56] | 65 | 6–35 Gy total dose HDR or IDR | 100% | | 1.5% | 8% | | 5% | 1.5% |
| Pisch *et al.* 1993 [48] | 39 | 10 Gy q 2w × 1–2 | 85% | 23% | 3% | | | | 6% |
| Bedwinek *et al.* 1992 [50] | 38 | 6 Gy q 1w × 3 | 100% | 22% | 32% | | 0% | 0% | 0% |
| Sutedja *et al.* 1992 [53] | 31 | 10 Gy q2w × 1–3 | 100% | 45% | 30% | | | 10% | |
| Gauwitz *et al.* 1992 [51] | 24 | 15 Gy @ 6 mm q2w × 3 | 100% | 0 | 4% | 4% | 4% | | |
| Aygun *et al.* 1992 [54] | 62 | 5 Gy q1w × 3–5 | 100% | | 15% | | | 0% | 1.7% |
| Khanavkar *et al.* 1991 [86] | 12 | 8 Gy @ 5 mm q1–2w × 2–8 | 92% | 42% | 50% | | | 17% | |

EBRT, external beam radiotherapy; Gy, gray; PDT, photodynamic therapy; IDR, intermediate dose rate; HDR, high dose rate; q, every; w, week.

*Treatment at 1 cm unless specified. Adapted from: Yao MS, Koh WJ. Endobronchial brachytherapy. *Chest Surg Clin North Am* 2001; **11**: 813–27 [10].

**Table 16.3** ABS modified grading of radiation bronchitis and stenosis

| Grade | Description |
|-------|-------------|
| Grade I | Mild mucosal inflammatory response with swelling characterized by a thin, whitish, circumferential membrane. No significant luminal obstruction. No intervention necessary. |
| Grade II | White fibrinous membrane with exudation causing symptoms such as cough and/or obstructive problems requiring therapeutic intervention. |
| Grade III | Severe inflammatory response with marked membranous exudates. Multiple debridement or other interventions required to reestablish full lumen of airway. |
| Grade IV | Greater degree of fibrosis with resulting circumferential stenosis leading to a decrease in luminal diameter. |
| Grade V | Necrosis, tracheal, and/or bronchial malacia, or massive hemorrhage related to the treatment without any evidence of invasion of the tumor. |

From: Nag S, Kelly JF, Horton JL, Komaki R, Nori D. Brachytherapy for carcinoma of the lung. *Oncology* 2001; **15**: 371–81 [12].

**Table 16.4** Potential treatments for radiation bronchitis

| Grade | Treatment |
|-------|-----------|
| Grade I | Observation |
| Grade II | Steroids—oral and/or inhaled<br>Bronchodilators<br>Narcotic cough suppressants |
| Grade III | Multiple bronchoscopic debridements |
| Grade IV | Debridement<br>Balloon or rigid dilation<br>Laser photoresection<br>Argon plasma coagulation/electrocautery resection<br>Cryotherapy<br>Stent placement |

Modified from: Speiser BL, Spratling L. Radiation bronchitis and stenosis secondary to the high dose rate endobronchial irradiation. *Int J Radiat Oncol Biol Phys* 1993; **25**: 598–97 [85].

three fractions, and 13% for those receiving 7.5 Gy at 1 cm for three fractions. Factors associated with increased risk included curative intent therapy, prior laser resection, concurrent external beam radiotherapy, and longer survival. A grading system proposed by Speiser and Spratling, with subsequent modifications from the American Brachytherapy Society, is presented in Table 16.3. Grade 3 or 4 radiation bronchitis was noted in 49% of the overall observed cases. In the analysis of complications by Gollins and colleagues, some degree of mucosal reaction was noted in 55% of follow-up bronchoscopic reactions [11]. Some degree of fibrosis was noted in the majority of bronchoscopic examinations at 6 months and beyond which found radiation-related changes. Only two patients out of 406 required bronchoscopic intervention, however. Hennequin and coworkers, in their series of 149 patients, observed radiation bronchitis in 13 cases (8.7%) [79]. Two cases were fatal secondary to complete obstruction of the trachea by fibrinous debris and subsequent infection. In univariate analysis, curative treatment, tumor location in the trachea or mainstem bronchi, brachytherapy dose, and tumor volume treated were associated with developing radiation bronchitis while in multivariate analysis only the tumor location retained statistical significance. In a study of 189 patients treated with three or four fractions of 8–10 Gy at 1 cm, Taulelle and colleagues noted bronchial stenosis in 12

patients (13%) [35]. In their comparison of different brachytherapy fractionation schemes in combination with external beam radiotherapy, Muto and coworkers observed grade 3 or 4 radiation bronchitis in 24% of patients receiving a single fraction of 10 Gy at 1 cm, 13% of patients receiving two fractions of 7 Gy at 1 cm, 17% of patients receiving three fractions of 5 Gy at 1 cm, and 8% of patients receiving three fractions of 5 Gy at 0.5 cm [20]. Potential treatments for radiation bronchitis and stenosis are listed in Table 16.4.

Other potential complications include airway fistulas, airway necrosis, tracheomalacia/bronchomalacia, pneumothorax, radiation pneumonitis, and bronchospasm [20,28,34, 35,39,40,41,44,52,53,55,59].

Based on the above discussions, it is clear that brachytherapy can be a useful modality in the palliation of symptoms related to endobronchial tumors. For those patients previously treated with external beam radiotherapy and who are symptomatic from endobronchial infiltration or obstruction as a result of recurrent disease, brachytherapy can be strongly considered. Based on the randomized trials by Huber and coworkers [26] and Langendijk and associates [27], the addition of brachytherapy to external beam radiation appears to confer no additional benefit in terms of symptom control, performance status, or survival. Based on the randomized trial conducted by Stout and colleagues comparing endobronchial brachytherapy to external beam radiotherapy [18], it appears that external beam radiation is superior to brachytherapy as initial treatment for symptoms related to non-small cell lung cancer. Treatment with Nd:YAG laser therapy with or without brachytherapy appears similar in terms of survival although symptom-free progression and need for additional bronchoscopic treatment is improved with the combined treatment.

Brachytherapy can be considered in the treatment of localized, endobronchial early stage lung cancer with curative intent. The data regarding the utility of brachytherapy in treating recurrent granulation tissue following stent placement are interesting, although further studies to define the role of such treatment would be helpful. With the advent of navigation bronchoscopy technologies, the possibility of treating peripheral lung cancers in medically inoperable patients is intriguing but, again, more data are needed. The optimal dose of brachytherapy and fractionation schedule is not clear given the small number of patients in randomized, controlled trials and differing doses and schedules used in the trials. Clinicians should be aware of the risk of fatal hemoptysis from brachytherapy as well as the possibility of developing airway obstruction in the short term from radiation bronchitis or long term from radiation-induced fibrosis and stenosis.

## Fiducial marker implantation

Many patients with early stage lung cancer are unable to undergo curative surgical resection due to respiratory impairment from underlying lung disease such as chronic obstructive pulmonary disease (COPD), severe cardiac disease, or other comorbidities, or are unwilling to undergo surgery due to personal preferences. Conventional external beam radiotherapy has been reported to have 5-year survival rates between 6 and 31%, with an average of 21% in one review [87]. Image-guided radiation therapy, including stereotactic body radiotherapy (SBRT) and intensity modulated radiation therapy (IMRT), allows for delivery of focused, high-dose radiation to localized cancers. Local control rates for SBRT for stage I lung cancers have ranged from 78 to 100% at 2–5 years and overall survival rates have ranged from 47 to 86% at 2–5 years [88]. A major obstacle to stereotactic radiotherapy and intensity modulated radiation therapy target delineation is respiration-induced target motion, also known as intrafractional tumor motion. Various techniques, including breathing control, respiratory gating, on-board imaging systems, and real-time tumor tracking, have been used to more accurately guide radiotherapy for lung cancer [88,89]. Some real-time tumor tracking systems, such as the CyberKnife with Synchrony technology (Accuray Inc., Sunnyvale, CA), utilize placement of dense metal gold or platinum markers, referred to as fiducials, in or near the tumor to allow for system tracking and beam adjustment [90–93]. Three fiducial markers are usually required, each 2 cm apart in different planes, although some clinicians may place an additional one or two markers in case of marker migration. Fiducial markers were initially placed percutaneously under CT-guidance. Given the multiple passes required for fiducial marker placement and the severe underlying emphysema in many patients undergoing such procedures,

reported pneumothorax rates between 6 and 25% are not surprising [91–93]. Given the problems with pneumothoraces from a percutaneous approach and the advent of navigation bronchoscopy technologies to assist in greater probability of successfully accessing small, peripheral lung cancers, significant interest in bronchoscopic placement of fiducial markers has arisen.

A variety of fiducial markers and methods of delivery for bronchoscopic implantation of fiducial markers have been utilized. Harada and colleagues used spherical gold markers from 1 to 2 mm in size with deployment through a polytetrafluoroethylene catheter, using a hard plastic wire inserted through the catheter, under fluoroscopic guidance alone [94]. Of the 20 patients, 16 with a peripheral lung cancer and four with a more central lung cancer, a marker could not be placed in one patient with a central type of cancer. Markers were held in place at the same position in 14 patients and dropped from inserted position in the remaining five patients, including the three remaining patients with central type tumors. In a follow-up study from the same investigators, 154 gold spherical fiducials were inserted into 57 patients with peripheral lung cancers using the same insertion technique [95]. Of the 154 placed fiducials, 122 (79%) were detected at CT planning 0–5 days after insertion; 115 of these markers were detected throughout the treatment period (range 6–15 days, median 10 days); 104 markers (68% of initial insertions) were detected at last follow-up (range 16–181 days, median 44 days). Several patients coughed up the markers and many dropped markers were noted on abdominal X rays. Less migration was observed with more peripherally placed fiducials. One patient developed a pneumothorax which resolved without intervention. Of note, a learning curve was observed in this study. The fixation rates were 58, 64, and 75% for physicians who had performed less than 20, between 20 and 50, and more than 50 insertions, respectively ($P = 0.05$).

Rectangular gold fiducial markers (item no. 351-1; Best Medical International Inc., Springfield, VA) were utilized by Reichner and coworkers [96]. The fiducial was placed in the 19-gauge needle of a 19/21-gauge Wang transbronchial needle (MW-319; CONMED Corp., Utica, NY). The needle tip was then dipped in sterile surgical lubricant to improve the fiducial's adherence to the needle. The 19-gauge fiducial-loaded needle was then retracted into the sheath and the sheath passed through the flexible bronchoscope. At the desired location, the 19-gauge needle was extended and inserted into the tumor through a jabbing method. The 21-gauge needle component was then tightened, deploying the fiducial. Placements were done under fluoroscopic guidance alone. A total of 54 fiducials, average 3.6 per patient, were placed in 15 patients with lung cancer or metastatic malignancies. Locations included the upper lobes, left lower lobe, station 2 and 4 paratracheal areas, subcarina, left hilum, left mainstem, and bronchus intermedius. Twelve fiducials were

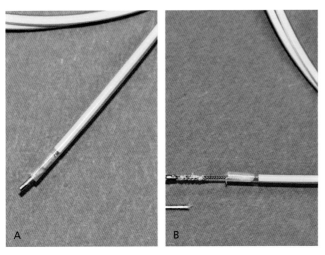

**Fig. 16.3** (A) Fiducial gold seed loaded on wax tip at end of a microbiology specimen brush. (B) Fiducial deployed when the brush is pushed out. From: Anantham D, Feller-Kopman D, Shanmugham LN, Berman SM, DeCamp MM, Gangadharan SP, Eberhardt R, Herth F, Ernst A. Electromagnetic navigation bronchoscopy-guided fiducial placement for robotic stereotactic radiosurgery of lung tumors: a feasibility study. *Chest* 2007; **132**: 930–5. Reproduced with permission of American College of Chest Physicians, Copyright 2007.

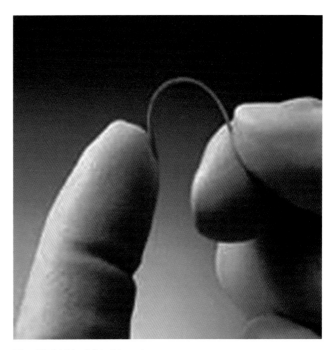

**Fig. 16.4** Visicoil fiducial marker.

dropped in the airways prior to deployment; seven were retrieved with biopsy forceps and the remainder were likely coughed out. No pneumothoraces occurred. One fiducial placed in a subcarinal node embolized through the pulmonary artery after deployment without adverse consequences.

Subsequent studies have utilized navigation bronchoscopy and/or peripheral radial EBUS for fiducial placement. Anantham and colleagues successfully implanted fiducials in eight of nine patients with peripheral T1/T2 lung primary or metastatic malignancies using the superDimension electromagnetic navigation bronchoscopy system [97]. Gold seeds with dimensions of 0.8 × 5 mm (model SMG0242-025; Alpha-Omega Services, Inc., Bellflower, CA) were used as the fiducials. The fiducials were wedged into the wax tip of a microbiology specimen brush (catalog No. 1650; Boston Scientific Corp., Natick, MA) (Fig. 16.3). After successful navigation to the tumor, the sensor probe was removed from the extended working channel and the loaded microbiology brush was placed through the extended working channel. When the brush catheter reached the distal end of the extended working channel, the brush was pushed through the wax tip to deploy the fiducial. The extended working channel was then navigated to a different area near the tumor and the process was repeated. Four to six fiducials were placed in each patient and in seven of the eight patients some fiducials were placed directly within the tumor. At the radiotherapy planning session 1 week later, 35 of the 39 inserted fiducials were still in place. One patient had a COPD exacerbation after placement and no pneumothoraces were observed.

Kupelian and coworkers described their experience with bronchoscopic fiducial placement using the superDimension navigation system in eight patients as well as percutaneous placement in 15 patients [98]. For bronchoscopic insertion, a double lumen Wang transbronchial aspiration was loaded with either 0.8 × 3 mm solid gold markers or 1 cm long Visicoil gold implants (IBA Dosimetry, Bartlett, TN) (Fig. 16.4). All patients were noted to have markers remain in place at 16–188 days. One patient who underwent bronchoscopic biopsy and fiducial placement during the same procedure developed a pneumothorax. Pneumothorax was noted in eight of the 15 patients who underwent percutaneous marker insertion. The authors note that they currently use 1–2 cm long Visicoil implants given the larger, flexible markers, which should be more stable as they will wedge in the airways or within tumors and their size and consistency will prohibit mobility.

The use of radial probe EBUS, with adjunct use of navigation bronchoscopy with the superDimension system for selected patients, in fiducial marker placement in 43 patients was reported by Harley and colleagues [99]. A 20-MHz EBUS radial probe (UM-S20-20R; Olympus Corp.) was inserted into a guide sheath and advanced as a unit into the bronchus of interest. When the peripheral lesion was localized, the probe was withdrawn, leaving the guide sheath within or close to the tumor. If a peripheral lesion was difficult to reach, electromagnetic navigation bronchoscopy was performed. Gold fiducials of sizes 0.8 × 5 mm or 0.8 × 3 mm (351-2, 351-1; Best Medical International, Springfield, VA) were loaded into the tip of a needle brush sheath (NB-120; CONMED Corp., Utica, NY) or a Wang 19/21-gauge transbronchial needle (MW-319; CONMED). The fiducial marker was sealed into the deployment systems using bone wax, preventing loss of the marker prior to deployment. The needle brush and transbronchial needles were inserted into the guide sheath or extended working channel and, once at the end, the marker was deployed using the brush or the inner needle of the Wang needle under fluoroscopic guidance. To ensure the fiducial was embedded in a distal airway or in the lung parenchyma, a cytology brush (Cellebrity 1601; Boston Scientific Corp., Natick, MA) was used under fluoroscopic guidance. Nine tumors were centrally located and 34 were peripheral, ranging in size from 0.9 to 6.5 cm. A total of 161 fiducials (average of 3.7 per patient) were deployed. At CT scan planning 2 weeks later, markers were in or on the tumor in 39 patients (90.6%) with 139 markers detected. No loss or appreciable movement of any of the fiducials was observed in 30 patients (69.7%). The markers that had become displaced were an average of 1.67 cm (range 0.5 to 4.56 cm) from the targeted tumor. A small pneumothorax requiring pigtail catheter placement occurred in one patient.

More recently, the use of coil spring fiducial markers has been described by Schroeder and coworkers [100]. The initial four patients in their series received 1 × 5 mm linear gold fiducial markers (CyberMark MT-NW-887-853; Civco Medical Solutions, Orange City, IA) (Fig. 16.5). The subsequent 56 fiducial marker placements were done using 3 × 3.3 mm diamond-shaped platinum vascular occlusion coils (VortX-18; Boston Scientific Corp., Natick, MA) (Fig. 16.6). After positioning the extended working channel of the superDimension electromagnetic navigation bronchoscopy system at the target, both markers were delivered using wax tip microbiology specimen brushes (catalog no. 130;

CONMED) through the extended working channel. The wax plug was removed before loading the delivery brush with the fiducials and then temporarily sealed with viscous sterile lubricant. After each placement, the extended working channel was navigated to a different area adjacent to the tumor. A total of 52 patients underwent 60 fiducial marker placements. Only eight (47%) of the 17 linear fiducials were still in place at radiotherapy planning 1–2 weeks after placement and two of the four patients receiving linear fiducials required an additional placement procedure. Of the 217 coil spring markers, 215 (99%) were still in place at radiotherapy planning (Fig. 16.7). The mean tumor diameter was 23.7 mm (range 8–53 mm). Three patients developed a pneumothorax, two of which were associated with transbronchial biopsy during the same procedure. The authors proposed that the coil spring markers have greater stability due to wedging themselves by recoil forces into the surrounding

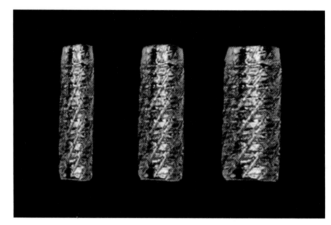

**Fig. 16.5** Civco fiducial markers. Photo courtesy of Civco.

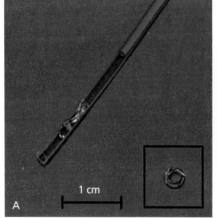 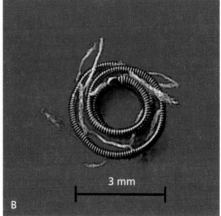

**Fig. 16.6** (A) Flattened platinum coil spring fiducial marker loaded in tip of microbiology specimen brush. (B) Magnified diamond-shaped deployed coiled spring fiducial marker with thrombogenic filament attachments. Reprinted from: Schroeder C, Hejal R, Linden PA. Coil spring fiducial markers placed safely using navigation bronchoscopy in inoperable patients allows accurate delivery of CyberKnife stereotactic radiosurgery. *J Thorac Cardiovasc Surg* 2010; **140**: 1137–42, with permission from Elsevier.

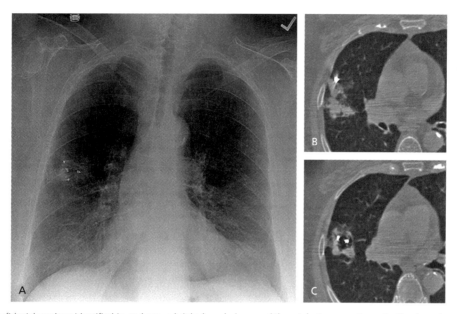

**Fig. 16.7** Radiopaque fiducial markers identified in and around right lung lesions on (A) postelectromagnetic navigation bronchoscopy chest radiograph; (B and C) corresponding CT scans. Reprinted from: Schroeder C, Hejal R, Linden PA. Coil spring fiducial markers placed safely using navigation bronchoscopy in inoperable patients allows accurate delivery of CyberKnife stereotactic radiosurgery. *J Thorac Cardiovasc Surg* 2010; **140**: 1137–42 with permission from Elsevier.

lung tissue and due to the dense polyester fibers attached to the metal coil, which promotes thrombosis and seating into the adjacent tissue.

McGuire and colleagues have described yet another set of methodologies for fiducial implantation [101]. The fiducial used by the authors was the 0.75-mm Visicoil coiled gold marker, typically a 20 mm length although lengths of 10 and 30 mm had also been used. In one approach, the MW-319 19/22-guage Wang transbronchial needle (CONMED) is used. Under navigation bronchoscopy guidance, the extended working channel is positioned at the lesion and Wang needle is advanced past the extended working channel and the needle inserted into the lesion under fluoroscopic guidance. The inner 21-gauge needle is completely removed, leaving the 19-gauge needle and sheath. The Visicoil marker is back loaded into the needle sheath and a 0.66-mm guidewire (ChoICE PT Extra Support; Boston Scientific Corp., Natick, MA) is used to push the marker through the length of the sheath. The needle is then slowly pulled back as pressure is maintained on the guidewire deploying the marker. In the second method, after positioning the extended working channel in the appropriate position, a 5-Fr JB1 angulated Benton–Hanafee–Wilson Glidecath catheter (Boston Scientific Corp., Natick, MA) is advanced through the extended working channel into the lesion. The Visicoil marker is loaded into the proximal end of the catheter and the 0.66-mm guidewire is placed through the catheter. Under fluoroscopic guidance the marker is then deployed by extrusion from the catheter with the guidewire. The Glidecath catheter can then be turned in different directions

allowing placement in different planes of the tumor owing to the angulated nature of the catheter. The authors note the latter approach is their preferred method. No data regarding success or migrations with either approach were provided in the report.

As can be surmised from the above publications, there is as yet no "gold standard" with regards to fiducials for image-guided radiation therapy for lung cancer and malignancies metastatic to the lung. Nor is there a standard method of fiducial implantation via bronchoscopy. The author has used an approach similar to that described by Harley and colleagues [99] for fiducial marker placement using a Wang transbronchial needle or the Olympus Guide Sheath (Olympus Co., Tokyo, Japan) and biopsy forceps in conjunction with the Broncus LungPoint virtual navigation bronchoscopy system (Broncus Technologies Inc., Mountain View, CA) and radial EBUS (Figs 16.8, 16.9, 16.10). Coil fiducials appear to have less migration than linear fiducials but are more expensive. The use of navigation bronchoscopy systems and/or peripheral EBUS to ensure more peripheral implantation of markers may lessen the migration rate of linear markers. Fiducial markers should be wedged in small peripheral airways or lung parenchyma to decreased dislodgement. For lymph nodes and central masses the markers may be directly placed into the node or mass with a standard transbronchial needle, with or without preceding localization with linear or radial EBUS. Markers which would be able to be directly deployed through EBUS transbronchial needles would be an attractive option for this application. As noted, three markers are typically placed, although some clinicians prefer to place more in case there is migration of one of the markers. CT planning should probably be done 1 week after fiducial placement to account for migrations given fibroblastic reactions to fiducials start approximately 5 days after implantation [102] and most marker loss seems to occur within the first week of placement. With better technologies to localize peripheral cancers and substantially less rates of pneumothoraces, bronchoscopic fiducial placement will likely supplant percutaneous placement at many institutions.

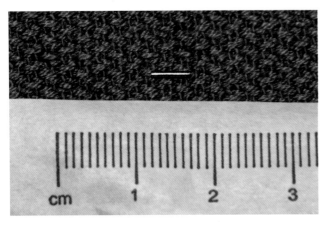

**Fig. 16.8** Alpha-Omega fiducial marker (model SMG0242-025; Alpha-Omega Services, Inc., Bellflower, CA).

# Radiofrequency ablation

Radiofrequency ablation (RFA) has recently emerged as an alternative therapy to surgery or radiotherapy for primary lung cancer in patients who are medically inoperable or for patients with malignancies metastatic to the lung [103,104]. During RFA, a radiofrequency generator produces an alternating current from an active electrode placed within the tumor to a ground electrode. The rapidly alternating current causes ions within the tissue to oscillate as they follow the changing direction of the alternating current. These high-speed ionic oscillations produce frictional heating of the tissue. Tissues heated to greater than 50°C undergo protein denaturation and coagulation necrosis. Tissues heated to more than 105°C will undergo charring and carbonization with production of small pockets of gas. Charring and cavitation as a result of tissue overheating can increase tissue impedance with resulting decrease in current flow and limitation of the coagulation necrosis. Temperatures of 60°C to 105°C within the tissue are thus preferred during RFA. Tumors within the lung may be well suited to RFA because of the so-called "oven effect" in which air-filled lung tissue surrounding an intraparenchymal tumor acts as an insulator and traps the delivered heat energy within the tumor as well as protecting normal structures that are nearby [105]. RFA is performed percutaneously under

**Fig. 16.9** Placement of fiducial marker in a hilar mass. (A) Fiducial marker in hilar mass and transbronchial needle extending into hilar mass (arrow). (B) Placement of second fiducial marker in hilar mass.

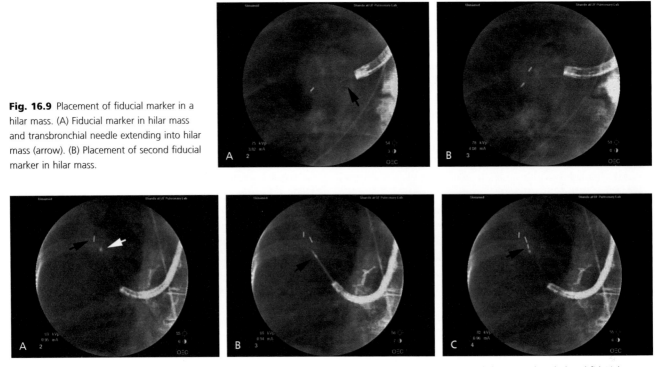

**Fig. 16.10** Placement of fiducial markers around a peripheral nodule. (A) End of the guide sheath near nodule (white arrow) and placed fiducial marker (black arrow). (B) Biopsy forceps and fiducial marker extending from end of the guide sheath (arrow) and two placed markers. (C) Third deployed fiducial marker near end of the guide sheath (arrow).

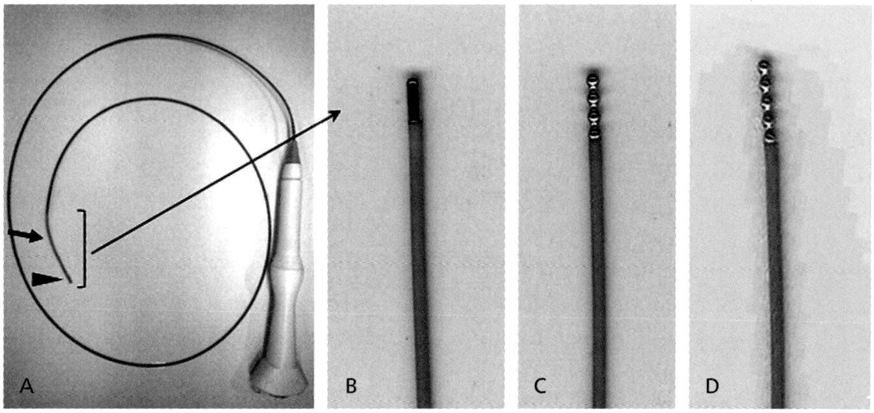

**Fig. 16.11** Internally cooled radiofrequency ablation (RFA) electrodes. The shaft (arrows) and tip of the electrode (arrowheads) are shown (A). The top electrode produced power output and measured the tip temperature and impedance. Three types of the tip were used: 5-mm cylindrical active tip (B); 8-mm active tip with four beads (C); and 10-mm active tip with five beads (D). From: Tanabe T, Koizumi T, Tsushima K, Ito M, Kanda S, Kobayashi T, Yasuo M, Yamazaki Y, Kubo K, Honda T, Kondo R, Yoshida K. Comparative study of three different catheters for CT imaging-bronchoscopy-guided radiofrequency ablation as a potential and novel interventional therapy for lung cancer. *Chest* 2010; **137**: 890–7. Reproduced with permission of American College of Chest Physicians, Copyright 2010.

CT-guidance with general anesthesia or heavy sedation. Currently available RFA systems use single needle electrodes, a cluster probe of three parallel needles, or probes with seven to nine expandable tines that increase surface area for treatment. The current RFA systems provide feedback regarding treatment effect during the procedure based upon temperature and/or impedance monitoring in the treated tissue. In a survey of the literature regarding RFA published in 2010, the overall survival rate was 58.3% over a mean follow-up of 40.4 months and the cancer-specific survival rate was 82.1% (range 58 to 100%) over a mean follow-up of 89.8 months in studies evaluating primary lung cancer alone [106]. For studies that included metastatic pulmonary disease alone, the overall survival rate was 65.5% over a mean follow-up of 25.4 months and cancer-specific survival was 75.2% (range 55–90%) with a mean follow-up of 72.3 months. The most common complications noted in the 2010 literature survey were pneumothorax with a rate of 28.3% (range 0–90%), pleural effusions (14.8%, range 0–87%), and chest pain (14.1%, range 0–100%) [106]. Other reported complications have included hemoptysis, pneumonia, lung abscesses, bronchopleural fistula, hemothorax, and acute respiratory distress syndrome (ARDS) [103,104,106].

Tsushima and colleagues conducted a feasibility study of bronchoscopy-guided RFA in sheep [107]. Self-designed standard non-cooled electrodes with a 4-mm active tip and internal-cooled electrodes with a 4-mm active tip were used. The cooled RFA electrode, with a power output setting of 30 W for 60 seconds and room temperature water, produced a 40 × 45 mm burn lesion while cold water cooling produced a 20 × 15 mm burn lesion. This was followed by a pilot study of CT-guided bronchoscopic RFA in 10 patients with T1 non-small lung cancers with subsequent standard surgical resection and analysis [108]. Three types of electrodes were used; an internal-cooled 5-mm active tip, an 8-mm active tip with four beads, and a 10-mm active tip with five beads, all with a diameter of 1.67 mm (Fig. 16.11). The position of the electrode tip within the tumor was confirmed with low-dose chest CT prior to RFA. Three RFA applications were performed in each patient. Satisfactory results were obtained with a 10-mm five-bead catheter tip at a power output of 20 W and delivery time of 50 seconds, producing ablated areas ranging from 13 × 8 mm to 16 × 12 mm. The peripheral zones did contain a few tumor cells when examined histologically, however.

At this time the potential for bronchoscopically delivered RFA is unclear. The advent of navigation bronchoscopy technologies, combined with radial EBUS, makes targeting of peripheral cancers with RFA an appealing idea. The complication rate, particularly for pneumothorax, would likely be much less with bronchoscopically placed RFA electrodes. Electrodes that are capable of delivering a sufficient area of treatment yet will still fit through the bronchoscope working channel or an extended working channel/guide sheath would need to be developed.

## References

1 National Cancer Institute. *SEER Stat Fact Sheets: Lung and Bronchus.* http://seer.cancer.gov/statfacts/html/lungb.html. (Accessed April 2011.)

2 Reddy SP, Marks JE. Total atelectasis of the lung secondary to malignant airway obstruction. Response to radiation therapy. *Am J Clin Oncol* 1990; **13**: 394–400.

3 Chetty KG, Moran EM, Sassoon CS, *et al*. Effect of radiation therapy on bronchial obstruction due to bronchogenic carcinoma. *Chest* 1989; **95**: 582–4.

4 Perez CA, Stanley K, Grundy G, *et al*. Impact of irradiation technique and tumor extent in tumor control and survival of patients with unresectable non-oat cell carcinoma of the lung: report by the Radiation Therapy Oncology Group. *Cancer* 1982; **50**: 1091–9.

5 Yankauer S. Two cases of lung cancer treated bronchoscopically. *NY Med J* 1922; **21**: 741–2.

6 Mehta M, Shahabi S, Jarjour N, *et al*. Effect of endobronchial radiation therapy on malignant bronchial obstruction. *Chest* 1990; **97**: 662–5.

7 Miller JI Jr, Phillips TW. Neodymium: YAG laser and brachytherapy in the management of inoperable bronchogenic carcinoma. *Ann Thorac Surg* 1990; **50**: 190–6.

8 Kohek PH, Pakisch B, Glanzer H. Intraluminal irradiation in the treatment of malignant airway obstruction. *Eur J Surg Oncol* 1994; **20**: 674–80.

9 Bastin KT, Mehta MP, Kinsella TJ. Thoracic volume radiation sparing following endobronchial brachytherapy: a quantitative analysis. *Int J Radiat Oncol Biol Phys* 1993; **25**: 703–7.

10 Yao MS, Koh WJ. Endobronchial brachytherapy. *Chest Surg Clin North Am* 2001; **11**: 813–27.

11 Gollins SW, Ryder WD, Burt PA, *et al*. Massive haemoptysis death and other morbidity associated with high dose rate intraluminal radiotherapy for carcinoma of the bronchus. *Radiother Oncol* 1996; **39**: 105–16.

12 Nag S, Kelly JF, Horton JL, *et al*. Brachytherapy for carcinoma of the lung. *Oncology* (Williston Park) 2001; **15**: 371–81.

13 Huber RM, Fischer R, Haǔtmann H, *et al*. Palliative endobronchial brachytherapy for central lung tumors. A prospective, randomized comparison of two fractionation schedules. *Chest* 1995; **107**: 463–70.

14 Huber RM, Fischer R, Hautmann H, *et al*. Does additional brachytherapy improve the effect of external irradiation? A prospective, randomized study in central lung tumors. *Int J Radiat Oncol Biol Phys* 1997; **38**: 533–40.

15 Langendijk H, de Jong J, Tjwa M, *et al*. External irradiation versus external irradiation plus endobronchial brachytherapy in inoperable non-small cell lung cancer: a prospective randomized study. *Radiother Oncol* 2001; **58**: 257–68.

16 Sur R, Ahmed SN, Donde B, *et al*. Brachytherapy boost vs teletherapy boost in palliation of symptomatic, locally advanced non-small cell lung cancer: preliminary analysis of a randomized, prospective trial. *J Brachy Intl* 2001; **17**: 309–15.

17 Sur R, Donde B, Mohuiddin M, *et al*. Randomized prospective study on the role of high dose rate intraluminal brachytherapy (HDRILBT) in palliation of symptoms in advanced non small cell lung cancer (NSCLC) treated with radiation alone. *Int J Radiat Oncol Biol Phys* 2004; **60** (Suppl 1): S205.

18 Stout R, Barber P, Burt P, *et al*. Clinical and quality of life outcomes in the first United Kingdom randomized trial of endobronchial brachytherapy (intraluminal radiotherapy) vs. external beam radiotherapy in the palliative treatment of inoperable non-small cell lung cancer. *Radiother Oncol* 2000; **56**: 323–7.

19 Mallick I, Sharma SC, Behera D, *et al*. Optimization of dose and fractionation of endobronchial brachytherapy with or without external radiation in the palliative management of non-small cell lung cancer: a prospective randomized study. *J Cancer Res Ther* 2006; **2**: 119–25.

20 Muto P, Ravo V, Panelli G, *et al*. High-dose rate brachytherapy of bronchial cancer: treatment optimization using three schemes of therapy. *Oncologist* 2000; **5**: 209–14.

21 Mallick I, Sharma SC, Behera D. Endobronchial brachytherapy for symptom palliation in non-small cell lung cancer—analysis of symptom response, endoscopic improvement and quality of life. *Lung Cancer* 2007; **55**: 313–8.

22 Skowronek J, Kubaszewska M, Kanikowski M, *et al*. HDR endobronchial brachytherapy (HDRBT) in the management of advanced lung cancer—comparison of two different dose schedules. *Radiother Oncol* 2009; **93**: 436–40.

23 Mantz CA, Dosoretz DE, Rubenstein JH, *et al*. Endobronchial brachytherapy and optimization of local disease control in medically inoperable non-small cell lung carcinoma: a matched-pair analysis. *Brachytherapy* 2004; **3**: 183–90.

24 Manali ED, Stathopoulos GT, Gildea TR, *et al*. High dose-rate endobronchial radiotherapy for proximal airway obstruction due to lung cancer: 8-year experience of a referral center. *Cancer Biother Radiopharm* 2010; **25**: 207–13.

25 Hauswald H, Stoiber E, Rochet N, *et al*. Treatment of recurrent bronchial carcinoma: the role of high-dose-rate endoluminal brachytherapy. *Int J Radiat Oncol Biol Phys* 2010; **77**: 373–7.

26 Ozkok S, Karakoyun-Celik O, Goksel T, *et al*. High dose rate endobronchial brachytherapy in the management of lung cancer: response and toxicity evaluation in 158 patients. *Lung Cancer* 2008; **62**: 326–33.

27 Hennequin C, Bleichner O, Trédaniel J, *et al*. Long-term results of endobronchial brachytherapy: A curative treatment? *Int J Radiat Oncol Biol Phys* 2007; **67**: 425–30.

28 Escobar-Sacristán JA, Granda-Orive JI, Gutiérrez Jiménez T, *et al*. Endobronchial brachytherapy in the treatment of malignant lung tumours. *Eur Respir J* 2004; **24**: 348–52.

29 Gejerman G, Mullokandov EA, Bagiella E, *et al*. Endobronchial brachytherapy and external-beam radiotherapy in patients with endobronchial obstruction and extrabronchial extension. *Brachytherapy* 2002; **1**: 204–10.

30 Anacak Y, Mogulkoc N, Ozkok S, *et al*. High dose rate endobronchial brachytherapy in combination with external beam radiotherapy for stage III non-small cell lung cancer. *Lung Cancer* 2001; **34**: 253–9.

31 Petera J, Spásová I, Neumanová R, *et al*. High dose rate intraluminal brachytherapy in the treatment of malignant airway obstructions. *Neoplasma* 2001; **48**: 148–53.

32 Harms W, Schraube P, Becker H, *et al*. Effect and toxicity of endoluminal high-dose-rate (HDR) brachytherapy in centrally located tumors of the upper respiratory tract. *Strahlenther Onkol* 2000; **176**: 60–6.

33 Kelly JF, Delclos ME, Morice RC, *et al*. High-dose-rate endobronchial brachytherapy effectively palliates symptoms due to airway tumors: the 10-year M. D. Anderson cancer center experience. *Int J Radiat Oncol Biol Phys* 2000; **48**: 697–702.

34 Marsiglia H, Baldeyrou P, Lartigau E, *et al*. High-dose-rate brachytherapy as sole modality for early-stage endobronchial carcinoma. *Int J Radiat Oncol Biol Phys* 2000; **47**: 665–72.

35 Taulelle M, Chauvet B, Vincent P, *et al*. High dose rate endobronchial brachytherapy: results and complications in 189 patients. *Eur Respir J* 1998; **11**: 162–8.

36 Ofiara L, Roman T, Schwartzman K, Levy RD. Local determinants of response to endobronchial high-dose rate brachytherapy in bronchogenic carcinoma. *Chest* 1997; **112**: 946–53.

37 Ornadel D, Duchesne G, Wall P, *et al.* Defining the roles of high dose rate endobronchial brachytherapy and laser resection for recurrent bronchial malignancy. *Lung Cancer* 1997; **16**: 203–13.

38 Nomoto Y, Shouji K, Toyota S, *et al.* High dose rate endobronchial brachytherapy using a new applicator. *Radiother Oncol* 1997; **45**: 33–7.

39 Pérol M, Caliandro R, Pommier P, *et al.* Curative irradiation of limited endobronchial carcinomas with high-dose rate brachytherapy. Results of a pilot study. *Chest* 1997; **111**: 1417–23.

40 Delclos ME, Komaki R, Morice RC, *et al.* Endobronchial brachytherapy with high-dose-rate remote afterloading for recurrent endobronchial lesions. *Radiology* 1996; **201**: 279–82.

41 Hernandez P, Gursahaney A, Roman T, *et al.* High dose rate brachytherapy for the local control of endobronchial carcinoma following external irradiation. *Thorax* 1996; **51**: 354–8.

42 Macha HN, Wahlers B, Reichle C, von Zwehl D. Endobronchial radiation therapy for obstructing malignancies: ten years' experience with iridium-192 high-dose radiation brachytherapy afterloading technique in 365 patients. *Lung* 1995; **173**: 271–80.

43 Trédaniel J, Hennequin C, Zalcman G, *et al.* Prolonged survival after high-dose rate endobronchial radiation for malignant airway obstruction. *Chest* 1994; **105**: 767–72.

44 Chang LF, Horvath J, Peyton W, Ling SS. High dose rate afterloading intraluminal brachytherapy in malignant airway obstruction of lung cancer. *Int J Radiat Oncol Biol Phys* 1994; **28**: 589–96.

45 Goldman JM, Bulman AS, Rathmell AJ, *et al.* Physiologic effect of endobronchial radiotherapy in patients with major airway occlusion by carcinoma. *Thorax* 1993; **48**: 110–14.

46 Gollins SW, Burt PA, Barber PV, Stout R. High dose rate intraluminal radiotherapy for carcinoma of the bronchus: outcome of treatment of 406 patients. *Radiother Oncol* 1994; **33**: 31–40.

47 Speiser BL, Spratling L. Remote afterloading brachytherapy for the local control of endobronchial carcinoma. *Int J Radiat Oncol Biol Phys* 1993; **25**: 579–87.

48 Pisch J, Villamena PC, Harvey JC, *et al.* High dose-rate endobronchial irradiation in malignant airway obstruction. *Chest* 1993; **104**: 721–5.

49 Nori D, Allison R, Kaplan B, *et al.* High dose-rate intraluminal irradiation in bronchogenic carcinoma: technique and results. *Chest* 1993; **104**: 1006–11.

50 Bedwinek J, Petty A, Bruton C, *et al.* The use of high dose rate endobronchial brachytherapy to palliate symptomatic endobronchial recurrence of previously irradiated bronchogenic carcinoma. *Int J Radiat Oncol Biol Phys* 1992; **22**: 23–30.

51 Gauwitz M, Ellerbroek N, Komaki R, *et al.* High dose endobronchial irradiation in recurrent bronchogenic carcinoma. *Int J Radiat Oncol Biol Phys* 1992; **23**: 397–400.

52 Mehta M, Petereit D, Chosy L, *et al.* Sequential comparison of low dose rate and hyperfractionated high dose rate endobronchial radiation for malignant airway occlusion. *Int J Radiat Oncol Biol Phys* 1992; **23**: 133–9.

53 Sutedja G, Baris G, Schaake-Koning C, van Zandwijk N. High dose rate brachytherapy in patients with local recurrences after radiotherapy of non-small cell lung cancer. *Int J Radiat Oncol Biol Phys* 1992; **24**: 551–3.

54 Aygun C, Weiner S, Scariato A, *et al.* Treatment of non-small cell lung cancer with external beam radiotherapy and high dose rate brachytherapy. *Int J Radiat Oncol Biol Phys* 1992; **23**: 127–32.

55 Burt PA, O'Driscoll BR, Notley HM, *et al.* Intraluminal irradiation for the palliation of lung cancer with the high dose rate micro-Selectron. *Thorax* 1990; **45**: 765–8.

56 Cotter, GW, Lariscy C, Ellingwood KE, Herbert D. Inoperable endobronchial obstructing lung cancer treated with combined endobronchial and external beam irradiation: a dosimetric analysis. *Int J Radiat Oncol Biol Phys* 1993; **27**: 531–5.

57 Mehta MP, Shahabi S, Jarjour NN, Kinsella TJ. Endobronchial irradiation for malignant airway obstruction. *Int J Radiat Oncol Biol Phys* 1989; **17**: 847–51.

58 Fuwa N, Kodaira T, Tachibana H, *et al.* Long-term observation of 64 patients with roentgenographically occult lung cancer treated with external irradiation and intraluminal irradiation using low-dose-rate iridium. *Jpn J Clin Oncol* 2008; **38**: 581–8.

59 Saito M, Yokoyama A, Kurita Y, *et al.* Treatment of roentgenographically occult endobronchial carcinoma with external beam radiotherapy and intraluminal low-dose-rate brachytherapy: second report. *Int J Radiat Oncol Biol Phys* 2000; **47**: 673–80.

60 Stranzl H, Gabor S, Mayer R, *et al.* Fractionated intraluminal HDR 192Ir brachytherapy as palliative treatment in patients with endobronchial metastases from non-bronchogenic primaries. *Strahlenther Onkol* 2002; **178**: 442–5.

61 Quantrill SJ, Burt PA, Barber PV, Stout R. Treatment of endobronchial metastases with intraluminal radiotherapy. *Respir Med* 2000; **94**: 369–72.

62 Chella A, Ambrogi MC, Ribechini A, *et al.* Combined Nd-YAG laser/HDR brachytherapy versus Nd-YAG laser only in malignant central airway involvement: a prospective randomized study. *Lung Cancer* 2000; **27**: 169–75.

63 Jang TW, Blackman G, George JJ. Survival benefits of lung cancer patients undergoing laser and brachytherapy. *J Korean Med Sci* 2002; **17**: 341–7.

64 Shea JM, Allen RP, Tharratt RS, *et al.* Survival of patients undergoing Nd: YAG laser therapy compared with Nd: YAG laser therapy and brachytherapy for malignant airway disease. *Chest* 1993; **103**: 1028–31.

65 Kohek PH, Pakisch B, Glanzer H. Intraluminal irradiation in the treatment of malignant airway obstruction. *Eur J Surg Oncol* 1994; **20**: 674–80.

66 Macha HN, Koch K, Stadler M, *et al.* New technique for treating occlusive and stenosing tumours of the trachea and main bronchi: endobronchial irradiation by high dose iridium-192 combined with laser cannalisation. *Thorax* 1987; **42**: 511–15.

67 Freitag L, Ernst A, Thomas M, *et al.* Sequential photodynamic therapy (PDT) and high dose brachytherapy for endobronchial tumour control in patients with limited bronchogenic carcinoma. *Thorax* 2004; **59**: 790–3.

68 Weinberg BD, Allison RR, Sibata C, *et al.* Results of combined photodynamic therapy (PDT) and high dose rate brachytherapy (HDR) in treatment of obstructive endobronchial non-small cell lung cancer (NSCLC). *Photodiagnosis Photodyn Ther* 2010; **7**: 50–8.

69 Allison R, Sibata C, Sarma K, *et al*. High-dose-rate brachytherapy in combination with stenting offers a rapid and statistically significant improvement in quality of life for patients with endobronchial recurrence. *Cancer J* 2004; **10**: 368–73.

70 Kobayashi T, Kaneko M, Sumi M, *et al*. CT-assisted transbronchial brachytherapy for small peripheral lung cancer. *Jpn J Clin Oncol* 2000; **30**: 109–12.

71 Imamura F, Ueno K, Kusunoki Y, *et al*. High-dose-rate brachytherapy for small-sized peripherally located lung cancer. *Strahlenther Onkol* 2006; **182**: 703–7.

72 Harms W, Krempien R, Grehn C, *et al*. Electromagnetically navigated brachytherapy as a new treatment option for peripheral pulmonary tumors. *Strahlenther Onkol* 2006; **182**: 108–11.

73 Becker HD, McLemore T, Harms W. Electromagnetic navigation and endobronchial ultrasound for brachytherapy of peripheral lung cancer-experience and long term results at two centers. *Am J Respir Crit Care Med* 2009; **179**: A6167.

74 Kennedy AS, Sonett JR, Orens JB, King K. High dose rate brachytherapy to prevent recurrent benign hyperplasia in lung transplant bronchi: theoretical and clinical considerations. *J Heart Lung Transpl* 2000; **19**: 155–9.

75 Halkos ME, Godette KD, Lawrence EC, Miller JI Jr. High dose rate brachytherapy in the management of lung transplant airway stenosis. *Ann Thorac Surg* 2003; **76**: 381–4.

76 Madu CN, Machuzak MS, Sterman DH, *et al*. High-dose-rate (HDR) brachytherapy for the treatment of benign obstructive endobronchial granulation tissue. *Int J Radiat Oncol Biol Phys* 2006; **66**: 1450–6.

77 Brenner B, Kramer MR, Katz A, *et al*. High dose rate brachytherapy for nonmalignant airway obstruction: new treatment option. *Chest* 2003; **124**: 1605–10.

78 Tendulkar RD, Fleming PA, Reddy CA, *et al*. High-dose-rate endobronchial brachytherapy for recurrent airway obstruction from hyperplastic granulation tissue. *Int J Radiat Oncol Biol Phys* 2008; **70**: 701–6.

79 Hennequin C, Tredaniel J, Chevret S, *et al*. Predictive factors for late toxicity after endobronchial brachytherapy: a multivariate analysis. *Int J Radiat Oncol Biol Phys* 1998; **42**: 21–7.

80 Hara R, Itami J, Aruga T, *et al*. Risk factors for massive hemoptysis after endobronchial brachytherapy in patients with tracheobronchial malignancies. *Cancer* 2001; **92**: 2623–7.

81 Carvalho H de A, Gonçalves SL, Pedreira W Jr, *et al*. Irradiated volume and the risk of fatal hemoptysis in patients submitted to high dose-rate endobronchial brachytherapy. *Lung Cancer* 2007; **55**: 319–27.

82 Langendijk JA, Tjwa MK, de Jong JM, *et al*. Massive haemoptysis after radiotherapy in inoperable non-small cell lung carcinoma: is endobronchial brachytherapy really a risk factor? *Radiother Oncol* 1998; **49**: 175–83.

83 Delclos ME, Komaki R, Morice RC, *et al*. Endobronchial brachytherapy with high-dose-rate remote afterloading for recurrent endobronchial lesions. *Radiology* 1996; **201**: 279–82.

84 Gustafson G, Vicini F, Freedman L, *et al*. High dose rate endobronchial brachytherapy in the management of primary and recurrent bronchogenic malignancies. *Cancer* 1995; **75**: 2345–50.

85 Speiser BL, Spratling L. Radiation bronchitis and stenosis secondary to high dose rate endobronchial irradiation. *Int J Radiat Oncol Biol Phys* 1993; **25**: 589–97.

86 Khanavkar B, Stern P, Alberti W, Nakhosteen JA. Complications associated with brachytherapy alone or with laser in lung cancer. *Chest* 1991; **99**: 1062–5.

87 Qiao X, Tullgren O, Lax I, *et al*. The role of radiotherapy in treatment of stage I non-small cell lung cancer. *Lung Cancer* 2003; **41**: 1–11.

88 Martin A, Gaya A. Stereotactic body radiotherapy: a review. *Clin Oncol* 2010; **22**: 157–72.

89 Chang JY, Dong L, Liu H, *et al*. Image-guided radiation therapy for non-small cell lung cancer. *J Thorac Oncol* 2008; **3**: 177–86.

90 Brown WT, Wu X, Fayad F, *et al*. Application of robotic stereotactic radiotherapy to peripheral stage I non-small cell lung cancer with curative intent. *Clin Oncol* 2009; **21**: 623–31.

91 van der Voort van Zyp NC, Prévost JB, Hoogeman MS, *et al*. Stereotactic radiotherapy with real-time tumor tracking for non-small cell lung cancer: clinical outcome. *Radiother Oncol* 2009; **91**: 296–300.

92 Collins BT, Vahdat S, Erickson K, *et al*, Anderson ED. Radical cyberknife radiosurgery with tumor tracking: an effective treatment for inoperable small peripheral stage I non-small cell lung cancer. *J Hematol Oncol* 2009; **2**: 1.

93 Le QT, Loo BW, Ho A, *et al*. Results of a phase I dose-escalation study using single-fraction stereotactic radiotherapy for lung tumors. *J Thorac Oncol* 2006; **1**: 802–9.

94 Harada T, Shirato H, Ogura S, *et al*. Real-time tumor-tracking radiation therapy for lung carcinoma by the aid of insertion of a gold marker using bronchofiberscopy. *Cancer* 2002; **95**: 1720–7.

95 Imura M, Yamazaki K, Shirato H, *et al*. Insertion and fixation of fiducial markers for setup and tracking of lung tumors in radiotherapy. *Int J Radiat Oncol Biol Phys* 2005; **63**: 1442–7.

96 Reichner CA, Collins BT, Gagnon GJ, *et al*. The placement of gold fiducials for CyberKnife stereotactic radiosurgery using a modified transbronchial needle aspiration technique. *J Bronchol* 2005; **12**: 193–5.

97 Anantham D, Feller-Kopman D, Shanmugham LN, *et al*. Electromagnetic navigation bronchoscopy-guided fiducial placement for robotic stereotactic radiosurgery of lung tumors: a feasibility study. *Chest* 2007; **132**: 930–5.

98 Kupelian PA, Forbes A, Willoughby TR, *et al*. Implantation and stability of metallic fiducials within pulmonary lesions. *Int J Radiat Oncol Biol Phys* 2007; **69**: 777–85.

99 Harley DP, Krimsky WS, Sarkar S, *et al*. Fiducial marker placement using endobronchial ultrasound and navigational bronchoscopy for stereotactic radiosurgery: an alternative strategy. *Ann Thorac Surg* 2010; **89**: 368–73.

100 Schroeder C, Hejal R, Linden PA. Coil spring fiducial markers placed safely using navigation bronchoscopy in inoperable patients allows accurate delivery of CyberKnife stereotactic radiosurgery. *J Thorac Cardiovasc Surg* 2010; **140**: 1137–42.

101 McGuire FR, Kerley M, Ochran T, *et al*. Radiotherapy monitoring device implantation into peripheral lung cancers: A therapeutic utility of electromagnetic navigational bronchoscopy. *J Bronchol* 2007; **14**: 189–92.

102 Imura M, Yamazaki K, Kubota KC, *et al*. Histopathologic consideration of fiducial gold markers inserted for real-time tumor-tracking radiotherapy against lung cancer. *Int J Radiat Oncol Biol Phys* 2008; **70**: 382–4.

103 Casal RF, Tam AL, Eapen GA. Radiofrequency ablation of lung tumors. *Clin Chest Med* 2010; **31**: 151–63.

104 Abbas G, Pennathur A, Landreneau RJ, Luketich JD. Radiofrequency and microwave ablation of lung tumors. *J Surg Oncol* 2009; **100**: 645–50.

105 Roy AM, Bent C, Fotheringham T. Radiofrequency ablation of lung lesions: practical applications and tips. *Curr Probl Diagn Radiol* 2009; **38**: 44–52.

106 Chan VO, McDermott S, Malone DE, Dodd JD. Percutaneous radiofrequency ablation of lung tumors: Evaluation of the literature using evidence-based techniques. *J Thorac Imaging* 2011; **26**: 18–26.

107 Tsushima K, Koizumi T, Tanabe T, *et al*. Bronchoscopy-guided radiofrequency ablation as a potential novel therapeutic tool. *Eur Respir J* 2007; **29**: 1193–200.

108 Tanabe T, Koizumi T, Tsushima K, *et al*. Comparative study of three different catheters for CT imaging-bronchoscopy-guided radiofrequency ablation as a potential and novel interventional therapy for lung cancer. *Chest* 2010; **137**: 890–7.

# 17

# Foreign Body Aspiration and Flexible Bronchoscopy

## Erik Folch[1] and Atul C. Mehta[2]

[1] Division of Thoracic Surgery and Interventional Pulmonology, Beth Israel Deaconess Medical Center, Harvard Medical School, Boston, MA, USA
[2] Respiratory Institute, Cleveland Clinic, Cleveland, OH, USA

## Introduction

The flexible bronchoscopy is the "gold standard" for the diagnosis of an airway foreign body and is the preferred instrument for its removal in adults [1].

Aspiration of foreign bodies occurs most commonly at the extremes of age—the young and the elderly. Although the symptoms are non-specific, a detailed history and physical exam, as well as chest X rays, are invaluable. Most often, the diagnosis can only be made through direct visualization with the flexible bronchoscope. In most cases in adults, the removal can be accomplished during the initial bronchoscopic procedure.

Each case of foreign body aspiration is different. The variables involved include type of object, reaction to the aspiration, and location. The physical characteristics of the object, the clinical presentation, and the expertise of the bronchoscopist will frequently determine the ultimate outcome. Foreign body removal can be a very rewarding procedure, as the success rate is high and the complication rate is frequently low. On the contrary, poor preparation prior to the procedure could lead to a disastrous outcome.

In children, the most common procedure performed for removal of foreign bodies is by the rigid bronchoscopy, with or without the use of adjuvant flexible bronchoscopy. However, in recent years data have emerged that support use of the flexible bronchoscope among pediatric patients as well. This chapter reviews the role of the flexible bronchoscope in foreign body removal as it stands today, in both adult as well as pediatric populations.

## Risk factors

Foreign body aspiration (FBA) is most common in early childhood (<5 years old) and amongst the elderly. The risk factors for the two groups are different. During childhood, aspiration usually results from the natural curiosity and tendency to mouth objects, but interestingly it is also due to the use of incisive teeth, which forcefully send the object to the back of the throat and cause a reflex of swallowing, thus causing aspiration.

Children also often laugh, talk, cry, or play with food in their mouth. In adults, on the other hand, the residents of nursing homes or mental health facilities, users of sedatives, and patients with parkinsonism are more prone to death from aspiration [2]. Unfortunately, death from asphyxiation still occurs, and usually occurs at home (41%), restaurants (29%), or in nursing homes or mental institutions (14%) [2]. Approximately 3700 (1.2 per 100,000 population) cases of death due to choking were reported in 2007 in the United States. This constitutes 3% of the accidental deaths reported in the US for the same year (National Safety Council. Injury Facts 2009. Information is available on line at www.nsc.org). Other risk factors for foreign body aspiration in adults are listed in Table 17.1. In children, approximately 80% of the FBA cases are under the age of 3 years, with a male:female ratio of 1.7 to 2.4:1, that is with a male predominance. Jackson in 1936, reported a decrease in mortality from FBA from 24 to 2% with the use of endoscopic techniques for foreign body removal [3].

## Clinical presentation

A high degree of suspicion is critical in identifying patients at risk; however, when in doubt, a proactive approach will prevent serious complications, particularly in children. The clinical presentation of foreign body aspiration is dependent upon the type of foreign body, site of impaction, and overall age and clinical status of the patient. Approximately one-third of all objects are proximal to the glottis after an episode of choking. These usually large objects can easily occlude the

*Flexible Bronchoscopy*, Third Edition. Edited by Ko-Pen Wang, Atul C. Mehta, J. Francis Turner.
© 2012 Blackwell Publishing Ltd. Published 2012 by Blackwell Publishing Ltd.

**Table 17.1** Risk factors for foreign body aspiration in adults

| |
|---|
| Alcohol intoxication |
| Sedative or hypnotic drug use |
| Poor dentition |
| Senility |
| Mental retardation |
| Parkinson's disease |
| Primary neurologic disorders with impairment of swallowing or mental status |
| Trauma with loss of consciousness |
| Seizure |
| General anesthesia |

**Table 17.2** Signs and symptoms of foreign body aspiration

| |
|---|
| History of choking episode |
| Chronic cough |
| Unilateral decrease in breath sounds |
| Atelectasis |
| Unilateral hyperinflation |
| Recurrent pneumonia |
| Unilateral or bilateral wheezing |
| Hemoptysis |
| Pneumothorax |
| Pneumomediastinum |
| Subcutaneous emphysema |
| Bronchiectasis |
| Lung abscess |
| Pleuritic chest pain |

larynx and present with severe coughing, choking, hoarseness, and gagging in the awake individual. In children, a witnessed or reported episode of choking is the most common presentation. Furthermore, children can present *in extremis*, and be found to have a radiopaque object or unilateral hyperinflation on the chest radiograph. In adults, in our experience and in some of the retrospective series reported to date, chronic aspiration of foreign bodies usually presents with chronic cough, and an absence of a history of choking [4]. In acute episodes, the patients present with sudden onset of choking and intractable cough, with or without vomiting, with less common symptoms being cough, fever, dyspnea, and wheezing (Table 17.2) [5]. It is important to remember that 39% of patients with a FBA will have no physical findings [6], and X rays may be normal in 6 to 38% of patients [6–12].

A significant, but unknown, number of patients expectorate the foreign body before presenting to the hospital, and some objects are even swallowed. In the presence of a suggestive clinical scenario of aspiration, approximately 50% of children with a history of choking have no foreign body in their airways. Whether this is the result of inadvertently coughing out the foreign body, never aspirated, or swallowing of the foreign body is unknown. Regarding the site of impaction, there is a predominance for the right lower lobe in adults. This is not seen in children as the size of the left main bronchus, and the angle of branching is not acute, as is the case in adults [13].

## Types of foreign body

Foreign bodies are frequently categorized as organic or inorganic. Organic foreign bodies tend to generate a significantly higher inflammatory response than inorganic materials. An example is peanuts or grass, which cause a vigorous host response within hours of the aspiration. This has clinical implications as the removal becomes harder and the rate of complications, such as bleeding and granulation tissue formation, increases. Among children, the most common foreign bodies are food particles, including peanuts, seeds, grains, and nuts [6,14]. Inorganic foreign bodies in children are usually toys or small pieces of plastic or metallic objects. These objects usually have minimal host reaction and can remain in place for several weeks to years. Interestingly, multiple case reports describe the incidental finding of a foreign body in children who underwent bronchoscopy for other reasons [15]. In adults, meat is the most common aspirated objects. However, approximately 30% of these cases have the foreign body in the glottic or subglottic space [2]. These type of foreign body are particularly risky, as they are large and can completely occlude the narrowest point of the upper airway, the subglottis. Fortunately, they can frequently be removed with postural drainage (Trendelenburg) and forceful cough from the patient. The use of Magill forceps and other direct laryngoscopic examination tools are also very effective.

Other common food particles aspirated by adults include: nuts, pumpkin seeds [16], melon seeds [17,18], and watermelon seeds [18]. Most common inorganic aspirated materials reported in the literature are: dental fixtures, dental fillings, coins, safety pins, ear plugs, glass, fragments of tracheostomy tubes [19], medication tablets, etc. Cultural, lifestyle, and dietary differences can lead to variations in the aspiration materials. For example, a recent case report in the Portuguese literature described the aspiration of a snail during a meal [20]. In the United States, the aspiration of nails and pins is seen in previously healthy young adults. The aspiration of blow gun darts has been described as well [21,22]. In Muslim countries, the aspiration of prayer beads, worry beads, and pins are relatively common among adults [18,23,24].

## Radiologic evaluation

The chest X ray (CXR) is often the initial diagnostic test whenever FBA is suspected. As previously described, most of the aspirated objects are not radiopaque. This limits the ability of standards X rays to diagnose FBA. However, the use of inspiratory and expiratory films may show subtle signs such as air trapping, atelectasis, mediastinal shift, or pulmonary infiltrates. In published studies, the operating characteristics of an abnormal CXR include a sensitivity of 70–82%, specificity of 44–74%, positive predictive value of 72–83%, and negative predictive value of 41–73% [8,9]. So we can conclude that the presence of a radio-opaque object is diagnostic, but the more common scenario is a normal CXR or subtle findings which should be interpreted with the clinical history. However, whenever the possibility of FBA is considered in the differential diagnosis, the bronchoscopic examination is the cornerstone of the diagnostic workup. The presence of pneumomediastinum in children is suggestive of the presence of foreign body aspiration [25]. Lateral neck films revealing a subglottic density or swelling may be suggestive of laryngotracheal foreign body [26]. The presence of a calcified foreign body on X rays suggests the possibility of a long-standing foreign object or a broncholith, as vegetable material can calcify over time [27] A broncholith is defined as the presence of calcified material within the bronchus, secondary to calcified lymph nodes compressing the adjacent airway or eroding into it. These lymph node calcifications are usually the result of histoplasmosis, tuberculosis, sarcoidosis, or fungal infection. (Fig. 17.1)

In chronic obstruction, the computed tomography (CT) of the chest can show the late complications of FBA, including bronchial stenosis, bronchiectasis, endobronchial masses, or granulation tissue. The use of magnetic resonance imaging (MRI) to identify peanut aspiration has been described [28–30]. The presence of fat within the peanut produces a high signal on T1-weighted imaging. Mucus on computed tomography appears as low attenuation, bubbly appearance, in the dependent airways, and frequently can be mobilized by forceful coughing [31]. The use of virtual bronchoscopy in the diagnosis of suspected foreign body aspiration in 60 children has been investigated [32]. The virtual bronchoscopy, or multidetector computed tomography-generated virtual bronchoscopy, demonstrated the presence of a lesion suggestive of foreign body in 40 cases. Thirty-eight underwent rigid bronchoscopy and 33 objects were identified and removed. Five patients had bronchial obstruction due to other causes, and two patients were observed with spontaneous resolution. The authors suggested the advantages of the virtual bronchoscopy include determination of presence

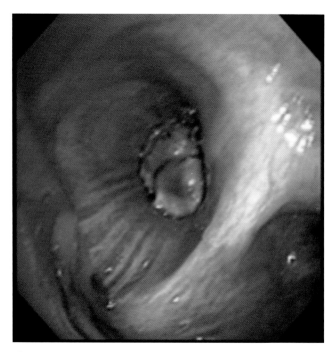

**Fig. 17.1** Broncholith seen during rigid bronchoscopy, in this case secondary to chronic histoplasmosis infection.

or absence of the foreign body, and pre-procedure localization of the foreign body. Furthermore, they describe seven negative rigid bronchoscopies in patients with a negative virtual bronchoscopy, thus raising the advantage of negative predictive value. Unfortunately, virtual bronchoscopy is not therapeutic, is not readily available in most hospitals, and may delay necessary interventions.

It is important to remember that aspirated foreign bodies are frequently misdiagnosed as croup, recurrent laryngitis, asthma, or primary airway tumors, leading to unnecessary delay and false treatment [33,34]. In adults, FBA has been confused with malignant tumors [35], asthma [36], tuberculosis, recurrent pneumonias, and various other entities.

## Complications of foreign body aspiration

The complications of FBA can be divided into acute and chronic. The acute complications include asphyxia, pneumothorax, pneumomediastinum, atelectasis, lung collapse, and even death. The chronic complications include postobstructive pneumonia, bronchiectasis, lung abscess, progressive respiratory failure, bronchial stenosis, granulation tissue, and hemoptysis. Due to the small caliber of the airways in children, the symptoms are usually more pronounced, and the diagnosis is reached earlier than in adults [5]. Nevertheless, there is a significant delay in diagnosis in 12–26% of children. [37]. These children are frequently misdiagnosed and treated for asthma, pneumonia, croup, or recurrent laryngitis [7,33].

## Therapeutic approach to the patient with foreign body aspiration

Whenever the diagnosis of foreign body aspiration has been evoked, the patient should remain under close observation until the diagnosis has been confirmed or excluded, and the foreign material has been removed. Even clinically stable patients can have a sudden change in their condition as a result of migration of the object, or occurrence of complications such as bleeding or pneumothorax [38,39].

The likelihood and the extent of tissue reaction increases the longer a foreign body remains in the airway [10,14,40]. The delay in removal in the foreign body should only be justified in order to coordinate the necessary personnel and equipment, or to promptly transfer to another institution with capabilities to deal with FBA. It is important to remember that during the first 24 hours the endobronchial mucosa suffers mild inflammation, erythema, and granulation tissue formation [10]. However, the degree of inflammatory response depends on the content of the foreign body aspirated. Nuts, peanuts, and grass are particularly irritative.

The management of the foreign body can be addressed by looking into three different approaches: postural drainage, rigid bronchoscopy, and flexible bronchoscopy.

### Postural drainage and other non-endoscopic therapies

Bronchodilator inhalation and postural drainage are not recommended in the initial management of foreign body aspiration; proximal migration of the object may lead to cardiopulmonary arrest in a small percentage of patients [41]. A delay in proceeding to bronchoscopy increases the risk of complications such as pneumonia, atelectasis, and cardiopulmonary arrest, while decreasing the likelihood of successful bronchoscopic removal. At least one clinical trial of bronchodilator inhalation and postural drainage for the treatment of FBA has described cardiopulmonary arrest, while others have reported extended hospital stay and more complications with the use of such protocols [40–42].

Another technique seldom employed is the use of therapeutic percussion while the patient coughs. Despite anecdotal reports of success, these efforts should not delay a clearly safer and more effective therapeutic maneuver such as rigid or flexible bronchoscopy.

### Rigid bronchoscopy

The rigid bronchoscope was developed as a result of the work of Dr Killian in 1897, who removed a pork bone while using a rigid endoscope. In 1936, Chevalier Jackson reported a decrease in mortality from 24 to 2% with a 98% success rate at removing foreign bodies [3]. In the most recent series, the reported success rate using rigid bronchoscopy for removal of aspirated foreign bodies is between 95 and 99% [14–18,38,43,44]. The rigid bronchoscope offers several advantages for the removal of foreign bodies including: adequate ventilation by using standard or jet ventilation, good visualization and suctioning capabilities, and a wide variety of instruments including optical forceps of different types, four-prong hooks, baskets, cryotherapy probes, and several types of balloons. The type of foreign body should be dictating the type of instrument employed, and depending on the location of the foreign body, more than one instrument is used. The rigid bronchoscope is also very useful in the removal of sharp objects. However, several series describe successful removal of pins with the flexible bronchoscope as well [23,24].

With appropriate technique and under general anesthesia, rigid bronchoscopy is safe. Unfortunately, rigid bronchoscopy is only regularly practiced by 7% of pulmonologists in the US.

### Flexible bronchoscopy

In 1968, Ikeda developed the flexible bronchoscope. The flexible system allows bronchoscopy to be performed under local anesthesia and better visualization of the distal airways. Initially, concerns about its safety and use were understandably raised [45]. However, with the development of expertise and experience, the flexible bronchoscope has become the most common diagnostic procedure performed by the pulmonologists [46]. In the evaluation of foreign body aspiration in adults, the flexible bronchoscope is the initial diagnostic tool. This diagnostic bronchoscopy should be exhaustive, as sometimes the foreign object is not obvious, is covered by blood or granulation tissue, or has been fragmented and is located in more than one distal airway.

Once the object type, size, and location have been identified, removal can be attempted.

Whenever removal is attempted, several instruments should be readily available, including a rigid bronchoscope. Instruments that have been developed for removal of FB through flexible bronchoscope include: flexible forceps, rat-tooth forceps, snares, Dormia basket, fishnet basket, cryotherapy probes, balloon catheters (Fogarty), magnet extractor, etc. These will be discussed below.

As is usually the case, in expert hands, a successful removal with the flexible bronchoscope spares the patient the inconveniences of rigid bronchoscopy, including, added costs and the risk of having to undergo a second procedure under general anesthesia. Several reports attest to the use of the flexible bronchoscope to remove foreign bodies. These reports show a success rate of greater than 90% in experienced hands [47–49]. Other reports of foreign bodies diagnosed and treated with the flexible bronchoscope have described the successful removal of teeth, windscreen glass,

**Table 17.3** Case series of airway foreign body removal by flexible bronchoscope

| Study | Total number of patients | Successful removal | % Success |
|---|---|---|---|
| Hiller *et al.* [59] | 7 | 6 | 86 |
| Cunanan [75] | 300 | 267 | 89 |
| Clark *et al.* [76] | 3 | 3 | 100 |
| Nunez *et al.* [77] | 17 | 12 | 71 |
| Lan *et al.* [74] | 33 | 32 | 97 |
| Limper *et al.* [43] | 23 | 14 | 61 |
| Chen *et al.* [78] | 43 | 32 | 74 |
| Moura e sa *et al.* [79] | 2* | 2* | 100 |
| Al-Ali *et al.* [24] | 16 | 9 | 56 |
| Gencer *et al.* [23] | 23 | 21 | 91 |
| Total | 426 + | 366 + | 86 + |

*Two cases of a series of 77 patients in which the foreign body could not be removed with rigid bronchoscopy.

ear plugs, pins, nails, fish bone, peanuts, and coins [23,24,50–55]. In Table 17.3, we list the series of foreign object removal with a flexible bronchoscope.

Intense debate surrounds the use of flexible or rigid bronchoscope for removal of the foreign bodies. This debate is understandable, as it is based on personal preference, individual expertise, and available instruments and technology at the time. Suffice to say that, what was thought to be contraindicated and almost impossible 30 years ago, is now routinely done. For example, transnasal flexible bronchoscopy was only recommended in conjunction with endotracheal intubation [45]. It is the opinion of the authors that flexible bronchoscopy has acquired paramount importance in the diagnosis and removal of foreign bodies in adults. However, self-control and understanding of the potential consequences of a failed procedure are very important. When in doubt, it is best to stabilize the patient and refer to an institution with expertise in flexible and rigid bronchoscopy. Not every pulmonologist who performs airway exams and transbronchial biopsies only occasionally is comfortable managing the potential consequences of a failed procedure. Regarding the rigid bronchoscope, the authors see its role as complementary and should be readily available whenever a foreign body removal is planned.

## Removing an airway foreign body with a flexible bronchoscope

To be successful in the removal of airway obstructions, the following basic bronchoscopic techniques are recommended.

### Rule one

Complications occur when a bronchoscopy is performed for unclear reasons or for the wrong indications. Prior to any bronchoscopic intervention, the objectives and the end point of the procedure should be carefully reviewed. Bronchoscopy performed for the wrong reasons will often lead to complications and mistakes. Mistakes beget mistakes. A grave mistake would be attempt foreign body removal in children via flexible bronchoscopy under local anesthesia [8,56]. Children's narrow airways make asphyxiation by the foreign body more likely. In addition, adequate moderate sedation and cooperation from the child is often difficult to obtain, making foreign body removal even more difficult. The flexible bronchoscope is useful as a diagnostic tool when the evidence of foreign body aspiration is not convincing. If a foreign body is found, the rigid bronchoscopy needs to be performed for extraction [8,57]. The flexible bronchoscope has been used to remove foreign objects successfully in children, but this is always with general anesthesia [48]. Additionally, in these instances, the rigid bronchoscope was always available for the possible conversion at a moment's notice. The flexible bronchoscope is only an adjunct and supplement to rigid bronchoscopy in the removal of foreign bodies in the pediatric age group [58].

### Rule two

Preparation ensures a 50% success rate. Adequate preparation is essential for a successful bronchoscopy. Problems and complications generally arise when one takes "short-cuts". All bronchoscopic accessories for foreign body removal should be ready and tested prior to the procedure. Multiple accessories may be needed to remove the object. One should always be ready to manage difficult and unexpected situations as impromptu and innovative adaptation of techniques may be needed in challenging airway obstructions [58,59].

Careful review of any radiologic studies is very important. On occasion, the review of radiologic studies with the thoracic radiologist results in a better, faster procedure.

### Rule three

Bronchoscopy is a three-handed procedure. A common mistake is to attempt bronchoscopy alone. An extra pair of hands (i.e. a trained assistant) is always needed to insert and manage the accessories of the bronchoscope (e.g. grasping forceps, basket, etc.) so as to allow the bronchoscopist to concentrate on maneuvering and manipulating the bronchoscope and its accessories to the desired position.

### Rule four

Superiorly trained personnel are necessary for a smooth and uneventful procedure. A skilled and experienced operator knows that a successful bronchoscopy is a team effort. Baharloo *et al.* report less time and stress for the participants when the usual team of experienced physicians and nurses performed the foreign body removal [5]. The bronchoscopic team must have well-defined roles. A nurse may be assigned to administer sedation and monitor vital signs. A bronchoscope assistant, trained in the use of all bronchoscopic accessories, helps the physician with the procedure. In addition, thoracic surgery and anesthesiology need to be within reach to help with any unplanned complications.

## Rule five

Time and commitment are essential. Most unsuccessful bronchoscopies occur because the clinician has other commitments and is in a hurry to finish the case. Patience should be practiced and the physician should be committed to take whatever time is necessary to remove the foreign body. A failed bronchoscopic procedure increases the risk of the patient having to undergo another procedure. Further, if the object is not removed within the first 24 hours, the likelihood and extent of tissue reaction increases the longer the foreign body remains in the airway [10,14,40]. However, in the absence of acute respiratory distress, a delay of several hours to ensure an organized, coordinated approach to removal is appropriate.

## Rule six

Know your limitations. Removal of a foreign object is probably the most challenging flexible bronchoscopic procedure, and this task may need to be delegated to a member of a group or to another institution with more experience and skill. Complications with foreign body removal have been shown to be higher in the hands of less-experienced physicians [5]. In the same way, the success rate of foreign body removal using either the rigid or the flexible bronchoscope will largely depend on the experience and skill of the operator rather than the instrument per se.

## Rule seven

Each case should be viewed as a teaching or training opportunity. More experienced and skilled operators need to pass on their skills to the junior staff. Pulmonary fellows and associate clinicians should be encouraged to actively participate in the removal of all airway obstructions. By doing so, the clinician is not only engaged in the care of the patient but is also ensuring the survival and refinement of the art of bronchoscopy.

## Anesthesia and analgesia

The flexible bronchoscope allows removal of the foreign body with local anesthesia under moderate sedation, unlike the rigid bronchoscope, which is performed under general anesthesia. An advantage of performing foreign body removal with conscious sedation is that it preserves the cough reflex, which can further facilitate the removal. An object brought forward to the trachea by bronchoscopic techniques described below can often be coughed out on

command given to the patient. The fact that foreign body removal by flexible bronchoscope is performed under moderate sedation and without a secure airway has led to much criticism. There has been much concern about the possibility of losing the object in a narrow subglottic area, leading to potential asphyxiation. To our knowledge, though, no incident of this kind has been reported in the literature. Notwithstanding, the rare event of this occurring, immediate intubation—either with bronchoscopic guidance or with a direct laryngoscope—can always be performed to secure the airway. Varying sizes of endotracheal tubes (ETT), as well as a laryngoscope, should always be available in the bronchoscopy suite for the rare happenstance of complications occurring with bronchoscopy. Extraction can then proceed via ETT. Another approach (aside from emergent intubation) would be to reintroduce the flexible bronchoscope to push the foreign body into the distal airways, thus clearing up the upper-airway obstruction.

In difficult cases, when moderate sedation cannot be achieved adequately, proceeding with rigid bronchoscopy under general anesthesia is the best option. In those instances where the object is too distal and inaccessible to remove with the rigid bronchoscope, the foreign body can be removed with a flexible bronchoscope via ETT. When the object is larger than the diameter of the tube, the ETT may need to be removed along with the bronchoscope and the secured foreign body [60,61]. Prompt reintubation can then be performed. An alternative to the use of ETT with general anesthesia is the use of laryngeal mask airway. Flexible bronchoscopy can be performed with reasonable airway control even with deeper sedation [62,63].

Experience with fospropofol, a prodrug of propofol, has been proven to be a safe and effective sedative during flexible bronchoscopy [64]. Interestingly, fospropofol is not a not a general anesthetic, and has distinct pharmacokinetic and pharmacodynamic characteristics and should not require anesthesia monitoring [65]. However, its use in therapeutic bronchoscopic procedures is yet to be described.

## Accessories for the flexible bronchoscope

Multiple instruments for the removal of foreign bodies with the flexible bronchoscope are available. The instrument of choice is largely dictated by the location, type of foreign body, and the accompanying host tissue reaction.

### Grasping forceps

The forceps is the most widely available and used instrument for the management of airway obstruction. The different designs include varying cup sizes and shapes, as well as rotation mechanisms, presence or absence of teeth, and accessories such as central fenestrations or needles. Among the grasping forceps are the W-shaped, alligator jaws, rat-tooth, shark-tooth, and covered tips forceps. The selected forceps should have a jaw size large enough to enclose the full

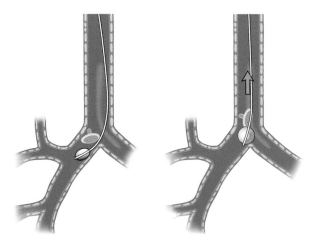

**Fig. 17.2** Balloon catheter (Fogarty) used as an aid to move a foreign body to proximal airways.

diameter of the foreign body. In cases where a firm grip is needed to prevent a hard object from slipping, the alligator jaws, rat-tooth, or shark-tooth forceps are recommended. For more delicate manipulations, a W-shaped or covered-tips forceps may be used. In general, grasping forceps are only used for the removal of flat or thin inorganic (e.g. coins, pins, screws, clips, etc.) or hard organic objects (e.g. bone), as attempted removal of a friable organic foreign body may cause it to fracture and disperse.

### Balloon catheters

Inflatable balloon catheters are probably the most useful, but clearly underutilized, tool available for removal of foreign objects. A Fogarty catheter (sizes 4 to 7) can be passed through the working channel of the bronchoscope and inflation of the balloon is achieved with injection of 1–3 ml of saline. The balloon is used to dislodge the foreign body and push it in a retrograde fashion from the distal to the proximal airways (Fig. 17.2). Other specially designed inflatable balloon catheters for use in conjunction with the broncho-scope are also available. We will describe step-by-step the use of the balloon catheters in the section on removal techniques below.

### Dormia basket

A modified version of the Dormia basket, used by gastroenterologists and urologists for the removal of calculi from the common bile duct and the ureter, is also available for the bronchoscopic removal of foreign bodies in the airway. The wings of the basket are normally retracted within a 1.6 mm diameter Teflon catheter. The basket is opened in the airway and maneuvered to allow its "wings" to surround and entrap the foreign body. The basket is most useful in the removal of large and bulky objects.

### Fishnet basket

The fishnet is a modified version of a polypectomy snare, in which a mesh of thin thread is attached to the snare wire for easy folding and unfolding. The net is normally retracted within the catheter for easy passage through the channel of the flexible bronchoscope. When the snare is advanced, the fishnet is slowly released to surround the object. The snare is then slowly retracted to enclose the foreign object within the fishnet. Once this is accomplished, the basket, the captured object, and the bronchoscope are then removed as a unit. The fishnet basket is also most useful in the removal of bulky objects.

### Three- or four-prong snares

The snares are usually squeezed together inside the catheter. Whenever they are deployed, the open wire of the snares are released, surrounding the foreign object. When the operator squeezes the handle of the device, the prongs distal ends come together, capturing the object. Once secured, the foreign body, snare, and flexible bronchoscope are withdrawn carefully as a single unit. Because the prongs are very flimsy, it is not advisable to use this accessory in the removal of hard, solid objects.

### Magnet extractor

A magnetic extractor consists of a flexible probe with a magnetic cylinder at its tip. This accessory is specially designed for passage through the working channel of the bronchoscope. Small and mobile metallic foreign bodies, such as broken forceps or cytology brushes, can be removed easily with this instrument [66,67].

### Cryotherapy catheter

Endobronchial cryotherapy is the application of extreme cold for the treatment of benign or malignant disease in the airways. However, the adhesive properties of the cryoprobe make it an ideal instrument for the removal of foreign bodies. The system has a cryogen tank (e.g. nitrous oxide or nitrogen) that by rapid gas-decompression or principle of Joule-Thompson, generates an extremely low temperature (−15 to −40°C) at the tip of the specially designed cryoprobe (Fig. 17.3). When the cryoprobe is placed in direct contact with the object, it becomes attached to the probe (cryoadhesion) and the operator then removes the flexible bronchoscope along with the cryoprobe and the foreign body once again as a single unit. This technique is extremely useful for the removal of blood clots, mucus plugs, organic materials, and small inorganic objects [68]. In our experience, this is one of the most useful instruments for the removal of organic materials. We recently removed a fragmented peanut from the airway of a 2-year-old through the combined use of rigid bronchoscope, pediatric flexible bronchoscope, and pediatric cryoprobe. The bronchoscopist should be careful to keep a clear field of view in order to prevent contact with

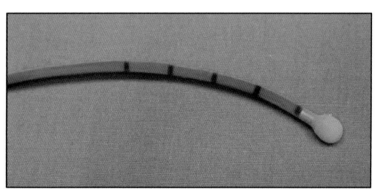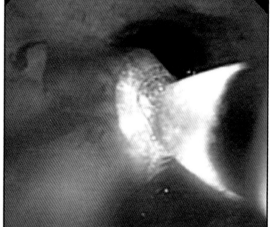

**Fig. 17.3** Cryoprobe application in benign airway disease.

the surrounding mucosa, and to inadvertently damage the normal tissue.

## Foreign body removal with the flexible bronchoscope

Extraction of the foreign body using the flexible bronchoscope is carried out in three steps: dislodgement, securing, and removal.

Whenever removal of a foreign body is planned, the flexible bronchoscopy is performed through the oral route, in order to avoid the narrow nasal passage [69]. Initially, a thorough airway examination is performed, starting with the suspected unaffected lung. The suspicious area of aspiration is examined last. The thorough and careful exam is performed to assure that there is only a single foreign object and that fragments have not been dispersed to other airways. When the object is visualized, the shape and structure of the foreign body in relation to the surrounding areas are carefully examined before an extraction attempt is made. The entire foreign body may not be visible bronchoscopically and a review of radiologic films may be necessary during the procedure to determine the position of the unseen portion. The appropriate bronchoscopic accessory is then determined, based on the size, shape, position, and density of the object.

Whenever the flexible bronchoscope is used, every care should be taken to not push the object farther down the airway. In general, our procedure has been to use the Fogarty balloon to dislodge the foreign body and to bring it proximally into the trachea, before attempting to secure it prior to its removal [50,70]. The Fogarty balloon catheter is positioned just distal to the object. The balloon is then inflated and the foreign body is pulled (retrograde push) out from the segments to the trachea (Fig. 17.2). Once in the trachea, the object is easily amenable to removal. We have often asked the patient to sit up and cough up the foreign body once it has been dislodged to the upper trachea. We usually employ this technique for small and soft objects. This has had successful results in approximately 90% of our cases.

A common misconception is that the foreign body is removed through the working channel of the bronchoscope. In fact, this is never the case. The key to removing foreign bodies lies in being able to adequately secure the object by either grasping or enclosing it with the bronchoscopic accessories. Once the object is snared or trapped, all three (bronchoscope, grasping instrument, and object) are removed simultaneously from the endobronchial tree as a single unit. During removal, the bronchoscopist must make every attempt to continuously visualize the object, always keeping it in the center of the airway.

Tissue reaction to the foreign body is also an important factor in object removal. In the event that the foreign body is concealed within a significant amount of granulation, extraction may be difficult. Sometimes the surrounding granulation tissue has to be cleared prior to the removal of the object. In these instances, bronchoscopic removal under general anesthesia may be necessary. Laser photoresection may be used in removing a large object by breaking it into small, manageable pieces [71,72] or by vaporizing surrounding granulation tissue [73]. Other modalities, such as bronchoscopic electrocautery, can also be used to similarly vaporize surrounding granulation tissue. Some authors suggest the use of a short course of steroids prior to removal procedures [11,57].

Hemoptysis is a rare complication of foreign body removal. Hemoptysis is better controlled with rigid bronchoscopy but, in careful hands, hemoptysis is rare. Rees described a single case of hemoptysis with foreign body removal from his review of 2500 similar cases [72]. There is no reason to favor rigid over flexible bronchoscopy in object retrieval for fear of massive hemoptysis [70,74].

Whenever hemoptysis does occur, our practice is to instill an epinephrine solution (1 : 10,000) through the bronchoscope to achieve topical vasoconstriction with decrease in blood flow and eventual thrombosis of the bleeding vessels. We also find cold saline (4°C) instillation to be effective in bleeding cessation. Cold saline causes hypothermic vasoconstriction and eventual thrombosis of the bleeding vessel.

Removal of a sharp object is an unmistakable challenge. The key to removing this type of foreign body is to locate the sharp end and to attempt its dislodgement. Once the sharp end is freed, the object can be grabbed and removed.

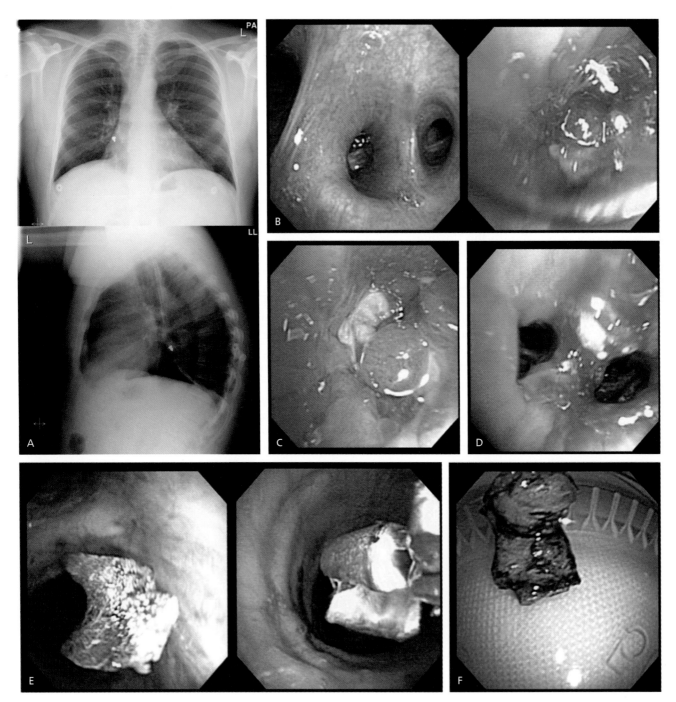

**Fig. 17.4** (A) PA and lateral chest X ray showing radio-opaque foreign body in the posterobasal right lower lobe. (B) Bronchoscopic view of posterobasal right lower lobe obstructed by granulation tissue in the area of the foreign body. (C) Bronchoscopic view of posterobasal right lower lobe obstruction with purulent drainage around the foreign body. (D) After removal of granulation tissue, the foreign body could be identified. (E) Foreign body mobilized proximally with a Fogarty balloon and held by biopsy forceps. (F) Foreign body was identified as a dental filling.

Grasping the shaft or the blunt end of a pointed instrument increases the difficulty in the removal because very likely the sharp end will get caught in the mucosa.

## Case presentation

For the purposes of describing how we approach a foreign body aspiration in practice, we will describe the latest foreign body removed at our institution.

A previously healthy 34-year-old male was referred from a local urgent care facility after the incidental finding of a radio-opaque foreign body on the CXR (Fig. 17.4A). The patient described a history of dry cough for the last 3 weeks, which correlated in time with a dental procedure. The dental procedure involved the complete removal of all teeth due to trauma during childhood, coupled with poor dental hygiene. The procedure was reported as uneventful and he was discharged home the same day. The cough had started the day after the procedure and continued for 3 weeks without significant change, so the patient decided to be checked at the local emergency room.

The bronchoscopy procedure was planned in a fully equipped bronchoscopy suite, under moderate sedation with intravenous midazolam and morphine, as well as local anesthesia with lidocaine with a maximum dose of 6 mg/kg.

The bronchoscopic exam started when the patient was appropriately sedated with a full airway exam, with the unaffected side examined first. Thereafter, the site of the aspiration was identified, but the object could not be seen, presumably due to granulation tissue (Fig. 17.4B). After probing the area with a Fogarty balloon #4, a small lumen around the granulation tissue was identified. We proceeded to remove some of the granulation tissue with biopsy forceps. This resulted in drainage of purulent material around the encased foreign body (Fig. 17.4C) The foreign body was identified (Fig. 17.4D) and after gentle proximal traction with the use of the Fogarty balloon, we were able to see the irregularly shaped foreign object, and grasp it with the use of biopsy forceps (Fig. 17.4E). The foreign body was removed uneventfully and confirmed to be a dental filling (Fig. 17.4F).

Finally, a bronchoscopic survey of the area confirmed that all purulent material was suctioned, and the obstruction was resolved. The patient was discharged home the same day.

## References

1 Rafanan AL, Mehta AC. Adult airway foreign body removal. What's new? *Clin Chest Med* 2001; **22**: 319–30.

2 Mittleman RE, Wetli CV. The fatal cafe coronary. Foreign-body airway obstruction. *JAMA* 1982; **247**: 1285–8.

3 Jackson C, Jackson CL. *Diseases of the Air and Food Passages of Foreign-body Origin*. Philadelphia: Saunders; 1936.

4 al-Majed SA, Ashour M, al-Mobeireek AF, *et al.* Overlooked inhaled foreign bodies: late sequelae and the likelihood of recovery. *Respir Med* 1997; **91**: 293–6.

5 Baharloo F, Veyckemans F, Francis C, *et al.* Tracheobronchial foreign bodies: presentation and management in children and adults. *Chest* 1999; **115**: 1357–62.

6 McGuirt WF, Holmes KD, Feehs R, Browne JD. Tracheobronchial foreign bodies. *Laryngoscope* 1988; **98**: 615–8.

7 Mantor PC, Tuggle DW, Tunell WP. An appropriate negative bronchoscopy rate in suspected foreign body aspiration. *Am J Surg* 1989; **158**: 622–4.

8 Martinot A, Closset M, Marquette CH, *et al.* Indications for flexible versus rigid bronchoscopy in children with suspected foreign-body aspiration. *Am J Respir Crit Care Med* 1997; **155**: 1676–9.

9 Hoeve LJ, Rombout J, Pot DJ. Foreign body aspiration in children. The diagnostic value of signs, symptoms and pre-operative examination. *Clin Otolaryngol Allied Sci* 1993; **18**: 55–7.

10 Wiseman NE. The diagnosis of foreign body aspiration in childhood. *J Pediatr Surg* 1984; **19**: 531–5.

11 Banerjee A, Rao KS, Khanna SK, *et al.* Laryngo-tracheobronchial foreign bodies in children. *J Laryngol Otol* 1988; **102**: 1029–32.

12 Pasaoglu I, Dogan R, Demircin M, *et al.* Bronchoscopic removal of foreign bodies in children: retrospective analysis of 822 cases. *Thorac Cardiovasc Surg* 1991; **39**: 95–8.

13 Cleveland RH. Symmetry of bronchial angles in children. *Radiology* 1979; **133**: 89–93.

14 Steen KH, Zimmermann T. Tracheobronchial aspiration of foreign bodies in children: a study of 94 cases. *Laryngoscope* 1990; **100**: 525–30.

15 Prakash UBS, ed. *Bronchoscopy*. New York, NY: Raven Press; 1994: 433–41.

16 Daniilidis J, Symeonidis B, Triaridis K, Kouloulas A. Foreign body in the airways: a review of 90 cases. *Arch Otolaryngol* 1977; **103**: 570–3.

17 Abdulmajid OA, Ebeid AM, Motaweh MM, Kleibo IS. Aspirated foreign bodies in the tracheobronchial tree: report of 250 cases. *Thorax* 1976; **31**: 635–40.

18 Elhassani NB. Tracheobronchial foreign bodies in the Middle East. A Baghdad study. *J Thorac Cardiovasc Surg* 1988; **96**: 621–5.

19 Yapici D, Atici S, Birbicer H, Oral U. Manufacturing defect in an endotracheal tube connector: risk of foreign body aspiration. *J Anesth* 2008; **22**: 333–4.

20 Santos Costa A, Afonso A. [Endobronchial *Helix pomatia*. A very rare foreign-body aspiration]. *Rev Port Pneumol* 2008; **14**: 415–19.

21 Clancy MJ. Bronchoscopic removal of an inhaled, sharp, foreign body: an unusual complication. *J Laryngol Otol* 1999; **113**: 849–50.

22 Vander Salm TJ, Ellis N. Blowgun dart aspiration. *J Thorac Cardiovasc Surg* 1986; **91**: 930–2.

23 Gencer M, Ceylan E, Koksal N. Extraction of pins from the airway with flexible bronchoscopy. *Respiration* 2007; **74**: 674–9.

24 Al-Ali MA, Khassawneh B, Alzoubi F. Utility of fiberoptic bronchoscopy for retrieval of aspirated headscarf pins. *Respiration* 2007; **74**: 309–13.

25 Burton EM, Riggs W Jr, Kaufman RA, Houston CS. Pneumomediastinum caused by foreign body aspiration in children. *Pediatr Radiol* 1989; **20**: 45–7.

26 Esclamado RM, Richardson MA. Laryngotracheal foreign bodies in children. A comparison with bronchial foreign bodies. *Am J Dis Child* 1987; **141**: 259–62.

27 Shepard JA. The bronchi: an imaging perspective. *J Thorac Imaging* 1995; **10**: 236–54.

28 Imaizumi H, Kaneko M, Nara S, *et al.* Definitive diagnosis and location of peanuts in the airways using magnetic resonance imaging techniques. *Ann Emerg Med* 1994; **23**: 1379–82.

29 Kitanaka S, Mikami I, Tokumaru A, O'Uchi T. Diagnosis of peanut inhalation by MRI. *Pediatr Radiol* 1992; **22**: 300–1.

30 O'Uchi T, Tokumaru A, Mikami I, *et al.* Value of MR imaging in detecting a peanut causing bronchial obstruction. *AJR Am J Roentgenol* 1992; **159**: 481–2.

31 Marom EM, Goodman PC, McAdams HP. Focal abnormalities of the trachea and main bronchi. *AJR Am J Roentgenol* 2001; **176**: 707–11.

32 Cevizci N, Dokucu AI, Baskin D, *et al.* Virtual bronchoscopy as a dynamic modality in the diagnosis and treatment of suspected foreign body aspiration. *Eur J Pediatr Surg* 2008; **18**: 398–401.

33 Atmaca S, Unal R, Sesen T, *et al.* Laryngeal foreign body mistreated as recurrent laryngitis and croup for one year. *Turk J Pediatr* 2009; **51**: 65–6.

34 Barben J, Berkowitz RG, Kemp A, Massie J. Bronchial granuloma—where's the foreign body? *Int J Pediatr Otorhinolaryngol* 2000; **53**: 215–9.

35 Oka M, Fukuda M, Takatani H, *et al.* Chronic bronchial foreign body mimicking peripheral lung tumor. *Intern Med* 1996; **35**: 219–21.

36 Matsuse H, Shimoda T, Kawano T, *et al.* Airway foreign body with clinical features mimicking bronchial asthma. *Respiration* 2001; **68**: 103–5.

37 Fitzpatrick PC, Guarisco JL. Pediatric airway foreign bodies. *J LA State Med Soc* 1998; **150**: 138–41.

38 Kosloske AM. Bronchoscopic extraction of aspirated foreign bodies in children. *Am J Dis Child* 1982; **136**: 924–7.

39 Kosloske AM. Tracheobronchial foreign bodies in children: back to the bronchoscope and a balloon. *Pediatrics* 1980; **66**: 321–3.

40 Law D, Kosloske AM. Management of tracheobronchial foreign bodies in children: a reevaluation of postural drainage and bronchoscopy. *Pediatrics* 1976; **58**: 362–7.

41 Bose P, El Mikatti N. Foreign bodies in the respiratory tract. A review of forty-one cases. *Ann R Coll Surg Engl* 1981; **63**: 129–31.

42 Cotton EK, Abrams G, Vanhoutte J, Burrington J. Removal of aspirated foreign bodies by inhalation and postural drainage. A survey of 24 cases. *Clin Pediatr* 1973; **12**: 270–6.

43 Limper AH, Prakash UB. Tracheobronchial foreign bodies in adults. *Ann Intern Med* 1990; **112**: 604–9.

44 Hsu W, Sheen T, Lin C, *et al.* Clinical experiences of removing foreign bodies in the airway and esophagus with a rigid endoscope: a series of 3217 cases from 1970 to 1996. *Otolaryngol Head Neck Surg* 2000; **122**: 450–4.

45 Zavala DC, Rhodes ML, Richardson RH, Bedell GN. Editorial: Fiberoptic and rigid bronchoscopy: the state of the art. *Chest* 1974; **65**: 605–6.

46 Colt H, Prakash UBS, Offord KP. Bronchoscopy in North America: Survey by the American Association for Bronchology, 1999. *J Bronchol* 2000; **7**: 8–25.

47 Debeljak A, Sorli J, Music E, Kecelj P. Bronchoscopic removal of foreign bodies in adults: experience with 62 patients from 1974–1998. *Eur Respir J* 1999; **14**: 792–5.

48 Swanson KL, Prakash UBS, McDougall JC. Airway foreign bodies in adults. *J Bronchol* 2003; **10**: 107–11.

49 Surka A, Chin R, Conforti J. Bronchoscopic myths and legends: airway foreign bodies. *Clin Pulm Med* 2006; **3**: 209–11.

50 Heinz GJ 3rd, Richardson RH, Zavala DC. Endobronchial foreign body removal using the bronchofiberscope. *Ann Otol Rhinol Laryngol* 1978; **87**: 50–2.

51 Mehta AC, Grimm M. Breakage of Nd-YAG laser sapphire contact probe inside the endobronchial tree. *Chest* 1988; **93**: 1119.

52 Fieselmann JF, Zavala DC, Keim LW. Removal of foreign bodies (two teeth) by fiberoptic bronchoscopy. *Chest* 1977; **72**: 241–3.

53 Klayton RJ, Donlan CJ, O'Neil TJ, Foreman DR. Letter: Foreign body removal via fiberoptic bronchoscopy. *JAMA* 1975; **234**: 806.

54 Lee M, Fernandez NA, Berger HW, Givre H. Wire basket removal of a tack via flexible fiberoptic bronchoscopy. *Chest* 1982; **82**: 515.

55 Rohde FC, Celis ME, Fernandez S. The removal of an endobronchial foreign body with the fiberoptic bronchoscope and image intensifier. *Chest* 1977; **72**: 265.

56 Nussbaum E. Flexible fiberoptic bronchoscopy and laryngoscopy in infants and children. *Laryngoscope* 1983; **93**: 1073–5.

57 Bolliger CT, Mathur PN. *Interventional Bronchoscopy*. Basel, New York: Karger; 2000.

58 Gibson WS Jr, Vrabec DP. Encounters with challenging bronchial foreign bodies: impromptu adaptation of technique. *Ann Otol Rhinol Laryngol* 2000; **109**: 86–8.

59 Hiller C, Lerner S, Varnum R, *et al.* Foreign body removal with the flexible fiberoptic bronchoscope. *Endoscopy* 1977; **9**: 216–22.

60 Downey RJ, Libutti SK, Gorenstein L, Mercer S. Airway management during retrieval of the very large aspirated foreign body: a method for the flexible bronchoscope. *Anesth Analg* 1995; **81**: 186–7.

61 Verea-Hernando H, Garcia-Quijada RC, Ruiz de Galarreta AA. Extraction of foreign bodies with fiberoptic bronchoscopy in mechanically ventilated patients. *Am Rev Respir Dis* 1990; **142**: 258.

62 Hirai T, Yamanaka A, Fujimoto T, *et al.* Bronchoscopic removal of bronchial foreign bodies through the laryngeal mask airway in pediatric patients. *Jpn J Thorac Cardiovasc Surg* 1999; **47**: 190–2.

63 McGrath G, Das-Gupta M, Clarke G. Bronchoscopy via continuous positive airway pressure for patients with respiratory failure. *Chest* 2001; **119**: 670–1.

64 Silvestri GA, Vincent BD, Wahidi MM, *et al.* A phase 3, randomized, double-blind study to assess the efficacy and safety of fospropofol disodium injection for moderate sedation in patients undergoing flexible bronchoscopy. *Chest* 2009; **135**: 41–7.

65 Jantz MA. The old and the new of sedation for bronchoscopy. *Chest* 2009; **135**: 4–6.

66 Saito H, Saka H, Sakai S, Shimokata K. Removal of broken fragment of biopsy forceps with magnetic extractor. *Chest* 1989; **95**: 700–1.

67 Mayr J, Dittrich S, Triebl K. A new method for removal of metallic-ferromagnetic foreign bodies from the tracheobronchial tree. *Pediatr Surg Int* 1997; **12**: 461–2.

68 Weerdt S De, Noppen M, Remels L, *et al*. Successful removal of a massive endobronchial blood clot by means of cryotherapy. *J Bronchol* 2005; **12**: 23–4.

69 Mehta AC, Dweik RA. Nasal versus oral insertion of the flexible bronchoscope: pro-nasal insertion. *J Bronchol* 1996; **3**: 224–8.

70 Mehta AC, Dasgupta A. Bronchoscopic approach to tracheo-bronchial foreign bodies in adults pro-flexible bronchoscopy. *J Bronchol* 1997; **4**: 173–8

71 Boelcskei PL, Wagner M, Lessnau KK. Laser-assisted removal of a foreign body in the bronchial system of an infant. *Lasers Surg Med* 1995; **17**: 375–7.

72 Rees JR. Massive hemoptysis associated with foreign body removal. *Chest* 1985; **88**: 475–6.

73 Hayashi AH, Gillis DA, Bethune D, *et al*. Management of foreign-body bronchial obstruction using endoscopic laser therapy. *J Pediatr Surg* 1990; **25**: 1174–6.

74 Lan RS, Lee CH, Chiang YC, Wang WJ. Use of fiberoptic bronchoscopy to retrieve bronchial foreign bodies in adults. *Am Rev Respir Dis* 1989; **140**: 1734–7.

75 Cunanan OS. The flexible fiberoptic bronchoscope in foreign body removal. Experience in 300 cases. *Chest* 1978; **73** (5 Suppl): 725–6.

76 Clark PT, Williams TJ, Teichtahl H, *et al*. Removal of proximal and peripheral endobronchial foreign bodies with the flexible fibreoptic bronchoscope. *Anaesth Intensive Care* 1989; **17**: 205–8.

77 Nunez H, Perez Rodriguez E, Alvarado C, *et al*. Foreign body aspirate extraction. *Chest* 1989; **96**: 698.

78 Chen CH, Lai CL, Tsai TT, *et al*. Foreign body aspiration into the lower airway in Chinese adults. *Chest* 1997; **112**: 129–33.

79 Moura e Sa J, Oliveira A, Caiado A, *et al*. Tracheobronchial foreign bodies in adults—experience of the Bronchology Unit of Centro Hospitalar de Vila Nova de Gaia. *Rev Port Pneumol* 2006; **12**: 31–43.

# 18

# The Role of Bronchoscopy in Hemoptysis

**Sunit R. Patel[1] and James K. Stoller[2]**

[1] UC Davis Medical Center, & Touro University and California Sleep Center Merced CA USA

[2] Cleveland Clinic Foundation, Cleveland, OH, USA

## Introduction

Hemoptysis is the coughing up of blood from a source below the glottis [1]. It is a common clinical symptom [2] that has been reported to be responsible for 6.8% of outpatient chest clinic visits [3], 11% of admissions to the hospital chest service [4], 38% of patients referred to a chest surgical practice [5], and up to 15% of all pulmonary consultations [6]. Hemoptysis poses a great diagnostic challenge, because it has been described in many cardiopulmonary diseases and some hematologic disorders [7–11]. Most episodes of hemoptysis are reportedly associated with chronic bronchitis, bronchiectasis, bronchogenic carcinoma, or tuberculosis [4,7,8,12–15]. However, over the years, the spectrum of leading causes of hemoptysis has been changing, perhaps contributing to the diagnostic dilemma [4,7,16,17].

The four major concerns in evaluating hemoptysis are to: rule out bronchogenic cancer; determine whether the underlying cause is treatable; localize the site of bleeding in case further therapeutic intervention is needed [6]; decide which treatment to implement if the bleeding persists, recurs, or is massive; and when to treat. In this regard, bronchoscopy (particularly flexible bronchoscopy) has assumed a central role in diagnosis and localization of bleeding and also in performing different therapeutic interventions to control bleeding [18]. Indeed, hemoptysis is one of the most frequent indications for bronchoscopy and accounts for 10 to 30% of bronchoscopic procedures in major medical centers [7,15,19,20]. For example, a 1989 survey of 871 bronchoscopists in North America, conducted by the American College of Chest Physicians (ACCP), reported that 81.1% of respondents listed hemoptysis as one of five most common indications for bronchoscopy. Overall, hemoptysis was the second most commonly cited indication for bronchoscopy [21].

With this background, this chapter reviews the definitions, pathogenesis, and differential diagnosis of hemoptysis and provides a systematic diagnostic approach to patients with hemoptysis, emphasizing the role of bronchoscopy in both diagnosis and therapy.

## Definitions and characterization of hemoptysis in the available literature

### Defining by severity: massive and non-massive hemoptysis

Hemoptysis may range from a small amount of blood-streaked sputum to a massive amount of bleeding that causes asphyxiation and exsanguination. Because the overall management of hemoptysis depends on the severity of bleeding, most authors distinguish between massive (e.g. potentially life-threatening) and non-massive hemoptysis [1,11,22,23]. Although no clear-cut definitions of non-massive hemoptysis are available, hemoptysis has been arbitrarily graded as small or mild when the amount ranges from blood-tinged sputum to less than 15–30 mL over 24 hours [1,23,24]. The term "gross" or "frank" hemoptysis is sometimes used to refer to a quantity of bleeding that is smaller than massive but greater than blood streaking [11].

Table 18.1 summarizes different available definitions of massive hemoptysis, which subsume definitions based on the volume of expectorated blood (e.g. at least 600 mL per 24 h) and those based on the magnitude of the clinical effect associated with hemoptysis (e.g. hemoptysis threatening asphyxia) [2,25–31]. The volume criteria cited for massive hemoptysis range from 100 to 1000 mL in a 24-hour period. However, volumes less than 100 mL in 24 hours are generally considered non-massive hemoptysis [26,27]. The most lenient volume definition of massive hemoptysis has been proposed by Amirana and colleagues [25] and Bobrowitz and coworkers [26] (expectorating 100 mL or more blood a day at least once). At the other extreme of volume definitions are those proposed by Crocco and associates [28] (more than 600 mL of expectorated blood in 48 hours) and

*Flexible Bronchoscopy*, Third Edition. Edited by Ko-Pen Wang, Atul C. Mehta, J. Francis Turner.
© 2012 Blackwell Publishing Ltd. Published 2012 by Blackwell Publishing Ltd.

**Table 18.1** Definitions of massive hemoptysis

Massive hemoptysis

    Spectrum of "volume" definitions

        ≥100 mL/24 h [25,26]

        >600 mL/48 h [27]

    Major (≥200 mL/24 h) versus massive (≥1000 mL/24 h) [28]

"Magnitude of effect" definitions [29]

    Presents risk of large aspiration

    Life-threatening by virtue of airway obstruction, hypotension, or anemia

Exsanguinating hemoptysis [30]

    Hemoptysis that threatens because of actual volume of blood lost

    Loss of ≥1000 mL total at rate of ≥150 mL/h

Commonly accepted definition [31–36]

    ≥600 mL over 24 h

Modified and reproduced with permission from: Stoller JK. Diagnosis and management of massive hemoptysis: a review. *Respir Care* 1992; **32**: 564–581.

Corey and Hla [29] (1000 mL or more of expectorated blood in 24 hours).

As an alternative to volume definitions, other authors have defined massive hemoptysis by the magnitude of the clinical consequences. For example, based on the fact that the anatomic dead space of the measured airways is 100–200 mL in most individuals, massive hemoptysis has been defined as the volume of expectorated blood that poses risk for lung aspiration or that is life-threatening by virtue of airway obstruction, hypotension, gas exchange abnormalities, or blood loss. Finally, an operational definition of massive hemoptysis has been proposed by Holsclaw and colleagues [27,30], who offer three criteria for massive hemoptysis: pulmonary bleeding that causes death or requires hospitalization, is large enough to give laboratory or clinical evidence of systemic blood loss, or requires blood or plasma transfusion.

Garzon and coworkers [27,31] distinguished "exsanguinating" hemoptysis as pulmonary bleeding that is brisk enough to threaten life not only by asphyxiation (i.e. from flooding the airways with blood), but also hypotension caused by blood loss itself, that is a volume of 1000 mL or greater at a rate of at least 150 mL/h. Although varying definitions have been proposed, a commonly accepted definition of massive hemoptysis is the expectoration of at least 600 mL over 24 hours [32–38]. The practical difficulty of measuring the volume of expectorated blood under

usual clinical circumstances limits the value of finer distinctions in defining massive hemoptysis [2]. Also, beyond the actual quantity of expectorated blood, the rate of bleeding appears to be clinically important [37,39]. In a study of 67 patients with at least 600 mL expectorated blood in 48 hours, Crocco and coworkers [28] showed that mortality was strikingly related to bleeding rate regardless of treatment. Specifically, patients expectorating 600 mL of blood over 4 hours had a combined mortality rate of 71%, those with more than 600 mL in 4–6 hours had a 45% mortality rate, and those with more than 600 mL in 16–48 hours had a 5% mortality rate.

## Defining by cause: idiopathic hemoptysis

Despite a careful work-up that includes flexible bronchoscopy, the cause of hemoptysis cannot be determined in some patients. This so-called idiopathic, essential, or cryptogenic hemoptysis has been reported in 2 to 18% of patients with hemoptysis [4,8–10,13,15,38]. The typical presentation and course of idiopathic hemoptysis is a single bout of bleeding with minimal or no respiratory symptoms, a normal chest radiograph, normal bronchoscopic findings, and bronchial washings without evidence of infection or malignancy [7,40]. Fortunately, the usual prognosis in "idiopathic hemoptysis" is favorable with resolution of bleeding within 6 months of evaluation [40].

## Defining by cause: pseudohemoptysis

Pseudohemoptysis is the expectoration of blood from a source other than the lower respiratory tract, causing diagnostic confusion, especially in patients who cannot clearly describe the source of the bleeding [11]. In addition to upper gastrointestinal bleeding (hematemesis), which can sometimes mimic true hemoptysis (when the blood is aspirated into the lungs), pseudohemoptysis may occur when blood from the oral cavity [41] or nasopharynx [41,42] drains to the back of the throat and initiates the cough reflex [8]. Pseudohemoptysis has also been described in patients with pneumonia from *Serratia marcescens*, when the red-pigment-producing bacteria imparts a red color to the phlegm [43]; and in patients with rifampin overdose, when the drug imparts a reddish color to sputum [44].

## Defining by frequency: recurrent hemoptysis

Recurrent hemoptysis is usually defined as bleeding episodes that recur at an interval of less than 1 year [45].

## Differential diagnosis of hemoptysis and massive hemoptysis

Table 18.2 presents the differential diagnosis of hemoptysis that has been amply described in several reviews [8–11,38,46]. Changing rates of disease occurrence (e.g.

**Table 18.2** Differential diagnosis of hemoptysis

**Pulmonary disorders**

*Infections*

    Lung abscess

    Pneumonia (bacterial or non-bacterial)*

    Mycetoma (e.g. aspergilloma)*

    Tuberculosis (active or inactive) and other mycobacterial infections*

    Parenchymal fungal infections (coccidioidomycosis, mucormycosis, histoplasmosis, cryptococcosis, etc.)

    Parasitic infections (amebiasis, ascariasis, clonorchiasis, echinococcosis, hookworm infestations, paragonimiasis, schistosomiasis, etc.)

    Others (actinomycosis, nocardiosis, viral, etc.)

*Neoplasms*

    Bronchogenic carcinoma*

    Pulmonary metastasis from extrapulmonary primary

    Bronchial adenoma (including carcinoid tumors)

    Others (sarcoma, hamartoma, hydatidiform mole, etc.)

*Tracheobronchial disease*

    Acute tracheobronchitis*

    Chronic bronchitis*

    Aspirated foreign body

    Tracheoesophageal or tracheovascular fistula

    Mucoid impaction of the bronchus

    Bronchiectasis (including cystic fibrosis)*

    Broncholithiasis

    Suture granuloma or airway dehiscence at airway anastomotic site (e.g. in lung transplant patients)

    Bronchial telangiectasia

*Congenital disease*

    Bronchopulmonary sequestration

    Bronchogenic cysts

*Pulmonary vascular disease*

    Pulmonary thromboembolism/ infarction

    Pulmonary venous varix

    Pulmonary artery aneurysms

    Fat/ tumor embolism

    Arteriovenous malformation (including Osler–Weber–Rendu syndrome)

    Pulmonary hemorrhage syndromes (Goodpasture's syndrome, idiopathic pulmonary hemosiderosis, Wegener's granulomatosis, etc.)

    Vasculitis (Behçet's syndrome, Churg–Strauss syndrome, Henoch–Schonlein purpura, systemic lupus erythematosus, rheumatoid arthritis, scleroderma, mixed cryoglobulinemia, mixed connective tissue disease, IgA nephropathy)

    Bronchial artery rupture

*Drug/ toxin related*

    Toxic / smoke inhalations

    Aspirin

    Anticoagulants

    Solvents

    Penicillamine

    Trimellitic anhydride

    Inhaled isocyanides

    Glycoprotein IIb/IIIa inhibitors

    Thrombolytic agents (Bevacizumab)

    Cocaine

*Traumatic*

    Blunt chest trauma (contusion, hematoma)

    Penetrating lung injury

    Fractured bronchus

*Miscellaneous*

    Amyloidosis

    Endometriosis (catamenial hemoptysis)

    Pneumoconiosis

    Extrinsic allergic alveolitis

    Aspiration of gastric contents

**Cardiovascular diseases**

    Left ventricular failure*

    Mitral stenosis*

    Superior vena cava syndrome

    Subclavian artery aneurysm

    Postmyocardial infarction syndrome

    Congenital heart disease

    Aortic and ventricular aneurysm

    Cardiac catheterization

    Coronary artery bypass grafting

**Hematologic disorders**

    Coagulopathy

    Thrombocytopenia

    Disseminated intravascular coagulation

    Leukemia

**Iatrogenic**

    Bronchoscopy including laser therapy

    Lung biopsy and surgery

    Cardiac catheterization

    Pulmonary artery catheter-related

    Intubation

**Idiopathic**

*Common causes.

declining rates of new onset bronchiectasis) and diagnostic advances (e.g. the advent of the flexible bronchoscope in the 1970s) likely account for a changing spectrum of the common causes of hemoptysis [2]. For centuries, hemoptysis was considered pathognomonic of pulmonary tuberculosis, an association highlighted by the Hippocratic aphorism: "Spitting of pus follows the spitting of blood, consumption follows the spitting of this and death follows consumption" [4]. Studies done in the 1940s and 1950s reported tuberculosis, bronchiectasis, and bronchogenic carcinoma as the most common causes of hemoptysis [5,12–15]. However, more recent series indicate that hemoptysis is now most commonly caused by bronchitis and less commonly by tuberculosis and bronchiectasis [16,17].

Massive hemoptysis accounts for a minority of patients with hemoptysis (4.8 to 6.7% of hospitalized patients with hemoptysis) [4,29], and the spectrum of causes of massive hemoptysis is narrower (Table 18.3). The most common causes of massive hemoptysis are bronchiectasis, TB (active and inactive), bronchogenic carcinoma, lung abscess, and mycetoma [2,28,31,33,34,47–49] and, unlike lesser hemoptysis (for which tuberculosis and bronchiectasis have become less frequent causes) [16,17], the spectrum of causes of massive hemoptysis has changed little among series that span three decades.

## Pathophysiology of hemoptysis

A rational approach to managing hemoptysis requires knowledge of the vascular anatomy of the lungs, which is summarized below. Sources of pulmonary bleeding include the pulmonary circulation, a low-pressure circuit (with normal pulmonary artery pressures of 15–20 mm Hg systolic and 5–10 mm Hg diastolic), and the bronchial circulation, consisting of the bronchial arteries (which branch from the aorta and have systemic arterial pressures), and the bronchial veins (which drain via systemic veins into the right heart) [2]. The bronchial arteries are the main vascular supply to the airways (from the mainstem bronchi to terminal bronchioles), and the supporting framework of the lung (i.e. the pleura, intrapulmonary lymphoid tissue, large branches of the pulmonary vessels, and nerves) [11,50]. The pulmonary arteries supply the pulmonary parenchymal tissue including the respiratory bronchioles [11,50]. As depicted in Figure 18.1, the bronchial and pulmonary circu-

**Table 18.3** Causes of massive hemoptysis in selected series

| Study | Patient | | | | | Cause of massive hemoptysis, % (No.) | | | | | |
|-------|---------|---|---|---|---|------|---|---|---|---|---|
| | Definition | Total | Active | Inactive | Lung cancer | Bronchiectasis | Abscess | Mitral | Fungoma | Unknown | Other |
| Crocco, 1968 [27] | > 600 mL/48 h | 67 | 49% (33) | 24% (16) | 8% (5) | 10% (7) | 9% (6) | — | — | — | — |
| Garzon, 1974 [32] | ≥ 600 mL/24 h | 62 | 26% (16) | 47% (29) | 3.2% (2) | 11.3% (7) | 6.5% (4) | — | — | — | 6.5% (4) |
| McCollum, 1975 [46] | Asphyxia threat | 15 | 33% (5) | | 6.7% (1)* | 20% (3) | — | — | 13.3% (2) | 6.7% (1) | 20% (3) |
| Yang, 1978 [47] | > 200 mL/24 h | 20 | 25% (5) | 25% (5) | 15% (3) | 15% (3) | — | 5% (1) | 5% (1) | 10% (2) | — |
| Garzon, 1982 [30] | > 1000 mL/6 h | 24 | 29% (7) | 17% (4) | 13% (3) | 17% (4) | 8% (2) | — | — | 8% (2) | 8% (2) |
| Conlan, 1983 [33] | NS | 123 | 38% (47) | 4.9% (6) | 30% (37) | 4.9% (6) | — | 3.3% (4) | — | 18.7% (23) | |
| Ulfacker, 1985 [45] | NS | 75 | 76% (57) | | — | 1.3% (1) | 2.6% (2) | — | 16% (12) | — | 3.9% (3) |

*Metastatic.
NS, not specified.
Modified and reproduced with permission from: Stoller JK. Diagnosis and management of massive hemoptysis: a review. *Respir Care* 1992; **32**: 564–581.

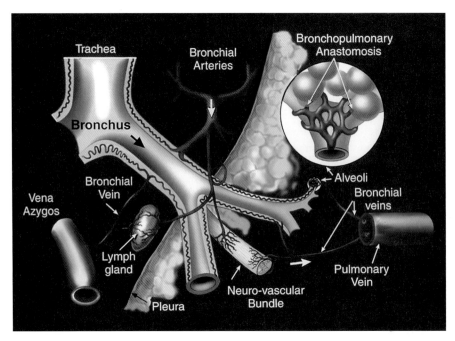

**Fig. 18.1** Diagram of the systemic blood supply to the lung. Note that flow from the extra pulmonary airways and supporting structures returns to the right heart, whereas intrapulmonary flow drains into the pulmonary veins and returns to the left heart. Reproduced by permission from Oeffebach ME, Charau NB, Lakshminarayan S. State of the art: the bronchial circulation-small but vitality tribute of the lung. *Am Rev Respir Dis* 1987; **135**: 467.

lations are normally connected; bronchial arterial blood feeding the proximal airways drains into the bronchial veins and empties into the right heart, whereas bronchial arterial blood perfusing the intrapulmonary airways and lung tissue drains through bronchopulmonary anastomoses into the pulmonary veins and left heart [2,51]. Anastomoses between bronchial arteries and tributaries of the pulmonary veins that account for the normal right-to-left shunt have been demonstrated in normal lungs at autopsy and may at times be a major source of massive hemoptysis [51]. Arteriographic studies in patients with active hemoptysis have demonstrated that the usual source of bleeding (92% of cases) is the systemic bronchial circulation [51]. Bronchial artery dilatation, ectasia, collateral formation, or active bleeding coinciding with the localized site of bleeding have been demonstrated during arteriography [51]. Still, the pulmonary circulation may be the source of hemoptysis. Examples of bleeding due to a pulmonary arterial source include rupture associated with placement of a Swan–Ganz pulmonary artery catheter, pulmonary artery aneurysms secondary to collagen vascular disease, and pulmonary artery vasculitis [27].

## Pathogenesis

The pathogenesis of hemoptysis depends on the type and location of the underlying disease [13]. Because a detailed discussion of the pathogenesis of hemoptysis in individual diseases is beyond the scope of this chapter, only the pathogenesis of some of the common causes of hemoptysis is discussed. The reader is referred to other published reviews for further information [10,11,13,37].

In tuberculosis, bleeding may result from several mechanisms [52]. First, an acute exudative pneumonia can cause necrosis of adjacent bronchial vessels or local mucosal ulceration [13]. In endobronchial tuberculosis, hemoptysis may result from ulceration of the bronchial mucosa or bronchiectasis [11]. In healed and fibrotic parenchymal disease, bleeding may arise from irritation of granulation tissue in the walls of bronchiectatic airways in the same areas [11]. A healed calcified lymph node may impinge on the bronchial wall and erode into a bronchial lumen; if a blood vessel lies in the path of a broncholith, hemoptysis may result, occasionally associated with coughing up gravel (lithoptysis) [53]. Chronic inactive fibrocaseous tuberculosis is a common setting for massive hemoptysis in tuberculosis. Although some controversy surrounds the precise source of the hemoptysis, it is commonly believed that the mechanism of this bleeding is rupture of Rasmussen's aneurysms [52–56], which are ectatic portions of the pulmonary artery traversing the thick-walled cavities caused by tuberculosis involvement of the adventitia and media vessels.

In bronchogenic carcinoma, pathologic studies have shown an increase in bronchial arterial supply to the region of the tumor [57]. Hemoptysis in cancer results from necrosis, mucosal invasion, or direct local invasion of a blood vessel [10,11,13]. About 10%, of patients with bronchogenic cancer experience massive hemoptysis during the course of their disease [58]. More than 80% of cases of massive hemoptysis in lung cancer are associated with squamous cell carcinomas that are generally located in the central airways and may cavitate in half the cases [37]. Up to 80% of lung cancer patients will develop tracheobronchial involvement over the course of their disease. These lesions are typically vascular and may bleed spontaneously or obstruct the airways [59].

Bronchiectasis is a frequent cause of massive hemoptysis (Table 18.3). In autopsy specimens from patients with bronchiectasis, Liebow and colleagues [60] report striking bronchial artery enlargement with tortuosity, marked by increased anastomoses with pulmonary arteries. These investigators postulate that budding capillaries in the granulation tissue of areas with organizing pneumonitis increase the capillary bed supplied by the bronchial arteries, leading to increased load and hypertrophy. In addition, the destruction of the pulmonary arterial capillary bed and local spasm in the pulmonary circulation from hypoxemia and inflammation may cause opening of bronchial-to-pulmonary artery communications and penetration of the high-pressure blood flow from the bronchial to the pulmonary circulation [37,61]. The enlarged ectatic vessels with extensive collaterals that lie in the wall of the bronchiectatic sacs are susceptible to further injury from the products of local inflammation and infection [37].

Mycetomas, most commonly caused by aspergillus, result from saprophytic colonization of pre-existing cavities from tuberculosis, sarcoidosis, lung abscess, infarction, or bronchiectasis. Putative causes of hemoptysis in this setting include mechanical trauma of the highly vascular–granular tissue of the cavity wall (from movement of a fungus ball), release of anticoagulant and trypsin-like proteolysis enzymes, aspergillus-associated endotoxin causing vascular injury, or a type III hypersensitivity reaction causing vascular damage [62,63].

In acute left ventricular failure and mitral stenosis, blood-streaked sputum is caused by rupture of pulmonary veins or capillaries, or anastomoses between bronchial and pulmonary arteries distended by elevated intravascular pressure or pulmonary venous hypertension [10,57,64]. In both acute and chronic bronchitis, bleeding results from irritation of friable and inflamed mucosa [10,13].

Finally, the pathogenesis of bleeding from a lung abscess is not entirely clear, but may be due to progression of local inflammatory processes causing necrosis of branches of both the bronchial and pulmonary circulations [27,65].

## Diagnostic approach to the patient with hemoptysis

All instances of hemoptysis require careful evaluation to determine the cause and to localize the bleeding source. Bronchoscopy is helpful in attaining both of these goals.

**Table 18.4** Routine prebronchoscopic evaluation*

History and physical examination ± nasopharyngeal evaluation

Complete blood count, urinalysis, coagulation profile (e.g. prothrombin time, partial thromboplastin time)

Chest radiographs (posteroanterior and lateral)

Sputum examination (cytology, acid-fast smear, and culture)

Electrocardiogram

Arterial blood gases (in moderate to massive hemoptysis)

*Evaluation can be individualized to each patient.

## Routine prebronchoscopy evaluation

The routine evaluation before bronchoscopy is outlined in Table 18.4. In patients with massive hemoptysis, localizing the site of bleeding and specific therapy (including airway maintenance, transfusion, and therapeutic interventions) should proceed simultaneously with diagnostic studies to determine the cause of bleeding [10].

A detailed history and physical examination should be performed to rule out hematemesis and other causes of pseudohemoptysis and to provide clues to the site and cause of hemoptysis. As outlined by Lyons [8], features of blood from the lung that may distinguish between hemoptysis and hematemesis are that blood from the lung is coughed versus vomited, partly frothy, alkaline versus acid (unless hematemesis is so massive that stomach acid is neutralized by blood), and mixed with pus, organisms, and macrophages versus sometimes mixed with food. Also, patients with hemoptysis sometimes report gurgling, a vague pressure sensation, tightness, and secretion accumulation in the chest and may even localize a bleeding site in the thorax versus experiencing nausea and vomiting, as is more typical in upper gastrointestinal bleeding [4,27]. Additional historical clues that may help establish true hemoptysis are reviewed in Table 18.5 [7,10,11,23,46,66].

Physical findings may also offer diagnostic clues (Table 18.6) [10,11,45,66]. Finally, routine laboratory studies may help identify the cause of hemoptysis [10,11,45]. The complete blood count may suggest the presence of an infection, chronic blood loss (e.g. idiopathic pulmonary hemosiderosis), or a hematologic disorder. Coagulation studies may suggest an underlying hematologic disorder. An electrocardiogram may suggest pulmonary hypertension, mitral stenosis, or ischemic heart disease as a marker of left ventricular dysfunction. Urinalysis may suggest a systemic disease or pulmonary–renal syndrome (e.g. Goodpasture's syndrome, Wegener's granulomatosis). Finally, collection of all expectorated sputum will allow both qualitative examination of the sputum (cytology, smear for acid-fast bacilli, and

**Table 18.5** Some historical clues that may help to establish cause of hemoptysis

| Clues | Diagnostic possibility |
|---|---|
| Young age | Adenoma, bronchiectasis, mitral stenosis, sequestration arteriovenous malformation |
| Age >40, smoking, abnormal chest X ray, small amounts of hemoptysis occurring daily for weeks | Bronchogenic carcinoma |
| Recurrence over months to years | Adenoma, bronchiectasis |
| Hematuria | Goodpasture's syndrome, Wegener's granulomatosis, polyarteritis nodosa |
| Occurrence during menses | Endometriosis (catamenial hemoptysis) |
| Fever, productive cough | Chronic bronchitis, bronchiectasis |
| | Tuberculosis, fungal disease, lung abscess |
| History of breast, colon, or renal cancer | Endobronchial metastasis |
| Dyspnea, acute pleuritic chest pain, calf tenderness | Pulmonary embolism with infarct or pneumonia |
| Associated with exertion, orthopnea or paroxysmal nocturnal dyspnea | Congestive heart failure, mitral stenosis |
| History of rheumatic fever | Mitral stenosis |
| History of anticoagulation | Coagulopathy from large dose or pulmonary embolism from too small a dose |
| History of deep venous thrombosis | Pulmonary embolism |
| Infertility, diabetes mellitus, malabsorption | Cystic fibrosis |
| Recent procedure | Iatrogenic (bronchoscopy, Swan–Ganz catheterization, etc.) |
| Sputum appearance | |
|   Mixed with gritty white material | Broncholithiasis |
|   Pink frothy | Left ventricular failure |
|   Rusty brown | Pneumonia |
|   Mixed with pus | Lung abscess, bronchiectasis |
| Travel history | |
|   Southwest USA | Coccidioidomycosis |
|   Midwest river valleys in USA | Histoplasmosis |
|   Far East | Paragonimiasis |
|   South America, Africa, Far East | Schistosomiasis |
| Prior drug intake | Aspirin, anticoagulant, clopidogrel, thrombolytics, antiangiogenic agents |

**Table 18.6** Physical findings that may help to establish the cause of hemoptysis

| Physical findings | Diagnostic possibility |
|---|---|
| Telangiectasia on lips, skin, and buccal mucosa | Osler–Weber–Rendu disease |
| Ecchymoses, petechiae | Hematologic disorder |
| Clubbing | Non-small cell bronchogenic carcinoma, bronchiectasis, lung abscess |
| Tachypnea, phlebitis, pleural rub | Pulmonary embolism with infarct |
| Ulceration of nasal septum | Wegener's granulomatosis |
| Diastolic rumble, opening snap, loud $S_1$, loud $P_2$ | Mitral stenosis |
| Loud $P_2$, holosystolic murmur tricuspid area | Pulmonary hypertension |
| Unilateral wheeze | Bronchial adenoma, carcinoma |
| Palpable cervical scalene | Bronchogenic carcinoma |
| Supraclavicular lymph node | Lymphoma |
| Localized wheezes, rhonchi, crackles | Area of hemorrhage, consolidation, bronchiectasis, or airway narrowed by blood clots |
| Flow murmur over the chest | Arteriovenous malformation |
| Lymph node enlargement, cachexia, violaceous lesions on skin | Kaposi's sarcoma |

cultures for tuberculosis, fungi, and bacteria) and measurement of the quantity of expectorated blood although, because sputum collection is often unappealing and cumbersome, it is not undertaken.

A chest radiograph can be useful to diagnose the site and cause of bleeding [7], and both standard posteroanterior and lateral chest radiographs should be obtained routinely before bronchoscopy [10,66]. As reviewed elsewhere [11,45, 66,67], both the characteristics of the infiltrate and the side and location of the infiltrate can suggest the cause of bleeding and its site. Specific disease entities such as malignancy, tuberculosis, mycetoma, bronchiectasis, and lung abscess may be strongly suspected from the chest radiograph [27]. Unilateral infiltrates usually indicate the side from which bleeding emanates [4], but chest radiographs showing bilateral infiltrates understandably offer little help in lateralization. Whenever abnormalities are found, obtaining older radiographs for comparison is advisable [45]. For example, abnormal findings can be obscured by aspirated blood or the changes may be chronic and unrelated to the recent hemoptysis [45]. Up to 30% of patients with hemoptysis will have normal chest radiographs [11], which should not discourage further investigation [10]. Examples of conditions that may cause hemoptysis with a normal (or minimally abnormal) chest radiograph include bronchitis, bronchiectasis, small areas of infection, angioma, infarction, broncholith, aortobronchial fistula, or any endobronchial lesion that is not large enough to cause occlusion of the bronchus [27,66].

Besides bronchoscopy, ancillary tests may also be useful. Examples include echocardiography when mitral stenosis or congenital heart disease is suspected, a ventilation/ perfusion lung scan or even pulmonary angiography when pulmonary embolism is suspected, antiglomerular basement membrane antibody, antineutrophilic cytoplasmic antibody, or renal biopsy in suspected pulmonary–renal syndromes.

## Localizing the bleeding: the role of bronchoscopy

Once the lung has been established as the cause of bleeding, attention turns to localizing the bleeding, particularly in recurrent or large-volume hemoptysis, because optimal treatment requires accurate knowledge of the bleeding site [2]. Localizing the bleeding source will also help guide further diagnostic techniques such as washings and biopsies. Using all available methods, overall success rates for specifically localizing bleeding have been 75 to 93% [38,68]. Lateralizing the bleeding source without more specific lobar localization has reportedly been accomplished in 95% of instances [69]. The yield of individual strategies for localizing the bleeding site has been assessed by Pursel and Lindskog [4] in a series of 105 patients with hemoptysis. Patients' self-assessments were least useful, offered by only 10% of patients, and inaccurate in 30% of these. Clinical examination correctly localized the bleeding source in 43% of patients but was inaccurate 2% of the time. Chest radiographs were correct in 60% of patients and no instance of inaccuracy was found. Finally, bronchoscopy during active bleeding was most accurate (86% of evaluations), but was possible in only a minority (20%) of all patients in that series.

Because bronchoscopy is widely considered the preferred initial procedure for localizing bleeding in hemoptysis (whether massive or non-massive) [11,46], an optimal diagnostic approach requires understanding the role of bronchoscopy.

### Indications for bronchoscopy

Although firm guidelines regarding bronchoscopy for hemoptysis are not available, it is generally agreed that bronchoscopy is indicated for patients with hemoptysis and parenchymal infiltrates confirmed on the chest radiograph (e.g. mass, infiltrate, cavity, or lobar atelectasis). In this setting, the diagnostic yield of bronchoscopy has been reported to be approximately 80% [20,70–76], with carcinoma comprising one-third of cases [70].

The indications for bronchoscopy in patients with hemoptysis and either a normal or non-localizing chest radiograph are more controversial. The yield of bronchoscopy may be increased in the presence of several clinical features (especially when cancer is suspected), including age over 40, bleeding duration exceeding 1 week, volume of expectorated blood greater than 30 mL, a smoking history over 40 pack-years, and male gender [69–71,77,78]. Whether to perform bronchoscopy in patients without these features remains a matter of individual discretion. Although some studies recommend that such patients may be observed following a negative sputum cytology and otolaryngologic examination [70–72,77–79], others have recommended bronchoscopy in all patients because bronchogenic carcinoma has been reported in 4 to 22% of patients with hemoptysis and normal or non-localizing chest radiographs [20,73,80–82]. As examples, Poe *et al.* performed bronchoscopy in 196 patients and found bronchogenic carcinoma in 6% and other abnormalities in 17% [78]. Also, O'Neil *et al.* bronchoscoped 119 patients and found 5% with malignancy [70]. In a retrospective review of 478 patients with hemoptysis and a normal chest radiograph, Lee *et al.* reported malignancy in 2.1% and an overall diagnostic yield of 4.2% [83]. Finally, Lederle and coworkers found bronchogenic carcinoma in 4.7% of 106 bronchoscopies performed in men over age 40 with normal and non-localizing chest radiographs [84]. Features associated with bronchogenic cancer in this series included smoking history greater than 20 pack-years and a centrally obscuring abnormality, but not a large volume of coughed blood. Although uncommon, bronchogenic cancer has been described in patients younger than age 40 and bronchoscopy should be considered in these patients as well. For example, Snider reports that 5% of 955 patients with bronchogenic carcinoma were less than 45 years of age [72]. Similarly, Cortese and colleagues report that 5.5% of patients with radiographically occult lung cancer was younger than age 50 [85]. Based on these considerations, the authors' view is that bronchoscopy should be performed in all cases to evaluate hemoptysis unless a clear cause is already established. For example, it would seem prudent to defer bronchoscopy if a small volume of expectorated blood develops in the setting of acute bronchitis. On the other hand, persistent or new-onset bleeding as the infection is resolving should be investigated.

Having performed bronchoscopy once for "cryptogenic hemoptysis," a controversial question is whether and when to repeat bronchoscopic examination if bleeding recurs. Adelman and coworkers [40] reviewed the clinical outcome of 67 patients with hemoptysis and a normal or non-localizing chest radiograph with a prior non-diagnostic fiber optic bronchoscopic examination. During a follow-up period up to 6 years, 85% of patients remained well without evidence of active tuberculosis or overlooked bronchogenic carcinoma, and nine patients died of non-pulmonary conditions. Only one patient developed bronchogenic carcinoma 20 months after bronchoscopy and resolution of symptoms.

Hemoptysis had resolved by 1 week in 57% of patients, and within 6 months in 90%. Only 4.5% of patients experienced recurrence of bleeding. The authors conclude that the prognosis for these patients is generally very good. In agreement with previous studies using rigid bronchoscopy [9,86], most of these studies have assessed the role of a single bronchoscopy in patients with recurrent hemoptysis. In contrast, the diagnostic role of multiple bronchoscopies in patients with recurrent hemoptysis was reviewed by Gong [87] in 14 patients over a 6-year period. Ten patients had two procedures, three patients underwent three procedures, and one patient had five bronchoscopies at various intervals. Definitive diagnosis was available in 17.6% of all bronchoscopies, all in patients with bronchogenic carcinoma. Although the optimal number of bronchoscopies and the optimal time between these procedures were not definitely identified in this series, a second diagnostic bronchoscopy did increase the diagnostic yield and caused subsequent changes in management compared to the first bronchoscopy. In another series, Balamugesh et al. reviewed 2220 bronchoscopies performed over a 3-year period, of which 132 procedures (6.3%) were repeat examinations. Of the 88 repeat bronchoscopies performed for diagnostic purposes, 41 (46.6%) yielded positive results either in the form of diagnostic histology or localization of the source of bleeding [88]. Based on these findings and the report by Adelman and associates that bleeding stops by 6 months in 90% of patients with cryptogenic hemoptysis [40], it seems justifiable to

repeat bronchoscopy in 6 months if hemoptysis recurs after an initial non-diagnostic examination. Although bronchoscopy is generally indicated for any significant or new hemoptysis, it may not be needed in some clinical situations. Examples include: patients with known chronic bronchitis with mild occasional blood streaking, particularly if associated with an exacerbation of acute tracheobronchitis [11,18]; patients with acute lower respiratory infections [11]; patients who have recent documentation of the site of bleeding by bronchoscopic examination [11]; and patients with obvious cardiac or pulmonary vascular disease such as congestive heart failure and pulmonary embolism [11]. Despite these broad indications, the decision to perform bronchoscopy should be individualized and depends on the degree of confidence assigned to the presumed cause of hemoptysis.

### Timing of bronchoscopy

Whether to perform bronchoscopy early (i.e. within 48 hours of acute bleeding) or remotely remains controversial. Table 18.7 presents the three available studies comparing early versus delayed bronchoscopy [4,20,89], all of which show a higher rate of successful localization with early bronchoscopy. However, careful analysis of the diagnostic impact of bronchoscopy has shown that although active bleeding and the site of bleeding are visualized more commonly with early versus delayed bronchoscopy (34 versus 11%, respectively), the timing of bronchoscopy rarely alters the suspected cause of bleeding or overall patient management [20]. Despite this controversy, we recommend early bronchoscopy because localizing the source can be critical if massive hemoptysis develops later, and because early bronchoscopy also lessens the chance that an old clot will be redistributed by coughing or that gravitational pooling from the true bleeding site will occur [46].

**Table 18.7** A summary of available studies of delayed versus immediate bronchoscopy for hemoptysis

| Study | No. | Yield of locating bleeding (%) | | |
| --- | --- | --- | --- | --- |
| | | Bronchoscopy | Delayed | Early |
| Pursel, 1961 [4] | 105 | Rigid | 52 | 86 |
| Smiddy, 1973 [66] | 71 (active) | Flexible | NS | 93 |
| Gong, 1981 [20] | 129 | Flexible | 11 | 34 |
| Bobrowitz, 1983 [26] | 25 | Flexible | NS | 86 |
| Rath, 1973 [73] | 31 | Flexible | NS | 68 |
| Corey, 1987 [28] | 59 | NS | NS | 39 |
| Saumench, 1989 [85] | 36 | Flexible | 50 | 91 |

NS, not stated.

Modified and reproduced by permission from: Stoller JK. Diagnosis and management of massive hemoptysis: a review. *Respir Care* 1992; **32**: 564–581.

## Choice of instruments

The flexible bronchoscope is the instrument of choice for non-massive hemoptysis, because flexible bronchoscopy can be performed in an outpatient setting or at the bedside under local anesthesia, is well tolerated by most patients, and provides an extended visual range into subsegmental bronchi including upper-lobe orifices [7,46,74].

Whether to use a rigid or flexible bronchoscope in massive hemoptysis is debated, but in the absence of a head-to-head comparison, no firm conclusion can be offered. Currently, the choice reflects the user's experience. Many surgeons advocate using a rigid instrument, whereas most pulmonologists favor a flexible bronchoscope. The important advantages of rigid bronchoscopy include improved suctioning capacity and a larger lumen to introduce tamponading materials, perform lavage, and allow continuous airway control [6].

However, the rigid bronchoscope is limited by reduced visual range and the need for general anesthesia and an operating room. As summarized by Neff, in cases of massive hemoptysis, the use of a rigid bronchoscope for emergency examinations seems more advantageous than using a flexible bronchoscope. The selection of which scope to use for hemoptysis seems less important, however, than the close communication between the experienced pulmonary physicians and skilled thoracic surgeon [90].

If the flexible bronchoscope is used and there has been recent massive bleeding, airway control should be maintained by inserting a large-caliber oral endotracheal tube, through which the bronchoscope can be passed [37]. Intubation also allows repeated easy removal and reinsertion in case the viewing lens needs to be cleaned after it is clouded by blood [37,91]. Besides providing airway control, a large-bore suction catheter can also be passed through the endotracheal tube to suction larger clots [92]. The flexible bronchoscope can be used to wash each segmental lobe orifice carefully for specimens, followed by close observation for the appearance of fresh blood [37].

Results of an updated poll of 230 attendees of a session on airway emergencies at the 1998 American College of Chest Physicians [92] showed that 79% of respondents favored use of the flexible bronchoscope through an endotracheal tube; advocates of this approach increased from 48% at a similar session 10 years earlier [32]. A larger-channel flexible bronchoscope (e.g. with a 2.6-mm channel or preferably even the newer therapeutic bronchoscopes with larger 3.2-mm aspiration channels) is recommended when a flexible instrument is used [91]. At times, when the rate of hemorrhage exceeds the suction capacity of the flexible bronchoscope, the flexible instrument can be passed via the rigid scope, thus combining safety (airway control and suctioning capacity) and maneuverability [36,44]. This practice is also used in laser treatment for tracheobronchial tumors [18,93,94].

In situations when uninterrupted ventilation is required, high-frequency jet ventilation can be used with either rigid or flexible bronchoscopy. The open system used in jet ventilation allows simultaneous bronchoscopy, ventilation, suctioning, and localization.

## Route of passing the flexible bronchoscope

If the source of bleeding is known to be subglottic, either the transnasal or transoral approach can be used. However, if doubt exists regarding the source of bleeding, the upper airways should be examined along with the standard evaluation of the tracheobronchial tree. Selecky [7] states that the transoral approach provides a unique view of the posterior nasopharynx and recommends flexing the tip of the bronchoscope cephalad 180° to view the posterior aspect of the nasal passages and turbinates. If an upper-airway source is suspected and the transnasal approach is selected, both sides of the nose should be examined.

## Bronchoscopic findings

Although bronchoscopy remains the best diagnostic and localizing modality in hemoptysis, it may not pinpoint the bleeding at a specific site. For example, Smiddy and Elliot [68] performed flexible bronchoscopy in 71 patients with active hemoptysis and identified a single bleeding point in 46.5%. Bleeding was localized to a bronchopulmonary segment in 38.0% of patients, multiple bleeding sites were identified in 8.45%, and the bleeding site could not be localized in 7.0%. To optimize the bronchoscopic yield, each bronchial orifice should be examined to its furthest extent, preferably to a subsegmental bronchus [18]. Sometimes, using a small-caliber or pediatric bronchoscope may enhance the diagnostic yield by allowing examination of the more distal bronchial tree [93]. Segmental lavage with sterile saline solution may also help identify the source of bleeding, as discussed earlier [37]. All abnormalities must be appropriately biopsied, brushed, or lavaged for adequate specimens, depending on the underlying clinical situation [7]. The bronchoscopist should pay special attention to the mucosa and visible vessels. Obvious vascular capillaries, bronchial inflammation, and subtle mucosal abnormalities are all considered valuable findings [18]. In the 1988 ACCP survey on hemoptysis [32], clinicians were asked to grade the clinical value of bronchoscopic findings and their impact on management in patients with normal or non-localizing chest radiographs. A specific diagnosis (e.g. lung cancer) was perceived to be more useful than a non-specific result, but more than 80% of respondents considered non-specific findings (objective bronchitis, normal airways, or either localized or diffuse tracheobronchial blood) valuable in clinical decision-making.

In the specific setting of patients with hemoptysis complicating renal insufficiency, Kallay and colleagues [95] assessed the role of flexible bronchoscopy. In the 34 patients evaluated, the etiology of hemoptysis was established in 41%; the source of bleeding was lateralized to one lung in 24%. The authors determined that the results of flexible bronchoscopy influenced therapy in 29% of patients, usually when infection was found. Overall, survival in these patients was 47% and did not differ between those in whom a specific etiology was found versus those where none was found; bleeding was lateralized versus not lateralized; or management was otherwise affected by bronchoscopic findings versus not at all affected. The investigators conclude that flexible bronchoscopy has limited impact in patients with hemoptysis complicating renal insufficiency; nonetheless, the possibility of impact on outcomes in even a few sick patients may endorse its early use.

## Diagnostic techniques other than bronchoscopy

When bronchoscopy does not indicate the source of bleeding, other diagnostic tests may be required, including bronchial arteriography, and chest CT. The comparative value of bronchial arteriography versus bronchoscopy has been examined in two studies. Saumench and associates [89] assessed the value of flexible bronchoscopy versus angiography for diagnosing the bleeding site in 36 patients with hemoptysis. Bronchial arteriography was performed in all 36 patients and the bleeding site was identified in 55.5%. Bronchoscopy was performed in 25 patients and the bleeding site was identified in 68%. Arteriography identified the bleeding site in only two of the eight patients with non-diagnostic bronchoscopies. In keeping with other studies, these authors conclude that the main advantage of arteriography is to plan bronchial artery embolization. In the second study, Katoh and coworkers [96] compared bronchoscopic findings to bronchial arteriography in seven patients with hemoptysis. The lesions were located in the second to fifth order bronchi and were either bulge lesions or mass lesions. Intrabronchial bulge was discovered by bronchoscopy in five patients. In one of these patients, the bulge corresponded to the site of an aneurysm in the bronchial arteriogram, whereas in the other four patients, the bulge corresponded to the site of hypervascularity on the bronchial arteriogram. An intrabronchial mass in two patients corresponded to obstruction with focal dilatation on one arteriogram and hypervascularity on the other. These intrabronchial lesions disappeared or diminished in size after bronchial artery embolization. However, some case reports suggest that some bronchial arterial lesions may resemble the bronchoscopic appearance of a tumor and thus predispose to serious hemorrhage if biopsy is attempted [97,98].

Dieulafoy's disease is a vascular anomaly characterized by the presence of a tortuous dysplastic artery in the submucosa [99–101]. Though more commonly seen in the gastrointes-tinal tract, Dieulafoy's disease has been described in the bronchial mucosa and should prompt caution because disruption of the lesion can lead to massive hemoptysis which may recur. Findings that should cause the bronchoscopist to suspect Dieulafoy's disease (and therefore avert biopsy) are a raised lesion of several millimeter diameter with normal overlying mucosa. Bleeding lesions may of course have surrounding blood or clot. Few reports of airway Dieulafoy's disease are available. In a recent series of 81 patients with cryptogenic hemoptysis, Dieulafoy's disease was observed in five of nine patients who underwent surgical resection to control the hemoptysis [100].

Several studies have compared the diagnostic impact of chest CT to bronchoscopy in patients with hemoptysis. Haponik and associates [102] performed plain chest radiographs, chest CT scans, and flexible bronchoscopy in 12 patients with hemoptysis of various causes. Chest CT scans provided unique imaging information in 15 (47%) of 32 patients, including 10 patients whose plain films were normal. However, in only two patients did CT provide diagnostic information not available after bronchoscopy, leading to alternative treatment in only one patient (3%). The authors conclude that although CT markedly enhances radiographic diagnostic yield, the management impact of CT is more meager and does not support its routine use in evaluating patients with hemoptysis [102]. Naidich and coworkers [103] retrospectively correlated chest CT and chest radiographic findings with those found at flexible bronchoscopy in 58 patients presenting with hemoptysis. Chest CT depicted focal abnormalities involving the central airways in 18 (31%) and bronchiectasis in 10 (17%). Focal abnormalities were seen at bronchoscopy in 18 cases (31%) and all were apparent with CT. Malignancy was diagnosed in 24 patients and CT was abnormal in all 24. Bronchoscopic examination was normal in three of these 24 patients (12.5%), but malignant cells were identified on transbronchial biopsy. In 11 (52%) of 21 patients with non-small cell lung cancer, CT allowed definitive staging by documenting either direct mediastinal invasion or metastatic disease. Bronchoscopy allowed definitive staging in only three patients by documenting tumor within 2 cm of the carina. In only six (25%) of 24 patients with malignancy, the CT failed to disclose new information compared to the plain chest radiograph and bronchoscopy. Because chest CT provided no false-negative results, the authors conclude that CT is effective in evaluating patients with hemoptysis. Only 10 patients in the series were evaluated using a specific high-resolution protocol, but results of this protocol or comparison with conventional techniques were not given. Millar and colleagues [104] performed chest CT in 40 patients with a history of hemoptysis and normal findings on both chest radiograph and bronchoscopy. Previously unsuspected abnormalities were detected in 20 patients (50%), seven of whom had evidence of bronchiectasis (18%). Using the contralateral lung of 93 patients undergoing CT for preoperative assessment of bronchogenic carcinoma as controls, the relative risk of having an abnormality on CT in the study group was 7.75. The authors concluded that chest CT scan was valuable in patients with unexplained hemoptysis and suggested that in patients with normal chest radiographs, CT should precede bronchoscopy to direct bronchoscopic techniques to areas of abnormality and to detect peripheral neoplasms and bronchiectasis not visible at bronchoscopy. In another series of 30 patients with a normal chest radiograph and hemoptysis, Magu *et al.* observed that a chest CT provided diagnostic information in 53% [105]. Also, Set *et al.* evaluated 91 patients with hemoptysis and compared CT scan with bronchoscopy for the diagnosis of lung cancer [106]; CT demonstrated all 27 tumors seen at bronchoscopy and an additional seven not seen bronchoscopically. Chest CT was insensitive for demonstrating mucosal abnormalities such as bronchitis, metaplasia, and papillomas. The authors concluded that bronchoscopy should be the first examination performed and that CT should be reserved for non-diagnostic bronchoscopic examination, especially when malignancy was considered [106]. Finally, McGuiness *et al.* [107] studied 57 patients with hemoptysis due to bronchiectasis (25%), tuberculosis (16%), lung cancer (12%), aspergilloma (12%), and bronchitis (12%). Chest CT and bronchoscopy were found to be complimentary, as CT was useful to demonstrate bronchiectasis and aspergilloma and bronchoscopy was useful in diagnosing mucosal lesions and bronchitis. In this study, flexible bronchoscopy localized bleeding in only 51% of the patients, making the CT a necessary adjunct to diagnosis and management.

More recently, multidetector row CT angiography has demonstrated high yield in identifying the source of hemoptysis [108]. For example, in a series of 22 patients with hemoptysis, Yoon *et al.* [108] showed that all 31 bronchial arteries felt to cause hemoptysis at bronchial arteriography were detected on 16-detector row CT angiography. Given the promise of multidetector CT and the fact that up to 41% of patients with hemoptysis whose plain chest radiographic are normal may have abnormalities on CT [109], we consider chest CT a routine testing in evaluating patients with hemoptysis with a normal chest radiograph [109].

The rapid evolution of multidetector row CT and three-dimensional volume rendering reconstruction allow a virtual trip down the airways by segmental computerized linking as in virtual bronchoscopy [110]. Preliminary experience suggests that virtual bronchoscopy has the potential to obviate the need for flexible bronchoscopy in a significant proportion of patients [111], though further evaluation is clearly needed to fully understand the role of virtual bronchoscopy.

Finally, bronchography (i.e. instilling lipophilic dye into the bronchi) can be performed to localize bleeding, but recent developments have rendered bronchography obsolete [112]. High-resolution CT has a high degree of sensitivity for diagnosing bronchiectasis and has essentially replaced bronchography where CT is available [103].

Overall, bronchoscopy and plain film radiography remain the mainstays for evaluating patients with hemoptysis. Chest CT is reserved to evaluate some patients with lung cancer or whose source of hemoptysis is elusive after initial work-up.

# Therapeutic role of bronchoscopy in hemoptysis

The development of several endobronchial topical treatments has revolutionized the role of bronchoscopy in managing hemoptysis [113]. These measures are used mainly to control massive or life-threatening hemoptysis and can be combined with surgical treatment. As adjunctive maneuvers, they help to "buy time" to restore clinical stability and to perform essential diagnostic and definitive management procedures such as embolotherapy or surgery. Treatments using the bronchoscope include lung isolation and airway control techniques, endobronchial balloon or direct bronchoscopic tamponade, cold saline lavage, laser therapy, electrocautery, brachytherapy, and application of topical vasoconstrictors or coagulants. Several of these techniques are discussed below. Others, such as laser and brachytherapy, are discussed elsewhere in this book.

## Lung isolation and airway control

Airway stabilization in focal hemoptysis ultimately relies on the ability of the physician to intubate, protect the "good lung," isolate the bleeding lung, and tamponade the source of bleeding or use different endobronchial or pharmacologic interventions to achieve hemostasis. Available techniques to achieve these goals are discussed below.

When there is active bleeding, the airway can be maintained during bronchoscopic localization by rigid bronchoscopy alone or by use of a flexible bronchoscope through a large-caliber endotracheal tube (ETT). The flexible bronchoscope can also be used to facilitate intubation, change ETTs, and extubate over the bronchoscope when edema or closure of upper-airway structures is a concern [114]. For airway management, the 5-mm outer diameter (OD) fiberoptic bronchoscope is optimal; to use this bronchoscope, an ETT with at least an 8-mm internal diameter (ID) has been recommended in adults [114]. This allows the remaining endotracheal ring size to approximate a 7-mm ID ETT even with the bronchoscope in place. The 6-mm OD flexible bronchoscope is not recommended for use with an ETT [114], except possibly when bleeding is controlled and bronchoscopy is being done only for intubation.

## Double-lumen endotracheal tube

Urgent management of massive hemoptysis must protect the uninvolved lung from aspiration of blood [115–120]. One method of isolating the lungs is to place a double-lumen ETT that can be guided over a flexible bronchoscope [115,116]. Available double-lumen ETTs include the Carlen's tube [115] (introduced in 1949 and less popular now because of the individual lumen's small caliber), the Robertshaw rubber tube [118] (right- and left-sided models), and disposable polyvinyl chloride variations of the Robertshaw tube, including the Mallinckrodt Broncho-Cath, the Rusch endobronchial tube, and the Sheridian Broncho-Trach [115]. Some recent double lumen tube models now have diaphragms on the ventilation adaptors which allows bronchoscopy without loss of airway pressure in patients undergoing mechanical ventilation [115]. Double-lumen tubes are currently available in five sizes: 28 F, 35 F, 37 F, 39 F, and 41 F. The size selection depends on the size of the patient. The largest possible tube through the glottis is preferred because it will have little chance of advancing too far down the left main stem bronchus and creates a better air seal. Using a smaller tube requires more endobronchial cut off pressure, increasing the chance of cuff herniation across the carina with resultant airway occlusion [115]. In general, most adult males can accommodate a 41 F double-lumen tube, whereas adult females more commonly accommodate a 39 F double-lumen tube [119]. The flexible bronchoscope has two roles with double-lumen tubes: (i) to facilitate difficult intubations, and (ii) to confirm correct tube placement and position. Diagnostic bronchoscopy through double-lumen tubes is difficult because of the small caliber of each lumen. Intubation over the bronchoscope usually requires shortening the double-lumen tube by 7 cm from the proximal end to allow an adequate working length for the bronchoscope [120]. A pediatric bronchoscope is recommended for use with double-lumen tubes smaller than 39 F [115,116] because the outside diameter of the smallest adult bronchoscope (4.9 mm) interferes with passage of the instrument through the smaller tubes [115].

The technique of double-lumen tube placement using a bronchoscope is well described by Dellinger [114]. The tube is first inserted into the trachea, either with a bronchoscope or by using direct laryngoscopy; the tracheal cuff is inflated, and mechanical ventilation begun or resumed. The bronchoscope is then advanced through the endobronchial lumen of the double-lumen tube and, for left-sided tube placement, advanced into the left mainstem bronchus (Fig. 18.2). In general, left-sided double-lumen tubes are preferred because adequate cuff seal is difficult to achieve on the right; the short distance between the main carina and the take off of the right main stem bronchus prevents easy placement of right-sided tubes or assurance of an adequate seal. After the bronchoscope is fixed in the left mainstem bronchus, the endobronchial tube is advanced into the left

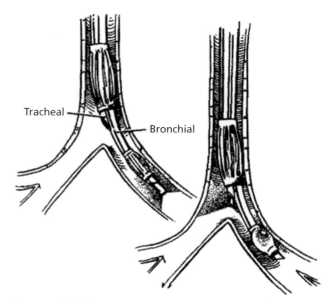

**Fig. 18.2** Flexible bronchoscopic insertion of the double-lumen endobronchial tube (left bronchial type). See text for details of technique. Reproduced by permission from Dellinger RP. Fiber optic bronchoscopy in adult airway management. *Crit Care Med* 1990; **18**: 884.

mainstem bronchus, using the bronchoscope as an obturator. The bronchoscope is then withdrawn and passed through the tracheal lumen. Once the bronchoscope passes out of the tracheal lumen, the left endobronchial tube can be visualized. The bronchial cuff is positioned and inflated in proper position. For correct double-lumen tube placement, the blue endobronchial cuff should be easily seen just beyond the carina, the cuff should not be herniating, and the double-lumen tube should not be too distal in the mainstem bronchus [113].

## Endobronchial balloon tamponade

Another catheter that can be placed using the bronchoscope is for endobronchial balloon tamponade, which has been used to control life-threatening hemoptysis in non-intubated patients [121–125]. Balloon tamponade involves occluding the bleeding airway by inflating a Fogarty embolectomy catheter (4 F for segmental bronchi and up to 14 F for the left mainstem bronchus), which is passed either through a fiberoptic or rigid bronchoscope, followed by removal of the bronchoscope over the catheter (Fig. 18.3) [2]. The balloon is deflated after 24–48 hours and then removed. An alternative approach is to pass the Fogarty catheter alongside the flexible bronchoscope [126].

In 1974, Hiebert [121] reported data on a patient with such brisk hemoptysis that visualization with a rigid bronchoscope could not be maintained. In desperation, a Fogarty catheter was passed into the right mainstem bronchus and inflated with successful tamponade of the bleeding, thus saving the patient's life. Thereafter, several others have

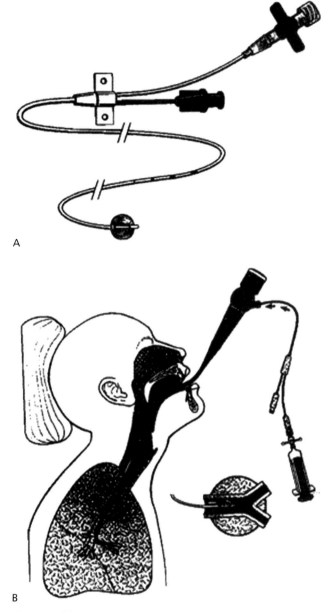

A

B

**Fig. 18.3** (A) Fogarty balloon embolectomycatheter with balloon inflated. (B) Fogarty balloon embolectomy catheter inserted through the channel of the flexible bronchoscope with balloon inflated after insertion.

reported successful use of this technique [122–125]. Saw and coworkers [123] report data on 10 patients in whom balloon tamponade successfully controlled acute bleeding. None of the patients died from hemoptysis or experienced recurrent bleeding (without surgical resection) for up to 9 months of follow-up. In four patients with cystic fibrosis and massive hemoptysis, Swersky and associates [125] achieved acute control of bleeding with balloon tamponade, although bleeding recurred in three of four patients. No complications of endobronchial tamponade were reported in either of these series.

More recently, Valipour *et al.* [127] have reported successful control of hemoptysis in 56 of 57 patients by topical hemostatic tamponade using an oxidized cellulose mesh that was inserted through the flexible bronchoscope.

Overall, although the reported experience is limited, the universal reported success with controlling acute bleeding and the lack of reported complications have caused endobronchial balloon tamponade to be widely used [2]. Balloon occlusion is a rapid method to isolate the bleeding from the good lung, allowing stabilization before more definitive treatment can be undertaken [37].

## Selective bronchial intubation

If the bleeding site can be localized only to the involved lung rather than to a specific lobe, Garzon and Gourin [128,129] recommend a technique of selective bronchial intubation or balloon catheter blockage of the bleeding bronchus. During right-sided bleeding, the endotracheal tube can be advanced into the left mainstem bronchus under bronchoscopic guidance to allow unilateral lung ventilation while simultaneously blocking spillover of blood to the left side (Fig. 18.4A). Because of normal anatomic asymmetry, selective intubation of the right lung carries a risk of occluding the right upper lobe bronchus, which generally rises just below the main carina [37]. Thus, a different approach is recommended for left-sided bleeding. An occluding Fogarty catheter can be placed into the left mainstem bronchus and the endotracheal tube is left in place in the trachea to ventilate the right side (Fig. 18.4B). Of 25 patients in Gourin and Garzon's series [128] in whom single-lung anesthesia was used, 18 patients underwent bronchial intubation or balloon catheter blockage. Only three patients showed contralateral aspiration on postoperative chest radiographs and only one died (of respiratory and renal failure). The effectiveness of selective bronchial intubation allows pulmonary resection or embolization therapy to be performed safely [113]. If medical therapy is indicated, supportive therapy can be maintained [113]. This technique can be combined with iced saline lavage to the bleeding site while aeration is maintained to the other lung and is also considered a first-line technique for managing a major bronchovascular fistula [113]. Another technique to isolate a bleeding lung regards placement of a single lumen Inoue endotracheal catheter with a self-contained balloon catheter. Such tubes are routinely used for single lung ventilation and lung collapse during thoracic surgery or thoracoscopy. The balloon catheter can be advanced blindly or under bronchoscopic guidance into the appropriate mainstem bronchus after intubation. This serves to isolate the bleeding lung and allows aspiration of blood [27].

## Direct tamponade with a bronchoscope

In the event of overwhelming hemoptysis occurring during the bronchoscopic evaluation, the flexible bronchoscope

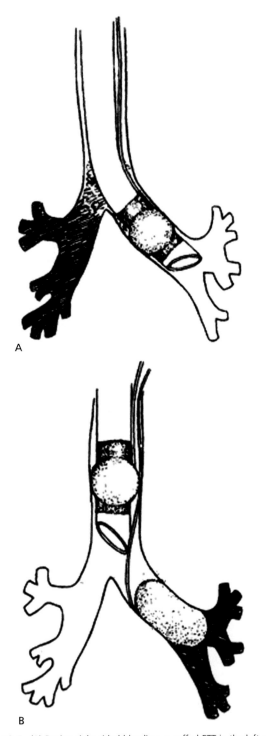

**Fig. 18.4** (A) During right-sided bleeding, a cuffed ETT in the left main bronchus protects the left lung from spillover. (B) During left-sided bleeding, a balloon occlusion catheter inflated below the carina in the left main stem isolates the left lung while an ETT in the trachea ventilates the right lung. Reproduced by permission from Gourin A, Garzon A. Control of hemorrhage in emergency pulmonary resection for massive hemoptysis. *Chest* 1975; **68**: 120–121.

can be advanced into the appropriate segmental or subsegmental bronchus under direct vision to act as an occlusive wedge [37,45]. This is a temporizing measure that allows the bleeding site to clot off while preventing spillage to normal areas. If the source of hemoptysis is proximal and a rigid bronchoscopy is being performed, the rigid instrument can also be used to directly tamponade the bleeding site using the side of the bronchoscope while maintaining the airway [18].

## Use of topical vasoconstrictors and coagulants

Instillation of epinephrine (1:20,000) through the bronchoscope is commonly used with the aim of achieving topical vasoconstriction with diminution of blood flow and thrombotic obstruction of the distal vessels [18,130,131]. Topical epinephrine is effective to control endobronchial hemorrhage after biopsy of a vascular tumor or severe bleeding from the mucosa [114,130]. Following balloon tamponade, regular endobronchial instillation of epinephrine through an irrigation catheter has also been proposed [125]. For example, in a retrospective review of 4273 patients, Poe *et al.* reported that topical application of epinephrine achieved universal success in controlling the bleeding following transbronchial biopsy that affected 2.8% of the patients [132]. However, the benefits of topical epinephrine in controlling massive hemoptysis are uncertain. Vasopressin is another topical vasoconstrictor used for controlling hemoptysis. Worth and colleagues [133] compared endobronchial versus intravenous vasopressin in lung bleeding during bronchoscopy. Eleven patients were treated with 1 mg of intravenous vasopressin and 16 patients received the same dose endobronchially at the site of bleeding. Endobronchial administration was equally efficacious to intravenous treatment, but lacked hemodynamic effects. Ramon *et al.* [134] have described successful acute control of severe hemoptysis in 14 of 20 patients using parenteral terlipressin. Finally, aerosolized vasopression has also been described to control hemoptysis in three palliative care patients with mild to moderate hemoptysis [135].

Instillation of topical coagulants through the bronchoscope has reportedly been useful to control hemoptysis and several coagulants, including bosmin [136], reptilase [137], thrombin [138], fibrinogen-thrombin [139,140], and fibrin precursors [119], have been described. Tsukamoto and coworkers [139] treated 19 patients with thrombin (5–10 mL of 1000 units/mL solution), and noted substantial efficacy (i.e. no recurrence within 14 days) in 14 (74%), partial efficacy (i.e. hemoptysis recurred between 24 hours and 14 days after treatment) in one patient, and failure to control bleeding in four patients (21%). In another 14 patients treated with fibrinogen–thrombin (5–10 mL of 2% fibrinogen solution), substantial efficacy was noted in 11 (79%) and partial efficacy in three (21%). A topical coagulant consisting of fibrin precursors (fibrinogen, fibronectin, factor XIII, and aprotinin) which is activated by adding calcium chloride and thrombin, is described by Bense [141]. With this approach, a four-channel catheter (OD 2 mm) is introduced into the bleeding bronchus with a flexible bronchoscope and the two main components, which together form a fibrin sealant, are mixed, heated to 370°C, and injected simultaneously but separately into two channels of the four-channel catheter. Using this technique, Bense safely arrested four episodes of hemoptysis that were resistant to other therapies [141]. Despite enthusiasm for using topical coagulants for even massive hemoptysis, lack of any controlled comparison and the paucity of available studies advise the reader to reserve judgment at this time. A further concern is that the continuous stream of blood in massive hemoptysis may flush away the fibrin glue before a stable clot forms [18].

### Cold saline lavage through the bronchoscope

In keeping with a time-honored treatment of upper-gastrointestinal bleeding, cold saline lavage has been used to stop bleeding in massive hemoptysis. For example, Conlan and Hurwitz [142] report that bronchial irrigation with 50 mL aliquots of cold (40°C) normal saline administered through a rigid bronchoscope successfully arrested bleeding in 12 patients with massive hemoptysis. The average volume of saline required was 500 mL (range 300–750 mL). The mechanism by which lavage arrests bleeding is presumably hypothermic vasoconstriction with diminution of blood flow and thrombotic obstruction of the distal vessels.

### Bronchoscopic laser therapy, electrocautery, and related interventions

As discussed in a previous chapter, the neodymium : yttrium aluminum–garnet laser (Nd : YAG), applied through either the flexible or rigid bronchoscope, has been used to achieve hemostasis in patients with hemoptysis from airway neoplasms. Also, endoscopic argon plasma coagulation, a non-contact form of electrocautery, has been found to control hemoptysis due to lung neoplasms [143]. For example, Morice et al. performed argon plasma coagulation in 60 patients whose endobronchial lesions caused hemoptysis and/or airway obstruction. Universal success was achieved in controlling hemoptysis with argon plasma coagulation over a mean follow-up period of 97 days [130].

Electrocautery is an alternative bronchoscopic treatment for hemoptysis. For example, Gerasin and Shafirovsky [143] performed endobronchial electrosurgery with the aid of a flexible bronchoscope and a diathermic snare in 14 patients with tracheal and bronchial tumors. Total tumor eradication was achieved in nine patients with benign tumors and airway potency was effectively established in three of five patients with malignant tumors. In one patient, emergent endobronchial electrosurgery successfully controlled massive hemorrhage caused by an endobronchial metastasis from thyroid carcinoma. Compared to laser, advantages of elec-

trocautery for treating hemoptysis through the bronchoscope include lower cost, availability, more rapid removal of tumor by diathermic snare, and the capability for excising tumors with cartilaginous and ostial components resistant to laser coagulation. A limitation of electrocautery with a diathermic snare is its inability to surround the tumor when the base is broad, when the bronchial lumen is tightly obstructed, or when the tumor is inaccessible (e.g. in a segmental bronchus) [144]. Two practical precautions about electrocautery should be noted: (i) contact of the diathermic snare with the tip of the bronchoscope should be avoided because the bronchoscope is not electrically grounded, and (ii) excessive current or pressure while closing the snare may lead to rapid cutting without cauterization of the vessel, resulting in further bleeding. Newer features of bronchoscopes, including improved grounding technology and innovative monopolar and bipolar probes, have made electrocautery a safe and inexpensive alternative to laser bronchoscopy in treating both malignant airway lesions and benign tumors [144].

Other, newer bronchoscopic interventions, like cryotherapy and photodynamic therapy, do not play a role in controlling bleeding because their airway effects are delayed.

### Endobronchial embolization with a silicon spigot as a temporary treatment for massive hemoptysis

A new bronchoscopic technique has been described that involves temporary placement (embolization) of a silicone spigot (blocker) through a flexible bronchoscope in order to prevent blood inundation preceding and during the time of bronchial artery embolism [145]. The spigot can then be removed following bronchial artery embolization. This reportedly inexpensive and simple technique requires a biopsy forceps for placement. More experience is needed before this technique can be recommended.

In summary, although many endobronchial treatments for hemoptysis are available, the paucity of comparative studies precludes a clear recommendation about which treatment to use first. For non-massive hemoptysis, our practice is to instill epinephrine topically, followed by bronchial balloon tamponade. For massive hemoptysis, immediate treatments would include intravenous vasopressin, placing the bleeding lung in the dependent position, and possibly selective bronchial intubation to stabilize the patient while bronchial embolization or surgery is planned.

## References

1 Marini J. Hemoptysis. In: *Respiratory Medicine for the House Officer*, 2nd edn. Baltimore: Williams and Wilkins; 1987: 223–5.
2 Stoller JK. Diagnosis and management of massive hemoptysis: a review. *Respir Care* 1992; **32**: 564–81.

3 Chaves AD. Hemoptysis in chest clinic patients. *Am Rev Tuberc* 1951; **63**: 144–201.

4 Pursel SE, Lindskog GE. Hemoptysis: a clinical evaluation of 105 patients examined consecutively on a thoracic surgical service. *Am Rev Respir Dis* 1961; **84**: 329–36.

5 Abbott OA. The clinical significance of pulmonary hemorrhage: a study of 1316 patients with chest disease. *Dis Chest* 1948; **14**: 824–42.

6 Johnston RN, Lockhart W, Ritchie RT, Smith DM. Hemoptysis. *Br Med J* 1960; **1**: 592–5.

7 Selecky PA. Evaluation of hemoptysis through the bronchoscope. *Chest* 1978; **73**: 741–5.

8 Lyons HA. Differential diagnosis of hemoptysis and its treatment. *ATS News* 1976; 26–30.

9 Barrett R J, Tuttle WM. A study of essential hemoptysis. *J Thorac Cardiovasc Surg* 1960; **40**: 468–74.

10 Wolfe JD, Simmons DH. Hemoptysis: diagnosis and management. *West Med* 1977; **127**: 383–90.

11 Irwin RS, Curley FJ. Hemoptysis. In: Rippe JM, Irwin RS, Alpert JS, *et al.*, eds. *Intensive Care Medicine*, 2nd edn. Boston: Little Brown; 1991: 513–24.

12 Jackson CR, Diamond S. Hemorrhage from the trachea, bronchi, and lungs of non-tuberculosis origin. *Am Rev Tuberc* 1942; **46**: 126–38.

13 Souders CR, Smith AT. The clinical significance of hemoptysis. *N Engl J Med* 1952; **247**: 790–3.

14 Heller R. *The significance of hemoptysis tubercule.* 1946; **26**: 70–4.

15 Moersch H J. Clinical significance of hemoptysis. *JAMA* 1952; **148**: 1461–5.

16 Johnston H, Reisz G. Changing spectrum of hemoptysis: underlying causes in 148 patients undergoing diagnostic flexible bronchoscopy. *Arch Intern Med* 1989; **149**: 1666–8.

17 Santiago S, Tobias J, William AJ. A reappraisal of the causes of hemoptysis. *Arch Intern Med* 1991; **151**: 2449–51.

18 Prakash UBS. Bronchoscopy. In: Bone RC, Dantzker DR, George RD, Matthay RA, Reynolds HY, eds. *Pulmonary and Critical Care Medicine*, Vol. 1. St. Louis: Mosby-Year Book; 1993: P(5), 1–18.

19 Kahn MP, Whitcomb ME, Snider GL. Flexible fiberoptic bronchoscopy. *Am J Med* 1976; **61**: 151–5.

20 Gong H, Salvatierra C. Clinical efficacy of early and delayed fiberoptic bronchoscopy in patients with hemoptysis. *Am Rev Respir Dis* 1981; **124**: 221–5.

21 Prakash UBS, Offord KP, Stubbs SE. Bronchoscopy in North America: the ACCP survey. *Chest* 1991; **100**: 1668–75.

22 Howard W, Rosario EJ, Calhoon SL. Hemoptysis: causes and practical management approach. *Postgrad Med* 1985; **77**: 53–7.

23 Karlinsky JB, Lau J, Goldstein RH. Hemoptysis. In: *Decision Making in Pulmonary Medicine*. Philadelphia: B. C. Decker; 1991: 10–11.

24 Clausen JL. Hemoptysis. In: Nordew RA, Moser KM, eds. *Manual of Clinical Problems in Pulmonary Medicine*. Boston: Little, Brown; 1991: 67–71.

25 Amirana M, Prater R, Tirschwell P, *et al.* An aggressive surgical approach to significant hemoptysis in patients with pulmonary tuberculosis. *Am Rev Respir Dis* 1968; **97**: 187–92.

26 Bobrowitz FD, Ramkrishna S, Shim YS. Comparison of medical vs. surgical treatment of major hemoptysis. *Arch Intern Med* 1983; **143**: 1343–6.

27 Comforti J. Management of massive hemoptysis. In: Simoff MJ, Sterman DH, Ernst A, eds. *Thoracic Endoscopy: Advances in Interventional Pulmonology.* Blackwell Future; 2006: 23, 330–43.

28 Crocco JA, Rooneyn, Pankushen DS, *et al.* Massive hemoptysis. *Arch Intern Med* 1968; **121**: 495–8.

29 Corey R, Hla RM. Major and massive hemoptysis: reassessment of conservative management. *Am J Med Sci* 1987; **294**: 301–9.

30 Holsclaw DS, Grand R J, Shuachman H. Massive hemoptysis in cystic fibrosis. *J Pediatr* 1970; **76**: 829–38.

31 Garzon AA, Cerruti MM, Golding ME. Exsanguinating hemoptysis. *Thorac Cardiovasc Surg* 1982; **84**: 829–33.

32 Haponik EP, Chin R. Hemoptysis: clinician's perspective. *Chest* 1990; **97**: 469–75.

33 Gourin A, Garzon AA. Operative treatment of massive hemoptysis. *Ann Thorac Surg* 1974; **18**: 52–60.

34 Conlan AA, Hurwitz SS, Krige L, *et al.* Massive hemoptysis: a review of 123 cases. *J Thorac Cardiovasc Surg* 1983; **85**: 120–4.

35 Bone RC. Massive hemoptysis. In: Sahn S, ed. *Pulmonary Emergencies*. New York: Churchill Livingston; 1982: 225–36.

36 Rogers RM (Moderator). The management of massive hemoptysis in a patient with pulmonary tuberculosis. *Chest* 1976; **70**: 519–26.

37 Winter SM, Ingbar DH. Massive hemoptysis: pathogenesis and management. *J Intensive Care Med* 1988; **3**: 171–88.

38 Ozgul MA, Turna A, Yildiz A, *et al.* Risk factors and recurrence patterns in 203 patients with hemoptysis. *Tuberk Toraks* 2006; **54**: 243–8.

39 Wedzicha JA, Pearson MC. Management of massive hemoptysis. *Respir Med* 1990; **84**: 9–12.

40 Adelman M, Haponik EP, Bleecker ER, Britt EJ. Cryptogenic hemoptysis. *Ann Intern Med* 1985; **102**: 829–34.

41 Steirnberg C. Hemoptysis of undetermined etiology. *Tex State Med* 1964; **60**: 630–3.

42 Thomson SC. Hemoptysis from the throat (hemoptysis not of pulmonary origin). *Ann Otol Rhinol Laryngol* 1928; **37**: 209–12.

43 Gale D. Overgrowth of *Serratia marcescens* in respiratory tract simulating hemoptysis. *JAMA* 1957; **164**: 1328–30.

44 Newton RW, Forest ARW. Rifmpicin over dosage—"the red man syndrome." *South Med J* 1975; **20**: 55–7.

45 Israel RH, Poe RH. Hemoptysis. *Clin Chest Med* 1987; **8**: 197–205.

46 Ingbar D. A systematic workup for hemoptysis. *Contemporary Int Med* 1989; (**Aug**): 60–70.

47 Uflacker R, Kaemmerer A, Picon PD, *et al.* Bronchial artery embolization in the management of hemoptysis: technical aspects and long-term results. *Radiology* 1985; **157**: 637–44.

48 McCollum WB, Mattox KL, Gninn GA, Beall AC. Immediate operative treatment for massive hemoptysis. *Chest* 1975; **67**: 152–5.

49 Yang CT, Berger HW. Conservative management of life-threatening hemoptysis. *Mt Sinai J Med* 1978; **45**: 329–33.

50 Remy J, Arnaud A, Pardou H, *et al.* Treatment of hemoptysis by embolization of bronchial arteries. *Radiology* 1977; **122**: 33–9.

51 Deffebach ME, Charau NB, Lakshminarayan S. State of the art: the bronchial circulation-small but a vital attribute of the lung. *Am Rev Respir Dis* 1987; **135**: 463–81.

52 Thompson JR. Mechanisms of fatal pulmonary hemorrhage in tuberculosis. *Dis Chest* 1954; **25**: 193–205.

53 Dixon GP, Donnerberg RL, Schonfeld SA, Whitcomb MI. Advances in the diagnosis and treatment of broncholithiasis. *Am Rev Respir Dis* 1984; **129**: 1028–30.

54 Auerhach O. Pathology and pathogenesis of pulmonary arterial aneurysm in tuberculosis cavities. *Am Rev Tuberc* 1939; **39**: 99–115.

55 Plessinger VA, Jolly PN. Rasmussen's aneurysms and fatal hemorrhage in pulmonary tuberculosis. *Am Rev Tuberc* 1949; **60**: 589–603.

56 Rasmussen V. Hemoptysis, especially when fatal, in its anatomical and clinical aspects. *Edinburgh Med J* 1868; **14**: 385–486.

57 Wood DA, Miller M. Role of dual pulmonary circulation in various pathologic conditions of the lungs. *J Thorac Surg* 1938; **7**: 649–54.

58 Miller RR, McGregor DH. Hemorrhage from carcinoma of the lung. *Cancer* 1980; **46**: 200–5.

59 American Cancer Society. *Cancer Facts and Figures 2002*. http: / www.cancer.org

60 Liebow AA, Hales MR, Lindskog GE. Enlargement of the bronchial arteries and their anastomoses with the pulmonary arteries in bronchiectasis. *Am J Pathol* 1949; **25**: 211–20.

61 Tadavarthy SM, KIngman J, Casjaneda-Zninga WR, *et al.* Systemic pulmonary collaterals in pathological states. *Radiology* 1982; **144**: 55–9.

62 Joynson DHM. Pulmonary aspergilloma. *Br J Clin Pract* 1977; **31**: 207–21.

63 Varkey B, Rose HD. Pulmonary aspergilloma: rational approach to treatment. *Am J Med* 1976; **61**: 626–31.

64 Ferguson PC, Kobilak RE, Deitrick JE. Varices of bronchial veins as a source of hemoptysis in mitral stenosis. *Am Heart J* 1944; **28**: 445–9.

65 Thoms NW, Wilson RF, Puro HE, Arbula A. Life-threatening hemoptysis in primary lung abscess. *Ann Thorac Surg* 1972; **14**: 347–57.

66 Strickland B. Investigating hemoptysis. *Br J Hosp Med* 1986; **35**: 246–51.

67 Soll B, Selecky PA, Chang R, *et al.* The use of the fiberoptic bronchoscope in the evaluation of hemoptysis. *Am Rev Respir Dis* 1977; **115**: 165–8.

68 Smiddy JR, Elliot RC. The evaluation of hemoptysis with fiberoptic bronchoscopy. *Chest* 1973; **64**: 158–62.

69 Shamji PM, Vallieres E, Todd ER, Sach H J. Massive or life-threatening hemoptysis. *Chest* 1991; **100**: 78S.

70 O'Neil KM, Lazarus AA. Hemoptysis: indications for bronchoscopy. *Arch Intern Med* 1991; **151**: 171–4.

71 Weaver L J, Solliday N, Cugell DW. Selection of patients for fiberoptic bronchoscopy. *Chest* 1979; **76**: 7–10.

72 Snider GL. When not to use the bronchoscope for hemoptysis. *Chest* 1979; **76**: 1–2.

73 Zavala DC. Diagnostic fiberoptic bronchoscopy. *Chest* 1975; **68**: 12–19.

74 Mitchell DM, Emerson C J, Collyer J, Collins JV. Fiberoptic bronchoscopy ten years on. *Br Med J* 1980; **281**: 360–3.

75 Rath GS, Schaff JT, Snider GL. Flexible fiberoptic bronchoscopy: techniques and review of 100 bronchoscopies. *Chest* 1973; **63**: 689–93.

76 Peters J, McClung H, Teague R. Evaluation of hemoptysis in patients with a normal chest roentgenogram. *West J Med* 1984; **141**: 624–6.

77 Jackson CV, Savage PJ, Quinn DL. Role of fiberoptic bronchoscopy in patients with hemoptysis and a normal chest roentgenogram. *Chest* 1985; **87**: 142–4.

78 Poe RH, Israel RH, Marin MG, *et al.* Utility of fiberoptic bronchoscopy in patients with hemoptysis and a non-localizing chest roentgenogram. *Chest* 1988; **92**: 70–5.

79 Heimer D, Bar-Ziv J, Scharf SM. Fiberoptic bronchoscopy in patients with hemoptysis and non-localizing chest roentgenographs. *Arch Intern Med* 1985; **145**: 1427–8.

80 Kallenbach J, Song E, Zwi S. Hemoptysis with no radiologic evidence of tumors: the value of early bronchoscopy. *S Afr Med J* 1981; **59**: 556–8.

81 Richardson RH, Zavala DC, Mukerjee PK, Bedell GN. The use of fiberoptic bronchoscopy and brush biopsy in the diagnosis of suspected pulmonary malignancy. *Am Rev Respir Dis* 1974; **109**: 63–6.

82 Heaton RW. Should patients with hemoptysis and normal chest x-ray be bronchoscoped? *Postgrad Med J* 1987; **63**: 947–9.

83 Lee CJ, Lee CH, Lan RS, *et al.* The role of fiberoptic bronchoscopy in patients with hemoptysis and a normal chest roentgenogram. *Changgeng Yi Zue Za Zhi* 1989; **12**: 136–40.

84 Lederle FA, Nichol KL, Parenti CM. Bronchoscopy to evaluate hemoptysis in older men with nonsuspicious chest roentgenograms. *Chest* 1989; **10**: 43–7.

85 Cortese DA, Parvolero PC, Bergstrach EJ, *et al.* Roentgenographically occult lung can a ten-year experience. *J Thorac Cardiovasc Surg* 1983; **86**: 373–80.

86 Douglas DE, Carr DT. Prognosis in idiopathic hemoptysis. *JAMA* 1952; **150**: 764–5.

87 Gong H Jr. Repeat fiberoptic bronchoscopy in patients with recurrent unexplained hemoptysis. *Respiration* 1983; **44**: 225–33.

88 Balamugesh T, Aggarwal AN, Gupta D, *et al.* Profile of repeat fiberoptic bronchoscopy. *Indian J Chest Disease Allied Sci* 2005; **47**: 181–5.

89 Saumench J, Escarrabil J, Padro I, *et al.* Value of fiberoptic bronchoscopy and angiography for diagnosis of the bleeding site in hemoptysis. *Ann Thorac Surg* 1989; **48**: 272–4.

90 Neff JA. Hemoptysis. *West J Med* 1977; **127**: 411–12.

91 Imgrund SP, Goldberg SK, Walkenstein MD, *et al.* Clinical diagnosis of massive hemoptysis using the fiberoptic bronchoscope. *Crit Care Med* 1985; **13**: 438–43.

92 Haponik EF, Fein A, Chin R. Managing life-threatening hemoptysis: has anything really changed? *Chest* 2000; **118**: 1431–5.

93 George PJM, Garrett CPO, Nixon C, *et al.* Laser treatment for tracheobronchial tumors: local or general anesthesia? *Thorax* 1987; **42**: 656–60.

94 Prakash UBS. The use of the pediatric fiberoptic bronchoscope in adults. *Am Rev Respir Dis* 1985; **132**: 715–17.

95 Kallay N, Dunagan D, Horman A, *et al.* Hemoptysis in patients with renal insufficiency: the role of flexible bronchoscopy. *Chest* 2001; **119**: 788–94.

96 Katoh O, Yamada H, Hiura K, *et al.* Bronchoscopic and angiographic comparison of bronchial arterial lesions in patients with hemoptysis. *Chest* 1987; **91**: 486–9.

97 Takeuchi Y, Namikawa S, Kusagawa M, *et al*. Bronchofiberscopic findings of bronchial artery lesions: a report of two cases. *J Jpn Soc Bronchology* 1985; **7**: 71–6.

98 Flick MK, Wasson K, Dunn LJ, Block AJ. Fatal pulmonary hemorrhage after transbronchial lung biopsy through the fiber optic bronchoscope. *Am Rev Respir Dis* 1975; **111**: 853–6.

99 Kuzucu A, Gurses I, Soysal O, *et al*. Dieulafoy's disease: a cause of massive hemoptysis that is probably under diagnosed. *Ann Thorac Surg* 2005; **80**: 1126–8.

100 Savale L, Parrot A, Khalil A, *et al*. Cryptogenic hemoptysis: From a benign to a life-threatening pathogenic vascular condition. *Am J Respir Crit Care* 2007; **175**: 1181–5.

101 Loschhorn C, Nierhoff N, Mayer R, *et al*. Dieulafoy's disease of the lung: A potential disaster for the bronchoscopist. *Respiration* 2006; **73**: 562–5.

102 Haponik EF, Britt EJ, Smith PI, Bleecker ER. Computed chest tomography in the evaluation of hemoptysis: impact on diagnosis and treatment. *Chest* 1987; **91**: 80–5.

103 Naidich DP, Font S, Ettenger NA, Arranda C. Hemoptysis: CT bronchoscopic correlations in 58 cases. *Radiology* 1990; **177**: 357–62.

104 Millar AB, Boothroyd AB, Edwards D, Hetzel M. The role of computed tomography (CT) in the investigation of unexplained hemoptysis. *Respir Med* 1992; **86**: 39–44.

105 Magu S, Malhotra R, Gupta KB, Mishra DS. Role of computed tomography in patients with hemoptysis and normal chest roentgenogram. *Indian J Chest Allied Sci* 2000; **42**: 101–4.

106 Set PA, Flower CD, Smith IE, *et al*. Hemoptysis: comparative study of the role of CT and fiberoptic bronchoscopy. *Radiology* 1993: **189**: 667–80.

107 McGuiness G, Beacher JR, Harkin TJ, *et al*. Hemoptysis: prospective high resolution CT/bronchoscopic correlation. *Chest* 1994; **105**: 982–3.

108 Yoon YC, Lee RS, Jeong YL, *et al*. Hemoptysis: bronchial and nonbronchial systemic arteries at 16-detector row CT. *Radiology* 2005; **234**: 292–8.

109 Tsoumakidou M, Chrysofakis G, Tsiligranni I, *et al*. A prospective analysis of 184 hemoptysis cases—Diagnostic impact of chest x-ray computed tomography, bronchoscopy. *Respiration* 2006; **73**: 808–14.

110 Yung RC, Lawler LP. Advances in diagnostic bronchoscopy and advanced airway imaging. In: *Thoracic Endoscopy: Advances in Interventional Pulmonology*. Blackwell Future 2006; 4, 44–75.

111 Kourelea S, Vontetsianos T, Maniatis V, *et al*. The application of virtual bronchoscopy in the evaluation of hemoptysis. Comparative evaluation with real fiberoptic bronchoscopy. *Information Technology Application in Biomedicine, 2000. Proceedings. IEEE EMBS International Conference*; 2000: 246–9.

112 Shephard JO, McLoud TC. Imaging the aneurysm: computed tomography and magnetic resonance imaging. *Clin Chest Med* 1991; **12**: 151–68.

113 Conlan AA. Massive hemoptysis: diagnostic and therapeutic implications. *Surg Ann* 1985; **17**: 337–55.

114 Dellinger RP. Fiberoptic bronchoscopy in adult airway management. *Crit Care Med* 1990; **18**: 882–7.

115 Strange C. Double-lumen endotracheal tubes. *Clin Chest Med* 1991; **12**: 497–506.

116 Shivaram U, Finch P, Nowak P. Plastic endobronchial tubes in the management of life-threatening hemoptysis. *Chest* 1987; **92**: 1108–10.

117 Bjork VO, Carlens E. The prevention of spread during pulmonary resection by the use of a double-lumen catheter. *J Thorac Surg* 1951; **20**: 151–4.

118 Robertshaw FL. Low resistance double-lumen endobronchial tubes. *Br J Anaesth* 1962; **34**: 576–9.

119 Brodsky JB. Isolation of the lungs. *Probl Anesth* 1990; **4**: 264–9.

120 Shulman MS, Brodsky JB, Levesque PR. Fiberoptic bronchoscopy for tracheal and endobronchial intubation with a double-lumen tube. *Can J Anaesth* 1987; **34**: 172–5.

121 Hiebert CA. Balloon catheter control of life-threatening hemoptysis. *Chest* 1974; **66**: 308–9.

122 Gottlieb LS, Hillberg R. Endobronchial tamponade therapy for intractable hemoptysis. *Chest* 1975; **67**: 482–3.

123 Saw EC, Gottlieb LS, Yokoyama T, Lee BC. Flexible fiberoptic bronchoscopy and endobronchial hemoptysis. *Chest* 1976; **70**: 589–91.

124 Faloney JP, Balchum OJ. Repeated massive hemoptysis: successful control using multiple balloon-tipped catheters for endobronchial tamponade. *Chest* 1978; **74**: 683–5.

125 Swersky RB, Chang JB, Wisoff BG, Gorvoy J. Endobronchial balloon tamponade of hemoptysis in patients with cystic fibrosis. *Ann Thorac Surg* 1979; **27**: 262–4.

126 Thompson AB, Teschler H, Rennard S. Pathogenesis, evaluation and therapy for massive hemoptysis. *Clin Chest Med* 1992; **13**: 69–82.

127 Valipour A, Kreuzer A, Koller H, *et al*. Bronchoscopy-guided topical hemostatic tamponade therapy for the management of life-threatening hemoptysis. *Chest* 2005; **127**: 2118.

128 Garzon AA, Gourin A. Surgical management of massive hemoptysis: a ten-year experience. *Ann Surg* 1978; **187**: 267–71.

129 Gourin A, Garzon AA. Control of hemorrhage in emergency pulmonary resection for massive hemoptysis. *Chest* 1975; **68**: 120–1.

130 Morice RC, Ece T, Ece F, Keus L. Endobronchial argon plasma coagulation for treatment of hemoptysis and neoplastic airway obstruction. *Chest* 2001: **19**: 781–7.

131 Zavala DC. Pulmonary hemorrhage in fiberoptic transbronchial biopsy. *Chest* 1976; **70**: 584–8.

132 Poe CA, Pacht ER. Complications of fiberoptic bronchoscopy at a university hospital. *Chest* 1995; **107**: 430–2.

133 Worth H, Breuer HWM, Charchut S, *et al*. Endobronchial versus intravenous application of Glypressin for the therapy and prevention of lung bleeding during bronchoscopy. *Am Rev Respir Dis* 1987; **135**: AI08.

134 Ramon PH, Wallaert B, Devollez M, *et al*. Traitement des hemoptysis graves par la terlipressine. *Rev Mal Resp* 1989; **6**: 365–8.

135 Anovar D, Schaad N, Mazzocato C. Aerosolized vasopressin is a safe and effective treatment for mild to moderate recurrent hemoptysis in palliative care patients. (letter). *J Pain Symptom Manage* 2005; **29**: 427–9.

136 Kaneko M, Ono R, Yoneyama T, Ikada S. A case of aortitis syndrome with massive hemorrhage following a transbronchial biopsy. *J Jpn Soc Bronchology* 1980; **3**: 73–80.

137 Nakano S. Use of Reptilase with an endoscope against bronchial hemorrhage. *Chin Rep* 1986; **20**: 229–35.

138 Kinoshita M, Shiraki R, Wagai F, *et al.* Thrombin instillation therapy through the fiberoptic bronchoscope in cases of hemoptysis. *Jpn J Thorac Dis* 1982; **20**: 251–4.

139 Tsukamoto T, Sasaki H, Nakamura H. Treatment of hemoptysis patients by thrombin and fibrinogen-thrombin infusion therapy using a fiber optic bronchoscope. *Chest* 1989; **96**: 473–6.

140 Takagi O, Kohda Y, Yamazaki K, *et al.* Effect on bronchial bleeding by local infusion of fibrinogen and thrombin solution. *J Jpn Soc Bronchology* 1983; **5**: 455–64.

141 Bense L. Intrabronchial selective coagulative treatment of hemoptysis. *Chest* 1990; **97**: 990–6.

142 Conlan AA, Hurwitz SS. Management of massive hemoptysis with the rigid bronchoscope and cold saline lavage. *Thorax* 1980; **35**: 901–4.

143 Gerasin VA, Shafirovsky BB. Endobronchial electrosurgery. *Chest* 1988; **93**: 270–4.

144 Jantz M, Silvestvi G. Fire and ice: Laser bronchoscopy, electrocautery and cryotherapy. In: Simoff MJ, Sterman DM, Ernst A, eds. *Thoracic Endoscopy: Advances in Interventional Pulmonology*. Blackwell Futura; 2006: 8, 134–54.

145 Dutau H, Palot A, Han A, *et al.* Endobronchial embolization with a silicon spigot as a temporary treatment for massive hemoptysis. A new bronchoscopic approach of the disease. *Respiration* 2006; **73**: 830–2.

# 19 Flexible Bronchoscopy and the Use of Stents

**Ko-Pen Wang,[1] Atul C. Mehta,[2] and J. Francis Turner Jr[3]**

[1] Chest Diagnostic Center and Lung Cancer Center at Harbor Hospital, Part-time Faculty of Interventional Pulmonology, Johns Hopkins Hospital, Baltimore, MD, USA

[2] Respiratory Institute, Cleveland Clinic, Cleveland, OH, USA

[3] Interventional Pulmonary and Critical Care Medicine, Nevada Cancer Institute and University of Nevada School of Medicine, Las Vegas, NV, USA

## Overview and history

Since the publication of the second edition of this text, there has been continued application of stents for both benign and malignant disease of the tracheobronchial tree. The basic precepts for the use of stents and their materials, however, have remained without significant change, and are as reviewed in this chapter. There has, however, been additional commentary regarding the indications for the utilization of stents in benign or malignant disease and the interaction and complications of various materials within the tracheobronchial tree, which is reviewed here, as well as our own experience during the intervening years.

Hippocrates (460–370 BC) first introduced the concept of stenting by placing a reed into the windpipe to aid a suffocating patient. Modern bronchologists now emulate Hippocrates' original work with the current techniques of stenting of the tracheobronchial tree. It would, however, be approximately 2000 years after Hippocrates before a British dentist, Charles R. Stent, would manufacture dental models and splints to provide support for grafts or anastomoses, with his name becoming the moniker for the concept that Hypocrites utilized many centuries before [1]. The subsequent insertion of airway prosthesis to aid the suffocating patient, and thus relieve suffering and improve functional status, has been detailed in the literature since the 1870s [2–6].

As the history of stenting has evolved, so too have the materials with which we have sought to aid the patient in respiratory distress. Early stents, fashioned from rubber or metals such as silver, have given way to the use of silicone, metallic alloys, and hybrid stents composed of both polymer and metallic alloys (Fig. 19.1). Montgomery pioneered the utilization of a rubber-silicone tube in 1965 when he described the use of a hollow tube with a side limb, which protruded through a tracheotomy site for the treatment of subglottic stenosis [7]. In 1990, Jon Franceau Dumon reviewed his experience in the development of a dedicated endobronchial stent in the treatment of external compression of the main airway [8]. In this breakthrough work he outlined his first use of a modified Montgomery T-tube, with subsequent development of a molded silicone tracheobronchial prosthesis. Other researchers have sought to improve upon Dumon's original design with the subsequent development of prosthesis from rubber silicone, medal alloys, or composite stents combining the materials from those previous utilized.

## Engineering and materials

As the history of the tracheobronchial stent has evolved so has understanding regarding the importance of the interaction between the airways and the utilized prosthetic materials and their inherent properties. The airways are elastic structures, which are impacted by the transmural pressure produced during the act of respiration [9].

As outlined in Chapter 4, on applied anatomy of the larynx and airways, the normal adult trachea extends approximately 10–14 cm until bifurcation into the left and right main stem bronchi. The trachea is supported by 18 to 22 "C" shaped cartilagenous rings, which are connected by the membranous portion of the trachea. The average tracheal diameter of 25 mm narrows upon bifurcation, with the average right and left main stem bronchi being around 16 mm and the right main stem bronchus being approximately 2 cm in length and left main stem bronchus approximately 5 cm in length. In addition to individual anatomic

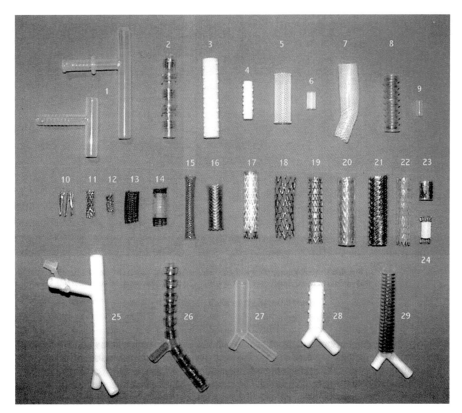

**Fig. 19.1** Selection of currently used airway stents.
(1) Montgomery T-tubes; (2) Orlowski tracheal stent; (3) Dumon tracheal stent; (4) Dumon bronchial stent; (5) Polyflex tracheal stent; (6) Polyflex bronchial stent; (7) Polyflex stump stent; (8) Noppen tracheal stent; (9) Hood bronchial stent; (10) Gianturco stent; (11) Palmaz stent; (12) Tantalum Strecker stent; (13) uncovered Ultraflex stent; (14) covered Ultraflex stent; (15) uncovered Wallstent; (16) covered Wallstent; (17–24) prototypes of stents; (25) Westaby T-Y stent; (26) bifurcated Orlowski stent; (27) Hood Y-stent; (28) bifurcated Dumon stent; (29) Rusch Dynamic stent.
Reproduced with permission from: Freitag L. Tracheobronchial stents. In: Bolliger CT, Mathur PN, eds. *Interventional Bronchoscopy*,. Basel, Switzerland: Karger; 2000: 176.

differences in the tracheobronchial tree and the impact of transmural pressure, the role of tracheobronchial mucociliary transport also needs to be considered [10].

Abnormalities in mucocilary clearance are implicated in a variety of disorders, with cough utilized as the mechanism to aid in the clearance of secretions and foreign bodies from the tracheobronchial tree [11]. This complex interaction of anatomic and physiological characteristics, with the increasing duration of time over which stents have been required to perform, has required advances in the engineering and use of materials for stents. Thus, the current development of stents is being undertaken with an understanding of certain biomechanical considerations, as outlined by Freitag [12].

**1 Airway stabilization.** Any design of a tracheobronchial stent should first have the ability to maintain patency of the airway in opposition to the stress that is imposed upon it by transmural airway pressure and additionally any extrinsic or intrinsic stenosis that necessitate its placement [12,13].

**2 Biocompatibility.** The material chosen should be non-irritating with the goals of easy insertion and possible redevelopment of the mucociliary escalator.

**3 Ease of insertion and deployment.** The stent should be self-expandable, resistant to migration, have the ability to conform to the irregular shape of the diseased tracheobronchial tree and be produced in differing lengths and diameters. It should also incorporate features allowing for manipulation and removal if necessary.

**4 Incorporation of treatment agents.** The design of the stent should allow customized incorporation of chemotherapeutic or radioactive agents for sustained treatment of malignancy.

As is quickly realized from the above list, the ideal stent has not yet been developed. Currently one of the arts of interventional pulmonology is the tailoring of the choice of stent material, size, and mode of implantation dependent on the individual patient's indications, contraindications, unique anatomy, and ability of the interventional pulmonologist.

# Indications

Stent placement is indicated in a variety of benign and malignant conditions. Indeed, 30% of patients with lung cancer will present with central airway obstruction owing to tumor at the time of diagnosis [14]. Prior to the insertion of any stent, careful consideration should be taken to ensure the patient does not have a surgically curable etiology for their airway abnormality [15].

Once assured that a surgically curable lesion is not present, the indications for insertion of stents are defined by the benign or malignant condition present as listed below and delineated by Mehta *et al.* in their review of airway stents (Table 19.1).

Benign obstruction
   Subglottic stenosis [16–19]
      Postinfection
      Postintubation
      Subglottic and laryngeal cysts or webs
      Tracheal rings
      Subglottic hemangioma
      Membranous web
      Tracheomalacia
      Closed first ring
      Trauma
      Systemic disease (collagen vascular diseases such as Sjögren's syndrome)

Tracheobronchial benign conditions
   Post-traumatic
   Postinfectious
   Systemic disease
   Postlung transplantation
   Tracheobronchial malacia
   Benign tumors
   Extrinsic compression from aortic aneurysms
   Tracheal distortion from kyphoscoliosis
   Large airway obstruction caused by esophageal stent
   Congenital tracheoesophageal fistula
Malignant neoplasm
   Extrinsic compression
   Intrinsic obstruction due to submucosal disease
   Tracheobronchial–esophageal fistula [20].

# Contraindications

Absolute and relative contraindications to stenting of the tracheobronchial tree are related to the underlying:
1 condition of the patient;
2 degree and duration of the obstruction;
3 location of the obstruction;
4 available personnel and equipment.

## Condition of the patient

Absolute contraindications to tracheobronchial stenting are few. The patient who is able to undergo surgical reconstruction and cure of the underlying benign or malignant condition should remain an absolute contraindication to the implantation of an artificial prosthesis. As well, those patients who are not mobile and are expected to survive only a brief period of time should be spared further intervention and considered for palliative care. This however does not preclude the use of stents, as well as combined modality therapy in seriously ill patients. In a retrospective review by Colt and Harrell, 32 patients requiring mechanical ventilation underwent combined modality therapy between 1994 and 1996 [21]. Of these 32 patients, 15 underwent stent insertion, (nine with malignant disease and six with benign disease). In this study, with stent insertion and combined therapy including rigid bronchoscopy, 52.6% of the patients were able to have mechanical ventilation immediately discontinued. In follow-up, stent migration or granulation tissue was noted to occur in only five patients, all with benign airway disease and high tracheal lesions. Additional studies have supported the concept that tracheobronchial stenting is applicable in patients with malignant airway obstruction and end-stage disease [22–25]. Monnier commented, in his study of 40 patients with inoperable tracheobronchial cancer, that clinical and endoscopic improvement were noted at follow-up at 1, 30, and 90 days in the dyspnea index, as well as improvement in the average Karnofsky

**Table 19.1** Palliative therapeutic options in major airway obstruction

| Neoplasia | Urgent | Endobronchial | Laser, stent |
|---|---|---|---|
| | | Submucosal | Stent |
| | | Extrinsic | Stent |
| | Elective | Endobronchial | |
| | | Exophytic | Laser, cryo, PDT, electrocautery |
| | | Submucosal | XRT, brachy, stent |
| | | Extrinsic | XRT, stent |
| Tracheal stenosis | | Fibrous stenosis | Laser, stent, dilatation |
| | | Non-fibrous stenosis | Stent |
| | | Postinflammatory | Systemic, stent |
| Tracheobronchomalacia | | | Stent |

Reproduced with permission from: Mehta AC, Dasgupta A. Airway stents. *Clin Chest Med* 1999; **20**: 139–151.

Performance Index from 40 to 70 [23]. A subsequent study by Vonk-Noordegraaf *et al.*, published in 2001, evaluated the palliative benefit of stent insertion in 14 patients with imminent suffocation due to central airways obstruction [24]. Although a small series, the objective of the study was to evaluate the limits of palliation in borderline clinical situations in the event of terminal care. Overall, the average length of survival for patients in this study was 11 weeks with 12 of the 14 surviving to discharge. Vonk-Noordegraff's study is noteworthy in that he included the evaluations of the patient's primary general practitioner to retrospectively judge the ultimate benefit of this palliative intervention. The conclusion was that although the patients presented with imminent suffocation, the use of stents allowed the majority of patients to die at home (80%) with the general practitioners, who were ultimately responsible for the terminal care of these patients at home. It was thus concluded that, in 58% of the patients, stent placement for terminal cancer patients with imminent suffocations was worthwhile. This study is notable for coming from the Netherlands, where the general practitioner is the key figure in home care of patients with a terminal illness and every patient may formally apply for euthanasia.

Relative contraindications are more dependent upon the patient condition and degree of obstruction. Those patients who are unable to tolerate conscious sedation or general anesthesia have a relative contraindication to the current techniques of stent insertion.

## Degree and duration of obstruction

When assessing the possibility of stent implantation, the degree and effect of obstruction must be assessed prior to attempted stent deployment. For successful deployment, an airway lumen with the potential to be expanded must have already have been identified prior to attempted stent deployment. This is determined by the interventional pulmonologists ability to pass a bronchoscope or probe distal to the obstruction to be opened. A proposed classification system for central airway stenosis was outlined by Freitag *et al.* published in the *European Respiratory Journal* in 2007. This suggests that stenosis may be described by the type of stenosis (structural or dynamic), degree of stenosis (percentage of lumen obstruction), and location in relation to position in the trachea or mainstem bronchi [26] (Tables 19.2 to 19.4; Fig. 19.2). The authors suggested this after review of the current stenosis grading systems that were structured primarily in consideration of laryngotracheal stenosis, particularly in the subglottic region [27–32]. The lumen, prior to attempted stent deployment, should already have been identified and balloon dilated or debulked. If a useful airway lumen cannot be identified or the degree of dilation will not permit placement of a stent, then the attempt should be abandoned [33]. It should also be recognized that the condition of the lung to which the newly patent airway leads

**Table 19.2** Stenosis groupings

| Stenosis | Type | Characteristics |
|---|---|---|
| Structural | 1 | Exophytic/ intraluminal |
| | 2 | Extrinsic |
| | 3 | Distortion |
| | 4 | Scar/ stricture |
| Dynamic or functional | 1 | Damaged cartilage/ malacia |
| | 2 | Floppy membrane |

Reproduced with permission from: Freitag L, Ernst A, Unger M, *et al.* A proposed classification system of central airway stenosis. *Eur Resp J* 2007; **30**: 7–12.

**Table 19.3** Numerical assignment of degree

| Code | Degree (%) |
|---|---|
| 0 | No stenosis |
| 1 | <25* |
| 2 | 26–50* |
| 3 | 51–75* |
| 4 | 76–90* |
| 5 | 90–complete obstruction |

*Decrease in cross-sectional area.
Reproduced with permission from: Freitag L, Ernst A, Unger M, *et al.* A proposed classification system of central airway stenosis. *Eur Resp J* 2007; **30**: 7–12.

**Table 19.4** Scoring system according to location

| | Location |
|---|---|
| I | Upper third of the trachea |
| II | Middle third of the trachea |
| III | Lower third of the trachea |
| IV | Right main bronchus |
| V | Left main bronchus |

Reproduced with permission from: Freitag L, Ernst A, Unger M, *et al.* A proposed classification system of central airway stenosis. *Eur Resp J* 2007; **30**: 7–12.

should be assessed prior to attempted lumen opening and stent placement. If the parenchyma distal to the occluded lumen has been atelectatic greater than 4 weeks, then re-expansion is less likely [34,35]. Should the intended lumen track into what is radiographically consistent with lung abscess then either reconsideration of the efficacy of re-opening the lumen or preparation for drainage of a lung abscess should be undertaken.

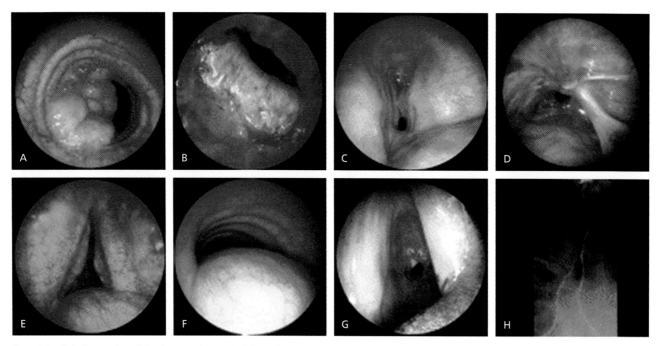

**Fig. 19.2** Clinical examples of the degrees of stenosis. (A) Intraluminar tumor or granulation; (B) distortion or buckling; (C) extrinsic compression; (D) scar stricture; (E) scabbard trachea; (F) floppy membrane; (G) abrupt transition (web stenosis); (H) tapered transition (hour glass stenosis). Reproduced with permission from: Freitag L, Ernst A, Unger M, *et al.* A proposed classification system of central airway stenosis. *Eur Respir J* 2007; **30**: 7–12.

## Location of obstruction

Although there are no absolute location contraindications, stent placement in the subglottic space may be more challenging, owing to close apposition of the vocal cords. Cotton, from Cincinnati, noted that ideally no stents in the subglottic space should be used owing to the fact that the initial insult leading to the stenosis most often resulted from an artificial airway. A stent, however, may be important to hold graphs or flaps in position to support a reconstructed laryngotracheal framework and prevent scar formation [36].

In contrast, Simpson *et al.* reported on the use of stents in 60 patients, with 84% of the patients having silastic stents placed in the subglottic space for internal support [37].

In addition, adaptations of the different stents have been utilized, with Colt *et al.* describing the technique of percutaneous external fixation of bronchoscopically placed subglottic stents [38], and Morris from the United Kingdom reporting on an adaptation of a Montgomery T-tube in the treatment of subglottic stenosis [39]. Also, Miyazawa has made use of some of the new hybrid stents in the subglottic region, as has our group (Fig. 19.3) [40].

Obstruction in the remainder of the tracheobronchial tree is often amenable to the use of a stent. The efficacy of segmental stenting, however, needs to be judged critically in view of the potential benefit or risk to the patient.

## Available personnel and equipment

The equipment necessary is dependent upon the type of obstruction, stent to be placed, and possibility of complica-

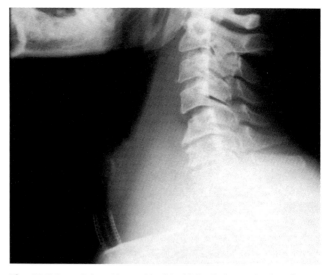

**Fig. 19.3** Lateral chest X ray with nitinol (Ultraflex) stent in place for subglottic obstruction.

tions. Appropriate equipment and personnel should be determined prior to attempted stent placement. The bronchoscopist and his team must be aware that even the planned routine implantation of a self-expandable metal stent may have attendant complications, requiring the immediate or subsequent use of re-positioning instruments such as forceps, balloons, up to and including a rigid bronchoscope and forceps. Regardless of the type of stent used, we therefore recommend stent placement be performed by a team that has been trained and drilled regarding stent placement and bronchoscopic delivery technique. This team should be familiar with potential adverse effects and schooled in the quick response to potential catastrophic complications such as airway obstruction, much as we previously recommended for the performance of laser bronchoscopy [34]. Although the advent of self-expandable metal stents has allowed for placement under conscious sedation, the degree of airway obstruction, particularly in the central airways may require deeper sedation, employing general anesthesia and muscle paralysis. Therefore, essential to this team is the anesthesiologist who understands the complex airway and co-management of the airway with the interventional pulmonologist. Conacher, writing in the *British Journal of Anesthesia*, suggested that TIVA (target-controlled total i.v. anesthesia) is recommended, particularly for those unfamiliar with the field [41]. Often combined anesthetic techniques, to include intravenous anxiolytics and opioids in addition to inhaled anesthetics combined with differing airways to include laryngeal mask airways (LMA), ventilating rigid bronchoscopes, spontaneous respiration, up to jet ventilation, are utilized.

## Stent types and insertion requirements

Because the ideal stent does not yet exist, due to the differing requirements of individual patients, types of obstructions and stenosis, varying personnel and expertise, and equipment, the over-riding principal recommended remains the realization of "different jobs—different stents." Therefore, the types of stents, techniques of insertion, and required personnel may vary dependent on individual patient's situations. The following description of the different techniques of insertion and stent types is intended to be an overview of indications and limitations of differing stent types and not a guide to the individual patient situation. This needs to be determined at the time of the bronchoscopists initial evaluation and treatment in a particular situation presented.

### Rubber and silicone stents

*The "Montgomery T-tube"*. In 1965 a T-tube was introduced as a treatment for subglottic stenosis [7]. Although early models were made of acrylic, these were later replaced by silicone rubber. The Montgomery T-tube has been used to treat stenosis up to the level of the vocal cords and requires a surgical tracheotomy. The stent is introduced at the time of the tracheotomy or subsequently through an existing tracheosotomy stoma. The distal limb of the T-tube is initially inserted through the stoma and then, with the "T" limb of the tube held with forceps, the proximal limb is pulled into place and positioned endoscopically (Figs 19.1(1) and 19.4).

The visible T-limb of the tube may be left open to allow for suctioning and ventilation. The T-limb may be plugged if a more proximal glottic obstruction is not present to allow phonation. This requires functioning vocal cords and oral pharynx to permit speaking. Migration is unlikely owning to the fixed T portion through the tracheotomy site. Obstructions from dried secretions, as well as recurrent stomal infections or granulation tissue, are possible (Fig. 19.5). Impaired vocal cord function may occur, particularly if the proximal proportion of the T abuts the vocal cords and glottic opening.

*The Hood stent* (Fig. 19.1(9)). The Hood stent is a silicone tube with flanges to try to prevent migration. These bifurcated silicone stents have a tracheal diameter of 14 mm and require the use of a rigid bronchoscope for insertion [41,42].

*Dumon stents* (Fig. 19.1(3, 4, 28)). Introduced in 1990, Dumon stents (Nova Tech, Abayone, France,) are now the most frequently utilized in the world. These silicone stents have been designed with external silicone studs to help prevent migration and are available in differing lengths and diameters. A bifurcated model of the Dumon stent is also available for tracheobronchial obstruction. The Dumon stent is very versatile, being held in place by contact pressure between the airway wall and the silicone studs [43]. Placement of the Dumon stent most commonly requires utilization of a rigid bronchoscope and dedicated Dumon stent deployment device; however, additional techniques involving the rigid bronchoscope with the use of a Hopkins telescope or a chest tube have been utilized. Placement without a rigid bronchoscope, using an endotracheal tube, has also been described [44].

Silicone stents for the trachea come in diameters of 14, 15, and 16 mm with lengths of 40, 50, and 60 mm. Left and right main stem bronchial stents also come in diameters from 10 to 13 mm and lengths of 20 to 40 mm. Complications from the Dumon stent are relatively uncommon, with Dumon's experience of 1574 stents placed between 1987 and 1994 notable for a migration rate of 9.5% and obstruction with secretions in 3.6% [45–48]. Additional, larger studies of silicone stents have revealed complications with retained secretions ranging from 3 to 4%, formation of granulation tissue from 6 to 20%, and migration in up to 17% [49–52].

Since the original development of the Montgomery T-tube and Dumon silicone stents, variations in design have occurred in the attempt to prevent complications such as migration. The Reynders–Noppen Tyron tracheal stent with screw threads was reported in comparison to the standard Dumon stent (Fig. 19.1(8))[53]. Their 46 patients with tracheal stenosis requiring the placement of 50 stents were studied and matched for ease of stent insertion and follow-up versus the standard Dumon stent. There was a

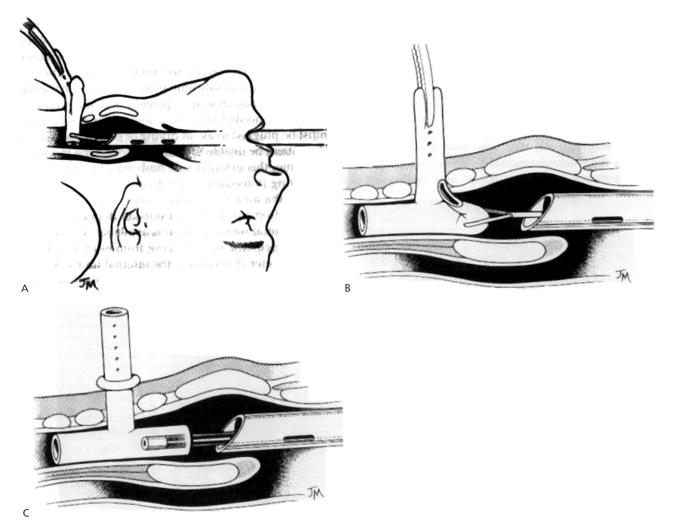

A

B

C

**Fig. 19.4** Montgomery T-tube. (A) Introduction of Montgomery T-tube through tracheostomy assisted with Kelly clamp and rigid forceps pushing distal limb downward. (B) Once the distal limb is in place forceps are used to pull the proximal limb upward while firmly maintaining the rigid bronchoscope in place within the subglottic space. (C) Once unfolded, the rigid bronchoscope is gently withdrawn to assess the distance between the proximal limb and the vocal cords. Reproduced with permission from: Colt HG. Silicone airway stents. In: Beamis JB, Mathur PN, eds. *Interventional Pulmonology*. New York, NY: McGraw-Hill; 1999:. 100.

statistically significant decrease in migration of the screw thread group versus the conventional Dumon stent (24 vs. 5%) seen in patients with benign tracheal stenosis.

## Metals and alloys

Use of metals in the stenting of the tracheobronchial tree is not new. Canfield and Norton implanted a silver tube with subsequent work by Harkins utilizing a chromium cobalt alloy popularizing the use of the metallic stents in the treatment of tracheal and bronchial stenosis [6,54]. Metallic stents made of alloy can be differentiated by underlying composition, biomechanical properties, or in regards their techniques of insertion, deployment, or complications. In this regard, the following metal stents are outlined as to their need for balloon dilation or self-expansion. Metallic and alloy stents have become increasingly utilized owing to their ability to be deployed by means of a guide wire or through the flexible bronchoscope in contrast to delivery using the rigid technique.

### Balloon-expandable metallic and alloy stents

*The Strecker stent (Boston Scientific National Natick, MA)*(Fig. 19.1(12)). The Strecker Stent is a tantalum wire mesh tube with origins as a vascular prosthesis [55]. The stent is deployed under fluoroscopy and when positioned at the site of stenosis is deployed by balloon inflation. Complications with the Strecker stent have included the development of granulation tissue and tumor in-growth.

*The Palmaz stent (Johnson & Johnson, Warren, NJ)*(Fig. 19.1(11)) is also a catheter-delivered and fluoroscopically positioned wire stent. The Palmaz steel stents also require

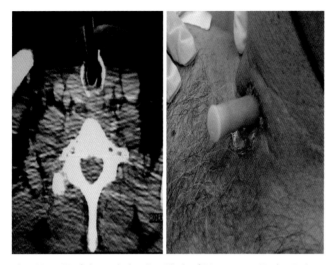

**Fig. 19.5** CT of the neck showing T-limb of Montgomery T-tube. Patient T-limb with formation of external granulation tissue and cellulitis.

balloon dilation and tend to be stiffer. Once deformed by changing respiratory pressure, as with a severe cough, they do not re-expand to their previous diameter and may cause additional obstruction [56,57].

### Self-expandable metallic and alloy stents

More recently, catheter delivered self-expanding metallic or alloy stents have been developed and are increasingly used due to their simplified delivery systems.

*The Gianturco stent (Cook, Bjaeverskov, Denmark)*(Fig. 19.1 (10)). A continuous loop of stainless steel with metal hooks at the end, the Gianturco stent is delivered in a cartridge with the ability for self-expansion when deployed. Difficulties with this stent include tumor in-growth and perforation. Also the metallic hooks make this particular stent difficult for manipulation or removal.

*The Wall stent (Boston Scientific, Natick, MA)*(Fig. 19.1 (15,16)). Constructed of woven filaments of a cobalt-based alloy, it is delivered by means of a guide wire and insertion device, or by means of a flexible bronchoscope through the instrument channel for some models. It has been used for both benign and malignant stenosis with Bolliger commenting on its particular use for hourglass-shaped stenosis [58,59]. The covered Wall stent incorporates the original design of the Wall stent with cobalt-based alloy filaments and a polyurethane cover. This had been designed to be delivered by means of a guide wire and with the ability for self-expansion. The polyurethane covering of the cobalt alloy does not diminish the stent's flexibility or ability to be placed. The polyurethane cover was developed to try to prevent in-growth of granulation tissue. Similar complications exist in placement but, in addition, should a covered Wall stent become dislodged, the possibility of tracheal or

bronchial occlusion exists. The Wall stent with pulmonary approval, which was available at the printing of the second edition of this text, is no longer available; however, some practitioners utilize those marketed for gastroenterology "off-label", although these are not manufactured or approved for pulmonary use.

*The nitinol stent (Boston Scientific, Natick, MA)*(Fig. 19.1(13, 14)). This marriage of titanium and nickel alloy has shape-memory properties, allowing for self-expansion upon deployment, and is also able to be delivered via guide-wire insertion and fluoroscopy [60] (Figs 19.6 and 19.7). The nitinol stent will expand to a preset diameter when inserted and is quickly incorporated into the surrounding epithelium, being covered with ciliated mucosa over a 3 to 4-month period. Although initially this stent can be manipulated by grasping a small loop with subsequent partial collapse of the stent, this becomes more difficult as the stent is incorporates into the tracheobronchial wall.

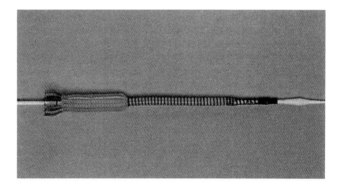

**Fig. 19.6** An Ultraflex stent is seen partially constrained on the delivery device. The stent continues to be deployed by pulling a release sting at the proximal end of the delivery device. The plastic delivery catheter is then removed.

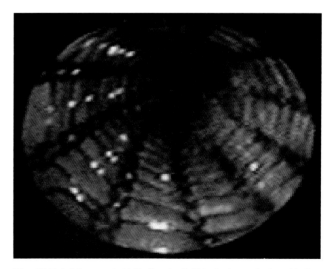

**Fig. 19.7** A full expanded Ultraflex stent. This stent was deployed in the subglottic space as in the chest X ray placement seen in Fig. 19. 3.

## Hybrid stents

Hybrid stents are those that incorporate both polymer and metal or alloy technology.

*Ultraflex (Microvasive Boston Scientific, Natick, MA).* The nitinol stent, constructed from tantalum filaments, also has a polyurethane-covered version. The purpose of the covering is similar to that of other covered stents, and have been placed in an attempt to prevent tumor in-growth (Figs 19.8 and 19.9). The Ultraflex stent may be placed by use of a

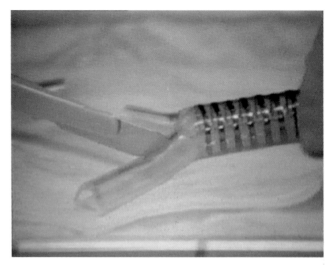

**Fig. 19.10** Left bronchial arm of a Dynamic stent being shortened.

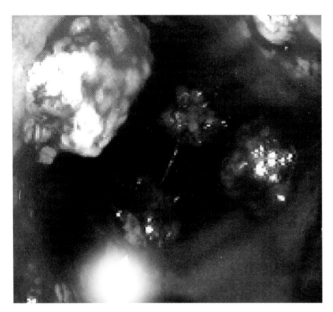

**Fig. 19.8** Multiple polypoid endotracheal metastasis with intrinsic, extrinsic obstruction. Courtesy of Dr David Brickey.

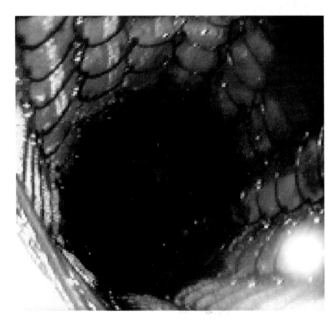

**Fig. 19.9** After argon plasma coagulation a covered Ultraflex stent was placed. Courtesy of Dr David Brickey.

guide wire through a flexible bronchoscope. Granulation tissue may still form on the end of the wire mesh.

*Polyflex stent (Boston Scientific, Natick, MA).* The Polyflex stent is a hybrid silicone and polyester stent. The stent's strength is derived from cross-woven polyester fibers inculcated in the stent's silicone cover. Insertion and deployment of a Polyflex requires rigid bronchoscopy or suspension laryngoscope for its deployment.

*Dynamic (Freitag) stent (Boston Scientific, Natick, MA).* The Dynamic stent is a bifurcated silicone stent with bands of stainless steel incorporated with silicone along the anterior and lateral surface to mimic tracheal cartilages. The posterior membrane is therefore flexible and mimics the motion of the posterior membranous trachea during respiration. The length of the stent may be modified by cutting the tracheal or bronchial limbs to the length desired (Fig. 19.10). The stent is placed by means of a rigid forceps delivery device, developed by Freitag, while visualizing the vocal cords by means of a laryngoscope. We have also been able to utilize a combined Hopkins telescope-rigid alligator biopsy forceps to hold, visualize, and place the Dynamic stent (Figs 19.11 and 19.12).

Silicone stents and hybrid stents with solid walls have been developed not only in order to maintain patency of airways but also to aid in sealing fistulas that have developed in the tracheobronchial wall. Figure 19.13 shows a barium swallow from a patient presenting with cough and shortness of breath, particularly after eating, which demonstrates barium in the tracheobronchial tree. Figure 19.14 shows the patient's bronchoscopy with a tracheoesophageal and left bronchoesophageal fistula seen. The stent shown had been previously placed in the esophagus. Figure 19.15 shows a Dynamic stent in place, sealing both the tracheal and left

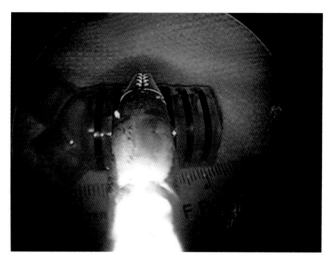

**Fig. 19.11** Rigid biopsy forceps seen with a Dynamic stent in view.

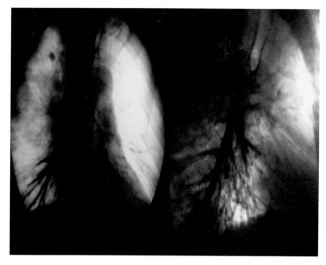

**Fig. 19.13** PA and lateral films from a barium swallow from a patient presenting with cough and shortness of breath particularly after eating, and demonstrating barium in the tracheobronchial tree.

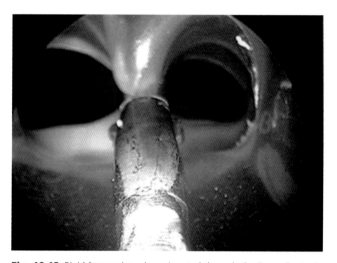

**Fig. 19.12** Rigid forceps have been inserted through the Dynamic stent with the bronchial arms grasped and closed. The view through the two bronchial arms is through the Hopkins 0-degree rigid telescope.

bronchial fistula. The patient was subsequently discharged home for palliative care.

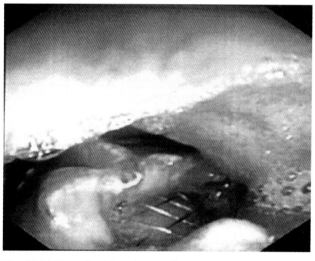

**Fig. 19.14** The patient's bronchoscopy demonstrated a tracheoesophageal and left bronchoesophageal fistula. The stent seen had been previously placed in the esophagus.

## Complications

Complications with stents center on unforeseen problems regarding:
1 choice of stent
2 insertion and deployment
3 migration
4 obstruction and infection
5 stent failure and perforation.

### Choice of stent

As earlier noted, the ideal stent had not yet been developed and therefore the principle of "different jobs, different stents" must be invoked. If the stent chosen for the patient's abnormality does not fit in terms of length and diameter, then the patient may have only partial relief of the obstruction, or may be more at risk from migration of the stent. Also, if an uncovered stent is used where tumor in-growth or a fistula exists then recurrence of the obstruction or continued aspiration may occur. In contrast to uncovered stents, where beating cilia have been noted to be visible through the stent walls, silicone stents and hybrid stents disrupt the normal transport of the mucociliary escalator and result in the collection of secretions. This buildup of mucous, with subsequent drying on the stent, can lead to obstruction and is best prevented with saline nebulization. Concern has also

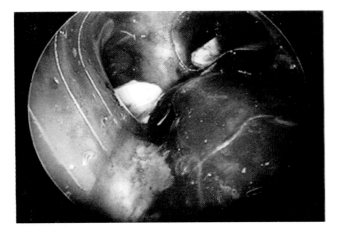

**Fig. 19.15** A Dynamic stent has been placed sealing both the tracheal and left bronchial fistula.

been expressed regarding the interaction of uncovered metal stents with the underlying mucosa. As these self-expanding metal stents exert permanent radial stent forces on the underlying mucosa and superficial tumor, Hauck *et al.* prospectively studied endobronchial histology before and 1 week after stent implantation. They reported a surprisingly low number of re-stenosis during a mean follow-up time of 122 days [61]. Also in their 1-week follow-up study, the pressure exerted by stents on adjacent tumor tissue caused a reduction in the amount of intact tumor cells, with more identification of necrosis or non-tumor cells in the sampled areas. This was most likely due to shear-stress forces causing decreased cell viability in superficial tumor areas, thus helping to maintain stent patency.

### Insertion and deployment

Although silicone stents are easily deployed and manipulated with the rigid bronchoscope, there are times when manipulation and balloon expansion are necessary. This manipulation may, however, be more difficult or not possible when self-expanding metallic or hybrid stents are utilized. Choice of the correct stent size therefore requires extra vigilance to assure proper placement. Figure 19.16 shows a metallic stent that needed to be removed. The forceps can be seen pulling an individual fiber loose in the foreground. The stent was removed successfully but the procedure required additional time as it could not be easily removed in one piece. In addition, the deployment of an incorrectly sized stent may precipitate increased granulation tissue and poststent re-stenosis. In a prospective study by Kim *et al.*, 38 patients had nitinol stents placed for benign tracheobronchial strictures [62]. These authors suggested that undersized stents resulted in excessive friction of the metallic stent on the airway wall and, conversely, an oversized stent caused excessive radial pressure, thus impairing the mucosal microcirculation; both may lead to excessive granulation tissue.

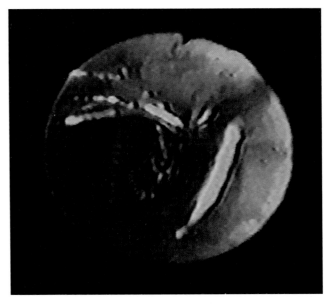

**Fig. 19.16** Pictured is a metallic stent that needed to be removed. The forceps can be seen to be pulling an individual fiber loose in the picture's foreground. The stent was removed successfully but required additional time as it could not be easily removed in one piece.

### Migration

Migration may commonly occur when the extrinsic force generated by the tumor mass is relieved with combined treatment. In benign conditions, such as tracheomalacia, migration rates up to 20% have been reported [44,46–48,63,64]. Migration has been particularly noted in benign disease, such as for post-tuberculosis tracheobronchial stenosis or expiratory central airway collapse, where migration has been noted in 51 and 10%, respectively [65,66]. A study with a hybrid silicone stent (Polyflex) in patients with benign tracheobronchial disease noted abandonment of this stent's use at the author's facility owing to overall incidence of complications (75%), specifically with migration occurring in 69% (11 of 16) patients [67].

### Stent obstruction and infection

With the interruption of the normal mucociliary escalator and drying of secretions, a stent may become obstructed. Colonization of the stent or secretions may occur leading to recurrent cough and mucous production. Nebulized saline may help to prevent the accumulation of secretions; however, routine use of antibiotics is not recommended unless an infection is suspected.

Tumor overgrowth or granulation tissue is possible with all types of stents. Granulation and tumor overgrowth may occur throughout the length of uncovered metal stents and also may occur at the uncovered ends of hybrid stents (Fig. 19.17). In a retrospective review of 40 patients by Thornton *et al.*, in whom stents were placed for benign tracheobronchial disease, 10 of 11 patients were identified by CT as

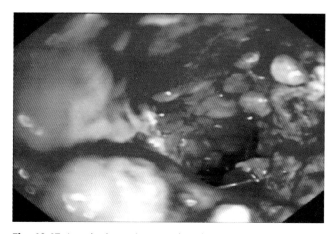

**Fig. 19.17** A tracheal stent is seen to have been compressed and overgrown by tumor. Some of the proximal and midtracheal metallic strands of the stent are seen.

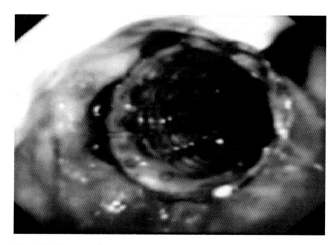

**Fig. 19.18** A metallic stent is seen protruding from a tracheocavitary fistula. See text for full details.

requiring re-intervention to optimize stent patency [68]. Primary patency for these stents, placed for benign disease, was 60% at 1 year, with loss of patency slowing subsequently and 46% maintaining primary patency at 6.8 years. Assisted patency was 90% at 6.8 years. Thornton concluded that metallic stents placed in the tracheobronchial tree are well tolerated for years and can be beneficial in patients treated for select benign indications.

The tracheobronchial tree is mobile and subjected to wide swings in pressure. With repeated movement the material of a stent may fracture, causing the integrity of the stent to fail. Also, repeated movement of the stent, particularly in those with sharp edges, may lead to perforation. This has been seen in a patient referred to our group after receiving a stent and adjuvant therapy (Fig. 19.18). The patient had received a metallic stent for intrinsic and extrinsic obstruction due to a paratracheal non-small cell carcinoma. Subsequent chemotherapy and radiation therapy caused the tumor mass to cavitate and a tracheocavitary fistula formed, with the stent being displaced into the mediastinal fistula.

## Stent failure and perforation

As noted above, the use of some stents, notably the Gianturco and Palmaz stents, were complicated by reports of perforation and breakage. Subsequent studies have noted stent failure is most often related to mucous plugging, re-stenosis due to granulation tissue, strut fracture, migration, and perforation [69,70].

## Stent removal

Silicone or fully covered hybrid stents may be removed by flexible or rigid bronchoscopy, generally without difficulty. Removal of self-expandable metallic stents (SEMS), however, may be challenging, depending on the type of stent and time the stent has been in place. Earlier models of SEMS, characterized by the Gianturco stent, were criticized for perforation due to the sharp metallic points at the stent ends. These same sharp points make removal difficult in conjunction with the epitheliazation that occurs with time, causing the stent struts to become embedded within the mucosa. Removal of SEMS may therefore require a coring-out with the distal end of the rigid bronchoscope or removal of individual struts with forceps, which may be time-consuming process. Newer SEMS, such as the covered nitinol stents, are designed with more-rounded ends, and in the case of the Ultraflex stent (Boston Scientific, Natick, Mass) have a purse string at the proximal stent end to allow the operator to grasp and partially collapse the stent for easier removal. Particular concern has been widely reported regarding the placement of SEMS in benign disease, due to the difficulty in removal, to the degree that the FDA have issued an advisory cautioning about their use in benign disease [71]. Noppen *et al.* described removal of these stents by grasping the extraction loop, advancing the rigid bronchoscope until the proximal end of the stent was within the distal rigid scope, and then pulling both out with a turning motion [70]. Difficulty in removing these stents may be enhanced by epithelial in-growth between the struts or granulation tissue overgrowth of the proximal or distal ends of the stent. Owing to stent epithelialization after 4–6 weeks, Rampey *et al.* described a combined endoscopic and open approach to SEMS removal in selected cases [72].

## Special comments

Stent placement for benign lesions have been described in a variety of conditions including cicatricial stenosis, postintubation, injury, or infection. Indeed, Wang's group described a patient who required multiple stents after falling into a vat of 35% hydrochloric acid with gross aspiration and resultant multilevel tracheobronchial stenosis [73]

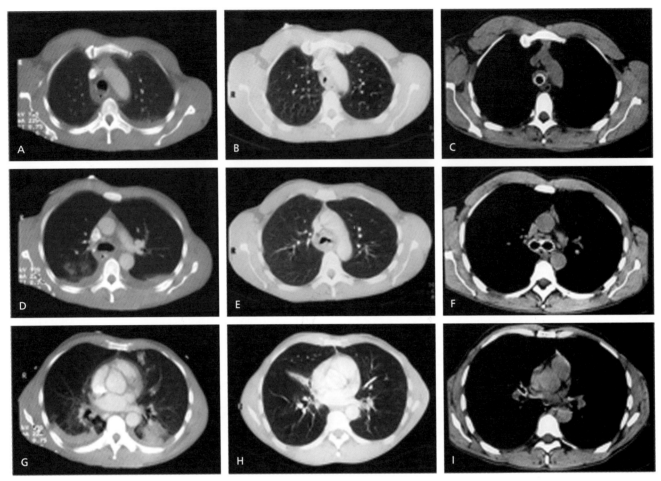

**Fig. 19.19** CT images immediately after the accident (A, D, G), on presentation 2 months after the accident (B, E, H), and status after placement of multiple stents (C, F, I). The representative images are taken at the levels of the distal trachea (A, B, C), the main carina (D, E, F), and the right middle/lower lobe bronchi (G, H, I). Note the pneumonitis present predominantly in the lower lobes immediately after the accident (G) that resolved subsequently (H, I). The marked narrowing of the airways are best seen at the trachea (B) and the carina (E) when compared to his initial presentation (A, D, respectively). The corrections of these strictures by stenting are seen in images C and F. Reproduced with permission from: Rubin AE, Wang KP, Liu MC. *Chest* 2003; **123**: 643–6.

(Fig. 19.19). The use of stents in benign disease has been commented on in lung transplant recipients and, as noted above, silicone stents have been frequently utilized due to their ease of removal. Mehta's group, from the Cleveland Clinic, reported a retrospective analysis of 112 SEMS, with 11 placed for airway complications following lung transplantation and 21 for miscellaneous benign conditions [74]. The median follow-up was 329 days for the lung transplant patients and 336 days for those with miscellaneous airway compromise. Subsequently, 27.3% of lung transplant patients and 47.6% of patients with benign miscellaneous conditions required further intervention for granuloma formation or to optimize airway patency. There were no cases of mucus plugging, chronic cough, fistula formation, or fatal hemoptysis noted. Their conclusion was that SEMS were an acceptable therapeutic alternative in patients with central airway obstruction who were not considered good surgical candidates. A subsequent retrospective study, by Gottlieb *et al.* from Hanover, Germany, detailed the use of SEMS in lung transplant patients. These authors reviewed 111 lung transplant patients, between January 1998 and February 2008, who had SEMS placed for symptomatic obstructive lesions with a diameter of less than 5 mm or extensive anastomotic dehiscence [75]. Eighty percent of patients experienced relief of clinical symptoms leading to stent insertion, with short-term (<30 days) complications related to mucus plugging (seven patients) and migration (two patients). Late complications, with a median time of follow-up of 777 days, were noted in 52 of 65 (80%) of patients. These were re-stenosis [34], bacterial colonization [26], stent fracture (six), hemoptysis (seven), and atelectasis (three). One patient died of fatal hemoptysis with autopsy revealing invasive *Aspergillus* at the graft site, without bleeding at the stent. The authors concluded that their re-stenosis rate of 52% was higher than in other studies (10–47% for benign and malignant disease) and attributed this to a longer follow-up and the use of mainly non-covered stents. These authors and other groups have reported a high rate of bacterial airway colonization—77% in the current study and 56% noted by Burns *et al.*, both utilizing SEMS in lung transplant patients [76]. In comparison, Noppen *et al.* reported an 80% incidence of bacterial colonization after placement of silicone stents in non-transplant patients [77]. Interestingly, in the report by Burns *et al.*, although airway colonization was noted as above, the incidence of pulmonary infection was actually reduced for up to 1 year after stent placement, which was thought to be due to patency of the airway and improved lung function.

Despite these complications, tracheobronchial stents are generally well tolerated and have remained in place for years without difficulty. Routine surveillance bronchoscopy was recently noted by Matsuo and Colt to be unnecessary after silicone stent insertion and repeat bronchoscopy should be performed dependent upon the patient's development of new symptoms [78].

Overall, the ideal stent has not yet been developed. Current placement techniques through the flexible bronchoscope with the aid of a guide wire are not suited to all situations and the use of a rigid bronchoscope in the placement of a stent or its removal may be required. Additional work in the area of biodegradable stents, as well as materials that can deliver chemotherapeutic or radioactive agents, are the subject of active research. As the ideal stent does not exist we return to a basic principal "different jobs, different stents". The bronchoscopist and team placing stents should critically evaluate the patient prior to any planned implantation and have the tools necessary for manipulation and rapid removal with protection of the airway if necessary. As such, a bronchoscopist should be available with training not only in stent placement, but also in rigid bronchoscopy and additional interventional techniques, such as laser or electrocautery if necessary. Also, prospective studies comparing these differing approaches, types of tracheobronchial stenosis, outcomes, and materials should be performed.

# References

1 *Taber's Cyclopedia Medical Dictionary*. Philadelphia: Davis Company; 1989.

2 Trendelenburg F. Beatrice zoo den Operationen an den Luftwegen. *Lange Becks Arch Chir* 1872; **13**: 335.

3 Bond CJ. Note on the treatment of tracheal stenosis by a new T-shaped tracheostomy tube. *Lancet* 1891; **i**: 539–40.

4 Burnings W, Albrecht W. *Directed Endoskopie der Loft- und Speisewege*. Stuttgart: Eke; 1915: 134–8.

5 Canfield N, Norton N. Bony stenosis of the larynx. *Ann Tool Rhino Laryngol* 1949; **58**: 559–65.

6 Harkins WB. An endobronchial metallic prosthesis in the treatment of stenosis of the Trachea. *Ann Otol Rhinol Laryngol* 1952; **61**: 663–75.

7 Montgomery WW. T-tube tracheal stent. *Arch Otolaryngol* 1965; **82**: 320–1.

8 Dumon JF. A dedicated tracheobronchial stent. *Chest* 1990; **97**: 328–32.

9 Rotate JR, Shardonofsky FR. Respiratory system mechanics. In: Murray JF, Navel JA, eds. *Textbook of Respiratory Medicine*, 3rd edn. Philadelphia, PA: WB Saunders and Co; 2000: 91–117.

10 Yeates DB, Bess Eris GJ, Wong LB. Physiochemical properties of mucous and its propulsion. In: Crystal RG, West JB, Weibel ER, *et al.*, eds. *The Lung: Scientific Foundations*. Philadelphia: Lippincott-Raven; 1997: 487–503.

11 Yates DB, Mortensen J. Deposition and clearance. In: Murray JF, Navel JA, eds. *Textbook of Respiratory Medicine*, 3rd edn. Philadelphia, PA: WB Saunders and Co; 2000: 349–79.

12 Freitag L. Tracheobronchial stents. In: Straus J, ed. *Pulmonary Endoscopy and Biopsy Techniques*. European Respiratory Monograph. Sheffield, UK: European Respiratory Society Journals; 1998: 79–105.

13 Freitag L, Eicker K, Donavan TJ, *et al*. Mechanical properties of airway stents. *J Bronchol* 1995; **2**: 270–8.

14 Dutau H, Toutblanc B, Lamb C, *et al*. Use of the Dumon Y-Stent in the management of malignant disease involving the carina. A retrospective review of 86 patients. *Chest* 2004; **126**: 951–8.

15 Grillo HC, Mathisen DJ. Surgical management of tracheal strictures. *Surg Clin North Am* 1988; **68**: 511–24.

16 Siegal PD, Katz J. Respiratory complications of gastroesophgeal reflux disease. Primary care. *Clin Office Pract* 1996; **23**: 433–41.

17 Cohen LF. Stridor and upper airway obstruction in children. *Pediatr Rev* 2000; **21**: 4–5.

18 Sano H, Kita Y, Nowata Y, *et al*. Case of Recurrent subglottic stenosis later followed by the development of Wegener's granulomatosis. *Nippon Naika Gakka Zasshi* 1999; **88**: 2469–70.

19 Freidman EM, Healy GB, McGill TJ. Carbon dioxide laser management of subglottic and tracheal Stenosis. *Otolaryngol Clin North Am* 1983; **16**: 871.

20 Mehta AC, Dasgupta A. Airway stents. *Clin Chest Med* 1999; **20**: 139–51.

21 Colt HG, Harell JH. Therapeutic rigid bronchoscopy allows level of care changes in patients with acute respiratory failure from central airways obstruction. *Chest* 1997; **112**: 202–6.

22 Sutedja G, Schrage F, van Kralingen K, *et al*. Stent placement is justifiable in end stage patients with malignant airway tumor. *Respiration* 1995; **62**: 148–50.

23 Monnier P, Muddy A, Stanzel F, *et al*. The use of the covered Wallstent for the palliative treatment of inoperable tracheabronchial cancers: a prospective, multicenter study. *Chest* 1996; **110**: 1161–8.

24 Vonk-Noordegraaf A, Postmus PE, Sutedja TG. Tracheobronchial stenting in the terminal care of cancer patients with central airways obstruction *Chest* 2001; **120**: 1811–14.

25 Chawla M, Finley D. Outcomes after airway stenting: how do we know it is the right move? *Am J Respir Crit Care Med* 2009; **179**: A6161.

26 Freitag L, Ernst A, Unger M, *et al*. A proposed classification system of central airway stenosis. *Eur Respir J* 2007; **30**: 7–12.

27 Cotton RT. Pediatric laryngotracheal stenosis. *J Pediatr Surg* 1984; **19**: 699–704.

28 Grundfast KM, Morris MS, Bentley C. Subglottic stenosis: retrospective analysis and proposal for standard reporting system. *Ann Otol Rhinol Laryngol* 1987; **96**: 101–5.

29 McCaffrey TV. Classification of laryngotracheal stenosis. *Laryngoscope* 1992; **102**: 1335–40.

30 Grille HC, Mark EJ, Mathisen DJ, *et al.* Idiopathic laryngotracheal stenosis and its management. *Ann Thorac Surg* 1993; **56**: 80–7.

31 Anand VK, Alomar G, Warren ET. Surgical considerations in tracheal stenosis. *Laryngoscope* 1992; **102**: 237–43.

32 Myer CM 3rd, O'Connor DM, Cotton RT. Proposed grading system for subglottic stenosis based on endotracheal tube sizes. *Ann Otol Rhinol Laryngeal* 1994; **103**: 319–23.

33 Hauck RW, Lembeck RM, Emslander HP, *et al.* Implantation of accuflex and strecker stents in malignant bronchial stenosis by flexible bronchoscopy. *Chest* 1997; **112**: 134–44.

34 Turner JF, Wang KP. Endobronchial laser therapy. *Clin Chest Med* 1999; **20**: 107–22.

35 Mehta AC, Lee FYW, DeBoer GE. Flexible bronchoscopy and the use of lasers. In: Wang KP, Mehta AC, eds. *Flexible Bronchoscopy*, 1st edn. Cambridge, MA: Blackwell Science; 1995: 247–74.

36 Cotton RT. Update on the pediatric airway. management of subglottic stenosis. *Otolaryngol Clin North Am* 2000; **33**: 111–30.

37 Simpson GT, Strong MS, Healy GB, *et al.* Predictive factors of success or failure in the endoscopic management of laryngeal and tracheal stenosis. *Ann Otol Rhinol Laryngol* 1982; **91**: 384–8.

38 Colt HG, Harrell J, Newman TR, *et al.* External fixation of subglottic tracheal stents. *Chest* 1984; **105**: 1653.

39 Morris DP, Malik T, Rothera MP. Combined 'trachea-stent': a useful option in the treatment of complex case of subglottic stenosis. *J Laryngol Otol* 2001; **115**: 430–3.

40 Miyazawa T, Yamakito M, Ikeda S, *et al.* Implantation of ultraflex nitinol stents in malignant tracheobronchial stenoses. *Chest* 2000; **118**: 959–65.

41 Conacher ID. Anesthesia and tracheobronchial stenting for central airway obstruction in adults. *Br J Anaesth* 2003; **90**: 367–74.

42 Acuff Tea E, Mack MJ, Ryan WH. Simplified placement of silicone tracheal y-stent. *Ann Thorac Surg* 1994; **57**: 496–7.

43 Freitag L. Tracheobronchial stents. In: Strausz J, ed. *Pulmonary Endoscopy and Biopsy Techniques. European Respiratory Monograph*, Vol. 3. European Respiratory Society; 1998: 79–105.

44 Nomori H, Horio H, Suemasu K. Dumon stent placement via endotracheal tube. *Chest* 1999; **115**: 582–3.

45 Dumon JF. A dedicated tracheobronchial stent. *Chest* 1990; **97**: 328–32.

46 Strausz J. Management of postintubation tracheal stenosis with stent implantation. *J Bronchol* 1997; **4**: 294–6.

47 Becker HD. Stenting the central airways. *J Bronchol* 1995; **2**: 98–106.

48 Dumon JF, Cavaliere S, Diaz-Jimenez JP, *et al.* Seven-year experience with the Dumon prosthesis. *J Bronchol* 1996; **3**: 6–10.

49 Colt HG, Dumon JF. Tracheobronchial stents: indications and applications. *Lung Cancer* 1993; **9**: 301–6.

50 Bolliger CT, Probst R, Tschopp K, *et al.* Silicone stents and the management of inoperable tracheobronchial stenosis: indications and limitations. *Chest* 1993; **104**: 1653–9.

51 Sonett JR, Keenan RJ, Ferson PF, *et al.* Endobronchial management of benign malignant and lung tranplantation airway stenosis. *Ann Thorc Surg* 1995; **59**: 1417–22.

52 Martinez-Ballarin JI, Diaz-Jimenez JP, Castro MJ, *et al.* Silicone stents in the management of benign tracheobronchial stenosis: tolerance and early results in 63 patients. *Chest* 1996; **109**: 626–9.

53 Noppen M, Meysman M, Claes I, *et al.* Screw-thread vs. Dumon endoprostheis in the management of tracheal stenosis. *Chest* 1999; **115**: 532–5.

54 Canfield N, Norton N. Bony stenosis of the larynx. *Ann Oto Rhino Laryngol* 1949; **58**: 559–65.

55 Strecker EP, Liermann D, Barth KH, *et al.* Expandable tubular stents for treatment of arterial occlusive diseases: Experimental and clinical results. *Radiology* 1990; **175**: 87–102.

56 Palmaz J. Balloon expandable intravascular stent. *AJR Am J Roentgenol* 1988; **150**: 1263–9.

57 Freitag L, Eicker K, Donavan TJ, *et al.* Mechanical properties of airway stents. *J Bronchol* 1995; **2**: 270–8.

58 Bolliger CT, Heitz M, Hauser R, *et al.* An airway Wallstent for the treatment of tracheobronchial malignancies. *Thorax* 1996; **51**: 1127–9.

59 Bolliger CT, Arnoux A, Oeggerli MB, *et al.* Covered Wallstent insertion in a patient with conical tracheobronchial stenosis. *J Bronchol* 1995; **2**: 215–18.

60 Buehler WF, Gilfrich JV, Wiley RC. Effect of low-temperature phase changes of the mechanical properties of alloys near composition TiNi. *J Appl Phys* 1963; **34**: 1475–7.

61 Hauck RW, Barbur M, Lembeck R. Cellular composition of stent-penetrating tissue. *Chest* 2002; **122**: 1615–21.

62 Kim JH, Shin JH, Song HY, *et al.* Benign tracheobronchial strictures: long-term results and factors affecting airway patency after temporary stent placement. *Am J Radiol* 2007; **188**: 1033–8.

63 Orlowski TM. Palliative intubation of the tracheobronchial tree. *J Thorac Cardiovasc Surg* 1987; **94**: 343–8.

64 Monnier P, Mudry A, Stanzel F, *et al.* The use of covered Wallstent for the palliative treatment of inoperable tracheobronchial cancers. A prospective multicenter study. *Chest* 1996; **110**: 1161–8.

65 Kim YJ, Yu CM, Choi JC, *et al.* Use of silicone stents for the management of post-tuberculosis tracheobronchial stenosis. *Eur Respir J* 2006; **28**: 1029–35.

66 Murgu SD, Colt HG. Complications of silicone stent insertion in patients with expiratory central airway collapse. *Ann Thorac Surg* 2007; **84**: 1870–7.

67 Gildea TR, Murthy SC, Sahoo D, *et al.* Performance of a self-expanding silicone stent in palliation of benign airway conditions. *Chest* 2006; **130**: 1419–23.

68 Thornton RH, Gordon RL, Kerlan RK, *et al.* Outcomes of tracheobronchial stent placement for benign disease. *Radiology* 2006; **240**: 273–82.

69 Chin CS, Little V, Yun J, *et al.* Airways stents. *Ann Thorac Surg* 2008; **85**: S792–6.

70 Noppen M, Stratakos G, D'Haese J, *et al.* Removal of covered self-expandable metallic airway stents in benign

disorders. indications, technique, and outcomes. *Chest* 2005; **127**: 482–7.

71 Lund ME, Force S. Airway stenting for patients with benign airway disease and the food and drug administration advisory. A call for restraint. *Chest* 2007; **132**: 1107–8.

72 Rampey AM, Silvestri GA, Gillespie MB. Combined endoscopic and open approach to the removal of expandable metallic tracheal stent. *Arch Otolaryngol Head Neck Surg* 2007; **133**: 37–41.

73 Rubin AE, Wang KP, Liu MC. Tracheobronchial stenosis from acid aspiration presenting as asthma. *Chest* 2003; **123**: 643–6.

74 Saad CP, Murthy S, Krizmanaich G. Self-expandable metallic airway stents and flexible bronchoscopy long-term outcomes analysis. *Chest* 2003; **124**: 1993–9.

75 Gottlieb J, Fuehner T, Dierich M. Are metallic stents really safe? A long-term analysis in lung transplant recipients. *Eur Respir J* 2009; **34**: 1417–22.

76 Burns KEA, Orons PD, Dauber JH. Endobronchial metallic stent placement for airway complications after lung transplantation: longitudinal results. *Ann Thorac Surg* 2002; **74**: 1934–41.

77 Noppen M, Peirard D, Meysman M. Bacterial colonization of central airways after stenting. *Am J Respir Crit Care Med* 1999; **160**: 672–7.

78 Matsuo T, Colt HG. Evidence against routine scheduling of surveillance bronchoscopy after stent insertion. *Chest* 2000; **118**: 1455–9.

# 20 Photodynamic Therapy in Lung Cancer

## Harubumi Kato,[1,2] Jitsuo Usuda,[2] and Yasufumi Kato[2]

[1]Department of Thoracic Surgery, Niizashiki Central General Hospital, Saitrama, Japan
[2]Department of Surgery, Tokyo Medical University, Tokyo, Japan

## Introduction

Lung cancer is the leading cause of death from cancer throughout the world, mainly because of the high prevalence of tobacco smoking and frequent detection of this cancer only at a late stage. Although surgical resection is the best therapeutic approach, surgery can prove to be difficult, as many patients also suffer from impaired lung function due to chronic obstructive pulmonary disease (COPD) caused by tobacco smoking. In addition, up to 10% of patients undergoing resection develop a second primary lung cancer over time, and a second resection might not be feasible at all. At present, there is a high demand for non-invasive, safe, and accurate therapies. Thus, therapeutic approaches that spare functional lung tissue, especially in conditions involving only the airways, are becoming increasingly attractive.

## Principle of photodynamic therapy

### Mechanism

Numerous reports on tissue destruction accomplished by photodynamic therapy (PDT) have been published since the 1980s [1–7]. When a photosensitizer localized in the target tissue is activated by light, it produces tissue destruction. On exposure to light of an appropriate wavelength, the photosensitized compound absorbs the light energy and becomes excited to the singlet status. Then, singlet oxygen can be produced in the tissue when the energy at the singlet status of the photosensitizer is transferred to the triplet status oxygen in the tissue. This reaction seems to depend mainly on the type II photo-oxidative process. In addition, the neovascular endothelium of tumors is highly susceptible to PDT, with loss of capillary integrity observed soon after treatment [8,9].

## Immunological aspects of photodynamic therapy

It has been reported that PDT induces direct tumor cell kill, and also acts indirectly on the tumor by changing the tumor microenvironment [9]. Sitnik et al. reported that the microvasculature damage induced by PDT is readily observable histologically, and that it is associated with a significant decrease in blood flow and severe hypoxia in the tumor [10]. Ferrario et al. reported that the reduction in vascular perfusion associated with PDT-mediated injury of the microvasculature produced tumor tissue hypoxia, which, in turn, induced vascular endothelial growth factor (VEGF) expression via activation of the hypoxia-inducible factor-1 (HIF-1) transcription factor [11]. Usuda et al. demonstrated, using VEGF-overexpressing cells (SBC-3/VEGF), that PDT using ATX-s10 (Na), a novel second-generation photosensitizer, prevents tumor recurrence despite induction of VEGF and promotion of tumor angiogenesis [12]. Usuda et al. previously reported that PDT using mono-L-aspartyl chlorine e6 (NPe6) induced the expressions of certain kinds of cytokines, for example IL-2, IL-6, IL-12 and TNF-alpha, in tumors [13]. Recently, we evaluated, both in vitro and in vivo, the role of cytokine expressions on the antitumor effects of PDT using cytokine-overexpressing cells, in order to elucidate the precise mechanisms underlying the effects of NPe6-PDT [14]. IL-2 expression may play an unfavorable role in attenuation of the antitumor effects of NPe6-PDT. It is suggested that the cell death caused by PDT was inhibited by induction of Gadd-45 alpha (growth arrest and DNA damage 45 alpha) expression and that tumor recurrence was

Flexible Bronchoscopy, Third Edition. Edited by Ko-Pen Wang, Atul C. Mehta, J. Francis Turner.

promoted by the enhancement of VEGF expression mediated by IL-2 upregulation.

## Photosensitizers

Numerous types of photosensitizers have been developed for PDT so far, including benz-porphyrin (BPD), mono-L-aspartyl chlorine e6 (NPe6), tetra (m-hydroxyphenyl) chlorine (m-THPC), and 5-amino-levulinic acid (5-ALA). BPD, m-THPC, and 5-ALA have already been approved for clinical use in certain countries [8]. A hematoporphyrin derivative (Photofrin, Axcan Pharmaceuticals, Canada) is the most commonly used photosensitizer in the world and its use has been approved in many countries [1,2]. Photofrin is a mixture of different porphyrin-based oligomers, and is commercially available. A standard dose of 2 mg/kg patient weight is slowly injected intravenously over 5 minutes. The drug is cleared from most organ systems within 72 hours, but is retained for longer periods of time in tumors, skin (up to 30 days), liver, and spleen. Patients become photosensitive and are therefore at a risk for sunburn immediately following the injection. Due to its better retention in tumor cells and the vascular endothelium, the cytotoxic action of Photofrin is somewhat selective against neoplastic cells. After a set time interval, the tumor is exposed to light energy, which triggers the cytotoxic reaction. Selection of the appropriate sensitizer for clinical use is important. Photosensitizers that efficiently absorb light of longer wavelengths are better, because light of longer wavelengths shows deeper penetration into cancer tissue.

The Soret band of Photofrin is 385–405 nm, and the Q band of the longest wavelength is 630 nm. For treatment taking into consideration the depth of tissue penetration, 630-nm red light is used, which produces tumor destruction up to a depth of 5–10 mm.

In Japan, Photofrin was approved by the government in 1994, for PDT in patients with early-stage lung cancer, esophageal cancer, gastric cancer, and cervical cancer. In 2004, mono-L-aspartyl chlorine e6, also known as talaporfin sodium (NPe6, Laserphyrin) was also approved in Japan as a second-generation photosensitizer for PDT in patients with early-stage lung cancer [15–17]. Talaporfin has been shown to exhibit the same degree of antitumor efficacy as Photofrin, but to be associated with a lower incidence of cutaneous photosensitivity than Photofrin on account of its more rapid clearance from the skin.

## Laser equipments

Several types of laser have been used over the past three decades. Although an argon dye-laser was widely used initially, gold vapor laser, copper vapor laser, excimer laser, yttrium aluminum garnet–optical parametric oscillated (YAG-OPO) laser, and potassium–titanol–phosphate (KTP)-pumped tunable dye laser have all been developed since. Recently, a compact, cheap and useful diode laser was developed and its use is becoming popular [16,17].

## Indications for photodynamic therapy in patients with lung cancer

There are three indications of PDT in patients with lung cancer: for complete cure, for palliative treatment, and as preoperative PDT for surgical candidates.

PDT affords the chance of complete cure in patients with early-stage central-type lung cancer. Sputum cytology is the best method to detect such cases.

PDT has been used for palliative treatment and improvement of the quality of life (QOL) of patients with airway stenosis caused by tumor obstruction. Preoperative PDT has been applied in some patients in order to reduce the resection volume or improve the scope for surgery [16,17].

### Early detection and diagnosis of lung cancer

Sputum cytology-detected squamous cell carcinoma is sometimes difficult to localize by bronchoscopy. Patients with early-stage central-type lung cancer, including carcinoma *in situ*, are good candidates for obtaining complete cure by PDT. However, the lesions are often invisible endoscopically. This has led to the development of the new technology of photodynamic diagnosis (PDD) using autofluorescence bronchoscopy for localizing invisible early lesions, and the Xillix LIFE system (Canada) and SAFE 3000 (HOYA Pentax, Japan) used for this purpose have been launched in the market [18,19] (Fig. 20.1). On the other hand, clarification of the depth of invasion of the bronchial wall is also an important issue. The authors are in the process of developing the new technology of optical coherence tomography (OCT) with the HOYA Pentax company [20] (Fig. 20.2). The mucosal structure can be seen much more clearly by this new technology than by ultrasonography (EBUS).

### Curative intent of photodynamic therapy

Several studies have demonstrated the safety and effectiveness of PDT in the treatment of lung cancer. In the United States, the technique is FDA-approved for the treatment of microinvasive endobronchial non-small cell lung cancer in patients who are not suitable candidates for surgery or radiotherapy.

In a study from Japan, 64 patients with superficial cancers were treated by PDT using Photofrin and an excimer laser. Of these, 58 patients (consisting of 21 with roentgenographically occult lung cancer, eight with stage I lung cancer, five with esophageal cancer, 12 with gastric cancer, eight with cervical cancer, and four with bladder cancer) were evaluable. Complete remission was obtained in 48 (82.8%) of the 58 cases. There were no serious complications, except for the development of skin photosensitivity in 13 patients [21].

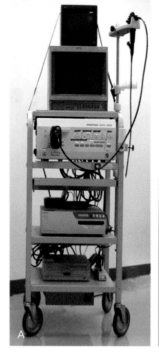

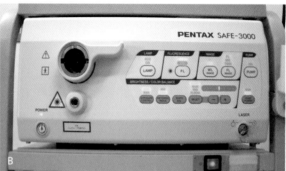

**Fig. 20.1** (A,B) The Pentax SAFE 3000, which consists of a color charge-coupled device (CCD) videoendoscopy based autofluorescence system with two light sources—a xenon lamp for white light and a diode laser (408 nm) as an autofluorescence-mode excitation light source.

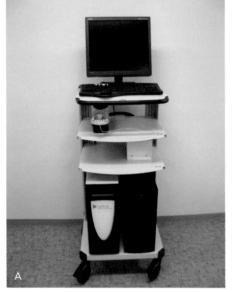

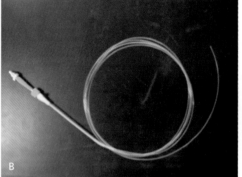

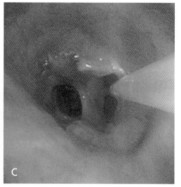

**Fig. 20.2** (A) The optical coherence tomography (OCT) control system. (B) OCT probe. (C) As the OCT probe is 1.5 to 0.75 mm in diameter, it is possible to insert it to the peripheral thin bronchus.

In Japan, a multicenter phase II clinical study was conducted from 1997 through 2000 to investigate the antitumor efficacy and safety of PDT using NPe6 and a diode laser in patients with early-stage lung cancer [22]. Forty patients with bronchoscopically superficial early-stage lung cancer with a normal chest X ray and CT and no lymph node or distant metastasis were treated. No skin photosensitivity was recognized in 84.8% of the patients and complete remission was obtained in 84.6% of the lesions. Thus, PDT using the new photosensitizer NPe6 and a diode laser

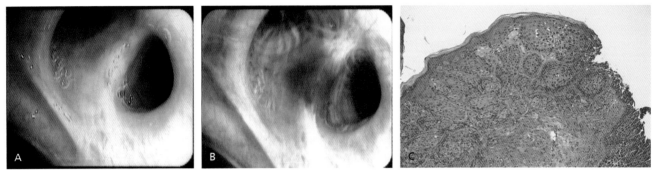

**Fig. 20.3** A 68-year-old-man with centrally located early lung cancer. This case is a rentogenologically occult lung cancer detected by sputum cytology. (A) Bronchoscopic finding is the invisible type. (B) SAFE 3000 showed the defect of autofluorescence at the tumor areas clearly. (C) The biopsy showed squamous cell carcinoma *in situ*.

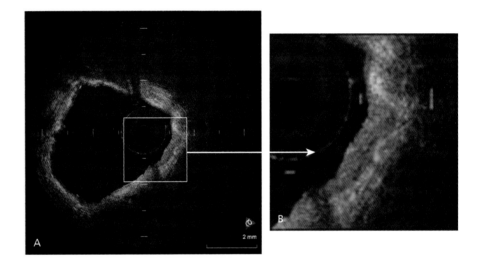

**Fig. 20.4** (A, B) Optical coherence tomography (OCT) showing thickening of the superficial layer. Carcinoma *in situ* was diagnosed by biopsy. OCT imaging shows clear intraepithelial invasion (A) and at higher magnification (B). A well-preserved basement membrane can be seen. This is a good example of a case indicated for photodynamic therapy for a complete cure.

demonstrated excellent antitumor effects and was also safe, particularly in terms of the low incidence of skin photosensitivity [22].

Several other studies evaluating the efficacy of PDT against various types of endobronchial cancer have been reported. Thus, PDT offers a chance for cure in patients with early-stage endobronchial cancer. Shown in Figure 20.3, a centrally located early lung cancer (squamous cell carcinoma) was localized at the bifuracation of rt $B^1_{a-b}$. The lesion was detected by SAFE-3000 (Fig. 20.3B) and OCT (Fig. 20.4A, B). The biopsy of the lesion identified carcinoma *in situ* (Fig. 20.3C).

## Therapeutic procedure

It is imperative to ensure that the laser is checked and found to be in working condition before a patient is injected with the photosensitizer for PDT, because no alternative treatment can be provided. Several different fibers are available. These fibers are flexible and easily passed through the working channel of a flexible bronchoscope. The most commonly used design is a "cylindrical diffuser". It differs from conventional laser fibers by emitting the light laterally over 360 degrees at the distal tip. The chosen length depends on the length of the lesion. The tip is also fairly rigid, allowing it to be embedded directly into the tumor. If a forward discharge of light is needed (as might be the case with small superficial tumors or a stump recurrence), a "microlens" can be employed. Fibers may be sterilized and reused for the same patient.

Because laser is non-thermal, the effects of PDT are not immediate. Energy delivery depends on the timing of treatment after injection and the energy delivered through the fiber. Light exposure should be scheduled approximately 48 hours after the injection of the photosensitizer; this allows for the sensitizer to be washed out of the normal mucosa, minimizing the risk of damage to non-malignant tissues. Application of $200 \, J/cm^2$ treated is recommended. Additional energy may be applied at the follow-up bronchoscopy that is performed 2 days later. It is also recommended that the dose of energy delivered does not exceed a total of 300–$400 \, J/cm^2$. In urgent cases, treatment may also be performed on the day of injection.

For elective procedures, a set schedule facilitates patient flow. Due to the intervals required between the interventions, we generally administer the injection to the patient as an outpatient on a Monday. The patient then returns in 48 hours for treatment and may be observed overnight. A follow-up bronchoscopy is scheduled for the Friday of the treatment week.

Instructions to patients focus on photosensitivity precautions. These effects last for 4–6 weeks and require the use of protective gear and eyewear whenever the patient is exposed to bright light. Shaded light—light from most artificial light sources and television sets—do not pose problems.

A fiber with the appropriate tip length is chosen. Longer lesions require longer tips. Before the procedure, the laser must be calibrated to ensure appropriate power output through the fiber. If the lesion is longer than the length of the chosen tip, the fiber is repositioned to the non-treated area and an additional light application is given.

Once the patient is sedated, the bronchoscope is introduced. Good topical anesthesia is mandatory to eliminate coughing. The nasal route is preferable, as the bronchoscope can be fixated more easily during the application time. Once the tumor is visualized, the fiber is introduced through the working channel. If possible, the rigid cylindrical tip should be embedded into the lesion; this not only protects the healthy surrounding mucosa from light exposure, but also delivers more energy to the tumor. Once the tip is in the desired position, the laser is activated and treatment initiated. We customarily suspend the light exposure at $100 \, J$ to check the tip position. This may be done as often as required, depending on the situation.

Additional areas are treated in the same fashion. If the tumor exceeds the length of the fiber tip, as may be the case in tracheal locations, we begin with the most distal segment first and advance proximally. We have treated up to four segments per session. After thorough suctioning of secretions, the bronchoscope is removed. A repeat bronchoscopy is planned for 48 hours later, when all the debris is removed. Additional energy may be applied if viable tumor tissue remains.

We often treat patients with advanced cancer by both PDT and external radiation therapy. Since both therapies may produce significant airway inflammation and edema, we provide an interval of 4–6 weeks between the treatments.

The main side effect of PDT using Photofrin is skin photosensitivity, whereas with the use of Laserphyrin, the incidence of photosensitivity is almost negligible. Immediate complications during the procedure are rare because the light is non-thermal, and no endobronchial smoke or immediate tumor necrosis develops. Cough with some blood-streaked sputum is not uncommon after the procedure and chest discomfort related to the inflammatory response may be noted.

Particularly in advanced cases, edema and secretions may lead to airway compromise within 24–48 hours of the treatment. This is especially worrisome if the procedure is performed in the trachea or at higher energy levels. Respiratory compromise may also occur after treatment in more distal areas, if the lung function is significantly compromised even to begin with. Patients at high risk for respiratory failure should be observed as inpatients. If problems develop, immediate therapeutic bronchoscopy must be scheduled.

## Guidelines for photodynamic therapy

In Japan, the criteria for early-stage lung cancer were strictly defined in 1975 [23]. Early-stage lung cancer can be divided into two categories: the central type or the peripheral type, according to the site of origin. In early-stage central-type lung cancer, most patients have symptoms such as cough, sputum production, or blood-tinged sputum [15–17]. To satisfy the definition of early-stage central-type lung cancer, the tumor must be located only as far as the segmental bronchi and be classified as carcinoma in situ or show only limited invasion into the bronchial wall. In 2003, the Japan Photodynamic Association and Japanese Society of Laser Surgery and Medicine established the therapeutic indications for PDT in patients with early-stage central-type lung cancer [15–17]:

1 Endoscopically evaluated early-stage lung cancer.
2 Normal chest X ray and CT imaging.
3 No evidence of metastasis to lymph nodes or distant metastasis.
4 Peripheral margin of the tumor visible endoscopically.
5 Tumor not more than 2 cm in diameter.

In the ACCP (American College of Chest Physicians) evidence-based clinical practice guidelines, PDT is recommended as an option of first choice for patients with centrally located early lung cancer who are not suitable surgical candidates [24]. Other endobronchial treatments, such as electrocautery, cryotherapy, and brachytherapy, are not as well studied. Use of high-power laser ablation, such as Nd : YAG laser, is not recommended because of the risk of perforation.

## Therapeutic method

PDT is performed using Photofrin or NPe6. Laser irradiation (630 nm) for Photofrin-PDT is transmitted via quartz fibers

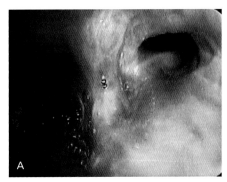 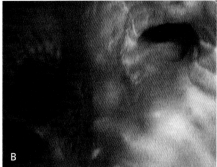

**Fig. 20.5** A 73-year-old man with centrally located early stage lung cancer. (A) Fiberoptic bronchoscopy revealed a superficial lesion. A thickened type squamous cell carcinoma can be visualized at the bifurcation of right B6 and basal bronchus. (B) Photodynamic diagnosis using SAFE-3000 and NPe6 was conducted before the photodynamic therapy. The red fluorescence excited by the diode laser (408 nm) from the SAFE-3000 system revealed the cancerous lesion.

inserted through the biopsy channel of the endoscope at 48 h after the administration of Photofrin (2 mg/kg). On the other hand, for NPe6-PDT, laser irradiation is accomplished 4 h after the administration of NPe6 using a PD laser (40 mg/m$^2$). The total energy of the laser irradiation is 100 J/cm$^2$, 150 mW/cm$^2$.

The Japanese Government approved the use of NPe6 for PDT against centrally located, early lung cancers in 2003, and the product became available in the Japanese market in June 2004 [15–17]. Just before PDT, PDD using SAFE-3000 is performed to define the tumor margin, based on the red fluorescence emitted from the tumor (Fig. 20.5) [17,19]. Figure 20.5 shows a centrally located, early stage lung cancer lesion. Fiberoptic bronchoscopy revealed a superficial lesion. A thickened type squamous cell carcinoma can be visualized at the bifurcation of right B6 and basal bronchus. PDD using SAFE-3000 and NPe6 was conducted before the PDT. The red fluorescence excited by the diode laser (408 nm) from the SAFE-3000 system revealed the cancerous lesion (Fig. 20.5).

Fiberoptic bronchoscopy with cytological and histological examination is performed at 1, 2, and 3 months after PDT, and thereafter at 3-month intervals during the first year and 6-month intervals during the second year after PDT. The antitumor effect of the initial treatment is rated based on endoscopic measurement of the tumor size using forceps, the morphologic appearance, and the pathological findings of the biopsy specimens, in accordance with the general rules of the Japan Lung Cancer Society and the Japan Society of Clinical Oncology. The antitumor effect is again evaluated at 3 months after the PDT. The tumors are then classified as showing complete response (CR) (no microscopically demonstrable tumor in the brushings and or biopsy specimens over a period of 4 weeks).

**Table 20.1** Characteristics of patients undergoing photodynamic therapy, Feb. 1980–Feb. 2005

| | |
|---|---|
| Total number of patients treated | 204 patients (264 lesions) |
| Gender | |
| Male | 198 patients (258 lesions) |
| Female | 6 patients (6 lesions) |
| Age (years) | |
| Range | 37–82 |
| Average | 67.5 |
| Histology | |
| Squamous cell carcinoma | 258 lesions |
| Severe dysplasia | 2 lesions |
| Carcinoid | 1 lesion |
| Adenocarcinoma | 3 lesions |
| Small cell carcinoma | 1 lesion |

## Therapeutic results at Tokyo Medical University

The efficacy of PDT for the treated lesions is shown in Table 20.1 [15]. CR and partial response (PR) were obtained in 224 (84.8%) and 40 (15.2%) lesions, respectively, out of the 264 lesions treated. Each of the lesions that showed PR was subsequently treated by other modalities, such as surgery, chemotherapy, or radiotherapy. Recurrence after CR occurred in 26 of the 224 (11.6%) lesions (Table 20.2). The 264 lesions were classified into four groups according to the maximum diameter in the longitudinal axis, as follows: less than 0.5 cm (56 lesions); 0.5–0.9 cm (124 lesions); 1.0–2.0 cm (50 lesions); greater than 2.0 cm (34 lesions). The CR rates in the above groups were 94.6, 93.5, 80, and 44.1%, respectively [15].

We have tried PDT in combination with surgery in locally advanced lung cancer. The example case shown in

Figure 20.6 suffered from dyspnea due to seriously poor pulmonary function. The tumor was located at the bifurcation with left upper and lower bronchus and swelling of no. 11 lymph node (Fig. 20.7A). We could not resect any part of the lung tissue due to pulmonary function. Therefore we planned to resect only a part of the bifurcation, with lymph node resection after PDT.

## Palliative photodynamic therapy for advanced lung cancer

Patients with advanced-stage central-type lung cancer often show stenosis and obstruction of the large airways with resultant dyspnea. The FDA has also approved the use of PDT for reducing the severity of obstruction and palliation of symptoms in patients with complete or partial obstruction caused by endobronchial non-small cell lung cancer. PDT shows excellent efficacy for the palliation of endobronchial obstruction [25]. With the FDA approval for palliative indications, more experience is expected to be accumulated on how PDT compares to conventional Nd:YAG laser treatment [26]. Non-pulmonary malignancies metastasizing to the airways have also been treated with success.

We believe that PDT has advantages over conventional Nd:YAG laser therapy. There is no endobronchial smoke during the procedure, the risk of bronchial perforation appears to be less, and there is evidence that the effects of PDT may be longer lasting than that of standard laser therapy. PDT may also be potentially useful in the treatment of stump recurrences and for preoperative treatment of advanced lung cancer, by reducing the resection volume, and also to improve the scope for surgery.

**Table 20.2** Results of photodynamic therapy

| Tumor size (cm) | No. of lesions | Complete response rate (%) | Partial response rate |
|---|---|---|---|
| <0.5 | 56 | 53 (94.6%) | 3 |
| 0.5 ≦ 1.0 | 124 | 116 (93.5%) | 8 |
| 1.0 ≦ 2.0 | 50 | 40 (80.0%) | 10 |
| 2.0≦ | 34 | 15 (44.1%) | 19 |
| Distal margin | | | |
| visible | 203 | 186 (91.6%) | |
| invisible | 61 | 38 (62.3%) | |
| Total | 264 | 224 (84.8%) | 40 |

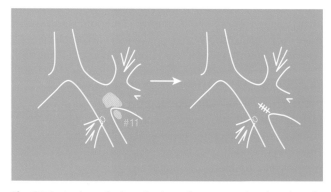

**Fig. 20.6** A schema for bronchoplasty after preoperative photodynamic therapy in patients with squamous cell carcinoma at the bifurcation between the left upper and lower bronchus.

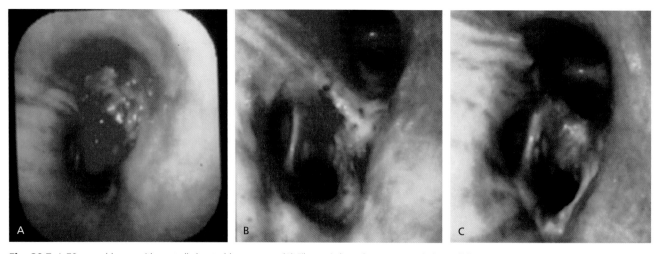

**Fig. 20.7** A 78-year-old man with centrally located lung cancer. (A) Fiberoptic bronchoscopy revealed a nodular type squamous cell carcinoma at the bifurcation between the left upper and lower bronchus. (B) Two months after photodynamic therapy. (C) Bronchoplasty was performed after photodynamic therapy.

# References

1 Dougherty TJ, Gomer CJ, Henderson BW, *et al.* Photodynamic therapy. *J Natl Cancer Inst* 1998; **90**: 889–905.

2 Dougherty TJ. An update on photodynamic therapy applications. *J Clin Laser Med Surg* 2002; **20**: 3–7.

3 Kato H, Horai T, Furuse K, *et al.* Photodynamic therapy for cancers: a clinical trial of porfimer sodium in Japan. *Jpn J Cancer Res* 1993; **84**: 1209–14.

4 McCaughan JS Jr, Photodynamic therapy of endobronchial and esophageal tumors: an overview. *J Clin Laser Med Surg* 1996; **14**: 223–38.

5 Kato H, Okunaka T, Shimatani H. Photodynamic therapy for early stage bronchogenic carcinoma. *J Clin Laser Med Surg* 1996; **14**: 235–8.

6 Cortese DA, Edell ES, Kinsey JH. Photodynamic therapy for early stage squamous cell carcinoma of the lung. *Mayo Clin Proc* 1997; **72**: 595–602.

7 McCaughan DA, Hawley PC, LaRosa JC, *et al.* Photodynamic therapy to control life-threatening hemorrhage from hereditary hemorrhagic telangiectasia. *Lasers Surg Mono* 1996; **19**: 492–4.

8 Oleinick NL, Morris RL, Belichenko I. The role of apoptosis in response to photodynamic therapy: what, where, why, and how. *Photochem Photobiol Sci* 2001; **1**: 1–21.

9 Gomer CJ, Ferrario A, Luna M, *et al.* Photodynamic therapy: combined modality approaches targeting the tumor microenvironment. *Lasers Surg Med* 2006; **38**: 516–21.

10 Sitnik TM, Hampton JA, Henderson BW. Reduction of tumor oxygenation during and after photodynamic therapy in vivo: effect of fluence rate. *Br J Cancer* 1998; **77**: 1386–94.

11 Ferrario A, von Tiehil KF, Rucker N, *et al.* Antiangiogenic treatment enhances photodynamic therapy responsiveness in a mouse mammary carcinoma. *Cancer Res* 2000; **60**: 4066–9.

12 Usuda J, Okunaka T, Ichinose S, *et al.* A possible relationship between the anti-cancer potency of photodynamic therapy using the novel photosensitizer ATX-s10-Na(II) and expression of the vascular endothelial growth factor in vivo. *Oncol Rep* 2007; **18**: 679–83.

13 Usuda J, Okunaka T, Furukawa K, *et al.* Increased cytotoxic effects of photodynamic therapy in IL-6 gene transfected via enhanced apoptosis. *Int J Cancer* 2001; **93**: 475–80.

14 Ohtani K, Usuda J, Ichinose S, *et al.* High expression of Gadd-45 alpha via upregulation of IL-2 after photodynamic therapy using NPe6. *Int J Oncol* 2008; **32**: 397–403.

15 Kato H, Usuda J, Okunaka T, Furukawa K. The history of the study of photodynamic therapy (PDT) and photodynamic diagnosis (PDD) in the department of Surgery, Tokyo Medical University. *Photodiagnosis Photodyn Ther* 2004; **1**: 107–10.

16 Kato H, Usuda J, Okunaka T, *et al.* Basic and clinical research on photodynamic therapy at Tokyo Medical University Hospital. *Lasers Surg Med* 2006; **38**: 371–5.

17 Usuda J, Kato H, Okunaka T, *et al.* Photodynamic therapy (PDT) for lung cancers. *J Thorac Oncol* 2006; **5**: 489–93.

18 Ikeda N, Honda H, Hayashi A, *et al.* Early detection of bronchial lesions using newly developed videoendoscopy-based autofluorescence bronchoscopy. *Lung Cancer* 2006; **52**: 21–7.

19 Usuda J, Tsutsui H, Honda H, *et al.* Photodynamic therapy for lung cancers based on novel photodynamic diagnosis using talaporfin sodium (NPe6) and autofluorescence bronchoscopy. *Lung Cancer* 2007; **58**: 317–23.

20 Tsuboi M, Hayashi A, Ikeda N, *et al.* Optical coherence tomography in the diagnosis of bronchial lesions. *Lung Cancer* 2005; **49**: 387–94.

21 Furuse K, Fukuoka M, Kato H, *et al.* A prospective phase II study on photodynamic therapy with photofrin II for centrally located early-stage lung cancer. *J Clin Oncol* 1993; **11**: 1852–7.

22 Kato H, Furukawa K, Sato M, *et al.* Phase II clinical study of photodynamic therapy using mono-L-aspartyl chlorine e6 and diode laser for early superficial squamous cell carcinoma of the lung. *Lung Cancer* 2003; **42**: 103–11.

23 Ikeda S. *Atlas of Early Cancer of Major Bronchi.* Tokyo: Igakushoin Publisher; 1975.

24 Mathur PN, Edell E, Sutedja T, Vergnon JM. Treatment of early non-small cell lung cancer. *Chest* 2003; **12** 3: 176–80.

25 Diaz-Jimenez JP, Martinez-Ballarin JE, Llunell A, *et al.* Efficacy and safety of photodynamic therapy versus Nd-YAG laser resection in NSCLC with airway obstruction. *Eur Respir J* 1999; **14**: 800–5.

26 Kvale PA, Selecky PA, Prakash UBS. Palliative care in lung cancer. *Chest* 2007; **132**: 368–403.

# 21 Balloon Bronchoplasty

## Sara R. Greenhill and Kevin L. Kovitz

Chicago Chest Center, Elk Grove Village, IL, USA

## Introduction

The presentation of tracheobronchial stenosis can range from minimal to no symptoms to dyspnea, infection, and life-threatening airway obstruction. Airway narrowing has been approached by many methods. It has been bypassed, such as a tracheostomy to create an airway beyond a sub-glottic stenosis. It has been surgically resected with reanastamosis, or surgically reconstructed, as with surgical bronchoplasty. Ideally, stenosis is best approached in the least invasive way possible, to minimize risk and maximize benefit to the patient. With that in mind, various endoscopic methods have been employed. Dilation has been part of the approach using rigid bronchoscopy, rigid dilators, endotracheal tubes, and balloons. Balloons are the focus of this chapter.

Interest in balloon dilation (i.e. bronchoplasty) grew with the development of angioplasty catheters. In the 1980s, angioplasty balloons were used by Groff and Allen to dilate a postintubation bronchial stenosis bronchus in an infant [1]. Cohen and colleagues used balloon bronchoplasty to dilate an infant's congenital stenosis [2]. Many other balloon options have developed since that time.

## Indications

The primary indication for balloon bronchoplasty is symptomatic airway stenosis. Typically, this is manifested as scarring of a segment or multiple segments of the airway. The resulting narrowed airway contributes to dyspnea or recurrent infection. Postintubation or postsurgical stenoses are the most common cause. Many other insults to the airway can be implicated (Table 21.1). Balloon dilatation has been reported for stenosis complicating tuberculosis [3,4], sarcoid and berylliosis [5,6], sleeve resection [7], lung transplantation [8–10], pill-induced trauma [11,12], radiation therapy, carcinoma, and Wegener's granulomatosis [13]. Acquired and congenital stenotic lesions have been dilated in both adult and pediatric populations [14–23].

Typical presenting symptoms include dyspnea or wheezing. Commonly, the patient is misdiagnosed with asthma and may be treated unsuccessfully for some time until a focal wheeze is recognized. The diagnosis of stenosis can be made by some combination of physical exam, flow-volume loops, tomograms, bronchograms, computed tomography (CT), magnetic resonance imaging (MRI), and/or bronchoscopic observation. Direct bronchoscopic observation is the most useful technique for diagnosing and planning the balloon bronchoplasty.

## Equipment and technique

Preoperative patient assessment is like that for any bronchoscopy. As with all procedures, adequate anesthesia and monitoring is required. Most patients require deeper sedation than the moderate sedation used for a standard bronchoscopy. Dilation of a major airway for up to 1 minute at a time is uncomfortable for the patient who is not under deep or general anesthesia. The degree of anesthesia, support, and monitoring should be appropriate for the clinical state of the patient. The airway can be stabilized using a rigid bronchoscope. Alternatively, the airway can be stabilized with an endotracheal tube or, for higher stenoses, a laryngeal mask airway (LMA), with a flexible bronchoscope introduced via these access points. Achieving an established airway allows for ease of reintroduction of scopes, wires, and balloons. Occasionally, for limited distal stenosis, the balloon can be introduced via a flexible bronchoscope through the mouth or nose, however, this is not the norm.

Balloon bronchoplasty can be done with a rigid or flexible bronchoscope, with or without fluoroscopic guidance.

*Flexible Bronchoscopy*, Third Edition. Edited by Ko-Pen Wang, Atul C. Mehta, J. Francis Turner.
© 2012 Blackwell Publishing Ltd. Published 2012 by Blackwell Publishing Ltd.

**Table 21.1** Indications for balloon deployment

Postintubation stenosis

Postsurgical anastomotic stenosis (i.e. post-transplant, postsleeve resection)

Postinfectious (i.e. tuberculosis)

Idiopathic

Postradiation

Postinhalational injury

Malignant stenosis

Inflammation (i.e. sarcoidosis, Wegener's)

Other therapeutic interventions:

Stent deployment

Tamponade of bleeding

Deliberate airway occlusion

Foreign body removal

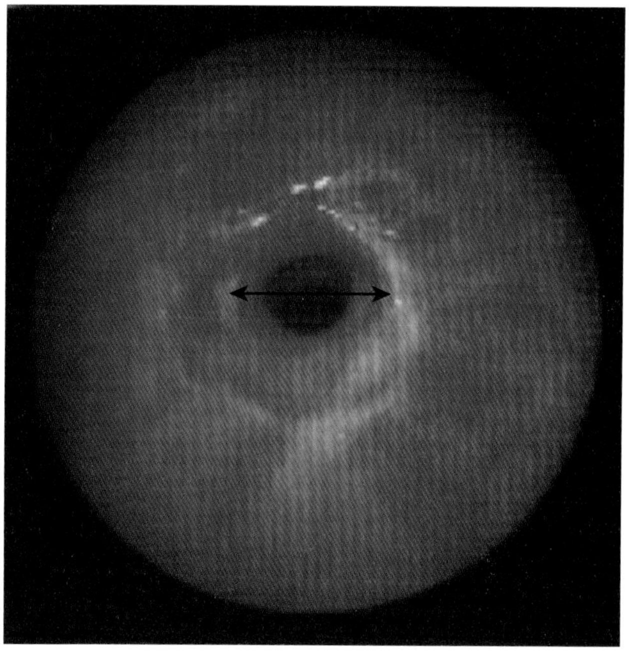

**Fig. 21.1** Representation of an airway stenosis due to intrinsic disease. Length of the stenosis is determined visually through the bronchoscope. Arrow perpendicular to the bronchus represents the desired postdilatation diameter.

Fluoroscopy without bronchoscopy can be used, but is not recommended. However, when using bronchoscopy, fluoroscopy is rarely if ever needed, as the airway is directly visualized. By performing the dilation under direct visualization, progress and complications may be readily assessed and treated. Even if one agrees that bronchoscopy is the method of choice, the approach can vary. A balloon can be passed directly through either a rigid or flexible bronchoscope. A working channel of 2.8 mm or greater is usually required, but one should verify the specifications of the balloon used. Alternatively, a guide wire can be placed first through the bronchoscope, which is then removed and reintroduced next to the wire. The balloon is passed over the wire into place. Each approach may or may not be guided by fluoroscopy. The approach should be individualized to the patient's needs, so a variety of options should be available so that each patient can have any other required interventions performed.

The diameter and length of the stenotic segment and desired end diameter are determined prior to dilation (Fig. 21.1). This is best done bronchoscopically. The balloon should be of adequate length to straddle the stenosis by at lease 1 cm above and below, if possible. It should be of a length that reaches the airway lesion. Proper straddling of the stenosis will help keep the balloon in place during inflation rather than "funneling" away when inflated.

Balloons are manufactured by many companies and, although bronchial specific balloons exist, most were developed for vascular or gastrointestinal (GI) use (Fig. 21.2). Balloons come in a fixed length with either a fixed diameter or a diameter that varies with inflation pressure. The GI and bronchial balloons are single or multiple uses, and are usually less costly than the vascular balloons. Inflation is done using a pressure syringe device. The balloon is typically filled with saline but can be filled with air or an iso-osmolar, non-ionic, dilute contrast medium. The atmospheres of pressure used are specific to each balloon used and should adequately achieve full deployment of the balloon at the narrow point according to its specifications. Balloons are designed to deploy throughout the length to the predetermined diameter and not merely comply with the vagaries of the airway. Brand choice is up to the operator. Inflation diameter ranges used are from 4 to 20 mm, and balloon lengths are typically 4–8 cm. Guide wire diameter is 0.035 inch and soft-tipped or as specified by the balloon used.

The chosen balloon should stretch the stenosis several millimeters (2–3 mm) beyond the desired end diameter. Usually, this requires several narrower balloons used to dilate up in intervals over the course of the procedure. The initial inflation diameter is selected to be several millimeters (2–3 mm) greater than the stenosis. The initial dilation can provide significant relief in and of itself, accommodating a more stable airway for the remainder of the procedure. The intervening diameters are chosen by the response of the stenosis to the preceding dilation. If possible, the final

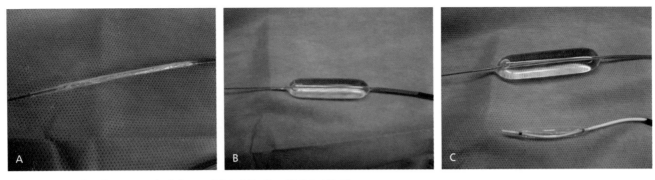

**Fig. 21.2** Examples of representative balloons, deflated (A, C) and inflated (B, C).

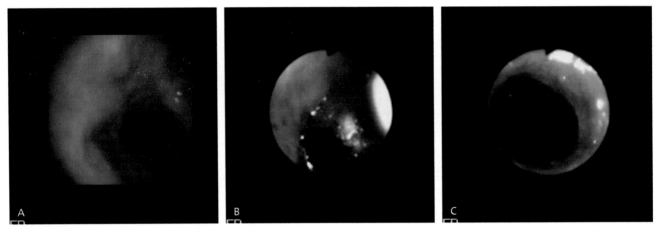

**Fig. 21.3** (A) Endoscopic view of a 6-mm diameter subglottic stenosis. (B) Endoscopic view of a balloon inflated in a subglottic stenosis. (C) Endoscopic view of a subglottic stenosis that is 14 mm in diameter postdilation.

balloon diameter chosen is several millimeters (2–3 mm) greater than the final desired diameter, as there may be some recoil of the airway. The maximum final desired diameter is determined by the diameter of the airway immediately proximal to the stenosis. Typical minimal desired ending diameters are 14–16 mm in the male trachea, 12–14 mm in the female, 12–14 mm in the male main bronchus, and 10–12 mm in the female. Actual end result or desired diameter, of course, may differ from those given.

The balloon is inflated and held at the pressure in atmospheres specific to the balloon and diameter desired using the syringe device described above attached to a manometer. The airway can be observed during the procedure and assessed and cleared between dilations (Fig. 21.3A–C). Each dilation is done for approximately 1 minute, typically repeated approximately three times at each diameter. However, the repetition frequency at each diameter depends on the ease of dilation at that stage. Dilation times have ranged from 15 to 150 seconds [24]. There is no definitive study of adequate dilation time, though, 60 seconds was chosen by experience and patient tolerance. Dilation

for deployment of a stent into place for dilation of a stenosis usually requires only a few seconds, and is distinct. Oxygen saturations should remain above 90%, and the patient should be well and even ventilated between inflations.

Antibiotics, systemic steroids, topical anti-inflammatory and topical antineoplastic agents have been used in conjunction with balloon bronchoplasty. These may or may not be useful but are commonly used. No trials exist to give specific guidance in this area. Finally, the operator and the team must be trained in the equipment's use and techniques. Planning and preparation allows the balloon bronchoplasty to achieve the desired result on its own or in conjunction with other aspects of the procedure, such as laser or stent.

## Complications

Complications are infrequent (Table 21.2). They fit into those that are seen with any bronchoscopy and

**Table 21.2** Complications of balloon bronchoplasty

As with any bronchoscopy
Airway tear
Malacia
Failure of dilation
Recurrence
Discomfort if anesthesia inadequate

those specific to the procedure. Potential complications include tracheobronchial rupture, pneumomediastinum, pneumothorax, airway obstruction, hemorrhage, mucus plugging, and respiratory insufficiency. The overall reported complication rate is approximately 5%. Tracheal rupture requiring thoracotomy and open surgical repair has been reported [24]. However, while airway tear is perhaps most feared, it is extremely rare and, when it occurs, is rarely clinically significant. Recurrences are not infrequent and multiple procedures may be required, as is discussed below.

## Outcomes

Balloon bronchoplasty is a safe and effective way to approach the treatment of airway stenosis. In the appropriate patient, it may be the only treatment necessary. It can also be used in conjunction with other forms of therapy. Balloon bronchoplasty can easily be repeated and does not preclude other options such as surgery if it becomes necessary. Most authors report improvement following the initial procedure. Hebra and colleagues report a 90% initial and 54% long-term positive result in children with a 15-year follow-up [19]. There were an average of four sessions. Ferretti and associates report 36 balloon bronchoplasties with a 68% initial and 56% long-term success rate. There were one to five repeat procedures in the 54% who restenosed in the first month [13]. Sheski and Mathur [21] had 10 of 14 dilations (71%) succeed with one procedure. The other four had multiple or adjunctive procedures, such as stenting or cryotherapy. At an extreme, one atypical patient had 30 dilations.

Hautmann and coauthors [22] demonstrate, in a much larger series, that 79% of stenoses had improved diameter after the first procedure, and most accomplished the goal (symptom relief, stenting) at that procedure; 43 to 52% maintained their results over time.

These studies are representative of outcomes in general. In essence, balloon bronchoplasty is an easy-to-perform, effective intervention for airway stenoses of many etiologies. It can be used alone or as an adjunct to other procedures and can be repeated if necessary.

## References

1 Groff DB, Allen JK. Gruentzig balloon catheter dilation for acquired bronchial stenosis in an infant. *Ann Thorac Surg* 1985; **4**: 379–81.
2 Cohen MD, Weber TR, Rao CC. Balloon dilatation of tracheal and bronchial stenosis. *Am J Roentgenol* 1984; **142**: 477–8.
3 Nakamura K, Terada N, Ohi M, *et al.* Tuberculosis bronchial stenosis: treatment with balloon bronchoplasty. *Am J Roentgenol* 1991; **157**: 1187–8.
4 Shim YS. New classification of endobronchial tuberculosis and balloon dilatation of bronchial stenosis. *Kekkaku* 1992; **67**: 353–7.
5 Ball JB, Delaney JC, Evans CC, *et al.* Endoscopic bougie and balloon dilatation of multiple bronchial stenosis: 10-year follow-up. *Thorax* 1991; **46**: 933–5.
6 Chapman JT, Mehta AC. Bronchoscopy in sarcoidosis: diagnostic and therapeutic interventions. *Curr Opin Pulm Med* 2003; **9**: 402–7.
7 Fowler CL, Aaland MO, Harris FL. Dilatation of bronchial stenosis with Gruentzig balloon. *J Thorac Cardiovasc Surg* 1987; **93**: 308–15.
8 Keller C, Frost A. Fiberoptic bronchoplasty. *Chest* 1992; **102**: 995–8.
9 Carre P, Rousseau H, Lombart L, *et al.* Balloon dilatation and self-expanding metal Wallstent insertion. *Chest* 1994; **195**: 343–8.
10 Santacruz JF, Mehta AC. Airway complications and management after lung transplantation: ischemia, dehiscence, and stenosis. *Proc Am Thor Soc* 2009; **6**: 79–93.
11 Carlin BW, Harell JH, Moser KM. The treatment of endobronchial stenosis using balloon catheter dilatation. *Chest* 1998; **93**: 1148–51.
12 Lee P, Culver DA, Farver C, Mehta AC. Syndrome of iron pill aspiration. *Chest* 2002; **121**: 1355–7.
13 Ferretti G, Jouvan FB, Thony F, *et al.* Benign noninflammatory bronchial stenosis: treatment with balloon dilation. *Radiology* 1995; **196**: 831–4.
14 Brown SB, Hedlung GL, Glasier CM, *et al.* Tracheobronchial stenosis in infants: successful balloon dilation therapy. *Radiology* 1987; **164**: 475–8.
15 Philippart AI, Long JA, Grennholz SK. Balloon dilatation of postoperative tracheal stenosis. *J Pediatr Surg* 1988; **23**: 1178–9.
16 Bagwell CE, Talbert JL, Tepas JJ. Balloon dilatation of long-segment tracheal stenosis. *J Pediatr Surg* 1991; **26**: 153–9.
17 Elkerbout SC, van Lingen RA, Gerritsen J, Roorda RJ. Endoscopic balloon dilatation of acquired airway stenosis in newborn infants: a promising treatment. *Arch Dis Child* 1993; **68**: 37–40.
18 Skedros DG, Siewers RD, Chan KH, Atlas AB. Rigid bronchoscopy balloon catheter dilation for bronchial stenosis in infants. *Ann Otol Rhinol Laryngol* 1993; **102**: 266–70.
19 Hebra A, Powell DD, Smith CD, Othersen HB. Balloon tracheoplasty in children: results of a 15-year experience. *J Pediatr Surg* 1991; **26**: 957–61.

20 Rivron A, Treguier C, Bourdiniere J, *et al.* [Acquired tracheo-bronchial stenosis of the premature infant under artificial respiration; value of bronchography and endoscopic balloon dilatation: apropros of 7 cases.] *Ann Otolaryngol Chir Cervicofac* 1992; **109**: 1–5.

21 Sheski FD, Mathur PN, Long-term results of fiberoptic broncho-scopic balloon dilatation in the management of benign tracheo-bronchial stenosis. *Chest* 1998; **114**: 796–800.

22 Hautmann H, Gamarra F, Pfeifer KJ, Huber RM. Fiberoptic bron-choscopic balloon dilatation in malignant tracheobronchial disease. *Chest* 2001; **120**: 43–9.

23 Edwards RD, Wilkinson LM, Turner MA. Benign bronchial ste-nosis treated with balloon bronchoplasty and metal stents. *Scottish Med J* 1995; **40**: 19–20.

24 Kovitz KL, Conforti JF. Balloon bronchoplasty: when and how. *Pulmonary Perspectives* 1999; **16**: 1–3.

# 4

# Special Considerations

# 22 Rigid Bronchoscopy

## J. Francis Turner Jr[1] and Ko-Pen Wang[2]

[1] Interventional Pulmonary and Critical Care Medicine, Nevada Cancer Institute and University of Nevada School of Medicine, Las Vegas, NV, USA

[2] Chest Diagnostic Center and Lung Cancer Center at Harbor Hospital, Part-time Faculty of Interventional Pulmonology, Johns Hopkins Hospital, Baltimore MD,USA

## Introduction

Gustav Killian has been called the "Father of Bronchoscopy," and although Rosenheim and Mikulicz had previously used esophagoscopes, it was Killian who first introduced a rigid scope into the trachea [1] (Fig. 22.1). The therapeutic potential of this innovation was demonstrated when on March 30, 1897 Killian successfully removed a piece of pork bone from the right main bronchus of a German farmer [2]. In the United States, the art of bronchoscopy continued with Chevalier Jackson constructing bronchoscopes based upon instruments being used for esophagoscopy at that time, with the subsequent development by H. H. Hopkins of the "Hopkins" telescope, allowing for improved visualization [3]. With the introduction of the flexible fiberoptic bronchoscope by Ikeda in 1970, the era of rigid bronchoscopy was thought by many to fade from importance. Thus, a generation of bronchoscopists in the United States and elsewhere have "grown up" without significant exposure to the instruments and art of rigid bronchoscopy. The decline in utilization so marked that approximately 92% of bronchoscopists never use the rigid scope in their clinical practice [4].

In certain circumstances, however, the rigid bronchoscope offers benefits over the flexible fiberoptic bronchoscope. The larger working channel of the rigid bronchoscope allows for easier control of massive hemoptysis and is advantageous in the removal of foreign bodies and placement of stents while maintaining a secure airway [5,6]. Although laser therapy is now frequently performed through the flexible fiberoptic bronchoscope, the rigid scope is preferred by some as the metallic construction of the rigid bronchoscope reduces the risk of endobronchial ignition as compared to the flexible

fiberoptic bronchoscope with its rubber housing [7]. In addition, the rigid scope can be used to core-out an obstructing lesion, thereby expediting removal of a mass. Also, mechanical ventilation can be provided through the rigid scope, making this technique more suitable for some patients with critical tracheobronchial stenosis. Colt and Harrell reviewed the use of emergency rigid bronchoscopy in patients presenting to an ICU in acute respiratory failure [8]. Of the 19 patients with central airways obstruction who underwent emergent therapeutic rigid bronchoscopy, 52.6% were able to have mechanical ventilation immediately discontinued. Of seven patients with no indwelling airway, 71.4% could be transferred to a lower level of care and overall 20 of the 32 patients (62.5%) could be immediately transferred to a lower level of care. The rigid scope also allows for the use of larger instruments, affording the ability to obtain larger samples. Finally, in case of mishap, the rigid scope is better suited to maintaining a clear airway and controlling hemorrhage.

Disadvantages to rigid bronchoscopy include more limited access to the distal airway compared to the flexible scope and the use of general anesthesia in most patients. In addition, the rigid scope cannot be used in patients with unstable necks, severely ankylosed cervical spines, or restricted temporomandibular joints [7].

## Equipment

A rigid bronchoscopy set is based around the main ventilating or "universal" bronchoscope. The metal tube selected varies dependent upon whether the subject is an infant or adult and may be up to 13.5 mm in internal diameter.

*Flexible Bronchoscopy*, Third Edition. Edited by Ko-Pen Wang, Atul C. Mehta, J. Francis Turner.
© 2012 Blackwell Publishing Ltd. Published 2012 by Blackwell Publishing Ltd.

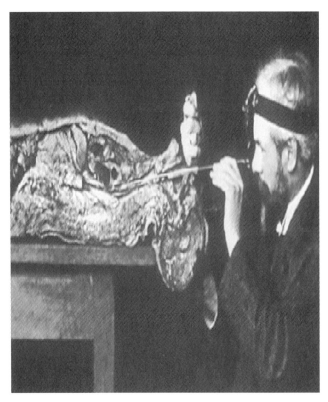

**Fig. 22.1** Gustov Killian positioning a rigid bronchoscope on a cadaver. Courtesy of Dr Heinrich Becker.

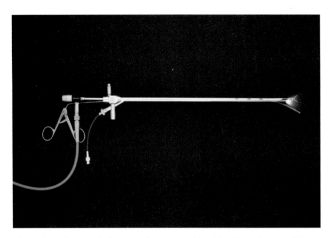

**Fig. 22.2** The ventilating bronchoscope with a Hopkins telescope, biopsy forceps, and suction catheter inserted. From: Turner JF, Ernst A, Becker HD. "How I do it" rigid bronchoscopy. *J Bronchol* 2000; **7**: 172.

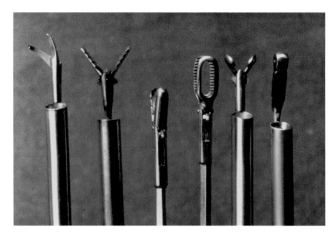

**Fig. 22.3** Additional biopsy forceps available for use with the bronchoscope. From: Turner JF, Ernst A, Becker HD. "How I do it" rigid bronchoscopy. *J Bronchol* 2000; **7**: 172.

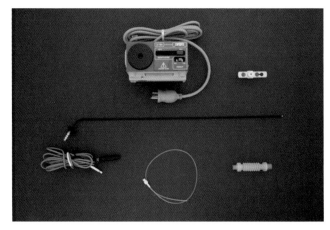

**Fig. 22.4** Clockwise, a portable light source, a "FLUVOG" adapter which may be attached to the proximal opening of the bronchoscope, a rigid electrocautery instrument with attached cord, a suction catheter, and a corrugated ventilation adapter. From: Turner JF, Ernst A, Becker HD. "How I do it" rigid bronchoscopy. *J Bronchol* 2000; **7**: 172.

Different manufacturers have developed modifications upon the original design with the most recent model introduced by Jean-Francois Dumon (Dumon–Harrell universal bronchoscope, Bryon Corp, Woburn, MA). Although the distal end of the tube is illuminated by means of a small light rod, a Hopkins telescope placed through the ventilating rigid tube is commonly utilized to provide adequate visualization. Figure 22.2 illustrates the stainless steel metal tube (Storz model, Karl Storz Endoscopy, Culver City, CA) with the Hopkins telescope, biopsy forceps, and suction catheter inserted through the ventilating bronchoscope with the brilliant light of the telescope seen at the distal end. Additional instruments (Fig. 22.3) allow for biopsies and interventional procedures to be performed. The Hopkins telescope may also be passed through and locked into different biopsy forceps, allowing for simultaneous viewing of the forceps and the intended target. Glass "windows" are available to occlude the proximal portion of the ventilating bronchoscope to help prevent loss of gasses and particulate matter. Some glass windows contain a small "keyhole" to allow passage of instruments. Figure 22.4 illustrates (clockwise) a portable light source, a "FLUVOG" adapter that may be attached to the proximal opening of the bronchoscope, a rigid electrocautery instrument with attached cord, a suction catheter, and a corrugated ventilation adapter. The FLUVOG adapter slides, placing one of three windows able to be selected over the proximal opening of the rigid scope. One selection is a glass lens, which allows distal visualization while occluding the proximal opening to help prevent escaped gas during ventilation. A notched lens allows for the insertion of an instrument, and a larger opening without a lens permits the working end of other devices (e.g. forceps, flexible bronchoscope) to be inserted.

## Indications and contraindications

The rigid bronchoscope is now often used in concert with the flexible bronchoscope. This blending of equipment offers the advantages of both instruments. There remain situations, however, where the rigid bronchoscope may be preferable, as discussed below.

The rigid bronchoscope has the ability to obtain larger biopsy specimens owing to the larger size of the working channel and available forceps. The rigid bronchoscope will not easily allow biopsy of upper lobe lesions, though, owing to the inflexibility of the scope and the combined use with the flexible bronchoscope is an advantage in this situation. Certainly, in keeping with the rigid scope's original use, the removal of foreign bodies in both children and adults continues to be an important indication [9,10]. Upon removal of the foreign body, the tracheal and laryngeal mucosa, as well as the vocal cords, are also protected as removal usually takes place through the ventilating bronchoscope.

Additional indications include the following:

*Massive hemoptysis.* Massive hemoptysis may quickly impair a patient's ability to ventilate and oxygenate. In this situation a properly used rigid scope is better able to maintain integrity of the airway and ventilate with improved visualization. The rigid scope's working channel also permits introduction of larger internal diameter suction catheters and the ability to pack a bleeding area with pledgets to tamponade the bleeding site or orifice.

*Central airway obstruction.* The rigid scope may be utilized as a mechanical coring device through the area of intrinsic obstruction of a central airway and has been used in the past for progressive dilation for subglottic stenosis (Fig. 22.5).

*Laser bronchoscopy.* Laser bronchoscopy is made safer owing to the absence of an ignitable endotracheal tube and improved ventilation of smoke and debris (Fig. 22.6).

*Stent placement and removal.* As the ideal stent does not yet exist owing to the differing requirements of individual patients, types of obstructions and stenosis, varying personnel and expertise, and equipment, the over-riding principal

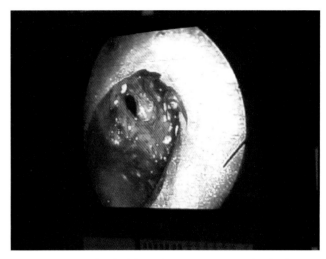

**Fig. 22.5** The distal end of the rigid scope is seen immediately above an area of subglottic stenosis.

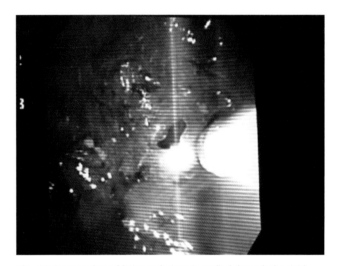

**Fig. 22.6** Laser photoablation technique is applied through the rigid bronchoscope to an area of subglottic stenosis.

recommended remains the realization of "different jobs–different stents" (Fig. 22.7). Therefore, the types of stents, techniques of insertion, and required personnel may vary dependent on the individual patient's situation. Owing to this, rigid bronchoscopy continues to be utilized in the placement and removal of both silicone and metallic stents.

Contraindications to rigid bronchoscopy include:

*Lack of adequately trained personnel.* As the primary tool for the bronchoscopist has become the flexible bronchoscope in conjunction with conscious sedation, the number of trained operators prepared to perform rigid procedures has decreased.

*Unstable cervical spine.* Instability of the cervical spine or a fixed cervical spine due to congenital malformations, arthritis, or mechanical fixation make passage of the rigid

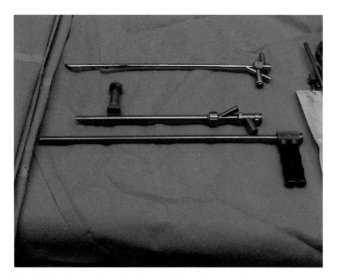

**Fig. 22.7** (top to bottom) Storz rigid bronchoscope, Dumon stent adaptor, Dumon rigid bronchoscope, Dumon stent introducer.

scope through the upper airway very challenging or not possible.

*Unstable cardiovascular status or hypoxemia not related to airway obstruction.* Patients with active cardiac ischemia, hemodynamically unstable, or otherwise at high risk for general anesthesia are also at increased risk for complications during rigid bronchoscopy. Rigid bronchoscopy, however, may be indicated if meant to relieve obstructing lesions causing hypoxemia or dependence on mechanical ventilation.

## Anesthesia

Rigid bronchoscopy is most often performed using deep conscious sedation or under general anesthesia. The techniques for ventilation available are dependent upon the procedural skill of the bronchoscopist, anesthesiologist, and available equipment. Although rigid bronchoscopy can be performed with topical anesthesia and conscious sedation, most often deep conscious sedation with assisted spontaneous ventilation or general anesthesia are utilized. After receiving an anxiolytic, or in the case of general anesthesia, an induction agent, the rigid bronchoscope is inserted into the trachea. When properly seated in the trachea a connection is established between one of the side ports and either an Ambu bag, anesthesia machine, or jet ventilator. Jet ventilation may be accomplished with a hand activated valve (100% $FiO_2$ at 50 psi) or high-frequency jet ventilator.

General anesthesia may be performed with either inhalational agents or intravenous medications. When ventilating by means of an Ambu bag or conventional circuit, care must be taken to avoid lack of adequate ventilation due to loss of gases through the nose, mouth, and proximal end of the

rigid instrument. Due to this, authors have described methods of intermittent insufflation with packing or compression of the nose and mouth [11]. We prefer to maintain ventilation by means of a jet ventilator, which allows the proximal portion of the scope to be open, permitting easy introduction of a flexible scope and other instruments as needed. The jet ventilator is familiar to most pulmonologists and achieves ventilation through the Venturi principle, with the oxygen saturation being monitored by the anesthesiologist. The concentration of oxygen used is of concern during therapeutic procedures, such as laser where the possibility of tracheal fire exists [12]. Additional methods of ventilation have been studied by examining different external modalities of ventilation with Natalini *et al.* describing the technique of rigid bronchoscopy with intermittent negative pressure ventilation and external high-frequency oscillation [13–15].

## Technique

Once the patient is properly relaxed, the head position is adjusted so that the neck is extended, creating a straight line from the oral cavity through the oropharynx to the vocal cords. The bronchoscope is then held in the right hand at the proximal portion with the distal flared lip of the bronchoscope being anterior. If the intubation is to be carried out with the Hopkins telescope already inserted (Fig. 22.2), then the image through the telescope must be oriented so as to assure it corresponds to the "clock face" of the distal portion of the rigid bronchoscope (i.e. the protruding distal lip should be at the 12 o'clock position) (Fig. 22.8). The tele-

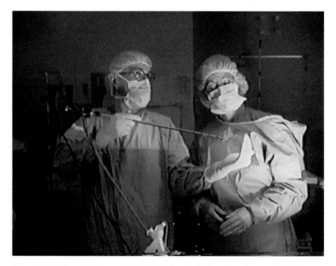

**Fig. 22.8** The rigid scope is held in the right hand at the proximal portion with the distal flared lip of the bronchoscope being anterior. The image through the telescope must be oriented so as to assure it corresponds to the "clock face" of the distal portion of the rigid bronchoscope.

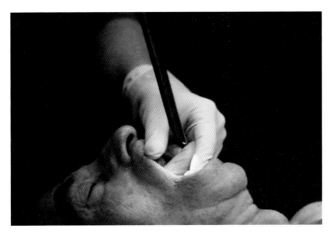

**Fig. 22.9** The ventilating bronchoscope is aimed vertically at a 90° angle to the opening of the mouth. From: Turner JF, Ernst A, Becker HD. "How I do It" rigid bronchoscopy. *J Bronchol* 2000; **7**: 174.

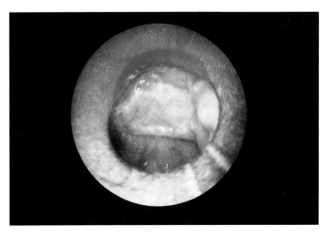

**Fig. 22.10** The bronchoscope is slowly advanced forward until the epiglottis is visualized. From: Turner JF, Ernst A, Becker HD. "How I do It" rigid bronchoscopy. *J Bronchol* 2000; **7**: 174.

scope is then held stationary in relation to the rigid bronchoscope with the right hand to maintain constant orientation. The distal end of the telescope must also always be inside the lip of the rigid bronchoscope to allow proper insertion. With the patients head in the proper "sniffing" position and the distal end of the rigid bronchoscope having the protruding lip in the 12 o'clock position, the left hand's second, third, and fourth fingers are inserted into the patients mouth. This allows positioning and stabilization of the patient's head that may be needed during intubation. The thumb and first finger of the left hand then serve as a guide though which to insert and pass the tube through the oropharynx. The forefinger will serve to protect the lower teeth and lip from direct contact with the rigid bronchoscope, with the thumb acting to protect the upper lip and teeth.

The tube is first aimed at a 90° angle to the opening of the mouth (Fig. 22.9). The rigid bronchoscope is then passed through the tunnel created by the thumb and forefinger of the left hand until the uvula is visualized. Once the uvula is reached the proximal portion of the rigid bronchoscope is angled downward gradually orienting the long axis of the tube more horizontally with the left thumb acting as a fulcrum against which the rigid bronchoscope moves. The forefinger of the left hand acts as the anterior guide for the bronchoscope as well as protecting the lower lip and teeth. The operator should not allow the bronchoscope to pivot on the upper teeth or lips, thereby causing lip trauma or fractured teeth. The rigid bronchoscope is advanced forward in the midline until the epiglottis is visualized with the protruding tip of the bronchoscope then used to elevate the epiglottis, much as a Miller or straight blade on an intubating laryngoscope is utilized (Fig. 22.10). The rigid bronchoscope is passed under the epiglottis and rotated 90° to permit easy passage of the lip of the tube through the vocal cords. The flared lip of the rigid bronchoscope may be used to gently

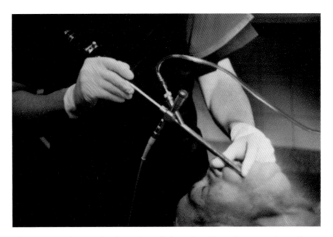

**Fig. 22.11** The proximal portion of the tube allowed to rest along the orobuccal fold and the operator is seen to be using a Hopkins telescope through the rigid bronchoscope. From: Turner JF, Ernst A, Becker HD. "How I do It" rigid bronchoscopy. *J Bronchol* 2000; **7**: 174.

push between the vocal cords, occasionally utilizing a slight corkscrewing motion. The bronchoscope should not, however, be forcefully pushed through the cords and, if the glottic opening is not large enough, consideration should be made for utilizing a smaller-diameter tube. Once the distal lip is past, the vocal cords the bronchoscope is rotated another 90° placing the protruding lip of the tube at the 6 o'clock position with the proximal portion of the tube allowed to rest along the orobuccal fold (Fig. 22.11). The teeth and gums may be cushioned with gauze or a rubber protector.

A second method of intubation with the rigid bronchoscope is to visualize the vocal cords with a laryngoscope and directly insert the rigid scope into the subglottic space in the same manner as endotracheal intubation is accomplished (Fig. 22.12).

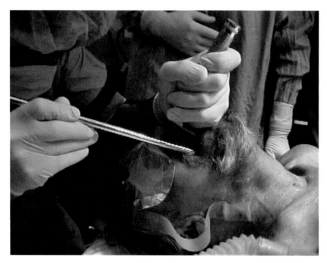

**Fig. 22.12** The laryngoscope is used to visualize the vocal cords and the patient is "intubated" with the rigid bronchoscope.

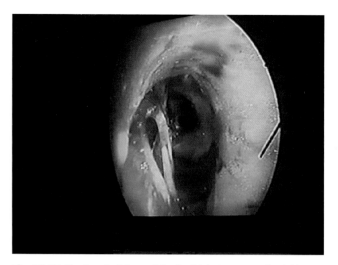

**Fig. 22.14** The "eye" of the endotracheal tube is seen as the rigid bronchoscope is slowly withdrawn.

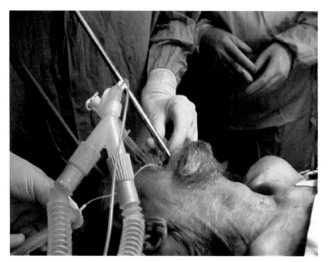

**Fig. 22.13** The rigid bronchoscope is inserted along the endotracheal tube, which is then slowly withdrawn while sliding the rigid tube forward between the vocal cords.

A third technique is to intubate the patient with a standard endotracheal tube prior to using the rigid scope. Intubation with the rigid scope is then accomplished by sliding the bronchoscope along the surface of the endotracheal tube until the glottic opening is visualized. The endotracheal tube is then slowly withdrawn while sliding the rigid tube forward between the vocal cords (Figs 22.13, 22.14).

If the operator has intubated the patient without the aid of the Hopkins telescope, this instrument is then inserted through the rigid bronchoscope until just proximal to the distal flared end of the rigid tube. Again, the distal flared end of the outer tube should be visible to prevent inadvertent perforation of the trachea or bronchi.

Once in the subglottic space, the rigid bronchoscope is slowly advanced forward carefully inspecting the trachea. The rigid bronchoscope is able to glide forward easily and should not be forced. When the main carina has been inspected the patient's head is rotated to permit intubation of the main bronchi and more distal inspection. Rotation of the patient's head to the right side positions the bronchoscope to intubate the left mainstem bronchi. Conversely, rotation of the patient's head to the left side allows intubation of the right mainstem bronchus. The upper and lower segmental orifices are generally easily identified. Complete examination to the subsegmental level is generally possible in the middle and lower lobe with a 0° telescope. The acute angle at which the right upper lobe branches from the right main bronchus will not allow full subsegmental inspection without the aid of a 90° lens. This acute angle will also prevent biopsies without the additional aid of a flexible fiberoptic bronchoscope. The left upper lobe segments and the lingula may be visualized with much the same technique as for the right upper lobe. After general inspection as needed, additional interventional procedures may be completed through the rigid bronchoscope.

Upon completion of the procedure, a flexible suction catheter is inserted through the rigid bronchoscope past the distal end. With continuous suction the rigid tube is then removed in the near horizontal plane in which it has been resting. This should be able to be accomplished with a smooth sliding motion unhampered by notable resistance.

## Complications

Complications are often related to the underlying pulmonary pathology requiring rigid bronchoscopy and result from:

**1** hypoxemia—inability to intubate and secure an airway or secondary to underlying pulmonary abnormality

**2** hemodynamic instability

**3** tracheal or esophageal perforation—the rigid instrument is forced or misdirected with resultant perforation of the upper airway, trachea, or esophagus

**4** dental trauma

**5** laryngeal edema.

Care must be taken not to insert the tube too quickly or with too great a force, thereby becoming disoriented and inadvertently entering a pyriform sinus, the esophagus, or pushing through the glottis without visualization. Proceeding in haste may also lead to improper positioning or avulsion of a vocal cord. This may happen particularly in those patients who have already undergone previous head and neck surgery. In these cases, careful advancement of the scope always using direct vision is essential in proper intubation. As with any type of intubation procedure the operator must be aware that the patient is apneic during this attempt and should permit the patient to be ventilated if prolonged or multiple intubation attempts are needed. Meticulous preoperative planning is essential with a clear understanding between the bronchoscopist and the anesthesiologist as to a primary plan for establishing ventilation with the rigid scope and consideration of alternative courses of action should the airway be "lost." Also, having a selection of varying sizes of rigid bronchoscopes, endotracheal tubes, LMAs, as well as, an emergent cricothyrotomy or tracheostomy kit should be part of every rigid operator's available equipment dependent upon the clinical problem.

## Training goals

All bronchoscopists, in our opinion, need not learn the technique and art of rigid bronchoscopy. The majority of bronchoscopic procedures can now be effectively performed through the use of the flexible bronchoscope. As noted above, however, there are circumstances where having the ability to use a rigid bronchoscope is desirable. As the number of bronchoscopic cases requiring rigid technique is small compared to the overall number of bronchoscopies performed in the United States, we propose that each major referral center should have at least one bronchoscopist who is skilled in both the rigid and flexible techniques. This is not to mean that the technique of rigid bronchoscopy is beyond the ability of the average bronchoscopist. On the contrary, as with any learned skill, the ability is dependent upon the training and individual ability. However, every operator understands that, as for any skill, a certain number of procedures are required to initially learn the technique and then maintain proficiency. Kvale proposed credentialling guidelines for laser bronchoscopy in 1990 [16], with at least 25 such procedures to be performed per physician per year to maintain proficiency. The American College of Chest Physician's formal bronchoscopic guidelines for the fiberoptic bronchoscope state that the minimal number of procedures to allow one to be able to anticipate problems and complications is 50 diagnostic bronchoscopies under supervision during the training program [17]. Trainees in rigid bronchoscopy, thus, should first practice on mannequins and be mentored through at least 50 supervised rigid bronchoscopy procedures before attempting the procedure alone.

## Summary

Rigid bronchoscopy continues to be a useful technique more than 100 years after its inception by Killian. The combination of a large-diameter tube in which to work with the advantage of controlled ventilation allows the performance of procedures not yet suitable for the smaller working channel of the fiberoptic scope. Continued training and mastery of this skill are needed for interventional bronchoscopists to carry on the therapeutic tradition into this new millennium.

## References

1 Zollner F. Gustav Killian: father of bronchoscopy. *Arch Otolaryng* 1965; **82**: 656–9.

2 Von Eiken C. The clinical application of the method of direct examination of the respiratory passes and upper alimentary tract. *Arch Laryngol Rhinol* 1904; 15.

3 Prakash UBS. Introduction. In: Prakash UBS, ed. *Bronchoscopy*. New York: Raven Press Ltd; 1994.

4 Prakash UBS, Offord KP, Stubbs SE. Bronchoscopy in North America: The ACCP Survey. *Chest* 1991; **100**: 1668–75.

5 Wedzicha JA, Pearson MC. Management of massive hemoptysis. *Respir Med* 1990; **84**: 9–12.

6 Freitag L. Flexible versus rigid bronchoscopic placement of tracheobronchial prosthesis (stents). Pro rigid bronchoscopy. *J Bronchol* 1995; **2**: 248–51.

7 Ayers ML, Beamis JF. Rigid bronchoscopy in the twenty-first century. *Clin Chest Med* 2001; **22**: 355–64.

8 Colt HG, Harrell JH. Therapeutic rigid bronchoscopy allows level of care changes in patients with acute respiratory failure from central airway obstruction. *Chest* 1997; **112**: 202–6.

9 Beamis J. Rigid bronchoscopy. In Beamis JF, Mathur PN, eds. *Interventional Pulmonology*. New York: McGraw-Hill; 1999: 17–28.

10 Kollofrath O. Entfernung eines Knochenstucks aus dem rechten Bronchus auf anturlichem Wege and Anwendung der directed Laryngoscopie. *MMW* 1897; **38**: 1038–9.

11 Ginsberg RJ. Rigid bronchoscopy. In: Feinsilver SH, Fein AM, eds. *Textbook of Bronchoscopy*. Baltimore: Williams & Wilkins; 1995: 486–93.

12 Turner JF, Wang KP. Endobronchial laser therapy. *Clin Chest Med* 1999; **20**: 107.

13 Natalini G, Cavaliere S, Seramondi V, *et al*. Negative pressure ventilation vs. external high-frequency oscillation during rigid bronchoscopy. *Chest* 2000; **118**: 18–23.

14 Natalini G, Vitacca M, Cavaliere S, *et al*. Negative pressure ventilation vs. spontaneous assisted ventilation during rigid bronchoscopy. *Acta Anaest Scand* 1998; **42**: 1063–9.

15 Natalini G, Vitacca M, Cavaliere S, *et al*. Use of Hayek oscillator during rigid bronchoscopy under general anesthesia [abstract]. *Br J Anaesth* 1997; **78** (Suppl 1): 23.

16 Kvale P. Training in laser bronchoscopy and proposal for credentialling. *Chest* 1990; **97**: 983–9.

17 American College of Chest Physicians, Section of Bronchoscopy. Guidelines for competency and training in fiberoptic bronchoscopy. *Chest* 1982; **81**: 739.

# 23 Pediatric Flexible Bronchoscopy for Adult Bronchoscopists

## Xicheng Liu,[1] Shunying Zhao,[1] and Peter Mogayzel[2]

[1] Center for Pediatric Bronchoscopy, Beijing Children's Hospital, Capital Medical University, Beijing, China
[2] Cystic Fibrosis Center, Johns Hopkins School of Medicine, Baltimore, MD, USA

## Introduction

The landmark article by Wood and Fink in 1978 describing the clinical utility of bronchoscopy in 127 children ushered in a revolutionary approach to evaluating pediatric lung disease [1]. Today, flexible fiberoptic bronchoscopy (FFB) is routinely used in children to diagnose airway abnormalities by visual inspection and evaluate infection and parenchymal disease through the use of bronchoalveolar lavage (BAL), bronchial brushing, and biopsy. Additionally, there is an ever increasing role for FFB in therapeutic interventions.

## Performing a pediatric flexible bronchoscopy

### Choosing a flexible fiberoptic bronchoscope

Flexible bronchoscopes are available in sizes that permit airway evaluation in even the smallest infants. Flexible pediatric bronchoscopes have an outer diameter of 2.8–4.0 mm, with a suction/instrument channel of 1.2–2.2 mm in diameter. Additionally, "ultrathin" instruments (2.2 mm in outer diameter) that do not possess a suction/instrument channel play an important role in the evaluation of premature infants and the distal airways of small full-term infants. Larger diameter (≥4.9 mm) bronchoscopes are appropriate for school-age and adolescent patients. Biopsy forceps are available for use in both 2.0–2.2 and 1.2-mm channels.

The choice of bronchoscope depends on the goals of the procedure and the size of the child. Airway diameter of a child can be approximated by the following calculation:

Airway caliber (mm) = 4 + (age in years)/4.

The choice of bronchoscope is critically important if it is going to be inserted via an endotracheal tube (ETT) since it will partially block the lumen [2]. The amount of the cross-sectional area blocked by the bronchoscope can be calculated from the formula:

$$1 - (\text{bronchoscope radius}^2/\text{ETT radius}^2) \times 100.$$

Therefore, placing a 2.8-mm bronchoscope into a 4.0-mm ETT will block 84% of the luminal diameter. For adequate spontaneous ventilation, the ETT internal diameter generally needs to be at least 1 mm greater than the external diameter of the bronchoscope. Assisted ventilation may be required when more than 50% of the ETT lumen is obstructed or for children who have with significant pre-existing gas exchange abnormalities.

## Preoperative preparation

The time immediately prior to the procedure can be difficult for both parents and children. There is often anxiety about the procedure itself as well as the potential of an unwanted discovery which may be revealed by FFB. Additionally, children are often fussy and anxious because they are hungry and in a foreign environment. Therefore, the preoperative area should be designed to minimize the level of anxiety associated with the FFB. This can be accomplished by providing distractions and minimizing painful procedures such as placing iv lines prior to the procedure. A sedative or anxiolytic premedication may benefit a very distressed or uncooperative child. Oral midazolam is well suited for this purpose.

## The bronchoscopy procedure
### Sedation and anesthesia

Sedating children for procedures can be challenging. Choosing the appropriate anesthetic approach is vital to achieving a successful procedure. There are several factors to consider including: safety of the child during the procedure; comfort of the child before, during, and after the

*Flexible Bronchoscopy*, Third Edition. Edited by Ko-Pen Wang, Atul C. Mehta, J. Francis Turner.
© 2012 Blackwell Publishing Ltd. Published 2012 by Blackwell Publishing Ltd.

procedure; preventing undue anxiety in both child and family; and establishing appropriate sedation to perform the procedure. Sedation for FFB is typically achieved by topical application of lidocaine in conjunction with intravenous sedatives or inhalational anesthetic agents. The depth of sedation and choice of sedative agents will be dictated by the goals for the FFB. Evaluation of the dynamic properties of the airway can be altered by changes in muscle tone and breathing induced by deep sedation or general anesthesia.

Current guidelines for sedation of pediatric patients require continuous monitoring of heart rate and oxygen saturation, and intermittent measurement of respiratory rate and blood pressure at a minimum, and observation by a competent, trained person with no other responsibility [3]. This individual must be trained in pediatric airway management and be familiar with the possible side effects of drugs being administered and have the skills to manage them.

### Topical agents

Flexible fiberoptic bronchoscopy has traditionally been performed in children by placing the bronchoscope into the airway via a nostril. Prior to insertion of the bronchoscope, viscous lidocaine can be applied into the nose using a cotton swab. A spray of a topical 1–2% lidocaine can also be applied to the nasopharynx. Once the bronchoscope has been introduced into the airway, several aliquots of 0.5–1% lidocaine should be instilled onto the vocal cords and the carina. Ensuring adequate local anesthesia will minimize the risk of laryngospasm and prevent coughing. In small children, care must be taken to avoid lidocaine toxicity, which can safely be administered up to a total dose of 7 mg/kg [4]. Atropine can be administered to infants to prevent vagally mediated bradycardia and dry secretions.

### Intravenous and inhalational agents

Examination of the upper airway in young infants can often be performed without sedation. However, deep sedation or general anesthesia is typically required for FFB of the lower airways. Traditionally, a combination of a narcotic and a benzodiazepine has been used for sedation. However, newer agents, such as propofol, are now widely used during FFB [5,6]. Propofol is an intravenous agent, which rapidly induces sleep that is of short duration. Propofol induces apnea in a dose-dependent fashion and can be used for the induction of general anesthesia. Propofol is approved in the USA for induction of anesthesia in pediatric patients aged 3 years and older and for the maintenance of anesthesia in children aged 2 months and older. Long-term therapy with propofol has been associated with deaths in the pediatric population [7]. However, propofol can be safely used in children for sedation for FFB [8].

Inhalational anesthetic agents can be used to induce general anesthesia, which may be appropriate for some patients, especially when dynamic airway changes are not being evaluated. Induction of anesthesia with an inhalational agent can also be used for placement of a laryngeal mask airway (LMA) or ETT or prior to the placement of an iv line for administration of medications.

### Airway management

Adequate management of the airway during the procedure is key to the success of a pediatric FFB. Hypoxemia resulting from airway obstruction by the bronchoscope leading to hypoventilation is probably the most frequent adverse event encountered during pediatric FFB. Hypoxemia is more likely to occur in younger children and those that require supplemental oxygen therapy at baseline [9]. The technique of airway management utilized during FFB will vary with the respiratory status of the child and the goals of the procedure [5,6,10]. Commonly used techniques include the following.

*Facemask.* This technique allows visualization of the entire upper and lower airways. Dynamic changes in the airway can be observed during normal respiration. Additionally, application of positive pressure can be used to evaluate dynamic airway lesions and treat upper airway obstruction [11]. The patient's breathing can also be assisted by the anesthetist if needed.

*Nasopharyngeal airway (prong).* The nasopharyngeal airway can prevent upper airway obstruction during sedation. The bronchoscope can be passed down the contralateral nostril of the nasopharyngeal airway so as not to limit the size of the bronchoscope used. This technique allows for inspection of the majority of the upper airway.

*Laryngeal mask airway.* Placement of an LMA provides better control of the airway than either a facemask or nasopharyngeal airway [12]. An LMA easily allows assisted ventilation in children that are at risk for significant gas exchange abnormalities during the procedure. Placement and maintenance of an LMA requires a greater depth of sedation or anesthesia than the use of a facemask. However, the depth of anesthesia required to maintain the LMA reduces the risk of both laryngospasm and bronchospasm. Laryngeal mask airways are available in a range of sizes that can fit even newborn infants (Table 23.1). If a single-use LMA is utilized then the grill at the aperture can be removed prior to placement to facilitate placement of the bronchoscope.

The downside to an LMA is that its placement may distort the upper airway anatomy. The aperture of the LMA can lie above the epiglottis, which may partially obstruct passage of the bronchoscope. Additionally, the depth of sedation required for LMA placement may alter airway dynamics and vocal cord movement.

**Table 23.1** Laryngeal mask airway (LMA) sizes

| LMA size | Child's weight (kg) |
|----------|---------------------|
| 1 | <5 |
| 1½ | 5–10 |
| 2 | 10–20 |
| 2½ | 20–30 |
| 3 | 30–50 |
| 4 | 50–70 |

Adapted from http://www.lmana.com.

**Table 23.2** Common airway anomalies that can be visualized during bronchoscopy

Laryngomalacia
Vocal cord paralysis
Posterior laryngeal cleft
Subglottic stenosis
Subglottic hemangioma
Subglottic cyst
Tracheal stenosis
Tracheal web
Tracheal cartilaginous sleeve
Complete tracheal rings
Tracheal diverticulum
Tracheal bronchus
Tracheomalacia and bronchomalacia
Tracheoesophageal fistula
Bronchial atresia/agenesis
Bronchial stenosis

*Endotracheal tube.* Placement of an ETT allows easy access to the lower airway for bronchoalveolar lavage (BAL) and other diagnostic procedures when evaluation of the upper airway is not required or in children at risk for significant respiratory comprise during the procedure. Effects of positive pressure on lower airway dynamics can also be studied. The main drawback to using an ETT is that the upper airway and proximal lower airway cannot be visualized. Additionally, dynamic abnormalities in the airway may be masked by the presence of the ETT and depth of anesthesia.

## Diagnosis and treatment of pediatric lung disease

### Visual examination
Flexible fiberoptic bronchoscopy allows for detailed examination of the pediatric airway anatomy including the dynamic movement of the glottis and vocal cords as well as changes in the lower airway with respiration and in some cases with the application of positive pressure. Dynamic abnormalities often visualized include airway collapse due to malacia or external compression by vascular structures. Bronchoscopy can identify airway obstruction by secretions and mucus plugs, blood, foreign bodies, and neoplasms. Additionally, there are many congenital airway abnormalities that can be detected using FFB (Table 23.2).

### Bronchoalveolar lavage
The technique for performance of BAL is similar in adults and children. The tip of bronchoscope is wedged into a segmental or subsegmental bronchus and one aliquot of normal saline is instilled and then aspirated back. The optimal volume for BAL is unclear [13]. Typically, saline aliquots of 1 mL/kg are instilled up to a maximum of 5 mL/kg. However, studies have suggested that adjusting the volume of saline instilled based on the child's age may be a better approach [14]. The usual fluid return from a BAL is approximately 30–60% of the instilled saline. The volume returned tends to increase with subsequent aliquots. Normal values for cellular components of BAL fluid from children are available [13,15]. Cellular components of the BAL are altered in disease states [16,17]. Bronchoalveolar lavage has also been used extensively in research studies to evaluate inflammatory mediators [18,19].

Therapeutic lavage can be used to treat atelectasis by removing inspissated secretions obstructing airways. Therapeutic lavage has also been used in the treatment of alveolar proteinosis [20].

### Brushing and biopsy
Bronchial brushing can be performed to: obtain epithelial cells for cytology or research purposes, identify intracellular pathogens, and evaluate cilia. The procedure, which involves the insertion of a soft cytology brush into the airway, is well tolerated by most children [21,22]. When using a smaller bronchoscope the brush must be removed from the protective plastic sheath. Therefore, after the brushing is performed the entire bronchoscope should be removed with the brush extended beyond the tip or just barely retracted into the bronchoscope.

Endobronchial biopsies have traditionally been performed using a rigid bronchoscope, especially when proximal airways are involved or if hemorrhage is anticipated. Recently, obtaining endobronchial biopsies via FFB has gained more widespread acceptance. Saglani *et al.* [23] demonstrated that endobronchial biopsies could be safely performed using FFB in children as young as 4 months of age. Further studies have demonstrated that this technique can be performed in children with significant cystic fibrosis lung disease [24]. Regamey *et al.* [25] demonstrated that adequate specimens can be obtained from 72–79% of children with asthma or cystic fibrosis. Biopsies can be used for histopathological and immunocytochemical analysis, microbiological culture, assessment of ciliary motility and architecture, and primary bronchial epithelial cell culture. Endobronchial biopsies have been utilized extensively to study the relationship between clinical signs and symptoms and structural abnormalities in children with both asthma [26–28] and cystic fibrosis [29].

Transbronchial biopsies can be used to diagnose a wide variety of infectious, immunologically mediated, and fibrotic pulmonary conditions [30]. Transbronchial biopsies are particularly useful in the management of patients following pulmonary transplantation. Many pediatric transplantation programs routinely perform surveillance transbronchial biopsies to detect occult allograft rejection [31,32]. The technique is performed in a similar manner in both children and adults. Excellent-quality biopsies can be obtained using 1.8-mm forceps that fit down a 2–2.2-mm working channel; and reasonable biopsies can also be obtained from the smaller 1-mm forceps that fit into a 1.2-mm channel [30]. These latter specimens are often quite small and require a skilled pathologist to make definitive diagnoses of parenchymal pathology.

Complications associated with biopsies include bleeding and pneumothorax. Bleeding can usually be controlled with lavage using cold saline or instillation of topical epinephrine. Occasionally, excessive bleeding will need control by rigid bronchoscopy. Isolating the contralateral lung with a rigid bronchoscope or ETT may be necessary in cases of massive hemorrhage, allowing adequate ventilation of one lung in order to adequately oxygenate the child. The risk of bleeding can be minimized by ensuring that clotting parameters and platelet count are optimized prior to bronchoscopy. The incidence of significant pneumothorax following biopsy is approximately 1%. The risk of pneumothorax may be increased in patients who require ventilatory support at the time of biopsy.

## Common indications for pediatric bronchoscopy

Common indications for pediatric FFB are listed in Table 23.3. The most common indications for FFB in children may be the definitive exclusion of anatomic anomalies or foreign body aspiration. The yield of diagnostic information from FFB is dependent on the indication for the bronchoscopy.

### Stridor

Laryngomalacia (Fig. 23.1) is by far the most common etiology of stridor in young children [33]. Other functional lesions, such as paralyzed vocal cord(s), can also be identified. Structural anomalies in the supraglottic or subglottic region can also lead to stridor. These include supraglottic

**Table 23.3** Common indications for bronchoscopy in children

Stridor
Persistent or recurrent wheezing
Chronic cough
Hemoptysis
Atelectasis
Suspected foreign body
Suspected airway anomaly, tracheoesophageal fistula or vascular ring
Pneumonia/lower respiratory tract infection
Cystic fibrosis
Lung transplantation
Airway evaluation after tracheostomy
Aid in intubation
To obtain specimens for research

cysts (Fig. 23.2) and subglottic stenosis (Fig. 23.3). Rigid bronchoscopy may be required to visualize some lesions, such as laryngeal clefts [34].

### Persistent wheezing

In a review of 1000 bronchoscopies, Wood [35] found relevant abnormalities in 70% of children with wheezing. The utility of FFB in evaluating persistent or recurrent wheezing may be improved when the results are interpreted in conjunction with other studies such as CT scans and fluoroscopy or tests for gastroesophageal reflux (GER) [36].

There are several anatomic abnormalities that can present as persistent wheezing. Dynamic lesions that lead to airflow limitation during expiration, such as bronchomalacia (Fig. 23.4), can be diagnosed using FFB. Other congenital lesions, such as complete tracheal rings, are much less common. Airway obstruction by masses, such as cysts or hemangiomas (Fig. 23.5), can also present as wheezing or persistent atelectasis. Although airway tumors are very rare in children, they can also be identified using FFB (Fig. 23.6). External airway compression by a pulsatile mass can indicate the presence of a vascular ring. Children with congenital heart disease can exhibit airway compression, which is frequently associated with significant malacia from abnormal vascular structures or cardiac enlargement.

Foreign bodies are occasionally the cause of persistent wheezing, which may or may not be localized on physical examination. Figure 23.7 shows the inflammatory response to remnants of an aspirated peanut. Foreign body removal is typically performed using rigid bronchoscopy. However, successful removal of foreign bodies from children using FFB has been described [37]. If a foreign body is unlikely, performing FFB first can be an effective approach to management [38].

Chronic aspiration associated with dysfunctional swallowing is a common cause of wheezing in infants, which often leads to edematous lower airway mucosa. Erythema and

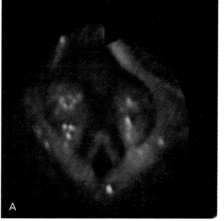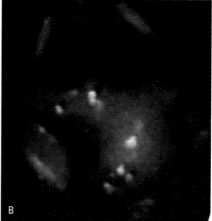

**Fig. 23.1** Laryngomalacia in a 5-month-old boy with stridor. (A) Larynx during expiration. (B) Airway collapse of airway during inspiration.

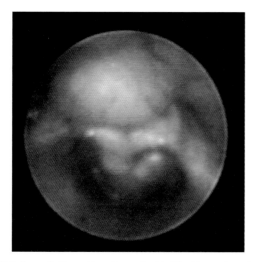

**Fig. 23.2** Supraglottic cyst in a 4-month-old girl with cough and stridor without hoarseness.

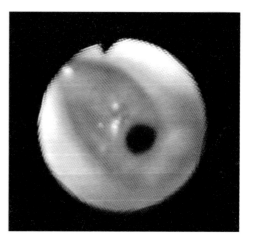

**Fig. 23.3** Subglottic airway stenosis in a 2-month-old boy with respiratory failure.

edema of upper airway structures suggests the presence of significant GER. However, the diagnosis of chronic aspiration cannot be made by FFB alone. The presence of lipid-laden macrophages (LLM) in BAL fluid can be an indication of aspiration. However, there is ample evidence that LLM are not a specific finding [39–41]. The finding of LLM in BAL fluid must be interpreted in conjunction with evaluation of the child's swallowing function, degree of GER, and severity of lung disease. The response to discontinuation of oral feedings is often the best way to diagnose chronic aspiration in infants. Identification of a tracheoesophageal fistula as a source of chronic aspiration may also be possible using FFB.

## Chronic cough

Bronchoscopy can frequently identify the etiologies of a chronic cough in a child. Wood [35] found relevant abnor-

malities in 55% of children evaluated for cough. Saito *et al.* [42] found lower airway abnormalities in 12/19 (63%) of 5–26–month-old infants with chronic cough. Both viral and bacterial pathogens were recovered frequently. Chronic bronchitis has also been implicated as a cause of chronic cough in a large series of patients with "wet" cough [43]. As with wheezing, chronic aspiration is a frequent cause of cough in infants.

## Atelectasis

The most common cause of atelectasis is airway obstruction by mucus plugs [35,44]. Therefore, removal of the secretions with therapeutic lavage can be an effective therapy for atelectasis. Other etiologies commonly encountered include: foreign bodies, airway stenosis, bronchomalacia, and extrinsic compression [44].

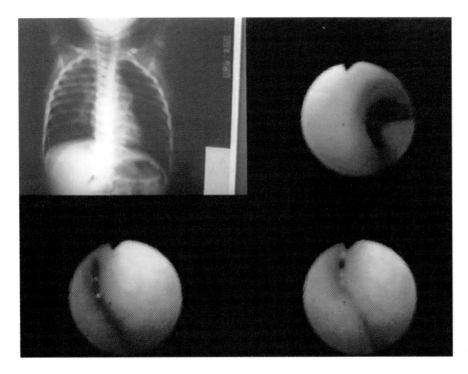

**Fig. 23.4** Bronchomalacia in a 5-month-old boy with persistent wheezing.

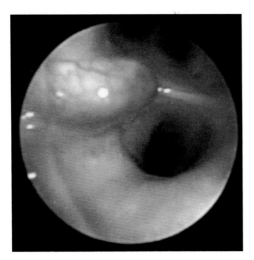

**Fig. 23.5** Bronchial hemangioma in a 12-year-old boy with chronic cough and hemoptysis for 2 years.

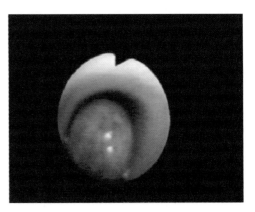

**Fig. 23.6** Right mainstem bronchus tumor in a 4-year-old boy with cough and recurrent pneumonia.

## Pneumonia and suspected infection

Since children often do not expectorate sputum, FFB can pay an important role in the identification of infectious pathogens in both immunocompetent and immunocompromised children. For example, the yield of BAL in detecting an organism in children with pneumonia following bone marrow transplantation ranges from 29 to 52% [45]. The likelihood of identifying a pathogen is increased by performing the FFB prior to extensive empiric antibiotic therapy. The use of FFB can also provide information, which cannot be gained from ETT aspirates, to direct therapy for ventilator-associated pneumonia [46]. Endobronchial infections such as tuberculosis can be easily identified by FFB (Fig. 23.8).

Pulmonary infection with organisms such as *Pseudomonas aeruginosa* has significant implications for children with cystic fibrosis. Surveillance oropharyngeal cultures are routinely performed in children with cystic fibrosis; however, these cultures may not provide a complete representation of

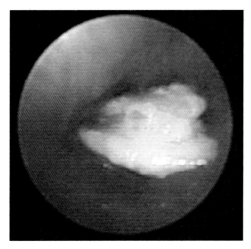

**Fig. 23.7** Peanut debris in a small airway of lower lobe in a 1.5-year-old boy with cough and pneumonia.

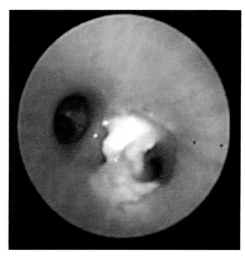

**Fig. 23.8** Bronchial tuberculosis in a 1-year-old boy with pulmonary hilar adenopathy.

the microbiology in the lower airway [47–49]. For this reason some cystic fibrosis centers perform FFB at diagnosis and routinely thereafter [48]. However, the value of routine bronchoscopy has recently been brought into question [50].

## Airway management

Flexible bronchoscopy can be utilized in the operating room and ICU to assist in difficult intubations. Routine visualization of the trachea every 6–12 months following tracheostomy "to assess the underlying airway pathology, detect and treat complications, assess tube size and position" is recommended by the American Thoracic Society [51]. The use of airway stents is controversial in young children. However, in properly selected patients, stent placement using FFB can successfully treat severe airway obstruction [52].

## Summary

Over the past 30 years FFB has become an indispensible part of the diagnosis and management of pediatric lung disease. Diagnostic procedures can be performed safely in even the smallest children. Additionally, there is an ever increasing array of therapeutic interventions that can be performed in children using FFB.

## References

1 Wood RE, Fink RJ. Applications of flexible fiberoptic bronchoscopes in infants and children. *Chest* 1978; **73** (5 Suppl): 737–40.

2 Balfour-Lynn IM, Harcourt J. Bronchoscopic equipment. In: Priftis KN, Anthracopoulos MB, Koumbourlis AC, Wood RE, (eds): *Pediatric Bronchoscopy*. Prog Respir res. Basel, Karger 2010; **38**: 12–21.

3 Cote CJ, Wilson S. Guidelines for monitoring and management of pediatric patients during and after sedation for diagnostic and therapeutic procedures: An update. *Pediatrics* 2006; **118**: 2587–602.

4 Amitai Y, Zylber-Katz E, Avital A, *et al.* Serum lidocaine concentrations in children during bronchoscopy with topical anesthesia. *Chest* Dec 1990; **98**: 1370–3.

5 Jaggar SI, Haxby E. Sedation, anaesthesia and monitoring for bronchoscopy. *Paediatr Respir Rev* 2002; **3**: 321–7.

6 Midulla F, de Blic J, Barbato A, *et al.* Flexible endoscopy of paediatric airways. *Eur Respir J* 2003; **22**: 698–708.

7 Kam PCA, Cardone D. Propofol infusion syndrome. *Anaesthesia* 2007; **62**: 690–701.

8 Hasan RA, Reddy R. Sedation with propofol for flexible bronchoscopy in children. *Pediatr Pulmonol* 2009; **44**: 373–8.

9 Schnapf BM. Oxygen desaturation during fiberoptic bronchoscopy in pediatric patients. *Chest* 1991; **99**: 591–4.

10 Niggemann B, Haack M, Machotta A. How to enter the pediatric airway for bronchoscopy. *Pediatr Int* 2004; **46**: 117–21.

11 Trachsel D, Erb TO, Frei FJ, Hammer J, on behalf of the Swiss Paediatric Respiratory Research Group. Use of continuous positive airway pressure during flexible bronchoscopy in young children. *Eur Respir J* 2005; **26**: 773–7.

12 Naguib ML, Streetman DS, Clifton S, *et al.* Use of laryngeal mask airway in flexible bronchoscopy in infants and children. *Pediatr Pulmonol* 2005; **39**: 56–63.

13 de Blic J, Midulla F, Barbato A, *et al.* Bronchoalveolar lavage in children. ERS Task Force on bronchoalveolar lavage in children. European Respiratory Society. *Eur Respir J* 2000; **15**: 217–31.

14 Ratjen F, Bruch J. Adjustment of bronchoalveolar lavage volume to body weight in children. *Pediatr Pulmonol* 1996; **21**: 184–8.

15 Brennan S, Gangell C, Wainwright C, *et al.* Disease surveillance using bronchoalveolar lavage. *Paediatr Respir Rev* 2008; **9**: 151–9.

16 Najafi N, Demanet C, Dab I, *et al.* Differential cytology of bronchoalveolar lavage fluid in asthmatic children. *Pediatr Pulmonol* 2003; **35**: 302–8.

17 Ratjen F, Costabel U, Griese M, *et al.* Bronchoalveolar lavage fluid findings in children with hypersensitivity pneumonitis. *Eur Respir J* 2003; **21**: 144–8.

18 Khan TZ, Wagener JS, Bost T, *et al.* Early pulmonary inflammation in infants with cystic fibrosis. *Am J Respir Crit Care Med* 1995; **151**: 1075–82.

19 Kim CK, Kim SW, Kim YK, *et al.* Bronchoalveolar lavage eosinophil cationic protein and interleukin-8 levels in acute asthma and acute bronchiolitis. *Clin Exp Allergy* 2005; **35**: 591–7.

20 Mahut B, Delacourt C, Scheinmann P, *et al.* Pulmonary alveolar proteinosis: Experience with eight pediatric cases and a review. *Pediatrics* 1996; **97**: 117–22.

21 Kicic A, Sutanto EN, Stevens PT, *et al.* Intrinsic biochemical and functional differences in bronchial epithelial cells of children with asthma. *Am J Respir Crit Care Med* 2006; **174**: 1110–18.

22 McNamara PS, Kicic A, Sutanto EN, *et al.* Comparison of techniques for obtaining lower airway epithelial cells from children. *Eur Respir J* 2008; **32**: 763–8.

23 Saglani S, Payne DN, Nicholson AG, *et al.* The safety and quality of endobronchial biopsy in children under five years old. *Thorax* 2003; **58**: 1053–7.

24 Molina-Teran A, Hilliard TN, Saglani S, *et al.* Safety of endobronchial biopsy in children with cystic fibrosis. *Pediatr Pulmonol* 2006; **41**: 1021–4.

25 Regamey N, Hilliard TN, Saglani S, *et al.* Quality, size, and composition of pediatric endobronchial biopsies in cystic fibrosis. *Chest* 2007; **131**: 1710–17.

26 Lex C, Ferreira F, Zacharasiewicz A, *et al.* Airway eosinophilia in children with severe asthma: Predictive values of noninvasive tests. *Am J Respir Crit Care Med* 2006; **174**: 1286–91.

27 Saglani S, Malmstrom K, Pelkonen AS, *et al.* Airway remodeling and inflammation in symptomatic infants with reversible airflow obstruction. *Am J Respir Crit Care Med* 2005; **171**: 722–7.

28 Barbato A, Turato G, Baraldo S, *et al.* Epithelial damage and angiogenesis in the airways of children with asthma. *Am J Respir Crit Care Med* 2006; **174**: 975–81.

29 Hilliard TN, Regamey N, Shute JK, *et al.* Airway remodelling in children with cystic fibrosis. *Thorax* 2007; **62**: 1074–80.

30 Visner GA, Faro A, Zander DS. Role of transbronchial biopsies in pediatric lung diseases. *Chest* 2004; **126**: 273–80.

31 Benden C, Harpur-Sinclair O, Ranasinghe AS, *et al.* Surveillance bronchoscopy in children during the first year after lung transplantation: Is it worth it? *Thorax* 2007; **62**: 57–61.

32 Faro A, Visner G. The use of multiple transbronchial biopsies as the standard approach to evaluate lung allograft rejection. *Pediatr Transplant* 2004; **8**: 322–8.

33 Zoumalan R, Maddalozzo J, Holinger LD. Etiology of stridor in infants. *Ann Otol Rhinol Laryngol* 2007; **116**: 329–34.

34 Wood RE. Evaluation of the upper airway in children. *Curr Opin Pediatr* 2008; **20**: 266–71.

35 Wood RE. The diagnostic effectiveness of the flexible bronchoscope in children. *Pediatr Pulmonol* 1985; **1**: 188–92.

36 Saglani S, Nicholson AG, Scallan M, *et al.* Investigation of young children with severe recurrent wheeze: Any clinical benefit? *Eur Respir J* 2006; **27**: 29–35.

37 Ramirez-Figueroa JL, Gochicoa-Rangel LG, Ramirez-San Juan DH, *et al.* Foreign body removal by flexible fiberoptic bronchoscopy in infants and children. *Pediatr Pulmonol* 2005; **40**: 392–7.

38 Righini CA, Morel N, Karkas A, *et al.* What is the diagnostic value of flexible bronchoscopy in the initial investigation of children with suspected foreign body aspiration? *Int J Pediatr Otorhinolaryngol* 2007; **71**: 1383–90.

39 Chang AB, Cox NC, Purcell J, *et al.* Airway cellularity, lipid laden macrophages and microbiology of gastric juice and airways in children with reflux oesophagitis. *Respir Res* 2005; **6**: 72.

40 Ding Y, Simpson PM, Schellhase DE, *et al.* Limited reliability of lipid-laden macrophage index restricts its use as a test for pulmonary aspiration: comparison with a simple semiquantitative assay. *Pediatr Dev Pathol* 2002; **5**: 551–8.

41 Rosen R, Fritz J, Nurko A, *et al.* Lipid-laden macrophage index is not an indicator of gastroesophageal reflux-related respiratory disease in children. *Pediatrics* 2008; **121**: e879–84.

42 Saito J, Harris WT, Gelfond J, *et al.* Physiologic, bronchoscopic, and bronchoalveolar lavage fluid findings in young children with recurrent wheeze and cough. *Pediatr Pulmonol* 2006; **41**: 709–19.

43 Marchant JM, Masters IB, Taylor SM, *et al.* Evaluation and outcome of young children with chronic cough. *Chest* 2006; **129**: 1132–41.

44 Wood RE. Spelunking in the pediatric airways: explorations with the flexible fiberoptic bronchoscope. *Pediatr Clin North Am* 1984; **31**: 785–99.

45 Collaco JM, Gower WA, Mogayzel PJ, Jr. Pulmonary dysfunction in pediatric hematopoietic stem cell transplant patients: overview, diagnostic considerations, and infectious complications. *Pediatr Blood Cancer* 2007; **49**: 117–26.

46 Bar-Zohar D, Sivan Y. The yield of flexible fiberoptic bronchoscopy in pediatric intensive care patients. *Chest* 2004; **126**: 1353–9.

47 Rosenfeld M, Emerson J, Accurso F, *et al.* Diagnostic accuracy of oropharyngeal cultures in infants and young children with cystic fibrosis. *Pediatr Pulmonol* 1999; **28**: 321–8.

48 Hilliard TN, Sukhani S, Francis J, *et al.* Bronchoscopy following diagnosis with cystic fibrosis. *Arch Dis Child* 2007; **92**: 898–9.

49 Armstrong DS, Grimwood K, Carlin JB, *et al.* Bronchoalveolar lavage or oropharyngeal cultures to identify lower respiratory pathogens in infants with cystic fibrosis. *Pediatr Pulmonol* 1996; **21**: 267–75.

50 Wainwright CE, Vidmar S, Armstrong DS, *et al.* Effect of bronchoalveolar lavage-directed therapy on *Pseudomonas aeruginosa* infection and structural lung injury in children with cystic fibrosis: a randomized trial. *JAMA* 2011; **306**: 163–71.

51 Sherman JM, Davis S, Albamonte-Petrick S, *et al.* Care of the child with a chronic tracheostomy. *Am J Respir Crit Care Med* 2000; **161**: 297–308.

52 Nicolai T. Airway stents in children. *Pediatr Pulmonol* 2008; **43**: 330–44.

# Bronchoscopy in the Intensive Care Unit

**Alex Chen and Marian H. Kollef**
Washington University School of Medicine, St Louis, MO, USA

## Introduction

The development of the flexible bronchoscope by Ikeda in the late 1960s significantly broadened the potential applications of bronchoscopy. One such adaptation has been its increasing use in the intensive care unit, where its diagnostic and therapeutic applications have made it an indispensible tool for the intensivist.

Critically ill patients can be defined as those who suffer from pathologic injury to one or more organ systems, resulting in significant impairment of bodily functions. These patients require careful monitoring and observation by personnel who are specifically trained in managing diseases and complications that can occur with critical illness.

Respiratory compromise may be the primary pathologic process or may occur as the progression of another illness. The tenuous nature of critically ill patients can render them unsuitable for transfer out of the intensive care unit; therefore, the ability to perform diagnostic as well as therapeutic procedures at the bedside in a fully monitored environment is advantageous.

## Indications

The indications for bronchoscopy in the intensive care unit are numerous, but can be broadly categorized as diagnostic or therapeutic. Some of the more common indications are summarized in Table 24.1.

Numerous reviews and studies have been published regarding the indications for bronchoscopy in the intensive care unit [1–6]. While indications vary somewhat between institutions and critical care settings (i.e. surgical, medical), the proportion of diagnostic and therapeutic bronchoscopy performed is generally balanced, with some procedures performed for both diagnostic and therapeutic processes.

## Equipment

A staff of medical personnel including physicians, nurses, technicians, and respiratory therapists is required when performing bronchoscopy in any setting. In critically ill patients, this staff must also be able and prepared to care for complications such as progressive respiratory failure, hemodynamic collapse, pneumothorax, and massive bleeding that may occur secondary to the severity of the underlying illness [7]. Further discussion of potential complications of bronchoscopy and considerations of bronchoscopy on mechanical ventilation will be addressed below.

When using the ICU room as a bronchoscopy suite, attention must be made such that continuous patient monitoring is available [8]. Measurements of continuous oxygen oximetry, end-tidal carbon dioxide level, blood pressure, and heart rate should be monitored as should all ventilator settings if the patient is supported on mechanical ventilation.

## Sedation and anesthesia

The majority of patients in the intensive care unit have orders for sedation, especially those on mechanical ventilation. Sedation in these patients usually consists of a short-acting benzodiazepine in addition to an opiate. Bronchoscopy can be performed using this combination, which will produce an anamnestic effect while providing analgesia. Alternatively, propofol, a hypnotic agent, may be used with the added benefit of rapid onset of action and short half-life.

---

*Flexible Bronchoscopy*, Third Edition. Edited by Ko-Pen Wang, Atul C. Mehta, J. Francis Turner.
© 2012 Blackwell Publishing Ltd. Published 2012 by Blackwell Publishing Ltd.

**Table 24.1** Major indications for bronchoscopy in the intensive care unit

| Diagnostic bronchoscopy | Therapeutic bronchoscopy |
|---|---|
| Airway inspection | Aspiration of secretions |
| Collection of respiratory specimens | Treatment of airway obstruction |
| Inspection of endotracheal tube position | Foreign body extraction |
|  | Endotracheal tube repositioning |
|  | Percutaneous dilational tracheostomy tube placement |
|  | Airway prosthetic placement |

**Table 24.2** Effect of bronchoscope in endotracheal tube on various respiratory mechanics

| Respiratory mechanic | Effect |
|---|---|
| Intratracheal pressure | Increased |
| Airway pressure | Increased |
| Functional residual capacity | Increased |
| Forced expiratory volume ($FEV_1$) | Decreased |
| Positive end expiratory pressure | Increased |
| Returned tidal volume | Decreased |

Topical anesthesia is achieved by the application of 2.5–5 mL aliquots of 1% lidocaine through the bronchoscope onto the tracheobronchial tree in intubated patients; in non-intubated patients, an atomizer can be used to apply topical lidocaine to the larynx and oropharynx. The nares may be anesthetized by spraying them with topical lidocaine or by applying lidocaine-soaked gauze onto the nasal mucosa.

## Bronchoscopy in patients on mechanical ventilation

Bronchoscopy can be performed safely in patients on mechanical ventilation, though certain considerations must be addressed [9]. The first of these is the impact of the flexible bronchoscope on both inspiratory and expiratory airflow through the endotracheal tube. Without an endotracheal tube, a bronchoscope occupies approximately 10% of the cross section of an adult trachea. A bronchoscope with a diameter of 5.7 mm occupies 51% of the cross section of an 8-mm endotracheal tube, resulting in a significant increase in airflow resistance [10]. The presence of a bronchoscope within an endotracheal tube also has significant influence on several other factors, as indicated in Table 24.2 [11]. Among these, increases in positive end-expiratory pressure (PEEP) can increase the risk for complications such as barotrauma.

To minimize these risks, it is advisable to perform bronchoscopy through endotracheal tubes no smaller than 8 mm when using a standard diagnostic bronchoscope. At our institution, a bronchoscope with an outer diameter of 4.9 mm is typically used, though bronchoscopes with an outer diameter of 5.2 mm would be acceptable as well. Additional recommendations for performing bronchoscopy on mechanically ventilated patients include pre-oxygenation at a fractional inspired oxygen ($FiO_2$) of 1.0 prior to insertion of the bronchoscope, increasing the tidal volume, decreasing or eliminating PEEP and decreasing the inspiratory flow rate to offset the high airway pressures caused by the bronchoscope within the endotracheal tube.

## Complications

Bronchoscopy is generally well tolerated, even in patients who are critically ill [12]. A review of more than 1000 bronchoscopies performed in the intensive care unit resulted in no deaths attributable to bronchoscopy. The safety of flexible bronchoscopy on mechanically ventilated patients has been specifically assessed as well. The use of bronchoalveolar lavage is associated with an increase in the alveolar–arterial gradient, though in one review did not result in complications necessitating premature termination of the procedure [13].

Transient hypoxemia commonly occurs during bronchoscopy, particularly in critically ill patients with pre-existing respiratory compromise, and usually returns to baseline following the procedure [14]. Maintaining an $FiO_2$ of 1.0 and avoiding unnecessary suctioning during bronchoscopy may help minimize the severity and degree of hypoxemia, though one should be prepared to remove the bronchoscope and manually ventilate the patient using an Ambu bag if necessary. Alternatively, it is possible to oxygenate patients directly through the suction channel of the bronchoscope if needed.

Bronchoscopy has several effects on the cardiovascular system, which may be augmented in the setting of critical illness. Cardiac arrhythmias can be seen in 3 to 11% of patients undergoing bronchoscopy, though cardiac arrest is highly unusual. Additional abnormalities such as elevation in heart rate, blood pressure, and cardiac output are likely due to surges of sympathetic activity. The likelihood of experiencing cardiac complications is augmented in those with underlying cardiovascular disease, particularly coronary artery disease. Continuous monitoring of heart rate, blood pressure, oxygen saturation, and telemetry (if available) are therefore advisable.

Bleeding associated with bronchoscopy is unusual unless coagulopathy is present and uncorrected. Patients with uremia may be pretreated with desmopressin given their qualitative platelet dysfunction. Thrombocytopenia is common among bone marrow transplant patients; additional platelets may be given prior to bronchoscopy, and uncontrollable bleeding even in this setting is rare when performing bronchoalveolar lavage (BAL) [15–21].

## Diagnostic bronchoscopy

### Airway inspection

Prior to the invention of the flexible bronchoscope, rigid bronchoscopy was used to examine the upper airways. Though rigid bronchoscopy remains useful and recommended in certain clinical scenarios, its limitations include the need for general anesthesia, lack of maneuverability resulting in the inability to thoroughly examine beyond central airways, and lack of widespread availability. In contrast, flexible bronchoscopy can be performed at the bedside under conscious sedation and is widely available to critical care personnel.

Indications for airway inspection in critically ill patients include the following:
• hemoptysis
• suspected traumatic airway injury
• following smoke inhalation
• aspiration of caustic substances
• persistent infiltrate on chest radiograph
• suspected tracheobronchial malacia or other airway abnormality
• concern for airway obstruction
• postoperative assessment of airway anastamosis following transplantation.

### Collection of respiratory specimens

Nosocomial pneumonia is the leading cause of death from hospital-acquired infections and ventilator-associated pneumonia (VAP) describes pneumonia developing in mechanically ventilated patients later than 48 hours following intubation. Numerous studies have demonstrated that patients with VAP receiving early inadequate antimicrobial therapy have higher mortality rates compared to patients receiving antibiotics to which the pathologic organisms are sensitive [22–32]. Therefore, early identification of pathologic organisms is desirable. BAL is a minimally invasive method to collect lower respiratory tract specimens that may subsequently be used to guide antimicrobial therapy in critically ill patients.

In one study of 130 patients, findings from BAL resulted in changes or discontinuation of antimicrobial therapy in nearly 60% of cases [33]. Among the most common indications for adjustment to the antimicrobial regimen was the

isolation of a resistant Gram-negative bacteria or the isolation of methicillin-resistant *Staphylococcus aureus* necessitating additional antibiotics.

## Technique for bronchoalveolar lavage in ventilated patients

A standardized approach to bronchoalveolar lavage in ventilated patients should be used when collecting respiratory specimens in critically ill patients. Table 24.3 lists the materials necessary to perform BAL in ventilated patients. This should include an inline adapter for the bronchoscope to the endotracheal tube, two sterile specimen containers, and saline.

With the patient in the supine position, the patient is given sedation, most often in the form of a benzodiazepine and opiate, or with propofol which has the added benefit of a very short half-life. A bite block is placed in the patient's mouth to protect the bronchoscope and an inline adapter for the bronchoscope is placed between the endotracheal tube and the ventilator tubing; 2.5–5 mL aliquots of 1% lidocaine can be administered through the endotracheal tube to provide topical anesthesia, and the bronchoscope is inserted through the inline adapter and advanced to the lobar bronchus that is to be sampled. Once the bronchoscope is wedged into position within a lobar or subsegmental bronchus, 50 mL of normal saline are injected through the suction channel of the bronchoscope into the wedged bronchus; suction is then applied and the aspirated fluid is collected in a sterile specimen container. The fluid aspirated following instillation of the initial 50 mL of normal saline is discarded as bronchial washing and the process is repeated with another 50 mL of normal saline. This fluid is then aspirated and is subsequently collected as bronchoalveolar lavage. Additional passes of 50 mL volumes may be instilled until the returned BAL amount is sufficient for submission of desired testing (i.e. microbiology, cytology). Arterial oxygenation has been shown to decrease following BAL in mechanically ventilated patients, though values seem to return to baseline within 12–15 hours following the procedure. One study demonstrated no significant difference in

**Table 24.3** Materials for bronchoalveolar lavage in ventilated patients

| |
|---|
| Inline adapter for bronchoscope |
| Sterile specimen containers × 2 |
| Normal saline |
| Bite block |
| 60 mL syringe |
| 4-way stop cock × 2 |
| Tubing |

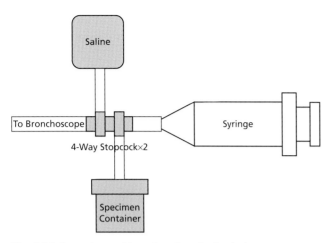

**Fig. 24.1** Apparatus used to perform bronchoalveolar lavage.

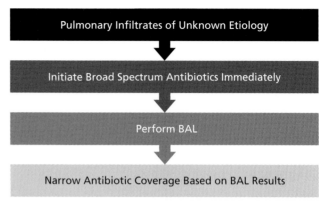

**Fig. 24.2** Algorithm for bronchoalveolar lavage in ventilator-associated pneumonia.

the decrease in oxygenation between instilled BAL volumes of 150 mL and 40 mL [34]. Figure 24.1 outlines the apparatus connected to the bronchoscope used at our institution to perform BAL.

## Timing of BAL in cases of suspected ventilator-associated pneumonia

If BAL is to be performed, it should be done early in the course of suspected VAP and should not delay the administration of appropriate antimicrobial coverage. Several studies have shown that the conversion of inadequate to adequate antimicrobial coverage following the results of BAL results in a similar rate of mortality to those who continued on inadequate therapy [33,35]. A suggested algorithm for BAL in VAP is outlined in Figure 24.2.

## Biopsy of lung tissue

Pulmonary infiltrates of uncertain etiology are often present or develop in critically ill patients requiring mechanical ventilation. While bronchoalveolar lavage provides a less invasive approach to sampling lower respiratory tract specimens, biopsy of lung tissue may be required to make certain diagnoses when BAL results are inconclusive. Open lung biopsy is a well established method for obtaining lung tissue, though may require transportation to an operating room, tube thoracostomy, and a surgical procedure, all of which can increase morbidity and mortality [36,37]. Bronchoscopic transbronchial lung biopsy in mechanically ventilated patients has subsequently been used in cases in which open lung biopsy is not desired. Previously, mechanical ventilation was felt to be a contraindication to transbronchial biopsy, though several studies have shown that it can be performed safely and successfully in this patient population [38,39].

One analysis reported that tissue examination obtained from transbronchial biopsy changed medical management in 60% of cases in mechanically ventilated patients, though this number was significantly lower for mechanically ventilated patients following lung transplantation [40]. Changes in medical management consisted of the initiation or discontinuation of antimicrobial agents, the initiation or discontinuation of corticosteroids, or the withdrawal of care following the diagnosis of lymphangitic carcinomatosis.

The incidence of pneumothorax following transbronchial lung biopsy in mechanically ventilated patients has been reported to be as much as three times higher than in those patients not on mechanical ventilation. In the aforementioned study, the overall pneumothorax rate was 14.3% though no deaths were directly attributable to this complication. While the result of transbronchial biopsy may alter medical management, the risk to benefit ratio must always be considered such that if the procedure is to be performed in a patient on mechanical ventilation, personnel and equipment needed for tube thoracostomy should be immediately available. Fluoroscopic guidance has been shown to decrease the risk of pneumothorax with transbronchial biopsy [41], and should therefore be used if available.

## Inspection of endotracheal tube position

Proper endotracheal tube position is an important component in the care of critically ill patients on mechanical ventilation. Studies have reported incorrect tube placement in up to 15% of ventilated patients [42,43], and fiberoptic bronchoscopy provides a quick and direct way of determining optimal positioning. Several factors may contribute to inadvertent movement of the endotracheal tube, such as turning or transport of the patient, and while chest radiographs may suggest inappropriate placement, direct visualization may be necessary to ensure a properly protected airway.

Fiberoptic bronchoscopy can also facilitate exchange of an endotracheal tube by loading a new endotracheal tube onto the bronchoscope which is then passed to the glottis alongside the pre-existing one which is slowly withdrawn under direct visualization. As the former endotracheal tube is removed, the bronchoscope is passed through the vocal cords and the new endotracheal tube is advanced into the trachea over the bronchoscope. This sequential method for endotracheal tube exchange allows direct visualization throughout the process, thereby decreasing the likelihood of esophageal intubation, or loss of the airway.

Fiberoptic intubation can also be performed electively, or in patients in which intubation with a laryngoscope is unsuccessful. Such patients may have limited neck mobility or upper airway pathology that renders a poor view using a standard laryngoscope [44]. In such cases the bronchoscope is loaded with an endotracheal tube and then advanced into the trachea. Once this position has been confirmed, the endotracheal tube is advanced over the bronchoscope into position. Success rates using this technique range from 95 to 98%.

Fiberoptic bronchoscopy can also be used to position double lumen endotracheal tubes and can also be used for selective left or right mainstem intubation in clinical scenarios such as hemoptysis [45–50].

## Therapeutic bronchoscopy

### Aspiration of secretions

Atelectasis is commonly seen in critically ill patients on mechanical ventilation. Traditionally, the focus of treatment for atelectasis has been on mobilization of secretions using physiotherapy, patient positioning, and inline suctioning through the endotracheal or tracheostomy tube. Flexible bronchoscopy is commonly used for the therapeutic aspiration of secretions and several studies report that this is its most common application in the intensive care unit [51,52]. In our experience, use of a large-caliber therapeutic bronchoscope can greatly facilitate the aspiration of large amounts of mucus, though endotracheal or tracheostomy tube size must still be considered to allow adequate inspiratory and expiratory airflow. Instillation of mucolytic agents can be performed directly through the bronchoscope, though this is seldom required.

Thick, tenacious mucus may form plugs that obstruct central airways or even the endotracheal tube lumen, resulting in significant hypoxemia due to airway obstruction. In such cases, even a large-caliber bronchoscope may be unable to successfully clear the obstruction. Cryotherapy applied through the flexible bronchoscope can be very helpful in relieving airway obstructions caused by material with a fluid component, such as mucus or blood clots. In this procedure, the cryotherapy probe is advanced through the bronchoscope to the obstructing material. Once the probe is touching the material, cryotherapy is applied which causes the material to contract around the probe and adhere to it. Once this has occurred, the bronchoscope with the cryotherapy probe

and adherent material can be removed *en bloc* through the endotracheal tube. This method is useful for removing large plugs of mucus and blood clots and can have significant clinical impact.

Bronchoscopic insufflation of atelectatic portions of the lung has also been described by wedging the bronchoscope into an airway of atelectatic lung and insufflating room air through the working channel of the bronchoscopic via connection to an Ambu bag [52]. Radiographic improvements as well as improvement in oxygenation have been reported using this method.

### Airway obstruction

Airway obstruction in critically ill patients may be caused by foreign bodies as in traumatic airway injury or by a neoplastic process in patients with underlying malignancy [53,54]. A variety of interventional procedures may be performed through the flexible bronchoscope such as wire basket retrieval of foreign bodies, cryotherapy, argon plasma coagulation, and electrosurgery for the removal of obstructing endobronchial lesions [55]. In cases such as removal of large foreign bodies or in instances of large, central airway obstruction, rigid bronchoscopy remains the preferred method for removal [56].

### Percutaneous dilational tracheostomy

Percutaneous dilational tracheostomy (PDT) has become a widespread method of performing tracheostomies in critically ill patients in intensive care units, largely because it can be performed at the bedside, thereby foregoing the need to transport patients who may be unstable. The use of flexible bronchoscopy to directly visualize cannulization of the trachea has improved the safety of this procedure and is now widely recommended [57].

### Airway prosthetics

Several studies have examined the efficacy of the placement of airway prosthetics, or stents, in patients with respiratory failure secondary to central airways disease [58]. Some have described successful weaning from mechanical ventilation in as many as 50% of critically ill patients following metallic stent placement in the trachea or mainstem bronchi. Airway stent placement can be performed at the bedside through a flexible bronchoscope with direct bronchoscopic visualization or with fluoroscopic assistance. Figure 24.3 shows improvement in airway caliber following metallic stent placement for extrinsic airway compression.

## Conclusion

The flexible bronchoscope is an indispensible tool for the modern day intensivist, allowing the physician to perform a range of diagnostic as well as therapeutic procedures at the

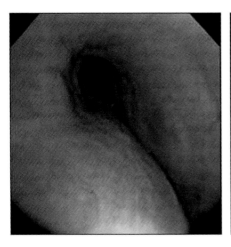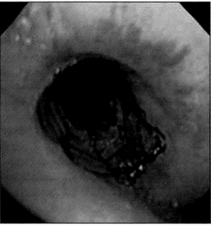

**Fig. 24.3** Improved airway caliber following metallic stent placement.

bedside. With the proper equipment and personnel, these procedures can be performed safely and can have a significant impact on the clinical course of critically ill patients.

## References

1 Raoof S, Mehrishi S, Prakash UB. Role of bronchoscopy in modern medical intensive care unit. *Clin Chest Med* 2001; **22**: 241–61.

2 Olopade CO, Prakash UB. Bronchoscopy in the critical care unit. *Mayo Clin Proc* 1989; **64**: 1255–63.

3 Jolliet PH, Chevrolet JC. Bronchoscopy in the intensive care unit. *Intensive Care Med* 1992; **18**: 160–9.

4 Turner JS, Willcox PA, Hayhurst MD, Potgieter PD. Fiberoptic bronchoscopy in the intensive care unit-A prospective study of 147 procedures in 107 patients. *Crit Care Med* 1994; **22**: 259–64.

5 Labbé A, Meyer F, Albertini M. Bronchoscopy in intensive care units. *Paediatr Respir Rev* 2004; **5** (Suppl A): S15–S19.

6 Bone RC, McElwee NE, Eubanks DH, Gluck EH. Analysis of indications for intensive care unit admission. Clinical efficacy assessment project: American College of Physicians. *Chest* 1993; **104**: 1806–11.

7 Krell WS. Pulmonary diagnostic procedures in the critically ill. *Crit Care Clin* 1988; **4**: 393–407.

8 Dunagan DP, Burke HL, Aquino SL, *et al.* Fiberoptic bronchoscopy in coronary care unit patients: indications, safety, and clinical implications. *Chest* 1998; **114**: 1660–7.

9 Anzuetto A, Levine SM, Jenkinson SG. The technique of fiberoptic bronchoscopy: Diagnostic and therapeutic uses in intubated, ventilated patients. *J Crit Ill* 1992; **7**: 1657–64.

10 Lindholm CE, Ollman JS, Millen EG, Grenvik A. Cardiorespiratory effects of flexible fiberoptic bronchoscopy in critically ill patients. *Chest* 1978; **74**: 362–8.

11 Matsushima Y, Jones R, King E, *et al.* Alterations in pulmonary mechanics and gas exchange during routine fiberoptic bronchoscopy. *Chest* 1984; **86**: 184–8.

12 Jin F, Mu D, Chu D, *et al.* Severe complications of bronchoscopy. *Respiration* 2008; **76**: 429–33.

13 Hertz MI, Woodward ME, Gross CR, *et al.* Safety of bronchoalveolar lavage in the critically ill, mechanically ventilated patient. *Crit Care Med* 1991; **19**: 1526–32.

14 Albertini RE, Harrell JH, Kurihara N, Moser KM. Arterial hypoxemia induced by fiberoptic bronchoscopy. *JAMA* 1974; **230**: 1666–7.

15 Dunagan DP, Baker AM, Hurd DD, Haponik EF. Bronchoscopic evaluation of pulmonary infiltrates following bone marrow transplantation. *Chest* 1997; **111**: 135–41.

16 Azoulay E, Mokart D, Rabbat A, *et al.* Diagnostic bronchoscopy in hematology and oncology patients with acute respiratory failure: prospective multicenter data. *Crit Care Med* 2008; **36**: 100–7.

17 Kim YH, Suh GY, Kim MH, *et al.* Safety and usefulness of bronchoscopy in ventilator-dependent patients with severe thrombocytopenia. *Anaesth Intensive Care* 2008; **36**: 411–17.

18 Rabbat A, Chaoui D, Lefebvre A, *et al.* Is BAL useful in patients with acute myeloid leukemia admitted in ICU for severe respiratory complications? *Leukemia* 2008; **22**: 1361–7.

19 Gruson D, Hilbert G, Valentino R, *et al.* Utility of fiberoptic bronchoscopy in neutropenic patients admitted to the intensive care unit with pulmonary infiltrates. *Crit Care Med* 2000; **28**: 2224–30.

20 White P, Bonacum JT, Miller CB. Utility of fiberoptic bronchoscopy in bone marrow transplant patients. *Bone Marrow Transpl* 1997; **20**: 681–7.

21 Kim YH, Suh GY, Kim MH, *et al.* Safety and usefulness of bronchoscopy in ventilator-dependent patients with severe thrombocytopenia. *Anaesth Intensive Care* 2008; **36**: 411–17.

22 Pereira Gomes JC, Pedreira Jr WL Jr, Araújo EM, *et al.* Impact of BAL in the management of pneumonia with treatment failure: positivity of BAL culture under antibiotic therapy. *Chest* 2000; **118**: 1739–46.

23 Fagon JY, Chastre J, Wolff M, *et al.* Invasive and noninvasive strategies for management of suspected ventilator-associated pneumonia. A randomized trial. *Ann Intern Med* 2000; **132**: 621–30.

24 Hayon J, Figliolini C, Combes A, *et al.* Role of serial routine microbiologic culture results in the initial management of ventilator-associated pneumonia. *Am J Respir Crit Care Med* 2002; **165**: 41–6.

25 Canadian Critical Care Trials Group. A randomized trial of diagnostic techniques for ventilator-associated pneumonia. *N Engl J Med* 2006; **355**: 2619–30.

26 Heyland DK, Cook DJ, Marshall J, *et al.* The clinical utility of invasive diagnostic techniques in the setting of ventilator-associated pneumonia. Canadian Critical Care Trials Group. *Chest* 1999; **115**: 1076–84.

27 Luna CM, Vujacich P, Niederman MS, *et al.* Impact of BAL data on the therapy and outcome of ventilator-associated pneumonia. *Chest* 1997; **111**: 676–85.

28 Timsit JF, Cheval C, Gachot B, *et al.* Usefulness of a strategy based on bronchoscopy with direct examination of bronchoalveolar lavage fluid in the initial antibiotic therapy of suspected ventilator-associated pneumonia. *Intensive Care Med* 2001; **27**: 640–7.

29 Fagon JY, Chastre J, Rouby JJ. Is bronchoalveolar lavage with quantitative cultures a useful tool for diagnosing ventilator-associated pneumonia? *Crit Care* 2007; **11**: 123.

30 Shorr AF, Sherner JH, Jackson WL, Kollef MH. Invasive approaches to the diagnosis of ventilator-associated pneumonia: a meta-analysis. *Crit Care Med* 2005; **33**: 46–53.

31 Bonten MJ, Bergmans DC, Stobberingh EE, *et al.* Implementation of bronchoscopic techniques in the diagnosis of ventilator-associated pneumonia to reduce antibiotic use. *Am J Respir Crit Care Med* 1997; **156**: 1820–4.

32 Mentec H, May-Michelangeli L, Rabbat A, *et al.* Blind and bronchoscopic sampling methods in suspected ventilator-associated pneumonia. A multicentre prospective study. *Intensive Care Med* 2004; **30**: 1319–26.

33 Kollef MH, Ward S. The influence of mini-BAL cultures on patient outcomes: implications for the antibiotic management of ventilator-associated pneumonia. *Chest* 1998; **113**: 412–20.

34 Bauer TT, Torres A, Ewig S, *et al.* Effects of bronchoalveolar lavage volume on arterial oxygenation in mechanically ventilated patients with pneumonia. *Intensive Care Med* 2001; **27**: 384–93.

35 Joffe AR, Muscedere J, Marshall JC, *et al.* The safety of targeted antibiotic therapy for ventilator-associated pneumonia: a multicenter observational study. *J Crit Care* 2008; **23**: 82–90.

36 Papazian L, Gainnier M. Indications of BAL, lung biopsy, or both in mechanically ventilated patients with unexplained infiltrations. *Eur Respir J* 2003; **21**: 383–4.

37 Baumann HJ, Kluge S, Balke L, *et al.* Yield and safety of bedside open lung biopsy in mechanically ventilated patients with acute lung injury or acute respiratory distress syndrome. *Surgery* 2008; **143**: 426–33.

38 Papin TA, Grum CM, Weg JG. Transbronchial biopsy during mechanical ventilation. *Chest* 1986; **89**: 168–70.

39 Ghamande S, Rafanan A, Dweik R, *et al.* Role of transbronchial needle aspiration in patients receiving mechanical ventilation. *Chest* 2002; **122**: 985–9.

40 O'Brien JD, Ettinger NA, Dhevlin D, Kollef MH. Safety and yield of transbronchial biopsy in mechanically ventilated patients. *Crit Care Med* 1997; **25**: 440–6.

41 White CS, Templeton PA, Hasday JD. CT-assisted transbronchial needle aspiration: usefulness of CT fluoroscopy. *AJR Am J Roentgenol* 1997; **169**: 393–4.

42 Weiss YG, Deutschman CS. The role of fiberoptic bronchoscopy in airway management of the critically ill patient. *Crit Care Clin* 2000; **16**: 445–1.

43 Schmidt U, Hess D, Kwo J, *et al.* Tracheostomy tube malposition in patients admitted to a respiratory acute care unit following prolonged ventilation. *Chest* 2008; **134**: 288–94.

44 Elizondo E, Navarro F, Pérez-Romo A, *et al.* Endotracheal intubation with flexible fiberoptic bronchoscopy in patients with abnormal anatomic conditions of the head and neck. *Ear Nose Throat J* 2007; **86**: 682–4.

45 Cahill BC, Ingbar DH. Massive hemoptysis. Assessment and management. *Clin Chest Med* 1994; **15**: 147–67.

46 Karmy-Jones R, Cuschieri J, Vallières E. Role of bronchoscopy in massive hemoptysis. *Chest Surg Clin N Am* 2001; **11**: 873–906.

47 Valipour A, Kreuzer A, Koller H, *et al.* Bronchoscopy-guided topical hemostatic tamponade therapy for the management of life-threatening hemoptysis. *Chest* 2005; **127**: 2113–18.

48 Fartoukh M, Parrot A, Khalil A. Aetiology, diagnosis and management of infective causes of severe haemoptysis in intensive care units. *Curr Opin Pulm Med* 2008; **14**: 195–202.

49 Ong TH, Eng P. Massive hemoptysis requiring intensive care. *Intensive Care Med* 2003; **29**: 317–20.

50 Shigemura N, Wan IY, Yu SC, *et al.* Multidisciplinary management of life-threatening massive hemoptysis: a 10-year experience. *Ann Thorac Surg* 2009; **87**: 849–53.

51 Kreider ME, Lipson DA. Bronchoscopy for atelectasis in the ICU: a case report and review of the literature. *Chest* 2003; **124**: 344–50.

52 Tsao TC, Tsai YH, Lan RS, *et al.* Treatment for collapsed lung in critically ill patients. *Chest* 1990; **97**: 435–8.

53 Dissanaike S, Shalhub S, Jurkovich GJ. The evaluation of pneumomediastinum in blunt trauma patients. *J Trauma* 2008; **65**: 1340–5.

54 Johnson SB. Tracheobronchial injury. *Semin Thorac Cardiovasc Surg* 2008; **20**: 52–7.

55 Folch E, Mehta AC. Airway interventions in the tracheobronchial tree. *Semin Respir Crit Care Med* 2008; **29**: 441–52.

56 Colt HG, Harrell JH. Therapeutic rigid bronchoscopy allows level of care changes in patients with acute respiratory failure from central airways obstruction. *Chest* 1997; **112**: 202–6.

57 Yuca K, Kati I, Tekin M, *et al.* Fibre-optic bronchoscopy-assisted percutaneous dilational tracheostomy by guidewire dilating forceps in intensive care unit patients. *J Otolaryngol Head Neck Surg* 2008; **37**: 76–80.

58 Lin SM, Lin TY, Chou CL, *et al.* Metallic stent and flexible bronchoscopy without fluoroscopy for acute respiratory failure. *Eur Respir J* 2008; **31**: 1019–23.

# 25 Bronchial Thermoplasty

**Samir Makani and Michael J. Simoff**

Henry Ford Hospital, Detroit, MI, USA

## Introduction

Asthma is a chronic lung disease characterized by episodic, reversible airflow obstruction and airway hyper-responsiveness (AHR). The major clinical symptoms include shortness of breath, wheezing, and cough. This chronic disorder has an enormous impact on the overall health of children and adults, and leads to significant morbidity. Exacerbations can lead to significant time lost from school, work, and other activities. For the 3-year period 2001–2003, an average annual 20 million persons in the United States had a diagnosis of asthma, requiring 12.3 million physician visits, 1.8 million emergency department visits, 504,000 hospital admissions, and leading to 4210 deaths [1]. Current available therapies can be divided into two main groups, namely, controller and rescue medications. Although these medications have provided relief for many asthmatic patients, a proportion remain refractory to therapy with persistent symptoms and recurrent exacerbations. Furthermore, current therapies are limited and may have significant side-effects, thus compelling investigation into innovative modalities of treatment and disease modification. The application of thermal energy to the bronchial airway wall with the intention of decreasing the amount of reactive airway smooth muscle has become an attractive investigative technique for the treatment of persistent asthma.

## Pathophysiology

Asthma is a complex immune-mediated disorder. The inflammatory response is characterized by infiltration of the airway wall with eosinophils, lymphocytes, and mast cells. Current data supports a CD4$^+$ T-cell cytokine release in a Th2 predominant pattern, which is essential to the pathogenesis of this disease. Cytokines, such as IL-4, IL-5, and IL-13, lead to

the recruitment and activation of primary effector cells of the allergic response, namely the eosinophil and mast cell. This in turn results in the release of a multitude of inflammatory mediators, which in combination induce changes in the airway wall and produce the symptoms seen clinically [2].

Chronic asthma is characterized by persistent airway inflammation leading to airway remodeling. The three main components of airway remodeling are goblet cell hyperplasia, increased collagen deposition, and hypertrophy and hyperplasia of airway smooth muscle. These changes lead to airway wall thickening and narrowing of the bronchial diameter, with airway smooth muscle playing a dominant role. Both large and small airways undergo remodeling in chronic asthma.

### Airway smooth muscle

Airway smooth muscle is present throughout the conducting airways to the level of the respiratory bronchioles. Its actual role in the respiratory tract has been postulated to include protective mechanisms, optimization of ventilation, and a peristaltic role for various purposes based on its common embryonic derivation of the gastrointestinal tract. Recently, its functional role has been brought under question. The possibility exists that the airway smooth muscle is similar to the appendix, and is merely a vestigial organ without current function, but maintains the ability to induce a serious state of chronic disease [3]. As stated above, airway smooth muscle hyperplasia and hypertrophy is central to airway remodeling and plays a dominant role in enhanced bronchoconstriction and airway hyper-responsiveness. The degree of smooth muscle change has been found to be proportionate to clinical disease severity [4,5].

Current pharmacotherapy has been shown to have an effect on airway smooth muscle through direct and indirect effects, demonstrated through *in vitro* models. Corticosteroids have been shown to decrease cytokine production, modulating airway smooth muscle function and proliferation. *In*

*Flexible Bronchoscopy*, Third Edition. Edited by Ko-Pen Wang, Atul C. Mehta, J. Francis Turner.
© 2012 Blackwell Publishing Ltd. Published 2012 by Blackwell Publishing Ltd.

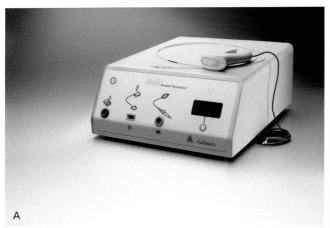
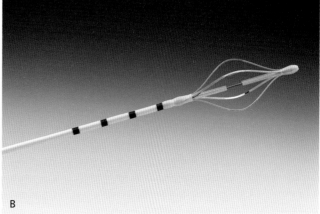

**Fig. 25.1** (A) The Alair generator system. (B) The expandable electrode basket for delivery of radiofrequency ablation energy to the airway for the Alair bronchial thermoplasty system. Reproduced with permission from Asthmatx Inc.

*vitro*, corticosteroids have also been shown to have a direct effect through cell cycle arrest and decreased contractile protein expression [6,7]. However, in murine models of asthma these effects have not been shown to decrease airway smooth muscle thickness [8]. Beta-agonists have also been shown to decrease smooth muscle proliferation [9]. Unfortunately, as in corticosteroid models, beta-agonist effects have also not been studied in humans. Bronchial thermoplasty is the first attempt at a procedural intervention designed to decrease airway smooth muscle mass with the goal of decreasing airway hyper-responsiveness and airway narrowing.

## Bronchial thermoplasty

Radiofrequency ablation (RFA) has been utilized for the treatment of cancer as well as the ablation of cardiac conduction abnormalities for several years with good success. RFA is a procedure in which an electrical generator originates alternating current delivered at high frequency by a needle electrode. Ions in the tissue follow the alternating current delivered by the needle. The ionic agitation causes frictional heating, resulting in protein denaturation and desiccation. The degree of thermal energy delivered can be precisely controlled. A similar concept, albeit with a different delivery device, has been adapted to deliver thermal energy to the bronchial airway wall—bronchial thermoplasty. These thermal applications lead to denaturation of the airway smooth muscle, which is replaced by fibroblasts, decreasing airway hyper-responsiveness and improving airway caliber.

## Procedure

The Alair system (Asthmatx, Mountain View, CA) is utilized to perform bronchial thermoplasty. It consists of a radiofrequency controller (Fig. 25.1A), which supplies energy via

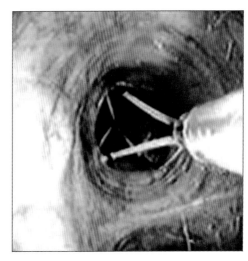

**Fig. 25.2** The expandable electrode basket as it appears deployed in the airway. Reproduced with permission from Asthmatx Inc.

the Alair catheter to heat the airway wall. The generator delivers monopolar radiofrequency energy at 460 kHz with active feedback mechanisms to maintain a continuous and exact treatment temperature for 10 seconds. The Alair catheter is a flexible tube with an expandable electrode basket at the tip (Fig. 25.1B) which allows for circumferential contact with the airway wall (Fig. 25.2).

The procedure is performed under moderate or deep sedation through a flexible bronchoscope with a 2.0-mm working channel. The complete procedure currently recommends three bronchoscopic treatment sessions performed at 3-week intervals. Each lower lobe is treated at independent sessions. Both the right and left upper lobes are treated at the third session. Due to its anatomy, the right middle lobe has been avoided. Each bronchoscopy session takes approximately 1 hour, with up to 85 treatments being performed in each lower lobe and up to 120 in both upper lobes. The optimal number of activations is yet to be determined and will be the subject of further research.

## Patient response

Bronchial thermoplasty is a well tolerated procedure. There is usually no gross evidence of treatment, except minimal mucosal blanching has been noted (Fig. 25.3). Adverse events were usually seen within 1 to 2 days of the procedure and were related to airway irritation and inflammation (cough, wheezing, chest discomfort, and chest pain). Most adverse events have been graded as mild to moderate with a minority of patients requiring hospitalization. Symptoms generally resolved within 1 week.

## Current supportive data

### Preclinical investigations

Bronchial thermoplasty was initially investigated by Danek *et al.* in 11 mongrel dogs. Each canine lung was divided into four regions (control and three treatment areas) and subjected to different temperatures (55, 65, and 75°C) in each region. The treatment temperatures were based on prior experience with radiofrequency electrosurgical tissue coagulation. Airway hyper-responsiveness was then measured using methacholine pre- and post-treatment. Histology up to 3 years postprocedure was also obtained. A total of 300 individual airway sites were examined from these 11 dogs. At 55°C, no significant difference was seen in AHR compared to control. At 65°C improvement in AHR was noted for all but one time point (week 12). At 75°C, a significant difference in AHR was also demonstrated at all time points, which were persistent over the 3-year study period. Histologically, altered airway smooth muscle was seen as early as 1 week postprocedure in all groups, and was most prominent in the 75°C group. At the 3-year time point, mature collagen was noted to have replaced airway smooth muscle, which was most prominently identified in the 75°C group (Fig. 25.4). At the study conclusion, a statistically significant inverse correlation was noted between the percentage of altered airway smooth muscle and airway responsiveness to methacholine [10].

### Clinical investigations

The first feasibility trial conducted in human subjects was performed in eight patients already scheduled to undergo lobectomy for suspected or proven lung cancer [11]. Each subject underwent bronchial thermoplasty during one bronchoscopic procedure and proceeded with their planned lobectomy 5 to 20 days later. During that period, no adverse events were noted. The first two subjects were treated with

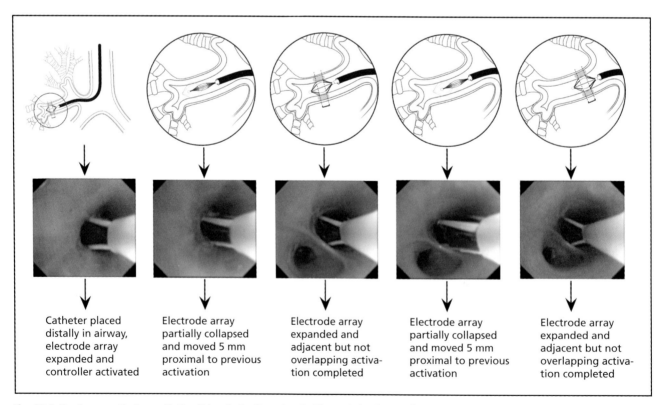

**Fig. 25.3** Contiguous activations with the Alair catheter. Reproduced with permission from Asthmatx Inc.

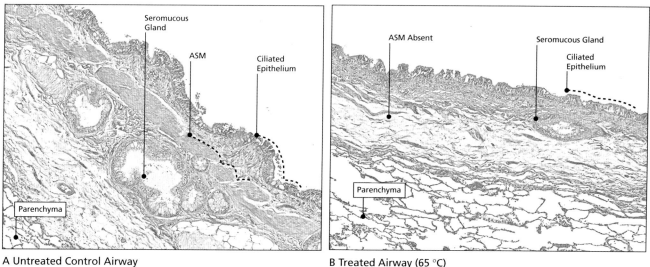

A Untreated Control Airway                 B Treated Airway (65 °C)

**Fig. 25.4** Histologic specimens of the airway wall without treatment and postbronchial thermoplasty, demonstrating the reduction in smooth muscle. Reproduced with permission from Asthmatx Inc.

55°C and the subsequent six with 65°C. Postlobectomy histology demonstrated that the epithelium remained normal. On average, approximately 50% alteration in airway smooth muscle was seen. The 65°C specimens overall appeared more significantly altered than the 55°C treatment group. This initial trial demonstrated that bronchial thermoplasty could be delivered safely in human subjects, reproducing the findings demonstrated in the animal models.

Cox *et al.* provided further safety data in 16 subjects prospectively studied in a non-randomized trial [12]. All subjects had "stable asthma" and were on an inhaled steroid, long acting beta-agonist, or both. Subjects were premedicated with systemic steroids prior to the procedure. Subjects underwent three to four treatment bronchoscopies scheduled at least 3 weeks apart. Subjects then were followed clinically for 2 years (12 weeks, 1 year, and 2 year visits). The majority of adverse events were noted to be mild, consisting of cough, dyspnea, and wheezing. Symptoms were mostly noted 1–2 days after the procedure and spontaneously resolved by day 5 postprocedure. All adverse events were managed on an outpatient basis. Although this study did not demonstrate improvements in $FEV_1$, there was improvement in airway hyper-responsiveness to methacholine challenge. This trial again demonstrated the ability to treat patients with bronchial thermoplasty safely.

The first randomized, prospective multinational trial was conducted by the Asthma Intervention Research (AIR) trial study group [13]. For this study 112 subjects were enrolled who met criteria for moderate to severe persistent asthma based on the Global Initiative for Asthma definition. All subjects were on moderate doses of inhaled corticosteroids and long acting beta-agonists (LABA). Per protocol, subjects were also required to demonstrate worsening asthma control

after discontinuation of their LABA for 2 weeks. This worsening of control was demonstrated by a decline of 5% in their morning peak expiratory flows (*PEF*) or an increase of 0.5 on the Asthma Control Questionnaire. Subjects were randomized to either a control or treatment group in an unblinded fashion. Subjects assigned to the treatment group underwent three bronchoscopy procedures scheduled at least 3 weeks apart. Control subjects similarly underwent three clinic visits, during which spirometry was performed. Both subjects and controls received pretreatment systemic corticosteroids. All subjects in the two groups were seen 2 weeks after each treatment visit. Follow-up visits were then conducted at 6 weeks, as well as 3, 6, and 12 months after the last treatment visit. Of note, at the 3-month visit, subjects were asked to discontinue their LABA unless required secondary to a severe exacerbation or judged by the investigator to have poor asthma control requiring the reinstitution of their LABA. During the follow-up period, patients maintained a daily diary recording *PEF*s, rescue medication use, symptom free days, and a symptom score which was based on day and night-time symptoms. Subjects were also questioned about potential adverse events at each interaction.

The primary outcome measure was the difference in exacerbations between the two groups. Exacerbations were identified as a decrease in *PEF* by 20% from previously identified average baseline, increased use of rescue inhalers, or nocturnal awakenings. The mean number of mild exacerbations was significantly less in the bronchial thermoplasty group compared with the control arm at both 3 and 12 months. These findings could be extrapolated to approximately 10 fewer mild exacerbations per subject per year in the thermoplasty group. No significant difference was identified between the two groups in regards to severe exacerbations, although overall, few episodes occurred. Analysis of secondary outcomes (*PEF*, AHR, use of rescue medications, asthma symptoms, and questionnaire scores) demonstrated statistically significant improvements in the thermoplasty group at 12 months in all criteria except AHR. This finding was different from data reported in previous trials. As seen in previous trials, adverse events were mainly noted approximately 1 day after the thermoplasty procedure, were mild in nature, and resolved by day 7. The most common symptoms were dyspnea, wheezing, and cough. There was also an increase in hospitalizations required for treatment of adverse events in the thermoplasty group, not seen in prior studies. Four patients required six hospitalizations, mainly for exacerbations of asthma. At 6 weeks post-treatment, adverse events were similar in both groups. This trial represented the first randomized effort to determine the efficacy of bronchial thermoplasty. The unblinded nature of the trial did lead to a concern of a placebo effect, although most significant findings were seen in objective data such as morning *PEF* and exacerbations. One surprising finding was the lack of decrease in AHR which had been previously reported. This could be attributed to the discontinuation of LABAs, or the degree of fixed obstruction seen in moderate and severe persistent asthmatic patients. Ongoing follow-up is planned and will be reported in future publications.

A second multinational, randomized, prospective, unblinded trial focused on severe persistent asthmatics. The Research in Severe Asthma trial (RISA) was primarily designed to evaluate the safety of bronchial thermoplasty in symptomatic severe persistent asthmatics [14]. Secondary outcomes to evaluate the effects of bronchial thermoplasty and daily medication requirements were also analyzed. Enrollment criteria included the use of high dose inhaled steroids and LABA, an *FEV₁* greater than 50%, and reversible airflow obstruction or airway hyper-responsiveness to methacholine; 34 subjects were randomized to either a treatment or control group. As previously reported, the treatment group underwent three bronchoscopic procedures at least 3 weeks apart. Once treatment had been completed, an attempt to taper either an oral corticosteroid or inhaled corticosteroid was performed per a predefined protocol. Subjects were initially subjected to a steroid stable phase (weeks 6–22), followed by a 14-week steroid wean phase (weeks 22–36), and finally a 16-week reduced steroid phase (weeks 36–52). The weaning process was discontinued if the subject experienced an exacerbation or worsening control; 32 patients completed the trial (15 treatment, 17 control). The primary outcome measure of safety demonstrated an increase in adverse events in the treatment group during the treatment period as reported in prior studies. Most adverse events were noted within 1 day of treatment and resolved on average within 1 week. The most common symptoms reported included wheezing, cough, dyspnea, and

chest discomfort. There was also a significant increase in the number of hospitalizations in the treatment group. Seven hospitalizations were required for four patients, mainly secondary to exacerbations of asthma. Two hospitalizations were secondary to mucus plugging and segmental collapse of the treated segment. This was also seen in one patient in the AIR I trial as well. In the post-treatment period, there was no difference in adverse events between the two groups. In regards to the secondary outcome measure of efficacy and medication reduction, during the steroid stable phase (weeks 6–22) the treatment group demonstrated a significant reduction in the use of rescue inhalers, improvement in prebronchodilator *FEV₁*, and asthma control questionnaire scores. During the weaning and reduced steroid phase (weeks 36–52), there were no significant differences is discontinuation or decreased dosing of corticosteroids between the two groups. Also, there were no significant differences noted in morning *PEFs*, AHR, and postbronchodilator *FEV₁* between groups. Beyond 52 weeks, the treatment group continued to demonstrate decreased rescue inhaler use as well as continued improvements in asthma control questionnaire scores.

In contrast to the AIR I trial subgroup analysis of high-dose inhaled steroid subjects, there was no improvement in morning *PEFs* or AHR, although these patients were not symptomatic as seen in the RISA trial. The RISA trial once again demonstrated the ability to perform bronchial thermoplasty safely even in the symptomatic, severe, persistent, asthmatic subject. Consistent with other studies, there was an increase in mild adverse events and hospitalizations associated with bronchial thermoplasty with the potential of decreasing exacerbations over the long term.

Most recently, the AIR trial study group conducted a second trial evaluating the safety and effectiveness of bronchial thermoplasty in stable severe persistent asthmatics (AIR II). This is the first multinational, randomized, prospective, double-blinded, sham-controlled trial evaluating bronchial thermoplasty. For this study 297 stable, severe, persistent asthmatics were randomized. Inclusion criteria included the use of high-dose oral corticosteroids and a LABA, AHR to methacholine, and a prebronchodilator *FEV₁* greater than 60% predicted. The primary outcome measure was the difference in Asthma Quality of Life Questionnaire (AQLQ) score. Secondary outcomes included rates of severe exacerbations, morning *PEFs*, and use of rescue inhalers. Both groups underwent three bronchoscopies scheduled 3 weeks apart by unblinded physicians (Bronchoscopy team). The procedure was performed as in prior publications. Sham procedures were performed using similar equipment providing audio and visual cues mimicking an actual procedure without delivering radio-frequency energy. Subjects were then evaluated at the end of the treatment period and again at 3-month intervals up to 1 year postintervention. Follow-up visits were performed by blinded physicians who were not present during the bronchoscopic procedure (Assessment team); 288 subjects completed the trial (190 treatment, 98 sham).

The primary outcome, measure of AQLQ scores, demonstrated a statistically significant improvement in the treatment group compared to the sham group. Significant reductions in the rate of severe exacerbations were also demonstrated in the treatment group compared to the sham group. Adverse events were similar to those reported in previous trials with the majority of adverse events being categorized as mild to moderate and occurred in the procedural phase of the trial. Similar rates were noted in both groups. Symptoms consisted of wheezing, dyspnea, cough, and chest pain. These symptoms were noted within 1 day of the procedure and resolved within 1 week. There was an increase in hospitalizations in the treatment group with 16 subjects requiring 17 hospitalizations compared to two hospitalizations in the sham group. In the postprocedural period, the treatment group had significantly less adverse events including exacerbations, emergency room visits, and hospitalizations. The AIR II trial again validated the safety of performing bronchial thermoplasty in severe persistent asthmatics. AQLQ scores were also significantly improved as demonstrated previously. Despite improvements in AQLQ scores and emergency room visits, decreased use of rescue inhalers or changes in morning *PEFs* was not seen as demonstrated in previous trials. To date, this was the largest sham-controlled trial in pulmonary medicine as it relates to device development for the treatment of severe asthmatics.

## The future for bronchial thermoplasty

Bronchial thermoplasty is an innovative technique, but several questions remain unanswered. Currently, the available catheter is capable of treating airways with a diameter of 3 mm or greater. Is this the airway diameter one should be treating, or should more peripheral, smaller-diameter airways, be targeted? Using alveolar nitric oxide measurements, van Veen *et al.* demonstrated a correlation between the degree of asthma and the contribution of peripheral airways inflammation [15]. This may suggest that the role of peripheral airways resistance in severe asthmatics is greater than in moderate or mild asthmatics and may contribute to the absence of changes in morning *PEFs* and AHR in some of the previously discussed trials. Severe asthmatics are a heterogeneous group of patients with varying degrees of peripheral airways disease, which adds to the difficulty of demonstrating a predominant physiological difference after bronchial thermoplasty. Among the trials discussed above, several primary outcome measures were utilized, predominantly rate of exacerbations and changes in asthma control scores. The difference noted in the trials speaks to the het-

erogeneity of the subjects studied. The AIR II trial was the first sham-controlled trial in relation to bronchial thermoplasty, but even in that trial the placebo effect noted by the authors was much higher than anticipated in the control group. The placebo effect could have been generated at many levels including frequent clinic visits and maintaining a daily diary. This would suggest that the true benefit of bronchial thermoplasty would be greater in a real-life setting.

Subgroup analysis in the AIR I trial did demonstrate an increased benefit over controls in the high-dose steroids group *post hoc* analysis. Further determination of which group of severe asthmatics would benefit would be beneficial. This could be related to the degree of airway inflammation, as this would not be treated by bronchial thermoplasty. Current published follow-up is up to 2 years. The long-term effects of bronchial thermoplasty have not yet been established, and results of the AIR I and AIR II trial long-term follow-up are awaited.

## Conclusions

Asthma is a complex disease process. The cascade of inflammatory mediators with subsequent pathophysiologic changes causing clinical symptoms for patients remains a global health issue leading to significant morbidity. Advances in therapy have led to improvements in morbidity, but many patients continue to have severe recurrent exacerbations. Bronchial thermoplasty is an innovative technique using radiofrequency ablation technology to treat the anatomical, and thus effect the pathophysiological, changes seen in asthma. Recent clinical trials have shown this technique to be a promising prospective therapy for uncontrolled, severe, persistent asthmatic patients. Bronchial thermoplasty is a new and exciting advance in the management of asthma. Despite the promising initial studies, further clinical trials are still needed to fully understand the use of this technology and answer several important questions prior to widespread use of this promising new therapeutic modality.

## References

1 Moorman J. National Surveillance for Asthma—United States, 1980–2004. *MMWR* 2007; **56**.
2 Wills-Karp M. Immunologic basis of antigen-induced airway hyperresponsiveness. *Ann Rev Immunol* 1999; **17**: 255–81.
3 Mitzner W. Airway smooth muscle: the appendix of the lung. *Am J Respir Crit Care Med* 2004; **169**: 787–90.
4 Carroll N, Elliot J, Morton A, James A. The structure of large and small airways in nonfatal and fatal asthma. *Am Rev Respir Dis* 1993; **147**: 405–10.

5 Benayoun L, Druilhe A, Dombret MC, *et al.* Airway structural alterations selectively associated with severe asthma. *Am J Respir Crit Care Med* 2003; **167**: 1360–8.

6 Fernandes D, Guida E, Koutsoubos V, *et al.* Glucocorticoids inhibit proliferation, cyclin D1 expression, and retinoblastoma protein phosphorylation, but not activity of the extracellular-regulated kinases in human cultured airway smooth muscle. *Am J Respir Cell Mol Biol* 1999; **21**: 77–88.

7 Fernandes DJ, Mitchell RW, Lakser O, *et al.* Do inflammatory mediators influence the contribution of airway smooth muscle contraction to airway hyperresponsiveness in asthma? *J Appl Physiol* 2003; **95**: 844–53.

8 Miller M, Cho JY, McElwain K, *et al.* Corticosteroids prevent myofibroblast accumulation and airway remodeling in mice. *Am J Physiol* 2006; **290**: L162–9.

9 Ammit AJ, Panettieri RA Jr. Airway smooth muscle cell hyperplasia: a therapeutic target in airway remodeling in asthma? *Prog Cell Cycle Res* 2003; **5**: 49–57.

10 Danek CJ, Lombard CM, Dungworth DL, *et al.* Reduction in airway hyperresponsiveness to methacholine by the application of RF energy in dogs. *J Appl Physiol* 2004; **97**: 1946–53.

11 Miller JD, Cox G, Vincic L, *et al.* A prospective feasibility study of bronchial thermoplasty in the human airway. *Chest* 2005; **127**: 1999–2006.

12 Cox G, Miller JD, McWilliams A, *et al.* Bronchial thermoplasty for asthma. *Am J Respir Crit Care Med* 2006; **173**: 965–9.

13 Cox G, Thomson NC, Rubin AS, *et al.* Asthma control during the year after bronchial thermoplasty. *New Engl J Med* 2007; **356**: 1327–37.

14 Pavord ID, Cox G, Thomson NC, *et al.* Safety and efficacy of bronchial thermoplasty in symptomatic, severe asthma. *Am J Respir Crit Care Med* 2007; **176**: 1185–91.

15 van Veen IH, Sterk PJ, Schot R, *et al.* Alveolar nitric oxide versus measures of peripheral airway dysfunction in severe asthma. *Eur Respir J* 2006; **27**: 951–6.

# Index

*Flexible Bronchoscopy*, Third Edition. Edited by Ko-Pen Wang, Atul C. Mehta, J. Francis Turner.
© 2012 Blackwell Publishing Ltd. Published 2012 by Blackwell Publishing Ltd.